WITHDRAWN

The embryonic ages for Streeter's stages XII–XXII have been altered
in accordance with the human data from Iffy, L., et al.: Acta Anat., *66*:178, 1967.

EXTREMITIES	HEART	GUT, ABDOMEN	LUNG	UROGENITAL	OTHER
					Early blastocyst with inner cell mass and cavitation (58 cells) lying free within the uterine cavity
		Yolk sac			Early amnion sac Extraembryonic mesoblast, angioblast Chorionic gonadotropin
	Merging mesoblast anterior to prechordal plate	Stomatodeum Cloaca		Allantois	Primitive streak Hensen's node Notochord Prechordal plate Blood cells in yolk sac
	Single heart tube Propulsion	Foregut		Mesonephric ridge	Yolk sac larger than amnion sac
Arm bud	Ventric. outpouching Gelatinous reticulum	Rupture stomato-deum Evaination of thyroid, liver, and dorsal pancreas	Lung bud	Mesonephric duct enters cloaca	Rathke's pouch Migration of myotomes from somites
Leg bud	Auric. outpouching Septum primum	Pharyngeal pouches yield parathyroids, lat. thyroid, thymus Stomach broadens	Bronchi	Ureteral evag Urorect. sept. Germ cells Gonadal ridge Coelom, Epithelium	
Hand plate, Mesench. condens. Innervation	Fusion mid. A-V canal Muscular vent. sept.	Intestinal loop into yolk stalk Cecum Gallbladder Hepatic ducts Spleen	Main lobes	Paramesonephric duct Gonad ingrowth of coelomic epith.	Adrenal cortex (from coelomic epithelium) invaded by sympathetic cells = medulla Jugular lymph sacs
Finger rays, Elbow	Aorta Pulmonary artery Valves Membrane ventricular septum	Duodenal lumen obliterated Cecum rotates right Appendix	Tracheal cartil.	Fusion urorect. sept. Open urogen. memb., anus Epith. cords in testicle	Early muscle
Clearing, central cartil.	Septum secundum			S-shaped vesicles in nephron blastema connect with collecting tubules from calyces	Superficial vascular plexus low on cranium
Shell, Tubular bone				A few large glomeruli Short secretory tubules Tunica albuginea Testicle, interstitial cells	Superficial vascular plexus at vertex

SMITH'S
Recognizable Patterns
of Human Malformation

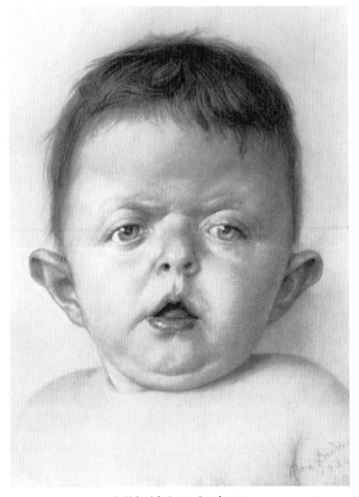

A Girl with Apert Syndrome
Original Max Brödel drawing No. 506. Property of the Johns Hopkins
University School of Medicine, Department of Art as Applied to Medicine.

SMITH'S
Recognizable Patterns of Human Malformation

Seventh Edition

Kenneth Lyons Jones, MD

*Professor of Pediatrics, Chief, Division of Dysmorphology and Teratology,
University of California, San Diego, School of Medicine, La Jolla, California*

Marilyn Crandall Jones, MD

*Professor of Clinical Pediatrics, Department of Pediatrics, University of California,
San Diego, School of Medicine, La Jolla, California; Clinical Service Chief,
Division of Genetics, Rady Children's Hospital, San Diego, California*

Miguel Del Campo, MD, PhD

*Assistant Professor, Ciències Experimentals i de la Salut, Universitat Pompeu Fabra;
Consultant in Clinical Genetics, Programa de Medicina Molecular I Genètica,
Hospital Vall d'Hebron, Barcelona, Spain*

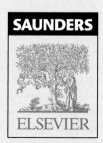

SAUNDERS

ELSEVIER

SAUNDERS

1600 John F. Kennedy Blvd.
Ste 1800
Philadelphia, PA 19103-2899

SMITH'S RECOGNIZABLE PATTERNS OF HUMAN MALFORMATION   ISBN: 978-1-4557-3811-3

Notices

Knowledge and best practice in this field are constantly changing. As new research and experience broaden our understanding, changes in research methods, professional practices, or medical treatment may become necessary.

Practitioners and researchers must always rely on their own experience and knowledge in evaluating and using any information, methods, compounds, or experiments described herein. In using such information or methods they should be mindful of their own safety and the safety of others, including parties for whom they have a professional responsibility.

With respect to any drug or pharmaceutical products identified, readers are advised to check the most current information provided (i) on procedures featured or (ii) by the manufacturer of each product to be administered, to verify the recommended dose or formula, the method and duration of administration, and contraindications. It is the responsibility of practitioners, relying on their own experience and knowledge of their patients, to make diagnoses, to determine dosages and the best treatment for each individual patient, and to take all appropriate safety precautions.

To the fullest extent of the law, neither the Publisher nor the authors, contributors, or editors assume any liability for any injury and/or damage to persons or property as a matter of products liability, negligence, or otherwise, or from any use or operation of any methods, products, instructions, or ideas contained in the material herein.

Library of Congress Cataloging-in-Publication Data
Jones, Kenneth Lyons, author.
  Smith's recognizable patterns of human malformation / Kenneth Lyons Jones, Marilyn C. Jones, Miguel Del Campo—Seventh edition.
      p. ; cm.
  Recognizable patterns of human malformation
  Includes bibliographical references and index.
  ISBN 978-1-4557-3811-3 (hardcover : alk. paper)
    I. Jones, Marilyn C., author.   II. Campo, Miguel del, author.   III. Title.   IV. Title: Recognizable patterns of human malformation.
  [DNLM: 1. Congenital Abnormalities. QS 675]
  RG627.5
  616'.043—dc23
                                                                              2013012502

Senior Content Strategist: Stefanie Jewell-Thomas
Content Development Manager: Lucia Gunzel
Content Development Specialist: Kelly McGowan
Publishing Services Manager: Anne Altepeter
Project Manager: Jessica Becher
Design Direction: Lou Forgione

Printed in the U.S.A.

Last digit is the print number: 9   8   7   6   5   4   3   2   1

Dedication to the First Edition

To my wife, Ann, beloved inspirational companion

*To my father, William H. Smith, accomplished engineer and
would-be physician*

*To my teachers, Dr. Lawson Wilkins, molder of clinicians and
humanist, and Professor Dr. Gian Töndury, complete anatomist,
who brings embryology into living perspective*

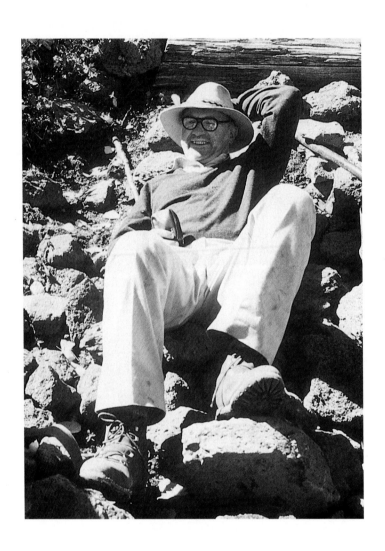

**Dedicated to the Memory of
David W. Smith, MD
1926–1981**

*"Far better it is to dare mighty things, to win glorious triumphs, even
though checkered by failure, than to take rank with those poor spirits
who neither enjoy much nor suffer much, because they live in the great
twilight that knows neither victory nor defeat."*

Theodore Roosevelt, in a speech before the Hamilton Club, Chicago,
April 10, 1899

Acknowledgments

The information set forth in this book represents an amalgamation of the knowledge, commitment, and hard work of many individuals. I would like to acknowledge a number of those who have made significant contributions to the development of the seventh edition:

Dr. Kurt Benirschke's breadth of knowledge, intellectual curiosity, and wisdom have acted as a continuing stimulus for me.

Dr. Christina D. Chambers' enthusiasm, creativity, and understanding of epidemiology have made me aware of a totally new approach to understanding the causes of birth defects.

Dr. Robert J. Gorlin and Dr. David L. Rimoin had a substantial influence on the thinking that went into this book. Both were great scientists and clinicians who had a significant impact on our field. We will miss them incredibly.

I am grateful to the following fellows in dysmorphology at the University of California, San Diego: Dr. H. Eugene Hoyme, Sanford School of Medicine, University of South Dakota; Dr. Luther K. Robinson, State University of New York, Buffalo; Dr. Ronald Lacro, Children's Hospital of Boston; Dr. Christopher Cuniff, University of Arizona; Dr. Rick Martin, Shire Human Genetic Therapies, Cambridge, Massachusetts; Dr. Leah W. Burke, University of Vermont; Dr. Stephen R. Braddock, St Louis University School of Medicine; Dr. Lynne M. Bird, University of California, San Diego; Dr. Kenjiro Kosaki, Keio University, Tokyo; Dr. Mary J. Willis, Balboa Naval Hospital, San Diego, and Dr. Keith Vaux, University of California, San Diego. Each has made his or her own significant contribution to the development of this book, and each has been a great inspiration to me.

Many colleagues have contributed photos, information, and expertise. Especially helpful have been Dr. John Carey, University of Utah School of Medicine; Dr. Michael Cohen, Jr., Dalhousie University, Halifax, Nova Scotia; Dr. Judith Hall, University of British Columbia, Vancouver; Dr. Jaime Frias, Centers for Disease Control and Prevention, Dr. Jon Aase, University of New Mexico; Dr. Bryan Hall, University of Kentucky, Lexington; Dr. James Hanson; University of Iowa; Dr. Sterling Clarren, University of Washington School of Medicine; Dr. John Graham, Cedars-Sinai Medical Center, Los Angeles; Dr. Margot Van Allen, University of British Columbia, Vancouver; Dr. Cynthia Curry, University of California, San Francisco; Dr. Roger Stevenson, Greenwood Genetic Center, Greenwood, South Carolina; Dr. Buzz Chernoff, Sacramento; Dr. Jeffrey Golden, Harvard Medical School; Dr. Mike Bamshad, University of Washington; Dr. David Weaver, Indiana University School of Medicine; Dr. Jules Leroy, Gent University Hospital, Ghent, Belgium; Dr. Mark Stephan, University of Washington School of Medicine; Dr. Margaret Adam, University of Washington; Dr. Art Aylsworth, University of North Carolina; Dr. Melanie Manning, Stanford University, Palo Alto; Dr. Angela Lin, Massachusetts General Hospital; Dr. Carol Clericuzio, University of New Mexico; Dr. Ian Krantz, Children's Hospital of Philadelphia; Dr. Maximilian Muenke, National Institutes of Health; and Dr. Kosuke Izumi, Children's Hospital of Philadelphia.

Special thanks go to Dr. Mark H. Paalman, senior editor at John Wiley and Sons, and Dr. John C. Carey, editor-in-chief of the American Journal of Medical Genetics who made it possible to publish many photographs initially published in the journal.

I am particularly grateful to Kathleen A. Johnson, my administrative assistant at the University of California, San Diego, for the past 25 years. The invaluable assistance of Robert Felix, Kelly Kao, Lyn Dick, Sonya Alvardo, Diana Johnson, Cesar Sanchez, and Yvonne O'Leary is also greatly appreciated.

Contents

Dysmorphology Approach and Classification

We ought not to set them aside with idle thoughts or idle words about "curiosities" or "chances." Not one of them is without meaning; not one that might not become the beginning of excellent knowledge, if only we could answer the question—why is it rare? or being rare, why did it in this instance happen?

JAMES PAGET, *Lancet* 2:1017, 1882

The questions set forth by Paget are still applicable. Every structural defect represents an inborn error in morphogenesis. Just as the study of inborn metabolic errors has extended our understanding of normal biochemistry, so may the accumulation of knowledge concerning defects in morphogenesis assist us in further unraveling the story of structural development. The major portion of this text is devoted to patterns of malformation, as contrasted with patterns of deformation due to mechanical factors, which is the subject of a separate text, *Smith's Recognizable Patterns of Human Deformation*. You will also find relevant chapters on normal and abnormal morphogenesis, genetics and genetic counseling, minor anomalies and their relevance, a clinical approach toward a specific diagnosis for particular categorical problems, and normal standards of measurement for a variety of features. It is hoped that the design of the book will lend itself to practical clinical application, as well as provide a basic text for the education of those interested in a better understanding of alterations in morphogenesis. Furthermore, many of the charts have been developed for direct use in the counseling of patients and parents.

Accurate diagnosis of a specific syndrome among the 0.7% of babies born with multiple malformations is a prerequisite to providing a prognosis and plan of management for the affected infant, as well as genetic counseling for the parents.

DYSMORPHOLOGY APPROACH

The following is the author's approach toward the evaluation of an individual with multiple defects:

I. Gather information. The family history is an essential aspect of such an evaluation. A question such as "Are there any individuals in the family with a similar type of problem?" may be helpful. The early history should usually include information about the onset and vigor of fetal activity, gestational timing, indications of uterine constraint, mode of delivery, size at birth, neonatal adaptation, and problems in postnatal growth and development. The physical examination should be complete, with the physician searching for minor as well as major anomalies. When possible, measurements should be taken to determine whether a given feature, such as apparent ocular hypertelorism or a small-appearing ear, is truly abnormal. The charts of normal measurements in Chapter 5 are provided for this purpose. An unusual feature ideally should be interpreted in relation to the findings in other family members before its relevance is determined.

II. Interpret the patient's anomalies from the viewpoint of developmental anatomy and strive to answer the following questions:

A. Which anomaly in the individual represents the earliest defect in morphogenesis? A table for this purpose is found in Chapter 2 (see Table 2-1). From such information, one can determine that the problem in development must have existed before a particular prenatal age and any factor after that time could not be the cause of that structural defect.

B. Can all the anomalies in the patient be explained on the basis of a single problem in morphogenesis that leads to a cascade of subsequent defects, as shown in Figure 1? These types of patterns of structural defects, referred to as *sequences,* may be divided into four categories from the developmental pathology viewpoint, as summarized in Figure 2. The first category is the *malformation sequence,* in which there has been a single, localized, poor formation of tissue that initiates a chain of subsequent defects. Malformation sequences occur in all gradation, the manifestations ranging from nearly normal to more severe, and have a recurrence risk that is most commonly in the 1% to 5% range.

The second category is the *deformation sequence,* in which there is no problem in the embryo or fetus (collectively referred to as fetus in this text), but mechanical forces such as uterine constraint result in altered morphogenesis, usually of the molding type. One example is the oligohydramnios deformation sequence, caused by chronic leakage of amniotic fluid; another is the breech deformation sequence, the manifold effects of prolonged breech position late in fetal life. The deformations and deformation sequences are the subject of a separate text, titled *Smith's Recognizable Patterns of Human Deformation.* Most deformations have a very good to excellent prognosis in contrast with many malformations. The recurrence risk for deformation is usually of very low magnitude, unless the cause of the deformation problem is a persisting one, such as a bicornuate uterus.

The third category is the *disruption sequence,* in which the normal fetus is subjected to a destructive problem and its consequences. Such disruptions may be of vascular, infectious, or even mechanical origin. One example of this is disruption of normally developing tissues by amniotic bands. The spectrum of consequences is set forth under *Amnion Rupture Sequence* in Chapter 1. In the final category, the *dysplasia sequence,* the primary defect is a lack of normal organization of cells into tissues. One example is the lack of migration of melanoblastic precursors from the neural crest. The spectrum of consequences is referred to as the *neurocutaneous melanosis sequence* (see Chapter 1), in which melanocytic hamartomas of the skin occur in conjunction with similar changes in the pia and arachnoid.

C. Does the patient have multiple structural defects that cannot be explained on the basis of a single initiating defect and its consequences but rather appear to be the consequence of multiple defects in one or more tissues? These are referred to as *malformation syndromes* and are most commonly thought to be due to a single cause. The known modes of etiology for malformation syndromes include chromosomal abnormalities, mutant gene

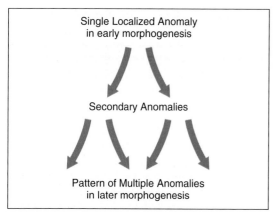

FIGURE 1. Sequence designates a single localized anomaly plus its subsequently derived structural consequences.

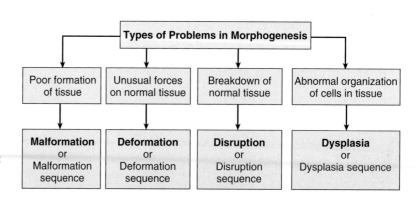

FIGURE 2. Four types of structural defects that can result in a chain of defects (sequence) by the time of birth.

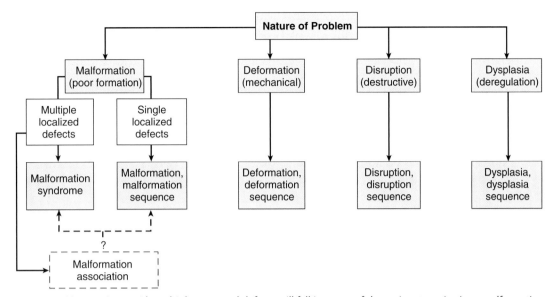

FIGURE 3. Most patients with multiple structural defects will fall into one of these six categories (e.g., malformation syndrome; malformation, malformation sequence; deformation, deformation sequence; disruption, disruption sequence; dysplasia; dysplasia sequence; and malformation association). The prognosis, management, and recurrence risk counseling may vary considerably among these categories.

disorders, and environmental teratogens. However, there are still many for which the mode of etiology has not been resolved.

III. Attempt to arrive at a specific overall diagnosis within the six categories (e.g., malformation syndrome; malformation, malformation sequence; deformation, deformation sequence; disruption, disruption sequence; dysplasia; dysplasia sequence; and malformation association) shown in Figure 3, confirm when possible, and counsel accordingly. When possible, counseling should include the following: an understanding of how the altered structures came to be, the natural history of the condition and what measures can be used to assist the child, and the mode of etiology and genetic counseling (recurrence risk).

IMPORTANT GENERAL PRINCIPLES

The following are some of the important principles and information that should be considered in the evaluation of a patient with multiple defects.

Nonspecificity of Individual Defects

With rare exceptions, a clinical diagnosis of a pattern of malformation cannot be made on the basis of a single defect, as is evident in the differential diagnosis in Appendix I. Even a rare defect may be a feature in several syndromes of variant etiology. A specific diagnosis usually depends on recognition of the overall *pattern of anomalies,* and the detection of minor defects may be as helpful as the detection of major anomalies in this regard.

Variance in Expression

Variance in extent of abnormality (expression) among individuals with the same etiologic syndrome is a usual phenomenon. Except for such nonspecific general features as mental deficiency and small stature, it is unusual to find a given anomaly in 100% of patients with the same etiologic syndrome. For example, in full 21 trisomy Down syndrome, only mental deficiency is ubiquitous; hypotonia is a frequent feature, but most of the other individual clinical features are found in less than 80% of such patients. However, a specific diagnosis of Down syndrome can generally be rendered, based on the *total pattern of anomalies.* It is especially important to appreciate that the environmentally determined disorders occur in all gradations of severity. Thus, as one example, prenatal exposure to alcohol leads to a spectrum of defects, including spontaneous abortion, the pattern of structural defects referred to as *fetal alcohol syndrome,* growth deficiency, and mental retardation.

Intraindividual variability in expression is also frequent, with variance in the degree of abnormality on the left versus the right side of the individual.

Heterogeneity

Similar phenotypes (overall physical similarity) may result from different etiologies. Only by finer discrimination of the phenotype or mode of etiology can such similar entities be distinguished. For example, the Marfan syndrome and homocystinuria were initially discriminated on the basis of homocystinuria, next by a difference in mode of etiology (autosomal dominant for the Marfan syndrome and autosomal recessive in homocystinuria), and finally by closer scrutiny of the phenotype. As another example, achondroplasia is frequently misdiagnosed among individuals who have chondrodystrophies that only superficially resemble true achondroplasia. A diagnosis should be rendered only when there is close resemblance in the overall pattern of malformation between the patient and the disorder under consideration.

Etiology

Most of the disorders described in this book have a genetic basis. Chapter 3 provides the background information relative to genetic counseling for these conditions.

Beyond the following established disorders, roughly one half of the individuals with multiple defects have conditions that have not yet been recognized as specific disorders. A small percentage of such patients have a structural chromosomal abnormality. In such cases, genetic counseling should be withheld until it has been determined whether either parent is a balanced translocation carrier of the chromosomal abnormality. In the absence of an evident chromosomal abnormality or familial data suggesting a particular mode of etiology, it is generally impossible to state any accurate risk of recurrence for unknown patterns of multiple malformations. It is presumptuous to inform the parents that "this is a rare condition and therefore unlikely to recur in your future children." Under these circumstances, the author's present approach is to inform the parents that the lowest recurrence risk is zero and the highest risk with each pregnancy is 25%. This figure is predicated on the possibility of recessive inheritance or a nondetectable chromosomal abnormality from a patient who carries a balanced translocation.

Nomenclature

Some of the recommendations of an international committee on "Classification and Nomenclature of Morphologic Defects," published in *Lancet* 1:513, 1975, are used in this text. The recommendations of a more recent international group, which met in Mainz, Germany, under the direction of Professor Jürgen Spranger in November 1979 and again in Seattle in February 1980, have also been used.

Most of the nomenclature has already been alluded to; the following recommendations pertain to the naming of single defects and patterns of malformation.

Naming of Single Malformations

An adjective or descriptive term should be used with the name of the structure or the classic equivalent in common use (e.g., small mandible or micrognathia).

Naming of Patterns of Malformations

1. When the etiology is known and easily remembered, the appropriate term should be used to designate the disorder.
2. Time-honored designations should be continued unless there is good reason for change.
3. In the absence of a reasonably descriptive designation, eponyms, some of them multiple, may be used until the basic defect for the disorder is recognized. However, use of an eponym should thereafter be limited to one proper name.
4. The use of the possessive form of an eponym should be discontinued, because the author neither had nor owned the disorder.
5. Designation of a disorder by one or more of its manifestations does not necessarily imply that they are either specific or consistent components of that disorder.
6. Names that may have an unpleasant connotation for the family or affected individual should be avoided.
7. The syndrome should not be designated by the initials of the originally described patients.
8. Names that are too general for a specific syndrome should be avoided.
9. Unless acronyms are extremely pertinent or appropriate, they should be avoided.

Nomenclature Used to Describe Chromosomal Syndromes

Many of the disorders set forth in this book are the result of chromosomal abnormalities. This section is intended to familiarize readers who are not versed in cytogenetics with some of the basic nomenclature used in describing chromosomal syndromes. Several shorthand systems have been devised. The examples shown use the "short system," which is the system most commonly used in the recent literature. By comparing the karyotype examples with those in the text, the reader can decipher the cytogenetic shorthand. No attempt has been made to include every possible abnormality. For a comprehensive discussion of nomenclature, the reader is referred to the following source: Mitelman M (ed): *ISCN (1995): An International System for Human Cytogenetic Nomenclature.* Basel: S Karger, 1995.

METHOD AND UTILITY OF PRESENTATION OF PATTERNS OF MALFORMATION

The arrangement of the disorders in this book is based predominantly on the similarity in overall features or in one major feature among the patterns of malformation, as set forth in the Contents. Thus, the order of presentation is designed to be of assistance in the diagnosis of the patient for whom a firm diagnosis has not been established. With the exception of the chromosomal abnormality syndromes, which share many features, and the disorders determined by an environmental agent, the conditions are not arranged in accordance with the mode of etiology. Each disorder has a listing of anomalies. The features that, together, tend to distinguish the syndrome from other known disorders are set in italic font. The main list consists of defects that occur in at least 25% and usually more than 50% of patients. Sometimes the actual percentage or number is stated for each anomaly. Below these are listed the occasional defects that occur with a frequency of 1% to 25%, most commonly 5% to 10%. The occurrence of these "occasional abnormalities" is of interest and has been ascribed loosely to "developmental noise." In other words, an adverse influence that usually causes a particular pattern of malformation may occasionally cause other anomalies as well. It is possible that differences in genetic background, environment, or both allow some individuals to express these "occasional" anomalies. The important feature is that they are not random for a particular syndrome. For example, clinicians who have seen a large number of children with Down syndrome are not surprised to see "another" Down syndrome baby with duodenal atresia, webbed neck, or tetralogy of Fallot.

The references listed for each disorder were selected to give the best account of that disorder, provide recent additional knowledge, or represent the initial description. They are arranged in chronological order.

A word of caution is indicated. This book does not contain a number of very rare syndromes. Furthermore, information that appeared after June 2012, regarding the identification of specific genes responsible for disorders set forth in this book, is not always included.

OTHER SOURCES OF INFORMATION

Information about parent support groups for specific disorders, as well as other general information that could be helpful to families, is available on the following website: www.geneticalliance.org.

Information on genetic testing and its use in diagnosis, management, and genetic counseling is available at http://genetests.org, and McKusick's Mendelian Inheritance in Man is available online at http://www.ncbi.nlm.nih.gov/entrez/query.fcgi?db=OMIM.

In addition to this text, many of the texts listed in the References may be of value in the recognition, management, and counseling of particular problems and patterns of malformation.

References

General

Benirschke K, Kaufmann P: Pathology of the Human Placenta, ed 5, New York, 2006, Springer-Verlag.

Cassidy SB, Allison JE: Management of Genetic Conditions, ed 2, New York, 2004, Wiley-Liss.

Epstein CJ, Erickson RP, Wynshaw-Boris A: Inborn Errors of Development: The Molecular Basis of Clinical Disorders of Morphogenesis, ed 2, New York, 2008, Oxford University Press.

Graham JM: Smith's Recognizable Patterns of Human Deformation, ed 2, Philadelphia, 1988, Saunders.

Hall JG, Allanson JE, Gripp KW, Slavotinek AM: Handbook of Physical Measurements, ed 2, New York, 2007, Oxford University Press.

Hennekam RCM, Kranz ID, Allanson JE: Gorlin's Syndromes of the Head and Neck, ed 4, New York, 2010, Oxford University Press.

Holmes LB: Common Malformations, New York, 2011, Oxford University Press.

Rimoin DL, Connor JM, Pyeritz RE, Korf BR: Emery and Rimoin's Principles and Practice of Medical Genetics, ed 5, New York, 2007, Churchill Livingstone.

Stevenson RE, Hall JG: Human Malformations and Related Anomalies, ed 2, New York, 2006, Oxford University Press.

Stevenson RE, Schwartz CE, Rogers RC: X-Linked Mental Retardation, New York, 2000, Oxford University Press.

Warkany J: Congenital Malformations, Chicago, 1971, Year Book Medical Publishers.

Chromosomal Abnormalities

Borgaonkar DS: Chromosomal Variation in Man: A Catalog of Chromosomal Variants and Anomalies, ed 8, New York, 1997, Wiley-Liss.

de Grouchy J, Turleau C: Clinical Atlas of Human Chromosomes, New York, 1984, John Wiley & Sons.

Schinzel A: Catalogue of Unbalanced Chromosome Aberrations in Man, New York, 2001, Walter de Gruyter.

Gardner RJM, Sutherland GR, Shaffer LG: Chromosome Abnormalities and Genetic Counseling, ed 4, New York, 2011, Oxford University Press.

Connective Tissue and Skeletal Dysplasias

Beighton P: McKusick's Heritable Disorders of Connective Tissue, ed 5, St. Louis, 1993, Mosby.

Ornoy A, Borochowitz A, Lachman R, et al: Atlas of Fetal Skeletal Radiology, Chicago, 1988, Year Book.

Spranger JW, Brill PW, Nishimura G, Superti-Furga A, Unger S: Bone Dysplasias: An Atlas of Genetic Disorders of Skeletal Development, ed 3, New York, 2012, Oxford University Press.

Staheli LT, Hall JG, Jaffe KM, et al: Arthrogryposis: A Text Atlas, New York, 1998, Cambridge University Press.

Wynne-Davies R, Hall CM, Apley AG: Atlas of Skeletal Dysplasias, New York, 1985, Churchill Livingstone.

Hereditary Deafness with Associated Anomalies

Toriello HV, Reardon W, Gorlin RJ: Hereditary Hearing Loss and Its Syndromes, ed 2, New York, 2004, Oxford University Press.

Overgrowth

Cohen MM, Neri G, Weksberg R: Overgrowth Syndromes, New York, 2002, Oxford University Press.

Craniosynostosis

Cohen MM, MacLean RE: Craniosynostosis: Diagnosis, Evaluation, and Management, ed 2, New York, 2000, Oxford University Press.

Skin

Sybert VP: Genetic Disorders of Skin, New York, 2010, Oxford University Press.

Teratology

Briggs GG, Freeman RK, Yaffe SJ: Drugs in Pregnancy and Lactation, ed 9, Baltimore, 2011, Lippincott, Williams & Wilkins.

Shepard TH: Catalog of Teratogenic Agents, ed 13, Baltimore, 2010, Johns Hopkins University Press.

REPROTOX. http://www.reprotox.org. Online information system on environmental hazards to human reproduction and development.

TERIS. http://depts.washington.edu/terisweb/teris/. Online database containing teratogen information in addition to online version of Shepard's Catalog of Teratogenic Agents.

CHAPTER 1

Recognizable Patterns of Malformation

A Chromosomal Abnormality Syndromes Identifiable on Routine Karyotype

DOWN SYNDROME (TRISOMY 21 SYNDROME)
Hypotonia, Flat Facies, Slanted Palpebral Fissures, Small Ears

Down's report in 1866 on the ethnic classification of idiots stated that a "large number of congenital idiots are typical Mongols," and he set forth the clinical description of the Down syndrome. The textbook by Penrose and Smith provides an overall appraisal of this disorder that has an incidence of 1 in 660 newborns, making it the most common pattern of human malformation.

ABNORMALITIES

General. Hypotonia with tendency to keep mouth open and protrude the tongue, diastasis recti, hyperflexibility of joints, relatively small stature with awkward gait, increased weight in adolescence.

Central Nervous System. Intellectual disability.

Craniofacial. Brachycephaly; mild microcephaly with upslanting palpebral fissures; thin cranium with late closure of fontanels; hypoplasia to aplasia of frontal sinuses, short hard palate; small nose with low nasal bridge and tendency to have inner epicanthal folds.

Eyes. Speckling of iris (Brushfield spots) with peripheral hypoplasia of iris; fine lens opacities by slit lamp examination (59%); refractive error, mostly myopia (70%); nystagmus (35%); strabismus (45%); blocked tear duct (20%); acquired cataracts in adults (30% to 60%).

Ears. Small; overfolding of angulated upper helix; sometimes prominent; small or absent earlobes; hearing loss (66%) of conductive, mixed, or sensorineural type; fluid accumulation in middle ear (60% to 80%).

Dentition. Hypoplasia, irregular placement, fewer caries than usual, periodontal disease.

Neck. Short with loose folds of skin.

Hands. Relatively short metacarpals and phalanges; hypoplasia of midphalanx of fifth finger (60%) with clinodactyly (50%), a single crease (40%), or both; simian crease (45%); distal position of palmar axial triradius (84%); ulnar loop dermal ridge pattern on all digits (35%).

Feet. Wide gap between first and second toes, plantar crease between first and second toes, open field dermal ridge patterning in hallucal area of sole (50%).

Pelvis. Hypoplasia with outward lateral flare of iliac wings and shallow acetabular angle.

Cardiac. Anomaly in approximately 40%; endocardial cushion defect, ventricular septal defect, patent ductus arteriosus, auricular septal defect, and aberrant subclavian artery, in decreasing order of frequency; mitral valve prolapse with or without tricuspid valve prolapse and aortic regurgitation by 20 years of age; risk for regurgitation after 18 years of age.

Skin. Cutis marmorata, especially in extremities (43%); dry, hyperkeratotic skin with time (75%); infections in the perigenital area, buttocks, and thighs that begin as follicular pustules in 50% to 60% of adolescents.

Hair. Fine, soft, and often sparse; straight pubic hair at adolescence.

Genitalia. Relatively small penis and decreased testicular volume; primary gonadal deficiency is common and progressive from birth to adolescence and is definitely present in adults. Although rare, cases of fertility in females have been reported; no male has reproduced.

OCCASIONAL ABNORMALITIES

Seizures (less than 9%); keratoconus (6%); congenital cataract (3%); low placement of ears; webbed neck; two ossification centers in manubrium sterni; funnel or pigeon breast; tracheal stenosis with hourglass trachea and midtracheal absence of tracheal pars membranacea; gastrointestinal tract anomalies (12%), including tracheoesophageal fistula; duodenal atresia; omphalocele, pyloric stenosis, annular pancreas, Hirschsprung disease, and imperforate anus. Incomplete fusion of vertebral arches of lower spine (37%); only 11 ribs; atlantoaxial instability (12%); posterior occipitoatlantal hypermobility (8.5%); abnormal odontoid process (6%); hypoplastic posterior arch C1 (26%). Hip abnormality (8%), including dysplasia, dislocation, avascular necrosis, or slipped capital femoral epiphyses; syndactyly of second and third toes; prune belly anomaly. The incidence of leukemia is approximately 1 in 95, or close to 1%. Thyroid disorders are more common, including athyreosis, simple goiter, and hyperthyroidism. Cholelithiasis in children and gallbladder disease in adults. Fatal perinatal liver disease has been reported.

PRINCIPAL FEATURES IN THE NEONATE

Hypotonia	80%
Poor Moro reflex	85%
Hyperflexibility of joints	80%
Excess skin on back of neck	80%
Flat facial profile	90%
Slanted palpebral fissures	80%
Anomalous auricles	60%
Dysplasia of pelvis	70%
Dysplasia of midphalanx of fifth finger	60%
Simian crease	45%

NATURAL HISTORY

Muscle tone tends to improve with age, whereas the rate of developmental progress slows with age. For example, 23% of a group of children with Down syndrome who were younger than 3 years had a developmental quotient above 50, whereas none of those in the 3- to 9-year group had intelligence quotients above 50. Although the IQ range is generally said to be 25 to 50, with an occasional individual above 50, the mean IQ for older patients is 24. Fortunately, social performance is usually beyond that expected for mental age, averaging 3⅓ years above mental age for the older individuals. Generally "good babies" and happy children, individuals with Down syndrome tend toward mimicry, are friendly, have a good sense of rhythm, and enjoy music. Mischievousness and obstinacy may also be characteristics, and 13% have serious emotional problems. Coordination is often poor, and the voice tends to be harsh. Early developmental enrichment programs for Down syndrome children have resulted in improved rate of progress during the first 4 to 5 years of life. Whether such training programs will appreciably alter the ultimate level of performance remains to be determined.

Sleep-related upper airway obstruction occurs in approximately one third of cases. Growth is relatively slow, and during the first 8 years, secondary centers of ossification are often late in development. However, during later childhood, the osseous maturation is more "normal," and final height is usually attained around 15 years of age. Adolescent sexual development is usually somewhat less complete than normal. Because thyroid dysfunction is common and can be easily missed, periodic thyroid function studies should be performed. Life expectancy is 58.6 years, and 25% live beyond 62.9 years. Alzheimer's disease is common. By 60 years of age, 50% to 70% of affected individuals develop dementia. The major cause for early mortality is congenital heart defects. Mortality from respiratory disease, mainly pneumonia, as well as other infectious diseases, is much higher than in the general population. Although leukemia has frequently appeared on death certificates of affected individuals, other neoplasms were listed less than one tenth as often as expected. Neutrophilia, thrombocytopenia, and polycythemia are common. Ten percent of newborns present with a transient myeloproliferative disorder characterized by a clonal population of megakaryoblasts. Low-grade problems that occur frequently are chronic rhinitis, conjunctivitis, and periodontal disease. Immunologic dysfunction, including both T-cell and B-cell derangement, has been demonstrated, as has the frequent occurrence of hepatitis B surface antigen carrier state. Therefore, HBV vaccination is advised.

Although asymptomatic atlantoaxial dislocation occurs in 12% to 20% of individuals with Down syndrome, symptoms referable to compression of the spinal cord are rare. Unfortunately, the literature regarding radiographic screening for this finding is controversial. No study to date has documented that radiographic findings can predict which children will develop neurologic problems. Any child with Down syndrome who develops changes in bowel or bladder function, neck posturing, or loss of ambulatory skills should be evaluated carefully with plain roentgenograms of the cervical spine. The majority of patients develop symptoms before 10 years of age, when the ligamentous laxity is most severe. The Committee on Genetics of the American Academy of Pediatrics has published health supervision guidelines for children with Down syndrome that offer recommendations for follow-up of affected children.

ETIOLOGY

The etiology of Down syndrome is trisomy for all of, or a large part of, chromosome 21. The combined results of 11 unselected surveys totaling 784 cases showed the following relative frequencies of particular types of chromosomal alteration for Down syndrome: Full 21 trisomy (94%), 21 Trisomy/ normal mosaicism (2.4%), Translocation cases (with about equal occurrence of D/G and G/G translocations) (3.3%).

Faulty chromosome distribution leading to Down syndrome is more likely to occur at older maternal age, as shown in the following figures of incidence for Down syndrome at term delivery for particular maternal ages: 15 to 29 years, 1 in 1500; 30 to 34 years, 1 in 800; 35 to 39 years, 1 in 270; 40 to 44 years, 1 in 100; and over 45 years, 1 in 50.

Although the general likelihood for recurrence of Down syndrome is 1%, the principal task in giving recurrence risk figures to parents is to determine whether the Down syndrome child is a translocation case with a parent who is a translocation carrier and thereby has a relatively high risk for recurrence. The likelihood of finding a translocation in the Down syndrome child of a mother younger than 30 years is 6%, and of such cases only one out of three will be found to have a translocation carrier parent. Therefore, the estimated probability that either parent of a baby with Down syndrome born of a mother younger than 30 years is a translocation carrier is 2% versus 0.3% when the baby with Down syndrome is born of a mother older than 30 years. Having excluded a translocation carrier parent, the risk for recurrence may be stated as about 1%. There is also the suggestion that the recurrence of a different trisomy subsequent to a previous trisomy 21 may also be increased. Although a low figure, it is enough to justify prenatal diagnosis for any future pregnancy. The recurrence risk for the rare translocation carrier parent will depend on the type of translocation and the sex of the parent. Mosaicism usually leads to a less severe phenotype. Any degree of intellectual ability from normal or nearly normal to severe retardation is found, and this does not always correlate with the clinical phenotype. Patients with the features of Down syndrome and relatively good performance are likely to have mosaicism (which is not always easy to demonstrate).

References

Down JLH: Observations on an ethnic classification of idiots. Clinical Lecture Reports, *London Hospital* 3:259, 1866.

Richards BW, et al: Cytogenetic survey of 225 patients diagnosed clinically as mongols, *J Ment Defic Res* 9:245, 1965.

Hall B: Mongolism in newborn infants, *Clin Pediatr* 5:4, 1966.

Penrose LS, Smith GF: *Down's Anomaly*, Boston, 1966, Little, Brown.

Davidson RG: Atlantoaxial instability in individuals with Down syndrome: A fresh look at the evidence, *Pediatrics* 81:857, 1988.

Pueschel SM: Atlantoaxial instability and Down syndrome, *Pediatrics* 81:879, 1988.

Pueschel SM: Clinical aspects of Down syndrome from infancy to adulthood, *Am J Med Genet Suppl* 7:52, 1990.

Ugazio AG, et al: Immunology of Down syndrome: A review, *Am J Med Genet Suppl* 7:204, 1990.

Pueschel SM, et al: A longitudinal study of atlantodens relationships in asymptomatic individuals with Down syndrome, *Pediatrics* 89:1194, 1992.

Cremers MJG, et al: Risks of sports activities in children with Down's syndrome and atlantoaxial instability, *Lancet* 342:511, 1993.

Bull MJ: American Academy of Pediatrics Committee on Genetics. Health supervision for children with Down syndrome, *Pediatrics* 128:393, 2011.

Yang Q, et al: Mortality associated with Down's syndrome in the USA from 1983 to 1997: A population-based study, *Lancet* 359:1019, 2002.

Tyler CV, et al: Increased risk of symptomatic gallbladder disease in adults with Down syndrome, *Am J Med Genet* 130A:351, 2004.

Wiseman FK, et al: Down syndrome—recent progress and future prospects, *Hum Mol Genet* 18:R75, 2009.

De Souza E, et al: Recurrence risks for trisomies 13, 18 and 21, *Am J Med Genet* 149:2716, 2009.

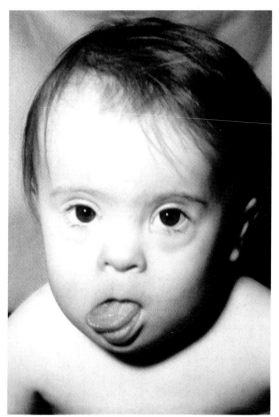

A

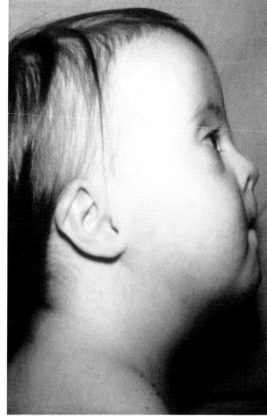

B

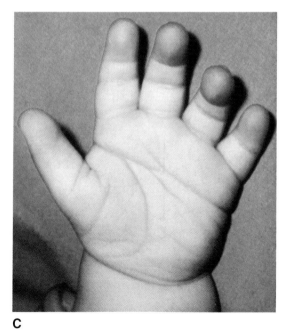

C

FIGURE 1. Down syndrome. **A–C,** Young infant. Flat facies, straight hair, protrusion of tongue, single crease on inturned fifth finger.

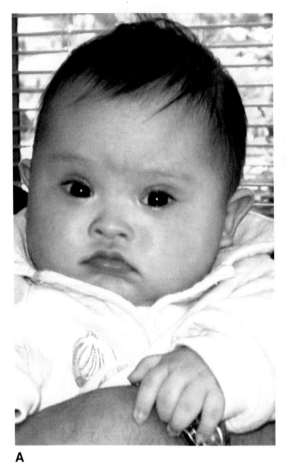

A

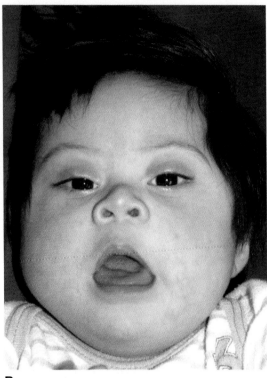

B

FIGURE 2.   A and B, Upslanting palpebral fissures. Low nasal bridge with upturned nares. (Courtesy Dr. Lynne M. Bird, Children's Hospital, San Diego.)

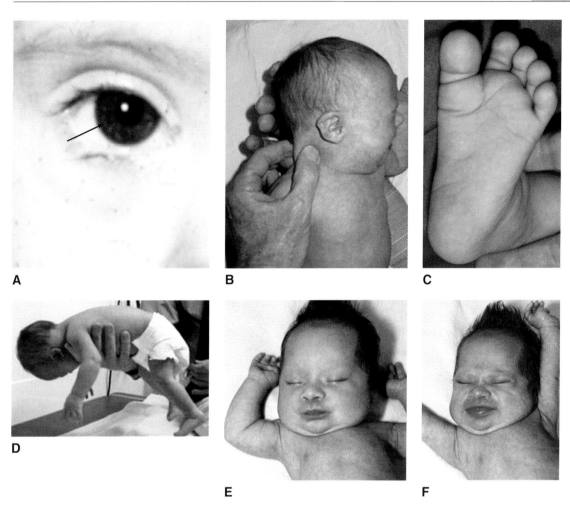

FIGURE 3.   A, Brushfield spots. B, Loose nuchal skin. C, Wide space between toes 1 and 2. D, Poor tone. E and F, Accentuation of typical face when crying.

TRISOMY 18 SYNDROME
Clenched Hand, Short Sternum, Low-Arch Dermal Ridge Patterning on Fingertips

This condition was first recognized as a specific entity in 1960 by discovery of the extra 18 chromosome in babies with a particular pattern of malformation (Edwards et al., Patau et al., and Smith et al.). It is the second most common multiple malformation syndrome, with an incidence of approximately 0.3 per 1000 newborn babies. There is a 3:1 preponderance of females to males. Several good reviews set forth a full appraisal of this syndrome. More than 130 different abnormalities have been noted in the literature on patients with the trisomy 18 syndrome, and therefore the listing of abnormalities has been divided into those that occur in 50% or more of patients, in 10% to 50% of patients, and in less than 10% of patients.

ABNORMALITIES FOUND IN 50% OR MORE OF PATIENTS

General. Feeble fetal activity, weak cry, altered gestational timing; one third premature, one third postmature; polyhydramnios, small placenta, single umbilical artery, growth deficiency; mean birth weight, 2340 g; hypoplasia of skeletal muscle, subcutaneous and adipose tissue; mental deficiency, hypertonicity (after neonatal period); diminished response to sound.

Craniofacial. Prominent occiput, narrow bifrontal diameter; low-set, malformed auricles; short palpebral fissures; small oral opening, narrow palatal arch; micrognathia.

Hands and Feet. Clenched hand, tendency for overlapping of index finger over third, fifth finger over fourth; absence of distal crease on fifth finger with or without distal creases on third and fourth fingers; low-arch dermal ridge pattern on six or more fingertips; hypoplasia of nails, especially on fifth finger and toes; short hallux, frequently dorsiflexed.

Thorax. Short sternum, with reduced number of ossification centers; small nipples.

Abdominal Wall. Inguinal or umbilical hernia and/or diastasis recti.

Pelvis and Hips. Small pelvis, limited hip abduction.

Genitalia. Male: cryptorchidism.

Skin. Redundancy, mild hirsutism of forehead and back, prominent cutis marmorata.

Cardiac. Ventricular septal defect, auricular septal defect, patent ductus arteriosus.

ABNORMALITIES FOUND IN 10% TO 50% OF CASES

Craniofacial. Wide fontanels, microcephaly, hypoplasia of orbital ridges; inner epicanthal folds, ptosis of eyelid, corneal opacity, retinal folds, retinal hypopigmentation, dysplasia and areas of hemorrhage and gliosis; cleft lip, cleft palate, or both.

Hands and Feet. Ulnar or radial deviation of hand, hypoplastic to absent thumb, simian crease; equinovarus, rocker-bottom feet, syndactyly of second and third toes.

Thorax. Relatively broad, with or without widely spaced nipples.

Genitalia. Female: hypoplasia of labia majora with prominent clitoris.

Anus. Malposed or funnel-shaped anus.

Cardiac. Bicuspid aortic and/or pulmonic valves, nodularity of valve leaflets, pulmonic stenosis, coarctation of aorta.

Lung. Malsegmentation to absence of right lung.

Diaphragm. Muscle hypoplasia with or without eventration.

Abdomen. Meckel diverticulum, heterotopic pancreatic and/or splenic tissue, omphalocele. Incomplete rotation of colon.

Renal. Horseshoe defect, ectopic kidney, double ureter, hydronephrosis, polycystic kidney.

ABNORMALITIES FOUND IN LESS THAN 10% OF CASES

Central Nervous System. Facial palsy, paucity of myelination, microgyria, cerebellar hypoplasia, defect of corpus callosum, hydrocephalus, Dandy-Walker malformation meningomyelocele.

Craniofacial. Wormian cranial bones, shallow elongated sella turcica; slanted palpebral fissures, hypertelorism, colobomata of iris, cataract, microphthalmos; choanal atresia.

Hands. Syndactyly of third and fourth fingers, polydactyly, short fifth metacarpals, ectrodactyly.

Other Skeletal. Radial aplasia, incomplete ossification of clavicle, hemivertebrae, fused vertebrae, short neck, scoliosis, rib anomaly, pectus excavatum, dislocated hip.

Genitalia. Male: hypospadias, bifid scrotum; female: bifid uterus, ovarian hypoplasia.

Cardiovascular. Anomalous coronary artery, transposition, tetralogy of Fallot, coarctation of aorta, dextrocardia, aberrant subclavian artery, intimal proliferation in arteries with arteriosclerotic change and medial calcification.

Abdominal. Pyloric stenosis, extrahepatic biliary atresia, hypoplastic gallbladder, gallstones, imperforate anus.

Renal. Hydronephrosis, polycystic kidney (small cysts), Wilms tumor.

Endocrine. Thyroid or adrenal hypoplasia.

Other. Hemangiomata, thymic hypoplasia, tracheoesophageal fistula, thrombocytopenia.

NATURAL HISTORY

Babies with the trisomy 18 syndrome are usually feeble and have a limited capacity for survival. Resuscitation is often performed at birth, and these babies may have apneic episodes in the neonatal period. Poor sucking capability may necessitate nasogastric tube feeding, but even with optimal management, these babies fail to thrive. Fifty percent die within the first week, and many of the remaining die in the next 12 months. Median survival time is 14.5 days. Only 5% to 10% survive the first year, typically with severe intellectual disability. Although most children who survive the first year are unable to walk in an unsupported fashion and verbal communication is usually limited to a few single words, it is important to realize that some older children with trisomy 18 smile, laugh, and interact with and relate to their families. All achieve some psychomotor maturation and continue to learn. There are at least 10 reports of affected children older than 10 years. Once the diagnosis has been established, limitation of extraordinary medical means for prolongation of life should be seriously considered. However, the personal feelings of the parents and the individual circumstances of each infant must be taken into consideration. Baty and colleagues documented the natural history of this disorder. For children who survived, the average number of days in the neonatal intensive care unit was 16.3, the average number of days on a ventilator was 10.1, and 13% had surgery in the neonatal period. There was no evidence for an increase in adverse reactions to immunizations. Growth curves for length, weight, and head circumference are provided in that study.

ETIOLOGY

The etiology of this disorder is trisomy for all of, or a large part of, the number 18 chromosome. The great majority of cases have full 18 trisomy, the result of faulty chromosomal distribution, which is most likely to occur at older maternal age; the mean maternal age at birth of babies with this syndrome is 32 years. Translocation cases, the result of chromosomal breakage, can be excluded only by chromosomal studies. When such a case is found, the parents should also have chromosomal studies to determine whether one of them is a balanced translocation carrier with high risk for recurrence in future offspring. There is an increased risk of trisomy 18 subsequent to a previous pregnancy with trisomy 18 (RR = 3.1), the increase being greater for women younger than age 35 at the previous trisomic pregnancy.

Mosaicism for an additional chromosome 18 leads to a longer survival and any degree of variation between a normal child and the full pattern of malformation. Recurrence risk for individuals with mosaic trisomy 18 has been variable. Four out of 12 affected individuals older than 20 years have given birth to or fathered a child with complete trisomy 18, and an additional 3 have had a combined total of 5 healthy children.

Partial trisomy 18: Trisomy of the short arm causes a very nonspecific clinical picture and mild or no intellectual disability. However, partial seizures have been seen. Cases with familial trisomy of the short arm, centromere, and proximal one third of the long arm show features of trisomy 18, although not the full pattern. Trisomy for the entire long arm is clinically indistinguishable from full trisomy 18. Trisomy for the distal one third to one half of the long arm leads to a partial picture of trisomy 18 with longer survival and less profound intellectual disability. In early childhood, the patients resemble trisomy 18 cases, whereas adolescents and adults display a more nonspecific pattern of malformation, including prominent orbital ridges, broad and prominent nasal bridge, everted upper lip, receding mandible, poorly modeled ears, short neck, and long, hyperextendible fingers. Muscular tone tends to be decreased, mental deficiency is severe, and about one third of the patients suffer from seizures.

References

Edwards JH, et al: A new trisomic syndrome, *Lancet* 1:787, 1960.

Patau K, et al: Multiple congenital anomaly caused by an extra autosome, *Lancet* 1:790, 1960.

Smith DW, et al: A new autosomal trisomy syndrome, *J Pediatr* 57:338, 1960.

Smith DW: Autosomal abnormalities, *Am J Obstet Gynecol* 90:1055, 1964.

Taylor A, Polani PE: Autosomal trisomy syndromes, excluding Down's, *Guys Hosp Rep* 13:231, 1964.

Warkany J, Passarge E, Smith LB: Congenital malformations in autosomal trisomy syndromes, *Am J Dis Child* 112:502, 1966.

Rasmussen S, Wong LY, Yang Q, et al: Population-based analysis of mortality in trisomy 13 and trisomy 18, *Pediatrics* 111:777, 2003.

Tucker ME, et al: Phenotypic spectrum of mosaic trisomy 18: Two new patients, a literature review, and counseling issues. *Am J Med Genet* 143A:505, 2007.

De Souza E, et al: Recurrence risk for trisomies 13, 18, and 21, *Am J Med Genet* 149A:2716, 2009.

Baty BJ, et al: Natural history of trisomy 18 and trisomy 13: I: growth, physical assessment, medical histories, survival and recurrence risk, *Am J Med Genet* 49:175, 1994.

Baty BJ, et al: Natural history of trisomy 18 and trisomy 13: II: psychomotor development, *Am J Med Genet* 49:189, 1994.

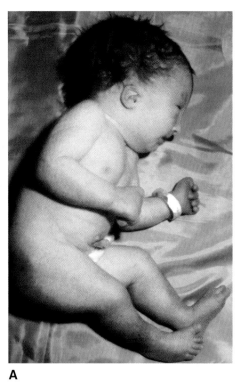

A

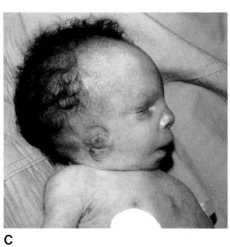

C

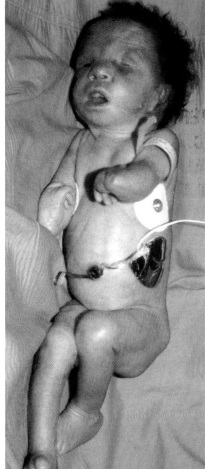

B

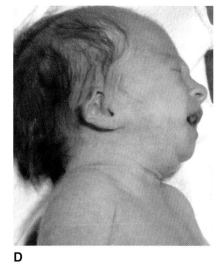

D

FIGURE 1. Trisomy 18 syndrome.
A and **B,** Note hypertonicity evident in the clenched hands and crossed legs; note the narrow pelvis. **C** and **D,** Hypoplastic supraorbital ridges; prominent occiput; low-set, slanted, malformed auricle.

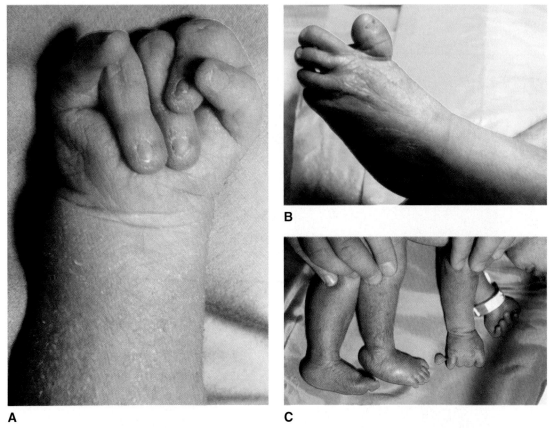

A

B

C

FIGURE 2.   A, Clenched hand with index finger overlying third; hypoplasia of fingernails. **B,** Dorsiflexed short hallux. **C,** Prominent calcaneus and postaxial polydactyly.

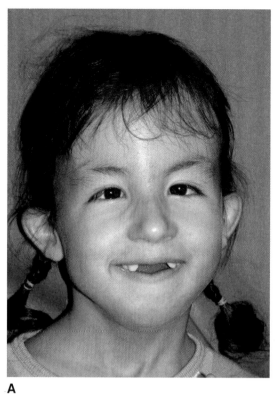

A

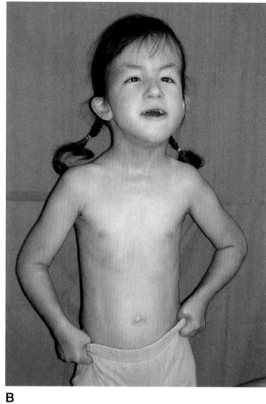

B

C

FIGURE 3. **A–C,** Older child with trisomy 18 syndrome. (Courtesy Dr. Lynne M. Bird, Children's Hospital, San Diego.)

TRISOMY 13 SYNDROME (PATAU SYNDROME)

Defects of Eye, Nose, Lip, and Forebrain of Holoprosencephaly Type; Polydactyly; Narrow Hyperconvex Fingernails; Skin Defects of Posterior Scalp

Apparently described by Bartholin in 1657, this syndrome was not generally recognized until its trisomic etiology was discovered by Patau and colleagues in 1960. The incidence is approximately 1 in 5000 births.

ABNORMALITIES FOUND IN 50% OR MORE OF PATIENTS

Central Nervous System. Holoprosencephaly type defect with varying degrees of incomplete development of forebrain and olfactory and optic nerves; minor motor seizures, often with hypsarrhythmic electroencephalography (EEG) pattern; apneic spells in early infancy; severe intellectual disability.

Hearing. Apparent deafness (defects of organ of Corti in the two cases studied).

Cranium. Moderate microcephaly with sloping forehead, wide sagittal suture and fontanels.

Eyes. Microphthalmia, colobomata of iris, or both; retinal dysplasia, often including islands of cartilage.

Mouth. Cleft lip (60% to 80%), cleft palate, or both.

Auricles. Abnormal helices with or without low-set ears.

Skin. Capillary hemangiomata, especially forehead, localized scalp defects in parieto-occipital area; loose skin, posterior neck.

Hands and Feet. Distal palmar axial triradii, simian crease, hyperconvex narrow fingernails, flexion of fingers with or without overlapping and camptodactyly, polydactyly of hands and sometimes feet, posterior prominence of heel.

Other Skeletal. Thin posterior ribs with or without missing rib, hypoplasia of pelvis with shallow acetabular angle.

Cardiac. Abnormality in 80% with ventricular septal defect, patent ductus arteriosus, auricular septal defect, and dextroposition, in decreasing order of frequency.

Genitalia. Male: cryptorchidism, abnormal scrotum; female: bicornuate uterus.

Hematologic. Increased frequency of nuclear projections in neutrophils, unusual persistence of embryonic and/or fetal type hemoglobin.

Other. Single umbilical artery, inguinal or umbilical hernia.

ABNORMALITIES FOUND IN LESS THAN 50% OF PATIENTS

Growth. Prenatal onset of growth deficiency; mean birth weight, 2480 g.

Central Nervous System. Hypertonia, hypotonia, agenesis of corpus callosum, hydrocephalus, fusion of basal ganglia, cerebellar hypoplasia, meningomyelocele.

Eyes. Shallow supraorbital ridges, upslanting palpebral fissures, absent eyebrows, hypotelorism, hypertelorism, anophthalmos, cyclopia.

Nose, Mouth, and Mandible. Absent philtrum, narrow palate, cleft tongue, micrognathia.

Hands and Feet. Retroflexible thumb, ulnar deviation at wrist, low-arch digital dermal ridge pattern, fibular S-shaped hallucal dermal ridge pattern, syndactyly, cleft between first and second toes, hypoplastic toenails, equinovarus, radial aplasia.

Cardiac. Anomalous pulmonary venous return, overriding aorta, pulmonary stenosis, hypoplastic aorta, atretic mitral and/or aortic valves, bicuspid aortic valve.

Abdominal. Omphalocele, heterotopic pancreatic or splenic tissue, incomplete rotation of colon, Meckel diverticulum.

Renal. Polycystic kidney (31%), hydronephrosis, horseshoe kidney, duplicated ureters.

Genitalia. Male: hypospadias; female: duplication and/or anomalous insertion of fallopian tubes, uterine cysts, hypoplastic ovaries.

Other. Thrombocytopenia, situs inversus of lungs, cysts of thymus, calcified pulmonary arterioles, large gallbladder, radial aplasia, flexion deformity of large joints, diaphragmatic defect.

NATURAL HISTORY

The median survival for children with this disorder is 7 days. Ninety-one percent die within the first year. Survivors have severe intellectual disability, often seizures, and fail to thrive. Only one adult, 33 years of age, has been reported. Because of the high infant mortality, surgical or orthopedic corrective procedures should be withheld in early infancy to await the outcome of the first few months. Furthermore, because of the severe brain defect, limitation of extraordinary medical means to prolong the life of individuals with this syndrome should be seriously considered. However, it is important to emphasize that each case must be taken on an individual basis. The individual circumstances of each child, as well as the personal feelings of the parents, must be acknowledged. Baty and colleagues documented the natural history of this disorder. For children who survived in their study, the average number of days in the neonatal intensive care unit was 10.8, average number of days on a ventilator was 13.3, and 23% had surgery in the neonatal period. There was no evidence for an increase in adverse reactions to immunizations. Growth curves are provided in that study. The Tracking Rare Incidence Syndromes (TRIS) project was established in 2007 to collect and analyze parent-provided data on a range of rare trisomy-related topics such as trisomy 13 and seeks to make this information available to families and interested educational, medical, and therapeutic professionals.

ETIOLOGY

The etiology for this disorder is trisomy for all of, or a large part of, chromosome 13. Older maternal age has been a factor in the occurrence of this aneuploidy syndrome. There is an increased risk of trisomy 13 subsequent to a previous pregnancy with trisomy 13 (RR = 9.5), the increase being greater for women younger than age 35 at the previous trisomic pregnancy. As with Down syndrome, chromosomal studies are indicated on 13 trisomy syndrome babies to detect the rare translocation patient having a balanced translocation parent for whom the risk of recurrence would be of major concern.

Cases with trisomy 13 mosaicism most often show a less severe clinical phenotype with every degree of variation, from the full pattern of malformation seen in trisomy 13 to a near-normal phenotype. Survival is usually longer. The degree of intellectual disability is variable.

Partial trisomy for the proximal segment (13pter→q14) is characterized by a nonspecific pattern, including a large nose, short upper lip, receding mandible, fifth finger clinodactyly, and, in most cases, severe intellectual disability. The overall picture shows little similarity to that of full trisomy 13, and survival is not significantly reduced.

Partial trisomy for the distal segment (13q14→qter) has a characteristic phenotype associated with severe intellectual disability. The facies is marked by frontal capillary hemangiomata, a short nose with upturned tip, and elongated philtrum, synophrys, bushy eyebrows and long, incurved lashes, and a prominent antihelix. Trigonocephaly and arrhinencephaly have occasionally been seen. Approximately

one fourth of the patients die during early postnatal life.

COMMENT

The defects of midface, eye, and forebrain, which occur in variable degree as a feature of this syndrome, appear to be the consequence of a single defect in the early (3 weeks) development of the prechordal mesoderm, which not only is necessary for morphogenesis of the midface but also exerts an inductive role on the subsequent development of the prosencephalon, the forepart of the brain. This type of defect has been referred to as holoprosencephaly or arrhinencephaly and varies in severity from cyclopia to cebocephaly to less severe forms.

References

Patau K, et al: Multiple congenital anomaly caused by an extra chromosome, *Lancet* 1:790, 1960.
Warburg M, Mikkelsen M: A case of 13–15 trisomy or Bartholin-Patau's syndrome, *Acta Ophthalmol* 41:321, 1963.
Smith DW: Autosomal abnormalities, *Am J Obstet Gynecol* 90:1055, 1964.
Warkany J, Passarge E, Smith LB: Congenital malformations in autosomal trisomy syndromes, *Am J Dis Child* 112:502, 1966.
Schinzel A: Autosomale Chromosomenaberationen, *Arch Genet* 52:1, 1979.
Goldstein H, Nielsen KG: Rates and survival of individuals with trisomy 13 and 18: Data from a 10-year period in Denmark, *Clin Genet* 34:366, 1988.
Baty BJ, et al: Natural history of trisomy 18 and trisomy 13: I. Growth, physical assessment, medical histories, survival and recurrence risk, *Am J Med Genet* 49:175, 1994.
Baty BJ, et al: Natural history of trisomy 18 and trisomy 13: II. Psychomotor development, *Am J Med Genet* 49:189, 1994.
Rasmussen SA, et al: Population-based analysis of mortality in trisomy 13 and trisomy 18, *Pediatrics* 111:777, 2003.
De Souza E, et al: Recurrence risks for trisomies 13, 18 and 21, *Am J Med Genet* 149A:2716, 2009.
Bruns D, et al: Birth history, physical characteristics, and medical survivors with full trisomy 13, *Am J Med Genet* 155A:2634, 2011.

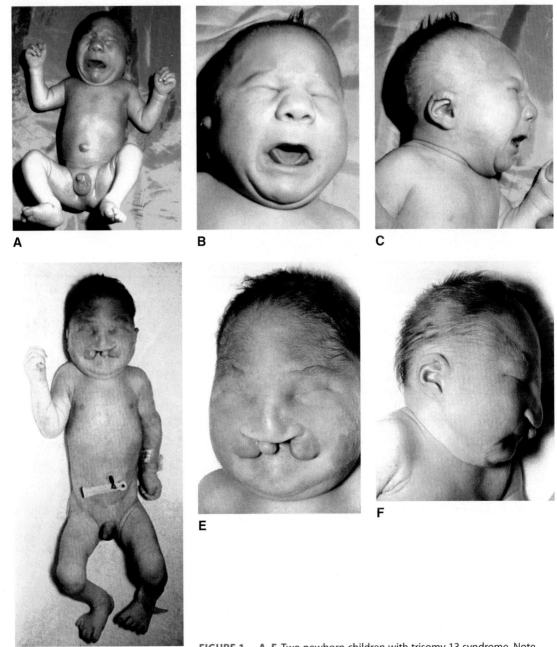

A

B

C

D

E

F

FIGURE 1.　**A–F,** Two newborn children with trisomy 13 syndrome. Note sloping forehead with variable defect in facial development.

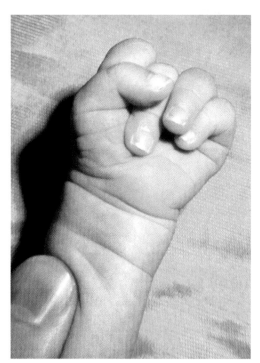

A

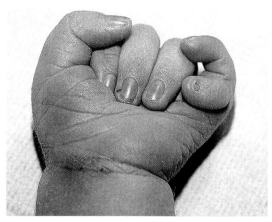

B

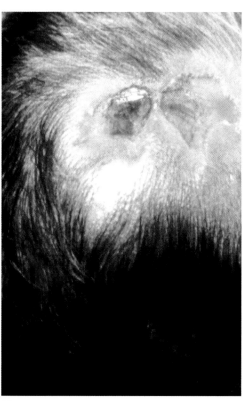

C

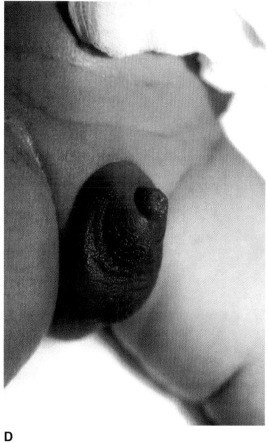

D

FIGURE 2.   A and **B,** Note hyperconvex nails and postaxial polydactyly. **C,** Aplasia cutis congenita over posterior occiput. **D,** Scrotalization of the phallus.

TRISOMY 8 SYNDROME (TRISOMY 8/NORMAL MOSAICISM)
Thick Lips, Deep-Set Eyes, Prominent Ears, Camptodactyly

Most cases are mosaic for trisomy 8/normal. More than 100 cases have been reported.

ABNORMALITIES

Growth. Variable, from small to tall.

Performance. Mild to severe intellectual disability with tendency toward poor coordination.

Craniofacial. Tendency toward prominent forehead, deep-set eyes, strabismus, hypertelorism with broad nasal root and prominent nares, full lips, everted lower lip, micrognathia, high-arched palate, cleft palate, and prominent cupped ears with thick helices.

Limbs. Camptodactyly of second through fifth fingers and toes, limited elbow supination, deep creases in palms and soles, single transverse palmar crease, major joint contracture, abnormal nails.

Other. Long, slender trunk; abnormal scapula, abnormal sternum, short or webbed neck; narrow pelvis; hip dysplasia; widely spaced nipples; ureteral-renal anomalies; cardiac defects.

OCCASIONAL ABNORMALITIES

Absent patellae, pili bifurcati, conductive deafness, seizures, vertebral anomaly (bifid vertebrae, extra lumbar vertebra, spina bifida occulta), scoliosis, cryptorchidism, uterus didelphys, jejunal duplication, agenesis of corpus callosum, hypoplastic anemia, leukopenia, coagulation factor VII deficiency, myelodysplastic syndrome and/or leukemia, Wilms tumor, nephroblastoma, mediastinal germ cell tumor, gastric leiomyosarcoma, placental-site trophoblastic tumor, Behcet syndrome (systemic inflammatory disease of unknown etiology characterized clinically by recurrent oral ulcers, genital ulcers, eye lesions, and skin lesions).

NATURAL HISTORY

The natural history is largely dependent on the severity of intellectual disability. There appears to be a lack of correlation between the phenotype and the percentage of trisomic cells.

ETIOLOGY

The etiology for this disorder is trisomy 8, the majority of patients being mosaics. Apparently, full trisomy 8 is, in most cases, an early lethal disorder.

References

Stalder GR, Buhler EM, Weber JR: Possible trisomy in chromosome group 6–12, *Lancet* 1:1379, 1963.

Schinzel A, et al: Trisomy 8 mosaicism syndrome, *Helv Pediatr Acta* 29:531, 1974.

Riccardi VM: Trisomy 8: An international study of 70 patients, *Birth Defects* XIII(3C):171, 1977.

Kurtyka ZE, et al: Trisomy 8 mosaicism syndrome, *Clin Pediatr* 27:557, 1988.

Breslau-Siderius LJ, et al: Pili bifurcati occurring in association with the mosaic trisomy 8 syndrome, *Clin Dysmorph* 5:275, 1996.

Becker K, et al: Constitutional trisomy 8 and Behcet syndrome, *Am J Med Genet* 149A:982, 2009.

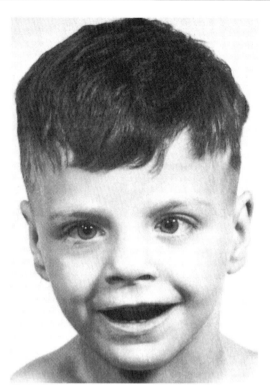

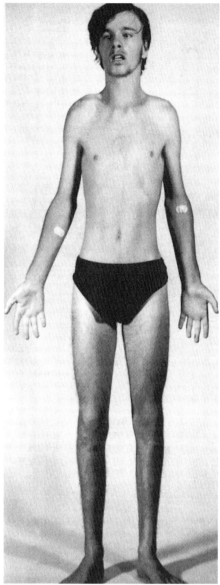

FIGURE 1. Amiable, tall individual at 4 years and at 16 years who has trisomy 8/normal mosaicism, with a normal karyotype from cultured leukocytes but trisomy 8 in skin fibroblast cells. He has a moderate hearing deficit and an IQ estimated in the 70s. He is quite active and skates, swims, and bowls. Note the facies, the small, widely spaced nipples, and the general body stance. There is some limitation of full extension of the fingers, which are partially webbed, and limited extension of the right elbow. There is hypoplasia of the supraspinatus, trapezius, and upper pectoral musculature. (Courtesy Dr. G. Howard Valentine, War Memorial Children's Hospital, London, Ontario.)

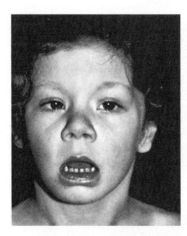
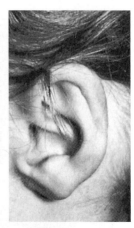
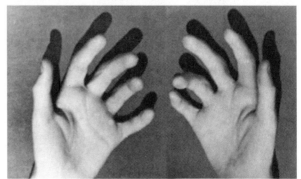

FIGURE 2.   Boy with trisomy 8/normal mosaicism. (From Riccardi VM, et al: *J Pediatr* 77:664, 1970, with permission.)

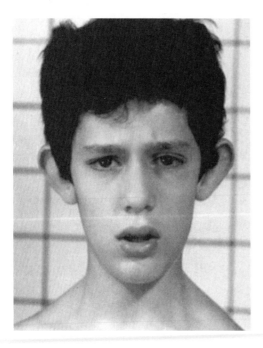

FIGURE 3.   Intellectually disabled 10-year-old boy with trisomy 8/normal mosaicism. Note the prominent ears. (From De Grouchy J, et al: *Ann Genet* 14:69, 1971, with permission.)

A

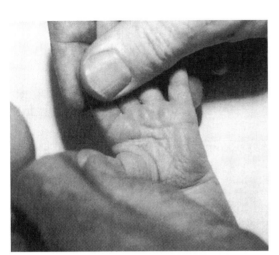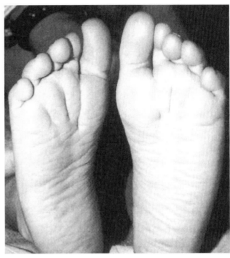

FIGURE 4. Note deep creases on palms and soles.

TRISOMY 9 MOSAIC SYNDROME
Joint Contractures, Congenital Heart Defects, Low-Set Malformed Ears

In 1973 Haslam and colleagues reported the first case of trisomy 9 mosaicism. In the same year, Feingold and colleagues reported the first example of a child with full trisomy 9 using blood lymphocytes.

ABNORMALITIES

Growth. Prenatal onset of growth deficiency.
Performance. Severe intellectual disability.
Craniofacial. Sloping forehead with narrow bifrontal diameter; upslanting, short palpebral fissures, deeply set eyes; prominent nasal bridge with short root, small fleshy tip, and slit-like nostrils; prominent lip covering receding lower lip; micrognathia, low-set, posteriorly rotated, and misshapen ears.
Skeletal. Joint anomalies, including abnormal position and/or function of hips, knees, feet, elbows, and digits; kyphoscoliosis; narrow chest; hypoplasia of sacrum, iliac wings, and pubic arch; hypoplastic phalanges of toes.
Other. Congenital heart defects in approximately two thirds of cases.

OCCASIONAL ABNORMALITIES

Subarachnoid cyst, choroid plexus cyst, cystic dilatation of fourth ventricle with lack of midline fusion of cerebellum, hydrocephalus, lack of gyration of cerebral hemispheres, meningocele, microphthalmia, corneal opacities, Peters anomaly, absence of optic tracts, preauricular tags, hearing loss, facial asymmetry, short neck, cleft lip and/or palate, velopharyngeal insufficiency, bile duct proliferation in absence of a demonstrable stenosis or atresia, gastroesophageal reflux, triphalangeal thumbs, punctate mineralization in developing cartilage, 13 ribs and 13 thoracic vertebrae. Diaphragmatic hernia. Nonpitting edema of legs, multiple pilomatricomas (benign neoplasms of hair matrix cells), simian crease, nail hypoplasia. Genitourinary anomalies, including hypoplastic external genitalia, XX sex reversal, cryptorchidism, cystic dilatation of renal tubules, diverticulae of bladder, hydronephrosis, and hydroureter.

NATURAL HISTORY

The majority of patients die during the early postnatal period. In those who survive, failure to thrive and severe motor and intellectual disability are the rule. However, several children walk unassisted, display social action skills, develop minimal speech and are able to care for some or all of their daily care needs (e.g. dressing, feeding).

ETIOLOGY

The etiology of this disorder is trisomy for chromosome 9. The incidence and severity of malformations and intellectual disability correlate with the percentage of trisomic cells in the different tissues.

References

Feingold M, et al: A case of trisomy 9, *J Med Genet* 10:184, 1973.

Haslam RHA, et al: Trisomy 9 mosaicism with multiple congenital anomalies, *J Med Genet* 10:180, 1973.

Bowen P, et al: Trisomy 9 mosaicism in a newborn infant with multiple malformations, *J Pediatr* 85:95, 1974.

Akatsuka A, et al: Trisomy 9 mosaicism with punctate mineralization in developing cartilages, *Eur J Pediatr* 131:271, 1979.

Frohlich GS: Delineation of trisomy 9, *J Med Genet* 19:316, 1982.

Kamiker CP, et al: Mosaic trisomy 9 syndrome with unusual phenotype, *Am J Med Genet* 22:237, 1985.

Levy I, et al: Gastrointestinal abnormalities in the syndrome of mosaic trisomy 9, *J Med Genet* 26:280, 1989.

Bruns D: Presenting physical characteristics, medical conditions, and developmental status of long-term survivors with trisomy 9 mosaicism, *Am J Med Genet* 155:1033, 2011.

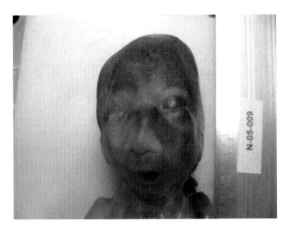

A

FIGURE 1. Facial features of a 22-week fetus with trisomy 9 syndrome. Note the sloping forehead, a broad and prominent nasal bridge, prominent upper lip covering receding lower lip, and micrognathia. (Courtesy Prof. JC Ferreres, Hospital Vall d'Hebron, Barcelona, Spain.)

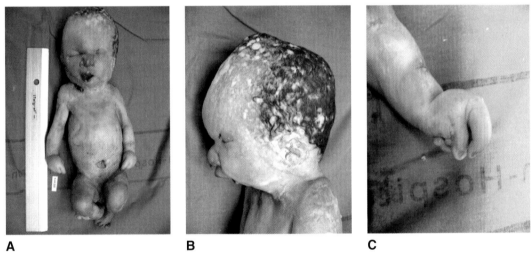

A   B   C

FIGURE 2.   **A,** Stillborn at term with mosaic trisomy 9. Note growth retardation as well as multiple contractures with extended elbows, flexed hips and knees. **A** and **B,** Facial features include short palpebral fissures, deeply set eyes; prominent nasal bridge with short root, small fleshy tip, and slit-like nostrils; prominent lip covering receding lower lip; micrognathia, low-set, posteriorly rotated, and misshapen ears. **C,** Note extended wrist with clenched hands and hypoplastic nails.

TRIPLOIDY SYNDROME AND DIPLOID/TRIPLOID MIXOPLOIDY SYNDROME

Large Placenta with Hydatidiform Changes, Growth Deficiency, Syndactyly of Third and Fourth Fingers

Triploidy, a complete extra set of chromosomes, is estimated to occur in approximately 2% of conceptuses. Most are lost as miscarriages, accounting for approximately 20% of all chromosomally abnormal spontaneous abortuses. Triploid pregnancies may be accompanied by varying degrees of toxemia. Fetal wastage may be due to hydatidiform placental changes or to specific cytogenetic characteristics, with only 3% of 69XYY conceptuses surviving to be recognized. Partial hydatidiform moles are usually associated with a triploid fetus and very rarely undergo malignant changes. Classic moles show more pronounced trophoblastic hyperplasia in the absence of a fetus. These moles show a diploid karyotype and are totally androgenic in origin.

Infrequently, triploid infants survive to be born after 28 weeks' gestation with severe intrauterine growth retardation. Instances of diploid/triploid mixoploidy are less frequent. Asymmetric growth deficiency with mild syndactyly and occasional genital ambiguity in 46,XX/69,XXY individuals are the important diagnostic features in mixoploid individuals.

ABNORMALITIES FOUND IN 50% OR MORE OF CASES

Placenta. Large, with tendency toward hydatidiform changes.

Growth. Disproportionate prenatal growth deficiency that affects the skeleton more than the cephalic region; in mixoploid individuals, skeletal growth may be asymmetric.

Craniofacial. Dysplastic calvaria with large posterior fontanel; ocular hypertelorism with eye defects, ranging from colobomata to microphthalmia; low nasal bridge; low-set, malformed ears; micrognathia.

Limbs. Syndactyly of third and fourth fingers, simian crease, talipes equinovarus.

Cardiac. Congenital heart defect (atrial and ventricular septal defects).

Genitalia. Male: hypospadias, micropenis, cryptorchidism, Leydig cell hyperplasia.

Other. Brain anomalies, including hydrocephalus and holoprosencephaly; adrenal hypoplasia; renal anomalies, including cystic dysplasia and hydronephrosis.

ABNORMALITIES FOUND IN LESS THAN 50% OF CASES

Aberrant skull shape; choanal atresia; cleft lip and/or palate; iris heterochromia; patchy cutaneous hyperpigmentation, hypopigmentation, or a mixture of both (referred to as pigmentary dysplasia); meningomyelocele; macroglossia; omphalocele or umbilical hernia; biliary tract anomalies, including aplasia of the gallbladder; incomplete rotation of colon; proximally placed thumb; clinodactyly of fifth finger; splayed toes.

NATURAL HISTORY

Partial hydatidiform molar pregnancies associated with a triploid fetus should not raise concern regarding the development of choriocarcinoma. All cases of full triploidy either have been stillborn or have died in the early neonatal period, with 5 months being the longest recorded survival. Individuals with diploid/triploid mixoploidy usually survive and manifest some degree of psychomotor retardation. Because of body asymmetry, patients with mixoploidy may require a heel lift for the shorter leg to prevent compensatory scoliosis, and some of these people may resemble those having Russell-Silver syndrome. Diagnosis of mixoploidy usually requires skin fibroblast cultures, since the triploid cell line may have disappeared from among peripheral blood leukocytes. The degree of skeletal asymmetry does not appear to correspond to the proportions of triploid cells present, and triploid cells in culture grow with the same variability as diploid cells, except for those with the XYY complement, which grow much more slowly.

ETIOLOGY

In 69% of cases, the extra set of chromosomes is paternally derived. However, the two most common mechanisms of origin are attributable to maternal factors: first, dispermy or double fertilization due to failure of the zone reaction, which normally prevents polyspermy, and second, a failure of meiosis II leading to a diploid egg. Approximately 60% of the cases have been XXY, with most of the remainder being XXX. It is not unusual for more than one X chromosome to remain active in triploidy. Older maternal age has not been a factor, and there are no data to indicate an increased risk of recurrence, such as that seen for chromosomal disorders due to nondisjunction. In several instances, a triploid pregnancy has been followed or preceded by a molar pregnancy.

References

Book JA, Santesson B: Malformation syndrome in man associated with triploidy (69 chromosomes), *Lancet* 1:858, 1960.

Ferrier P, et al: Congenital asymmetry associated with diploid-triploid mosaicism and large satellites, *Lancet* 1:80, 1964.

Niebular E: Triploidy in man: Cytogenetical and clinical aspects, *Humangenetik* 21:103, 1974.

Wertelecki W, Graham JM, Sergovich FR: The clinical syndrome of triploidy, *Obstet Gynecol* 47:69, 1976.

Jacobs PA, et al: The origin of human triploids, *Ann Hum Genet* 42:49, 1978.

Poland BJ, Bailie DL: Cell ploidy in molar placental disease, *Teratology* 18:353, 1978.

Jacobs PA, et al: Late replicating X chromosomes in human triploidy, *Am J Hum Genet* 31:446, 1979.

Graham JM, et al: Diploid-triploid mixoploidy: Clinical and cytogenetic aspects, *Pediatrics* 68:23, 1981.

Wulfsberg EA, et al: Monozygotic twin girls with diploid/triploid chromosome mosaicism and cutaneous pigmentary dysplasia, *Clin Genet* 39:370, 1991.

Zaragoza MV, et al: Parental origin and phenotype of triploidy in spontaneous abortions: Predominance of diandry and association with the partial hydatidiform mole, *Am J Hum Genet* 66:1807, 2000.

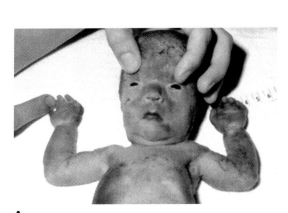 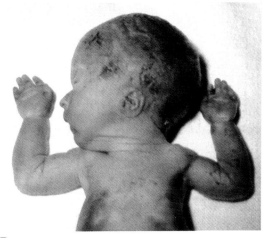

A **B**

FIGURE 1. **A** and **B,** Stillborn infant with triploidy showing relatively large-appearing upper head in relation to very small face and 3-4 syndactyly of the fingers.

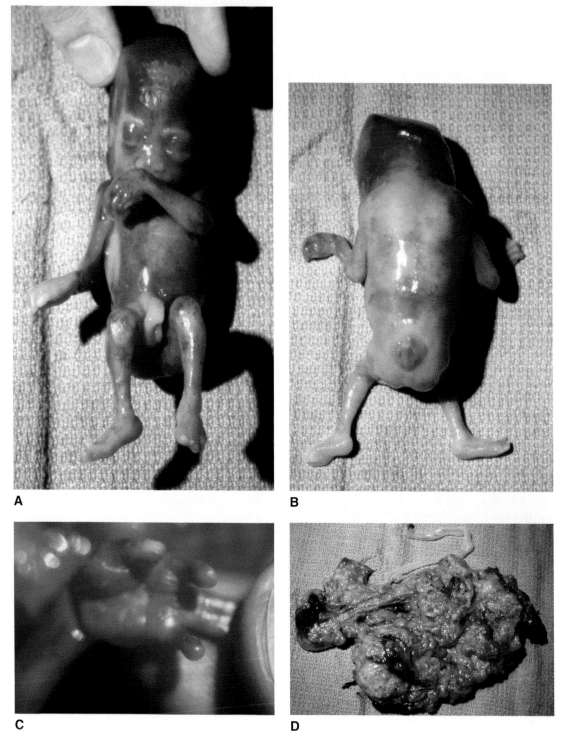

FIGURE 2.   A–D, Severely growth-retarded 20-week fetus with 69,XXY karyotype. Note the meningomyelocele and 3-4 syndactyly. This phenotype is consistent with two paternal chromosomal copies and one maternal chromosomal copy. It is the most common form of triploidy and typically results in a growth-retarded fetus with a large hydatidiform placenta.

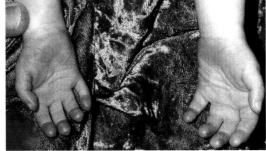

B

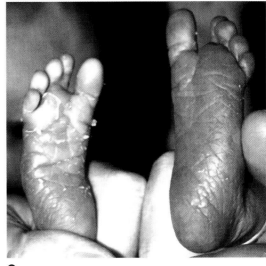

C

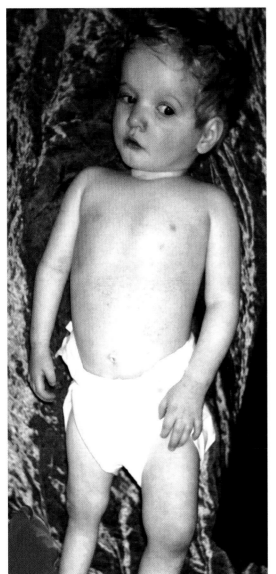

A

FIGURE 3.   A–C, Infant with asymmetric growth deficiency (right side smaller), syndactyly of third and fourth fingers, and mild developmental delay who has triploid/diploid mixoploidy syndrome that is evident only in cultured fibroblasts. (Courtesy Dr. John M. Graham, Cedars-Sinai Medical Center, Los Angeles.)

DELETION 3P SYNDROME
Mental and Growth Deficiency, Ptosis, Postaxial Polydactyly

Partial deletion of the distal part of the short arm of chromosome 3 was first reported by Verjaal and De Nef in 1978. Many cases have subsequently been reported. In most cases the disorder has arisen de novo. Although typically a terminal deletion with breakpoints at chromosome band 3p25, more recent molecular studies have shown the location of the 3p breakpoint to be variable.

ABNORMALITIES

Growth. Prenatal onset of growth deficiency, most striking postnatally.
Performance. Severe to profound intellectual disability, hypotonia.
Craniofacial. Microcephaly with flat occiput, synophrys, epicanthal folds, ptosis, short palpebral fissures, prominent nasal bridge, small nose with anteverted nares, long philtrum, malformed ears, micrognathia, downturned corners of mouth.
Other. Postaxial polydactyly of hands and, less frequently, of the feet.

OCCASIONAL ABNORMALITIES

Trigonocephaly with prominent metopic sutures, agenesis of corpus callosum, upslanting palpebral fissures, ocular hypertelorism, preauricular pits or fistula, cleft palate; cardiac defects, including ventricular septal defect (two patients) and one patient with double mitral valve, atrioventricular canal defect and tricuspid atresia; inguinal and/or umbilical hernia, hiatal hernia, common mesentery, anteriorly placed anus; renal anomalies, including pelvic and/or cystic kidney; cryptorchidism; scoliosis.

NATURAL HISTORY

Nasogastric tube feeding because of poor suck is often required. Persistent central and obstructive apnea is common with frequent pneumonia. Gastroesophageal reflux and profound failure to thrive often occur. Limited life span is typical; however, survival into adulthood has been reported. Many survivors are blind and deaf and interact only minimally with their environment. Many are blind and deaf and interact only minimally with their environment.

ETIOLOGY

The cause of this disorder is partial deletion of the short arm of chromosome 3. Most cases are terminal deletions with breakpoints at 3p25. However, the 3p breakpoint has recently been shown to be variable. In one case an interstitial deletion at 3p25-p26, thought to be the smallest 3p deletion associated with the characteristic phenotype, was reported. In the vast majority of cases, the deletion has occurred de novo.

References

Verjaal M, De Nef J: A patient with a partial deletion of the short arm of chromosome 3, *Am J Dis Child* 132:43, 1978.

Higginbottom MC, et al: A second patient with partial deletion of the short arm of chromosome 3: Karyotype 46,XY,del(3)(p25), *J Med Genet* 19:71, 1982.

Tolmie JL, et al: Partial deletion of the short arm of chromosome 3, *Clin Genet* 29:538, 1986.

Schwyzer U, et al: Terminal deletion of the short arm of chromosome 3, del(3pter-p25): A recognizable syndrome, *Helv Paediatr Acta* 42:309, 1987.

Nienhaus H, et al: Infant with del(3)(p25-pter): Karyotype-phenotype correlation and review of previously reported cases, *Am J Med Genet* 44:573, 1992.

Mowrey PN, et al: Clinical and molecular analysis of deletion 3p25-pter syndrome, *Am J Med Genet* 46:623, 1993.

Cargile CB, et al: Molecular cytogenetic characterization of a subtle interstitial del(3)(p25.3p26.2) in a patient with deletion 3p syndrome, *Am J Med Genet* 109:133, 2002.

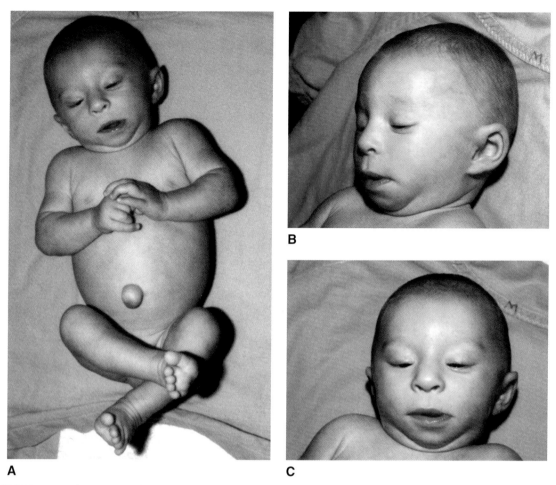

FIGURE 1.   Deletion 3p syndrome. **A–C,** Photograph of affected 5-month-old boy. Note the bilateral ptosis, long philtrum, micrognathia, and umbilical hernia. (From Higginbottom MC, et al: *J Med Genet* 19:71, 1982, with permission.)

DUPLICATION 3Q SYNDROME
Mental and Growth Deficiency, Broad Nasal Root, Hypertrichosis

First described by Falek and colleagues in 1966, this disorder initially was confused with the Brachmann–de Lange syndrome. Hirschhorn and colleagues performed chromosome banding studies in 1973 that associated duplication of the 3q21→qter region with a distinct phenotype that Francke and Opitz subsequently emphasized can be clinically distinguished from Brachmann–de Lange syndrome.

ABNORMALITIES

Growth. Postnatal growth deficiency (100%).

Performance. Intellectual disability with brain anomalies/seizures.

Craniofacial. Abnormal head shape, frequently due to craniosynostosis; hypertrichosis and synophrys; upslanting palpebral fissures; broad nasal root; anteverted nares; prominent maxilla; long philtrum; downturned corners of mouth; high-arched palate; cleft palate; micrognathia; malformed ears; short, webbed neck.

Limbs. Fifth finger clinodactyly, hypoplastic nails, simian crease, talipes equinovarus arch dermal ridge pattern or digital pattern with low ridge counts.

Other. Cardiac defects, chest deformities, renal or urinary tract anomalies, genital anomalies (primarily cryptorchidism), umbilical hernia.

OCCASIONAL ABNORMALITIES

Microphthalmia, glaucoma, cataract, coloboma, strabismus, agenesis of corpus callosum; decreased white matter; conductive hearing loss; central apnea; syndactyly, polydactyly, camptodactyly, short limbs, cubitus valgus, dislocated radial head, ulnar or fibular deviation of hands or feet, omphalocele, hemivertebrae.

NATURAL HISTORY

Death before 12 months occurs in about one third of cases, primarily related to infections and cardiac defects. For survivors, intellectual disability, growth retardation, and pulmonary infections are the rule.

ETIOLOGY

The etiology of this disorder is duplication for 3q21→qter. Seventy-five percent of cases arise from a segregation of a parental rearrangement. Only nine cases with pure dup3q have been reported. A gene or genes at 3q26.31-q27.3 are most likely essential for the characteristic phenotype.

COMMENT

Although superficial resemblance exists between the duplication 3q syndrome and the Brachmann–de Lange syndrome, they are clearly distinct disorders that can be differentiated clinically.

References

Falek A, et al: Familial de Lange syndrome with chromosome abnormalities, *Pediatrics* 37:92, 1966.

Hirschhorn K, et al: Precise identification of various chromosomal abnormalities, *Ann Hum Genet* 36:3875, 1973.

Francke U, Opitz J: Chromosome 3q duplication and the Brachmann-de Lange syndrome (BDLS), *J Pediatr* 95:161, 1979.

Steinbach P, et al: The dup(3q) syndrome: Report of eight cases and review of the literature, *Am J Med Genet* 10:159, 1981.

Wilson GN, et al: Further delineation of the dup(3q) syndrome, *Am J Med Genet* 22:117, 1985.

Van Essen AJ, et al: Partial 3q duplication syndrome and assignment of D3S5 to 3q25→3q28, *Hum Genet* 87:151, 1991.

Aqua M, et al: Duplication 3q syndrome: Molecular delineation of the critical region, *Am J Med Genet* 55:33, 1995.

Battaglia A, et al: Familial complex 3q;10q rearrangement unraveled by subtelomeric FISH analysis, *Am J Med Genet* 140A:144, 2006.

Shanske AL, et al: Delineation of the breakpoints of pure duplication 3q due to a de novo duplication event using SOMA, *Am J Med Genet* 152A:3185, 2010.

A

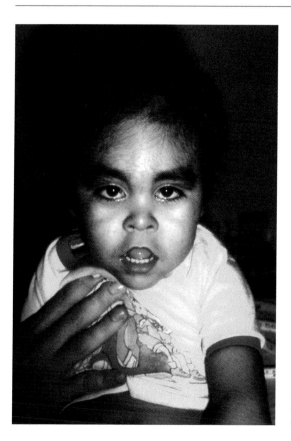

FIGURE 1. Duplication 3q syndrome. An affected 3-month-old boy. Note the hypertrichosis, long philtrum, and downturned corners of the mouth.

DELETION 4P SYNDROME (WOLF-HIRSCHHORN SYNDROME)

Ocular Hypertelorism with Broad or Beaked Nose; Microcephaly and/or Cranial Asymmetry; and Low-Set, Simple Ear with Preauricular Dimple

After delineation of the cri du chat syndrome, a few patients with deletions of the short arm of a B-group chromosome were found who lacked the typical cry and some other features of that condition. Autoradiographic labeling studies revealed that the deficit chromosome was a number 4 rather than a number 5.

ABNORMALITIES

Growth. Marked growth deficiency, of prenatal onset.

Performance. Feeble fetal activity, hypotonia, severe intellectual disability, seizures.

Craniofacial. Microcephaly, "Greek warrior helmet" appearance of nose, high forehead, prominent glabella, highly arched eyebrows, strabismus, eye or optic nerve defects, upper lid/iris/chorioretinal coloboma, ocular hypertelorism, epicanthal folds, cleft lip and/or palate, downturned "fishlike" mouth, short upper lip and philtrum, micrognathia, posterior midline scalp defects, cranial asymmetry, preauricular tag or pit.

Extremities. Hypoplastic dermal ridges, low dermal ridge count, simian creases, talipes equinovarus, hyperconvex fingernails.

Skin. Cutis marmorata, dry skin, dimples.

Other. Hypospadias, cryptorchidism, clitoral hypoplasia, sacral dimple or sinus; cardiac anomalies, including atrial septal defect, pulmonary stenosis, ventricular septal defect, and patent ductus arteriosis; scoliosis.

OCCASIONAL ABNORMALITIES

Exophthalmos, ptosis, microcornea, Rieger anomaly, nystagmus, glaucoma, low-set ears, fused teeth, taurodontism, defect of the medial half of the eyebrows, hearing loss, hypodontia of permanent teeth, low hairline with webbed neck, metatarsus adductus, polydactyly, ectrodactyly, clinodactyly, hip dislocation, accessory ossification centers in proximal metacarpals, absence of pubic rami, bladder exstrophy, diaphragmatic hernia, delayed bone age, abnormalities in sternal ossification centers, "bottle opener" deformity of clavicles, precocious puberty, renal anomaly, malrotation of small bowel, cavum or absent septum pellucidum, interventricular cysts, tethered cord, myelodysplastic syndrome, autism spectrum disorder.

NATURAL HISTORY

Although severe intellectual disability is the rule, 45% of patients in one study became ambulatory, 18% could help with dressing and undressing and performing simple household tasks, and 10% became toilet trained. Seizures, initially difficult to control, tend to disappear with age. Expressive language is extremely limited, although 6% were able to pronounce simple sentences. Major feeding difficulties, often requiring gastrostomy, are a major problem in infancy. Routine care in infancy should include cardiac, ophthalmologic, and audiologic evaluations, renal ultrasound, EEG, swallowing studies, and developmental testing. In childhood, continued developmental testing, appropriate school placement, and follow-up EEG are indicated. Slow but continued progress in all areas should be anticipated.

ETIOLOGY

The cause of this disorder is partial deletion of the short arm of chromosome 4. The clinical phenotype is determined by 4p deletions that include the terminal 4p16.3 region. A newly defined critical region within an interval of 300–600 kb between the loci D4S3327 and D4S98-D4S168 has been discovered. The size of the deletion, the occurrence of complex chromosome anomalies, and the severity of seizures are prognostic factors. Eighty-seven percent of cases represent de novo deletions, while in 13% of cases, one of the parents is a balanced translocation carrier. In the cases in which there is a familial translocation, there is a 2-to-1 excess of maternally derived 4p deletions, while in the de novo deletions, the origin of the deleted chromosome is paternal in approximately 80% of cases. In those cases in which the disorder is suspected clinically but standard chromosome studies are normal, molecular approaches can be utilized.

References

Leão JC, et al: New syndrome associated with partial deletion of short arms of chromosome no. 4, *JAMA* 202:434, 1967.

Wolf U, Reinwein H: Klinische und cytogenetische Differentialdiagnose der Defizienzen an den kurzen Armen der B-Chromosomen, *Z Kinderheilkd* 98:235, 1967.

Guthrie RD, et al: The 4p- syndrome, *Am J Dis Child* 122:421, 1971.

Lurie IW, et al: The Wolf-Hirschhorn syndrome, *Clin Genet* 17:375, 1980.

Katz DS, Smith TH: Wolf syndrome, *Pediatr Radiol* 21:369, 1991.

Quarrell OWJ, et al: Paternal origin of the chromosomal deletion resulting in Wolf-Hirschhorn syndrome, *J Med Genet* 28:256, 1991.

Estabrooks LL, et al: Molecular characterisation of chromosome 4p deletions resulting in Wolf-Hirschhorn syndrome, *J Med Genet* 31:103, 1994.

Fagan-Bagric K, et al: A practical application of fluorescent in situ hybridization to the Wolf-Hirschhorn syndrome, *Pediatrics* 93:826, 1994.

Sharathkumar A, et al: Malignant hematological disorders in children with Wolf-Hirschhorn syndrome, *Am J Med Genet* 119:164, 2003.

Battaglia A, et al: Update on the clinical features and natural history of Wolf-Hirschhorn (4p-) syndrome: Experience with 87 patients and recommendations for routine health supervision, *Am J Med Genet* 148C:246, 2008.

Zollino M, et al: On the nosology and pathogenesis of Wolf-Hirschhorn syndrome: Genotype-phenotype correlation analysis of 80 children and literature review, *Am J Med Genet* 148C:257, 2008.

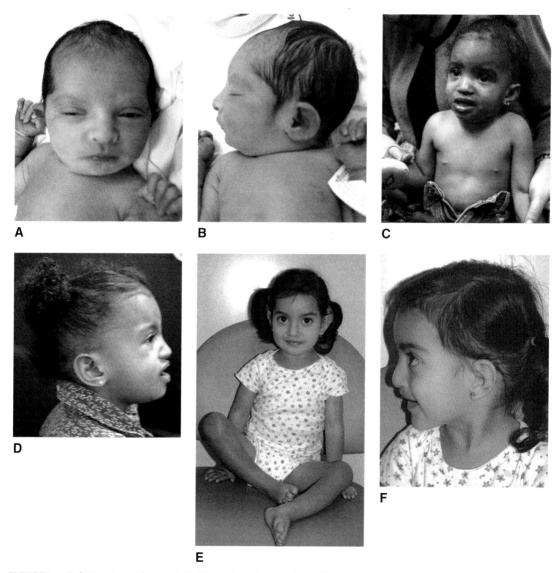

FIGURE 1. Deletion 4p syndrome. **A–F,** Affected children at three different ages. Note the ocular hypertelorism, prominent glabella, supraorbital ridge continuous with the nasal bridge, short philtrum, micrognathia, and simple ears. (**E** and **F,** Courtesy Dr. Lynne M. Bird, Children's Hospital, San Diego.)

DELETION 4Q SYNDROME
Mental and Growth Deficiency, Cleft Palate, Limb Anomalies

Partial deletion of the long arm of chromosome 4 was initially reported by Ockey and colleagues in 1967. Townes and colleagues proposed the existence of a 4q- syndrome in 1981. The phenotype was further delineated by Mitchell and colleagues in 1981 and by Lin and colleagues in 1988.

ABNORMALITIES

Growth. Postnatal onset of growth deficiency (83%)

Performance. Moderate to severe mental deficiency (92%), hypotonia (28%), seizures (17%)

Craniofacial. Ocular hypertelorism (56%), short nose (67%), broad nasal bridge (94%), cleft palate (94%), micrognathia (94%), low-set, posteriorly rotated ears (56%), abnormal pinnae (67%)

Limbs. Fifth finger clinodactyly (44%), tapering fifth finger (50%), pointed/duplicated fifth fingernail (33%), absent to hypoplastic flexion creases on fifth fingers (56%), abnormal thumb/hallux implantation (44%), simian crease (61%), overlapping toes (22%)

Cardiac. Ventricular septal defect, patent ductus arteriosus, peripheral pulmonic stenosis, aortic stenosis, tricuspid atresia, atrial septal defect, aortic coarctation, tetralogy of Fallot; genitourinary defects (50%); gastrointestinal defects (22%).

OCCASIONAL ABNORMALITIES

Asymmetric face (17%), small, upslanting palpebral fissures (22%), epicanthal folds (39%), anteverted nares (33%), cleft lip (39%), Robin sequence (28%), camptodactyly (17%), missing digits (11%), genitourinary defects (50%), gastrointestinal defects (22%)

NATURAL HISTORY

Fifty percent of patients with a terminal deletion (q31→qter) died before 15 months of age of cardiopulmonary difficulties including asphyxia, apnea, and congestive heart failure. The Robin sequence needs careful consideration and management. Of those who survived, moderate to severe intellectual disability occurred in the vast majority. One child who is at least 15 years old has profound mental deficiency, behavioral disorder, and seizures.

ETIOLOGY

The cause of this disorder is deletion of 4q31→qter. Virtually all cases represent de novo defects.

COMMENT

Deletions at 4q32 seem to be similar to deletions at 4q31. More distal deletions at 4q33 and 4q34 are associated with a less severe clinical phenotype. Patients with interstitial deletion of 4q differ completely from those with terminal deletions.

References

Ockey CH, et al: A large deletion of the long arm of chromosome no. 4 in a child with limb abnormalities, *Arch Dis Child* 42:428, 1967.

Townes PL, et al: 4q- syndrome, *Am J Dis Child* 133:383, 1979.

Davis JM, et al: Brief clinical report: The del(4) (q31) syndrome—a recognizable disorder with atypical Robin malformation sequence, *Am J Med Genet* 9:113, 1981.

Mitchell JA, et al: Deletions of different segments of the long arm of chromosome 4, *Am J Med Genet* 8:73, 1981.

Lin AE, et al: Interstitial and terminal deletions of the long arm of chromosome 4: Further delineation of phenotypes, *Am J Med Genet* 31:533, 1988.

Taub PJ, et al: Mandibular distraction in the setting of chromosome 4q deletion, *J Plast Reconstr Aesthet Surg* 65:e95, 2012.

A

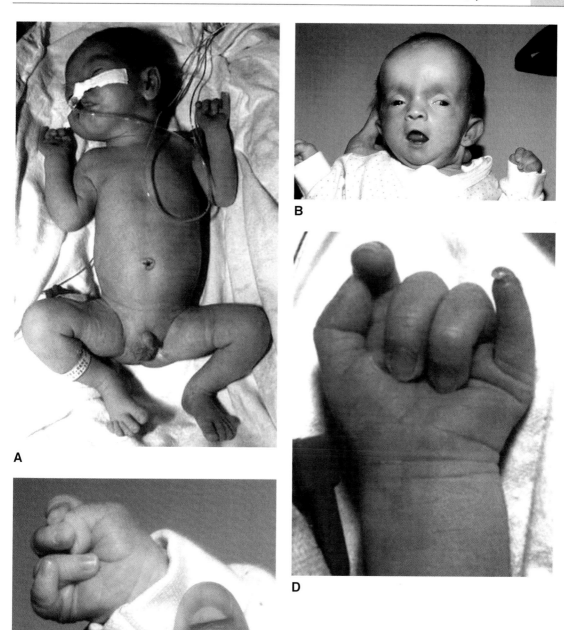

A

B

C

D

FIGURE 1. Deletion 4q syndrome. **A–D,** Affected newborn infants. Note the ocular hypertelorism, abnormal pinnae, and pointed fifth fingernail.

DELETION 5P SYNDROME
(CRI DU CHAT SYNDROME, PARTIAL DELETION OF THE SHORT ARM OF CHROMOSOME NUMBER 5 SYNDROME, 5P- SYNDROME)
Cat-Like Cry in Infancy, Microcephaly, Downward Slant of the Palpebral Fissures

Lejeune and colleagues first described this condition in 1963. The incidence of this condition is estimated between 1:15,000 and 1:50,000.

ABNORMALITIES

Growth. Pre- and postnatal growth deficiency with respect to length, weight, and head circumference.

Performance. Intellectual disability; cat-like cry at birth, throughout the first year of life, and later; timbre of voice (shrill, sometime hoarse) abnormal in most adolescents; hypotonia in infancy, replaced later by hypertonia; hyperactivity.

Craniofacial. Round face, metopic ridging, hypertelorism, epicanthal folds, downslanting palpebral fissures, strabismus, downturned corners of mouth, short philtrum, micrognathia, low-set poorly formed ears, facial asymmetry.

Cardiac. Most commonly ventricular and atrial septal defects, patent ductus arteriosus.

Hands. Simian crease, distal axial triradius, slightly short metacarpals.

OCCASIONAL ABNORMALITIES

Agenesis of corpus callosum, cerebral atrophy, cerebellar hypoplasia. Cleft lip and cleft palate, myopia, optic atrophy, preauricular skin tag, bifid uvula, dental malocclusion, short neck, clinodactyly, inguinal hernia, cryptorchidism, absent kidney and spleen, hemivertebra, scoliosis, flat feet, premature graying of hair. Renal anomalies, including renal agenesis or hypoplasia, renal ectopia, horseshoe kidney, and hydronephrosis. Congenital megacolon.

NATURAL HISTORY

In one study 6.4% of affected children died (9 within the first 6 months of life). As babies, the patients tend to be unusually squirmy in their activity. The mewing cry, ascribed to abnormal laryngeal development, becomes less pronounced with the increasing age of the patient. Sucking and feeding problems are common in the first year, as are respiratory difficulties. A study by Wilkins and colleagues of 65 children with cri du chat syndrome reared in the home suggests that a much higher level of intellectual performance can be achieved than was previously suggested from studies performed on institutionalized patients. With early special schooling and a supportive home environment, some affected children attained the social and psychomotor level of a normal 5- to 6-year-old child. One half of the children older than 10 years had a vocabulary and sentence structure adequate for communication. Scoliosis is a frequent occurrence.

ETIOLOGY

The underlying chromosomal aberration is partial deletion of the short arm of chromosome number 5. Approximately 85% of cases result from sporadic de novo deletions, while 15% arise secondary to unequal segregation of a parental translocation. Although the size of the deletion is variable, a critical region for the high-pitched cry maps to 5p15.3, while the chromosomal region involved in the remaining features maps to 5p15.2. There is variability in expression of the clinical phenotype related to the size and type of the deletion. Thus, for example, individuals with deletion involving just 5p15.3 have the cat-like cry, but the facial features and degree of developmental delay are much less severe.

References

Lejeune J, et al: Trois cas de deletion partielle du bras court du chromosome 5, *C R Acad Sci [D] (Paris)* 257:3098, 1963.

Berg JM, et al: Partial deletion of short arm of a chromosome of the 4 and 5 group (Denver) in an adult male, *J Ment Defic Res* 9:219, 1965.

Breg WR, et al: The cri-du-chat syndrome in adolescents and adults, *J Pediatr* 77:782, 1970.

Wilkins LE, Brown JA, Wolf B: Psychomotor development in 65 home-reared children with cri-du-chat syndrome, *J Pediatr* 97:401, 1980.

Overhauser J, et al: Molecular and phenotypic mapping of the short arm of chromosome 5: Sublocalization of the critical region of the cri-du-chat syndrome, *Hum Mol Genet* 3:247, 1994.

Gersh M, et al: Evidence for a distinct region causing a cat-like cry in patients with 5p deletions, *Am J Med Genet* 56:1404, 1995.

Mainardi PC, et al: The natural history of cri du chat syndrome. A report from the Italian Register, *Eur J Med Genet* 49:363, 2006.

Cerruti Mainardi P: Cri du Chat syndrome, *Orphanet J Rare Dis* 1:33, 2006.

A

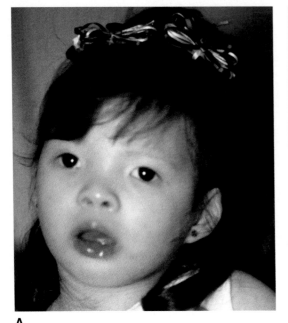

A

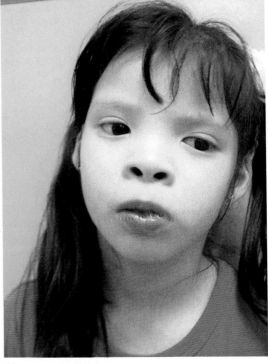

B

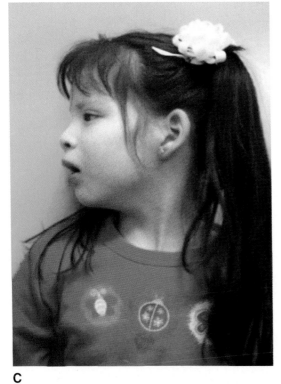

C

FIGURE 1.   Deletion 5p syndrome. **A–C,** Affected child at 3 and 5 years of age. Note the round face, ocular hypertelorism, and epicanthal folds. (Courtesy Dr. Lynne M. Bird, Children's Hospital, San Diego.)

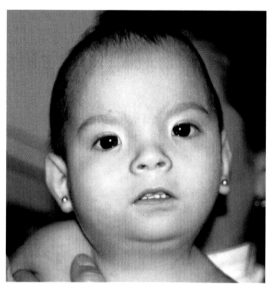 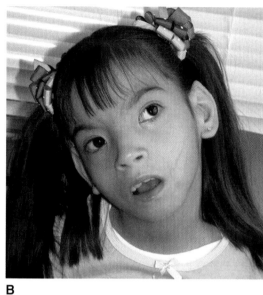

A   **B**

FIGURE 2.   **A** and **B,** Affected child at 13 months and 8 years of age. Note the round face, ocular hypertelorism, and epicanthal folds. (Courtesy Dr. Lynne M. Bird, Children's Hospital, San Diego.)

DELETION 9P SYNDROME (9P MONOSOMY, 9P- SYNDROME)
Craniostenosis with Trigonocephaly, Upslanting Palpebral Fissures, Hypoplastic Supraorbital Ridges

Since the initial delineation of this disorder in 1973 by Alfi and colleagues, more than 100 similarly affected patients with 9p- as the sole chromosomal anomaly have been reported.

ABNORMALITIES

Growth. Usually normal.

Performance. Mean intelligence quotient (IQ) is 49, with a range from 33 to 73; motor delay; hypotonia; speech delay; learning difficulties; behavioral problems, including low concentration, temper tantrums with head banging, and sleep problems; social adaptation is often good.

Craniofacial. Craniosynostosis involving the metopic suture leading to trigonocephaly; flat occiput; short, upslanting palpebral fissures; epicanthal folds, prominent eyes secondary to hypoplastic supraorbital ridges; highly arched eyebrows; midfacial hypoplasia with a short nose, depressed nasal bridge, anteverted nares, and long philtrum; small mouth, micrognathia; posteriorly rotated, poorly formed ears with hypoplastic, adherent ear lobes; short broad neck with low hairline.

Limbs. Long middle phalanges of the fingers with extra flexion creases; short distal phalanges with short nails; excess in whorl patterns on fingertips; foot positioning defects; simian crease.

Cardiovascular. Ventricular septal defects, patent ductus arteriosus, and/or pulmonic stenosis in one third to one half of patients.

Other. Scoliosis, widely spaced nipples, diastasis recti, inguinal and/or umbilical hernia, micropenis and/or cryptorchidism in males; hypoplastic labia majora in females.

OCCASIONAL ABNORMALITIES

Ptosis; cleft palate; choanal atresia; congenital glaucoma; postaxial polydactyly; diaphragmatic hernia; omphalocele; hydronephrosis; radiographic anomalies of ribs, clavicles, and vertebrae; male-to-female sex reversal; melanoma, gonadoblastoma.

NATURAL HISTORY

Mean age for sitting without support is 13 months, for walking without support is 27.6 months, for acquisition of first words is 20 months, and for speaking two-word sentences is 39 months. The majority of children learn to ride a bike. All have learning difficulties varying from mild to severe. Behavioral problems are common. Despite the delay in language acquisition, following development of sufficient speech, these children's abilities are often overestimated because of fluent language development and social skills.

ETIOLOGY

The critical region for the consensus clinical phenotype of the deletion 9p syndrome is localized in a ~300 kb region on 9p22.3. However, it is important to realize that del 9p is heterogeneous and is associated with variable deletion sizes. The candidate region for sex reversal, an occasional feature of deletion 9p syndrome, has been narrowed down to the 9p24.3 region. The neurodevelopmental features are independent of the size of the deletion.

References

Alfi OS, et al: Deletion of the short arm of chromosome 9(46,9p-): A new deletion syndrome, *Ann Genet* 16:17, 1973.

Huret JL, et al: Eleven new cases of del(9p) and features from 80 cases, *J Med Genet* 25:741, 1988.

Onesimo R, et al: Chromosome 9 deletion syndrome and sex reversal: novel findings and redefinition of the critically deleted regions, *Am J Med Genet* 158A:2266, 2012.

Chilosi A, et al: Del (9p) syndrome: Proposed behavior phenotype, *Am J Med Genet* 100:138, 2001.

Swinkels MEM, et al: Clinical and cytogenetic characterization of 13 Dutch patients with deletion 9p syndrome, *Am J Med Genet* 146A:1430, 2008.

Barbaro M, et al: Characterization of deletions at 9p affecting the candidate regions for sex reversal and deletion 9p syndrome by MLPA, *Eur J Hum Genet* 17:1439, 2009.

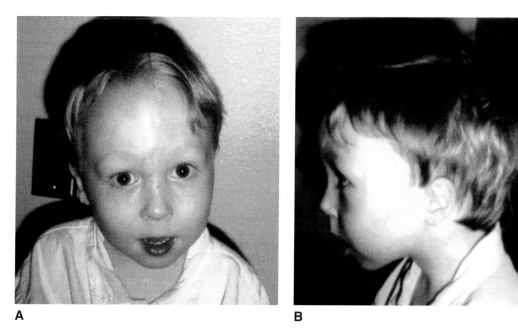

A   **B**

FIGURE 1.   Deletion 9p syndrome. **A** and **B,** Note the prominent forehead with metopic ridge, trigonocephaly, frontal hair upsweep, short nose with anteverted nares, and low-set ears.

DUPLICATION 9P SYNDROME (TRISOMY 9P SYNDROME)
Distal Phalangeal Hypoplasia, Delayed Closure of Anterior Fontanel, Ocular Hypertelorism

First reported in 1970 by Rethoré and colleagues, the pattern of malformation was set forth by Centerwall and Beatty-DeSana in 1975. More than 150 individuals with complete or partial dup9p have been reported.

ABNORMALITIES

Growth. Growth deficiency, primarily of postnatal onset; delayed puberty such that some patients continue to grow up to the middle of their third decade.

Performance. Severe mental deficiency; language tends to be most significantly delayed.

Craniofacial. Microcephaly, hypertelorism, downslanting palpebral fissures, deep-set eyes, prominent nose, downturned corners of the mouth, cup-shaped ears.

Limbs. Short fingers and toes with small nails and short terminal phalanges; fifth finger clinodactyly with single flexion crease; single palmar crease.

Other Skeletal. Kyphoscoliosis, usually developing during the second decade; hypoplasia of periscapular muscles with deep acromial dimples; defective ossification of the pubic bone, broad ischial tuberosity; pseudoepiphysis of metacarpals, metatarsals, and middle phalanges of fifth fingers; delayed closure of cranial sutures and fontanels.

OCCASIONAL ABNORMALITIES

Normal intelligence (1 patient); micrognathia, epicanthal folds, short or webbed neck; partial 2-3 syndactyly of toes and 3-4 syndactyly of fingers, congenital heart defects in 5% to 10% of cases and cleft lip and/or palate in 5%; hydrocephalus, agenesis of corpus callosum, renal malformations, micropenis, cryptorchidism, hypospadias, talipes equinovarus, and congenital hip dislocation.

NATURAL HISTORY

Approximately 5% to 10% of reported patients died in early childhood.

ETIOLOGY

Partial duplication of 9p. The 9p22 region is responsible for the observed phenotype. However, there are a number of cases reported with various duplicated areas. Although intellectual disability occurs in virtually all of these patients, the severity of the clinical phenotype correlates with the extent of the triplicated material. Partial trisomy 9pter→p21 is associated with mild craniofacial features and rare skeletal or visceral defects. Partial trisomy 9pter→p11 is associated with the typical craniofacial features, while partial trisomy 9pter→q11-13 is associated not only with the typical craniofacial features but also with skeletal and cardiac defects. Partial trisomy 9pter→q22-32 is associated with the typical craniofacial features, intrauterine growth deficiency, cleft lip/palate, micrognathia, cardiac anomalies, and congenital hip dislocation. If the trisomic segment is larger than that (9pter→9q31 or 32), the clinical findings no longer fit into the trisomy 9p syndrome but rather resemble trisomy 9 mosaic syndrome.

References

Rethoré MO, et al: Sur quatre cas de trisomie pour le bras court du chromosome 9. Individualisation d'une nouvelle entité morbide, *Ann Genet* 13:217, 1970.

Centerwall WR, Beatty-DeSana JW: The trisomy 9p syndrome, *Pediatrics* 56:748, 1975.

Schinzel A: Trisomy 9p, a chromosome aberration with distinct radiologic findings, *Radiology* 130:125, 1979.

Wilson GN, et al: The phenotypic and cytogenetic spectrum of partial trisomy 9, *Am J Med Genet* 20:277, 1985.

Zou YS, et al: Further delineation of the critical region for the 9p-duplication syndrome, *Am J Med Genet* 149A:272, 2009.

Bouhjar IB, et al: Array-CGH study of partial trisomy 9p without mental retardation, *Am J Med Genet* 155A:1735, 2011.

Trisomy 9p
Main hand x-ray findings at age 9 years

Trisomy 9p
Main feet x-ray findings at age 9 years

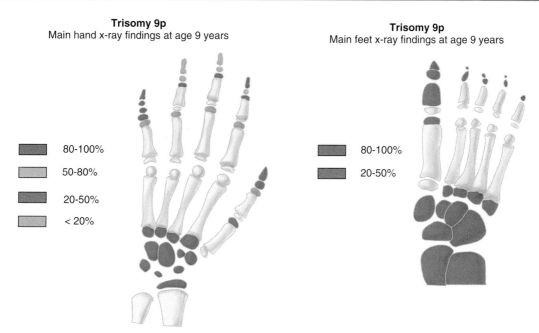

80-100%

50-80%

20-50%

< 20%

80-100%

20-50%

FIGURE 1. Duplication 9p syndrome. Diagram of major radiologic findings in hand and foot of a 9-year-old patient. Pseudoepiphyses on metacarpals and metatarsals 2 to 5; notches on metacarpal 1, metatarsal 1, and proximal and middle phalanges of fingers; hypoplasia of the middle phalanx of fifth finger, terminal phalanges of fingers, and middle and terminal phalanges of toes; thick epiphyses, especially of terminal phalanges of big toe, thumb, and little finger; and clinodactyly of fifth finger. (From Schinzel A: *Radiology* 130:125, 1979, with permission.)

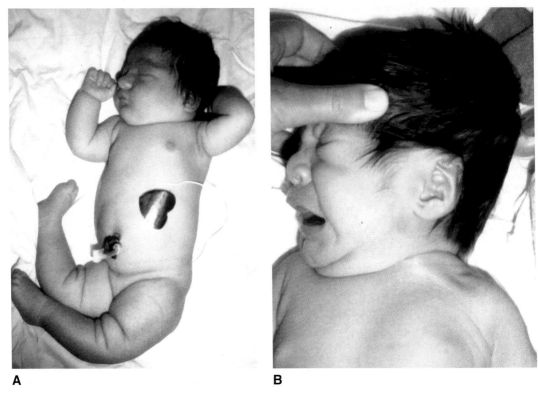

A   B

FIGURE 2.   A and B, Affected newborn.

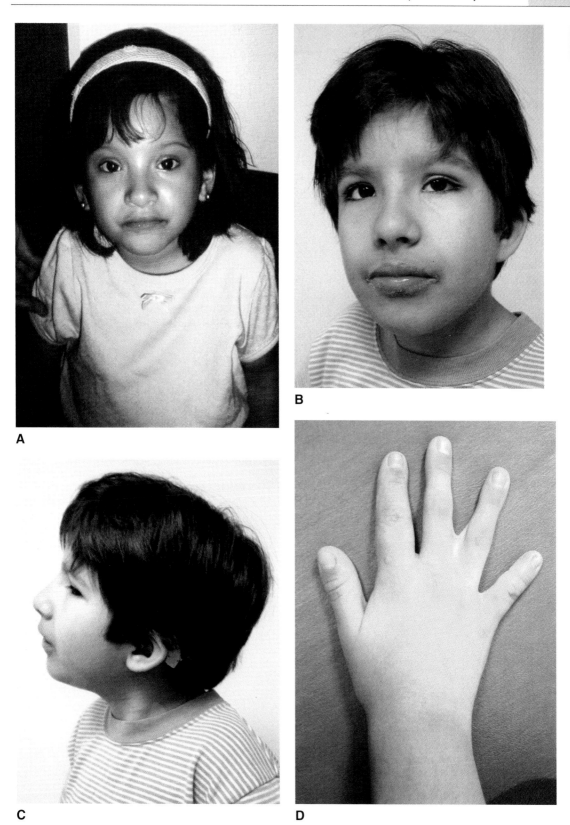

FIGURE 3. **A–D,** Note the ocular hypertelorism, prominent nose, downturned corners of mouth, cup-shaped ear, short fingers, and 3-4 syndactyly.

DUPLICATION 10Q SYNDROME
Ptosis, Short Palpebral Fissures, Camptodactyly

First set forth as a specific phenotype by Yunis and Sanchez in 1974, this disorder was further delineated by Klep-de Pater and colleagues in 1979.

ABNORMALITIES

Growth. Prenatal onset of growth deficiency; mean birth weight, 2.7 kg.

Performance. Severe to moderate intellectual disability, hypotonia.

Craniofacial. Microcephaly; flat face with high forehead and high, arched eyebrows; ptosis; short, downslanting palpebral fissures; microphthalmia; broad and depressed nasal bridge, anteverted nares, bow-shaped mouth with prominent upper lip; cleft palate; malformed posteriorly rotated ears.

Limbs. Camptodactyly, proximally placed thumbs, syndactyly between second and third toes, foot position anomalies, hypoplastic dermal ridge patterns.

Other. Heart and renal malformations, each of which occurs in approximately one half of affected patients; kyphoscoliosis; pectus excavatum; 11 pairs of ribs; congenital hip dislocation; cryptorchidism.

OCCASIONAL ABNORMALITIES

Brain malformations, ocular anomalies, malrotation of the gut, hypospadias, vertebral malformations, postaxial polydactyly of hands, streak gonads.

NATURAL HISTORY

Approximately one half of reported patients died within the first year of life, usually from congenital heart defects and other malformations. Surviving children showed marked mental deficiency and usually are bedridden without the ability to communicate.

ETIOLOGY

This disorder is caused by duplication 10q24→qter, the distal segment of the long arm of chromosome 10. Individuals with dup10q25→qter lack major malformations, and the prognosis is more favorable.

References

Yunis JJ, Sanchez O: A new syndrome resulting from partial trisomy for the distal third of the long arm of chromosome 10, *J Pediatr* 84:567, 1974.

Klep-de Pater JM, et al: Partial trisomy 10q. A recognizable syndrome, *Hum Genet* 46:29, 1979.

Briscioli V, et al: Trisomy 10qter confirmed by in situ hybridization, *J Med Genet* 30:601, 1993.

Aglan MS, et al: Partial trisomy of the distal part of 10q: A report of two Egyptian cases, *Genet Couns* 19:199, 2008.

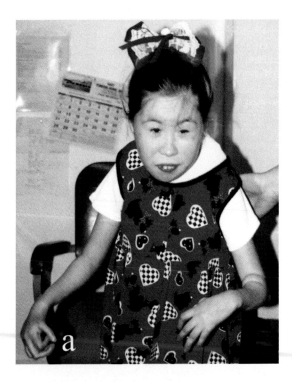

FIGURE 1. Note the ptosis, high-arched eyebrows, and proximally placed thumbs. (Courtesy Dr. Bryan D. Hall, University of Kentucky, Lexington.)

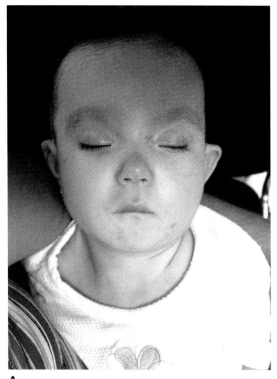

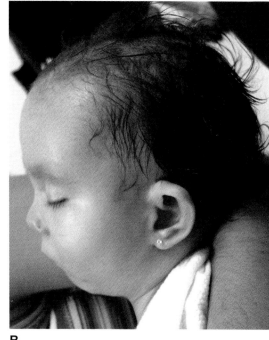

FIGURE 2.   Duplication 10q syndrome. **A–C,** Six-month-old infant. Note the flat face with high forehead; broad nasal bridge; anteverted nares; malformed, posteriorly rotated ears; camptodactyly; and proximally placed thumbs.

ANIRIDIA–WILMS TUMOR ASSOCIATION (WAGR SYNDROME)

Numerous cases of the association of Wilms tumor and aniridia have been reported, and it is estimated that 1 in 70 patients with aniridia also has Wilms tumor. In 1978 Riccardi and colleagues identified an interstitial deletion of 11p in a group of patients with aniridia and Wilms tumor, who also had genitourinary anomalies and intellectual disability, a pattern of malformation referred to as WAGR syndrome. The features of that disorder are set forth below.

ABNORMALITIES

Performance. Moderate to severe intellectual disability in most patients, attention-deficit/hyperactivity disorder, autism spectrum disorder.
Growth. Growth deficiency and microcephaly in at least 50% of patients.
Craniofacial. Prominent lips, micrognathia, poorly formed ears.
Eyes. Aniridia; congenital cataracts, glaucoma, nystagmus, optic nerve hypoplasia.
Genitourinary. Wilms tumor in 50% of patients; cryptorchidism.
Other. Obesity.

OCCASIONAL ABNORMALITIES

Ptosis, blindness, anterior segment anomaly, macular/foveal hypoplasia, microphthalmia, retinal detachment, micrognathia, kyphoscoliosis, metatarsus adductus, hemihypertrophy, talipes equinovarus, syndactyly/clinodactyly, inguinal hernias, obesity, ambiguous external genitalia, sex reversal, hypospadias, streak ovaries, bicornate uterus, hypoplastic uterus, ureteral duplication, renal cysts, gonadoblastoma, fifth finger clinodactyly, ventricular septal defects, patent ductus arteriosis, tetralogy of Fallot, atrial septal defects, chronic pancreatitis, hyperlipidemia, diabetes.

ETIOLOGY

Most cases represent a de novo deletion of 11p13 that encompasses, among a number of contiguous genes, the aniridia gene, *PAX6,* and the Wilms tumor suppressor gene, *WT1.* Differences in the size of the deleted segment (especially distal to 11p13) in individual cases may account for the observed variability in concomitant features and in the degree of growth and mental deficiency. A subset of patients with WAGR syndrome in which the deletion includes brain-derived neurotrophic factor (BDNF) have childhood-onset obesity and hyperphagia. In one study, by 10 years of age, 100% of WAGR patients with heterozygous BDNF mutations were obese as opposed to 20% without that mutation. Deletions of segments in 11p, not including 11p13, do not cause the aniridia–Wilms tumor association. Familial occurrence resulting from unbalanced transmission of a balanced insertional translocation has been recorded. An interstitial deletion in 11p should be particularly sought in the cytogenetic investigation of intellectually disabled patients with Wilms tumor and/or aniridia.

COMMENT

It has been estimated that Wilms tumor develops in one third of patients with sporadic aniridia and in 50% of patients with aniridia, genitourinary anomalies, and intellectual disability. The risk of Wilms tumor in patients with aniridia who have a cytogenetically detectable deletion of 11p13 increases to 60%. FISH using a probe spanning *PAX6* and *WT1* is available to determine if a risk for Wilms tumor exists for patients with sporadic aniridia who have normal chromosomes and an otherwise normal phenotype. Ultrasound screening for Wilms tumor should be continued until age 6. However, a case can be made for frequent abdominal examination and periodic testing into adulthood with frequent screening for hypertension and proteinuria. Fifty-three percent of patients with WAGR syndrome develop renal failure.

References

Anderson SR, et al: Aniridia, cataract and gonadoblastoma in a mentally retarded girl with deletion of chromosome 11, *Ophthalmologica* 176:171, 1978.

Riccardi VM, et al: Chromosomal imbalance in the aniridia-Wilms' tumor association: 11p interstitial deletion, *Pediatrics* 61:604, 1978.

Francke U, et al: Aniridia-Wilms' tumor association: Evidence for specific deletion of 11p13, *Cytogenet Cell Genet* 24:185, 1979.

Yunis JJ, Ramsay NKC: Familial occurrence of the aniridia-Wilms tumor syndrome with deletion 11p13-14.1, *J Pediatr* 96:1027, 1980.

Clericuzio CL: Clinical phenotypes and Wilms' tumor, *Med Pediatr Oncol* 21:182, 1993.

Pavilack MA, Walton DS: Genetics of aniridia: The aniridia-Wilms' tumor association, *Int Ophthalmol Clin* 33:77, 1993.

Breslow NE, et al: Renal failure in the Denys-Drash and Wilms' tumor-aniridia syndromes, *Cancer Res* 60:4030, 2000.

Fischbach BV, et al: WAGR syndrome: A clinical review of 54 cases, *Pediatrics* 116:984, 2005.

Han JC, et al: Brain-derived neurotrophic factor and obesity in the WAGR syndrome, *N Eng J Med* 359:918, 2008.

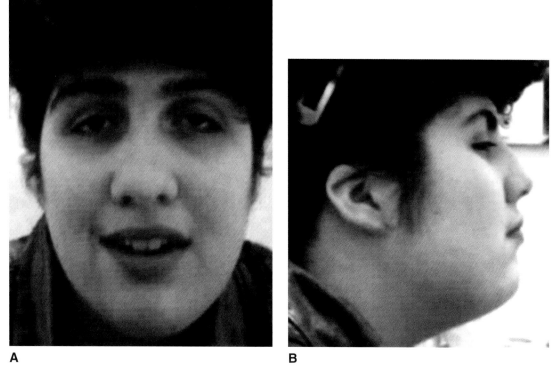

A   B

FIGURE 1.   A and **B,** Prominent lips and poorly formed ears in a female with aniridia–Wilms tumor association. (Courtesy Dr. Carol Clericuzio, University of New Mexico, Albuquerque.)

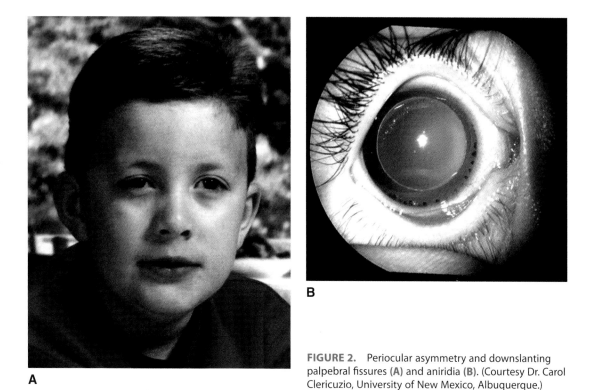

B

A

FIGURE 2.   Periocular asymmetry and downslanting palpebral fissures **(A)** and aniridia **(B)**. (Courtesy Dr. Carol Clericuzio, University of New Mexico, Albuquerque.)

DELETION 11Q SYNDROME
Ocular Hypertelorism; Large, Carp-Shaped Mouth; Cardiac Defects

Described initially by Jacobsen and colleagues in 1973, more than 200 cases of this disorder have been reported. In the majority of cases, the deletion involves band 11q23→qter. However, it appears that the clinical phenotype is due to deletion of subband 11q24.1.

ABNORMALITIES

Growth. Prenatal onset of growth deficiency (76%).

Performance. Intellectual disability (96%). Although all degrees have been reported, approximately one half have been in the moderate range, and most of the remaining are more severely affected. A small percentage of children are in the normal range. Hypotonia in infancy, frequently progressing toward spasticity, hearing loss, speech impairment.

Craniofacial. Prominent forehead (62%), microcephaly (40%), epicanthal folds (60%), ocular hypertelorism (70%), ptosis (67%), strabismus (75%), depressed nasal bridge (93%), short nose with upturned nasal tip (91%) and long philtrum, large, carp-shaped mouth (78%) with thin upper lip, micrognathia (77.7%), low-set and/or malformed ears (85%).

Other. Joint contractures (65%); cardiac defect (60%), primarily ventricular septal defect and left-sided obstructive defect, hypospadias and/or cryptorchidism (50%); Paris-Trousseau syndrome (defect in platelet development characterized by neonatal thrombocytopenia and persistent platelet dysfunction).

OCCASIONAL ABNORMALITIES

Trigonocephaly, macrocephaly, hydrocephalus, holoprosencephaly, cerebral atrophy, and agenesis of corpus callosum cerebellar hypoplasia; seizures; bipolar affective disorder; cataract, ocular coloboma, optic atrophy, retinal reduplication, and retinal dysplasia; short neck; dental anomalies; tetralogy of Fallot; digital anomalies, including hammer position of great toes, 2-3 syndactyly of toes, fifth finger clinodactyly, and brachydactyly; pyloric stenosis, imperforate anus, inguinal hernia, and renal malformations; vesico-vaginal fistula, hypoplasia of labia and clitoris; eczema; hypoplastic left heart; IGF-1 deficiency.

NATURAL HISTORY

About 20% of children who have deletion 11q syndrome die in the first year. For those who survive, life expectancy is unknown. Cardiac defects and bleeding are the major causes of morbidity and mortality. Feeding difficulties are common, and chronic constipation occurs in almost 50% of these children. Recurrent episodes of otitis media and/or sinusitis are frequent. Common variable immunodeficiency has been described,

ETIOLOGY

This disorder is caused by partial deletion of the long arm of chromosome 11 involving 11q23→qter, most commonly a simple deletion and occasionally as part of a ring-11 chromosome. Larger deletions extending into 11q23 or q24.1 are associated with moderate degrees of intellectual disability and significant speech impairment while those with small terminal deletions are more mildly affected with some having normal intelligence.

References

Jacobsen PH, et al: An (11;21) translocation in four generations with chromosome 11 abnormalities in the offspring, *Hum Hered* 23:568, 1973.

Schinzel A, et al: Partial deletion of long arm of chromosome 11[del(11)(q23)]: Jacobsen syndrome, *J Med Genet* 14:438, 1977.

O'Hare AE, et al: Deletion of the long arm of chromosome 11 [46,XX,del(11)(q24.1→qter)], *Clin Genet* 25:373, 1984.

Fryns JP, et al: Distal 11q monosomy. The typical 11q monosomy syndrome is due to deletion of subband 11q24.1, *Clin Genet* 30:255, 1986.

Penny LA, et al: Clinical and molecular characterization of patients with distal 11q deletions, *Am J Med Genet* 56:676, 1995.

Grossfeld PD, et al: The 11q terminal deletion disorder: A prospective study of 110 cases, *Am J Med Genet* 129:51, 2004.

Mattina T, et al: Jacobsen syndrome, *Orphanet J Rare Diseases* 4:9, 2009.

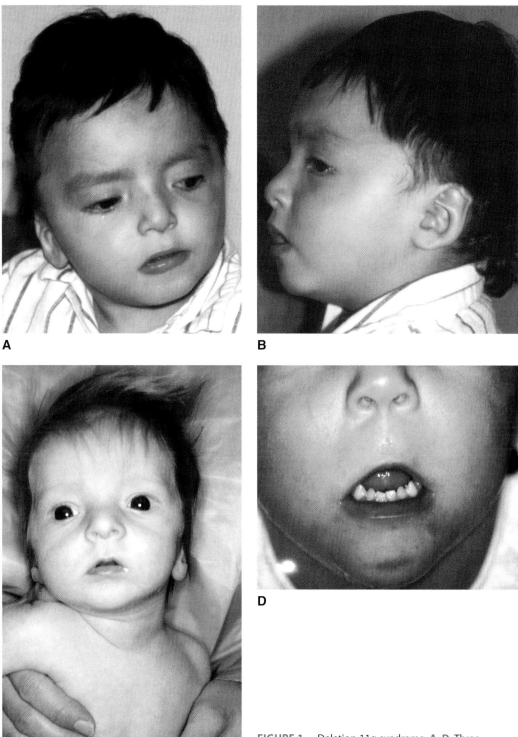

FIGURE 1. Deletion 11q syndrome. **A–D,** Three affected children. Note the ocular hypertelorism, malformed ears, and carp-shaped mouth.

DELETION 13Q SYNDROME (13Q- SYNDROME)
Microcephaly with High Nasal Bridge, Eye Defect, Thumb Hypoplasia

Partial deletion of the long arm of one of the D-group chromosomes was initially reported in 1963 by Lele and colleagues in an intellectually disabled and growth-deficient patient with retinoblastoma. Subsequently, more than 130 cases have been recorded, and the deleted chromosome has been considered number 13. Although the phenotype is variable, it can be divided into three clusters based on the specific deleted segment of 13q. A similar phenotype has been noted in 13 ring chromosome patients who are missing part of the short arm as well as part of the long arm of chromosome 13.

ABNORMALITIES

Growth. Growth deficiency, usually of prenatal onset.
Central Nervous System. Mental deficiency, microcephaly with tendency toward trigonocephaly- and holoprosencephaly-type brain defects.
Facial. Prominent nasal bridge, hypertelorism, ptosis, epicanthal folds, microphthalmia, colobomata, retinoblastoma (usually bilateral), prominent maxilla, micrognathia, prominent, slanting, low-positioned ears.
Neck. Short, webbing.
Limbs. Small to absent thumbs, clinodactyly of fifth finger, fused metacarpal bones 4 and 5, talipes equinovarus, short big toe.
Cardiac. Cardiac defect.
Genitalia. Hypospadias, cryptorchidism.
Other. Focal lumbar agenesis.

OCCASIONAL ABNORMALITIES
Optic nerve and retinal dysplasia, facial asymmetry, posterior auricular pits, narrow palate, imperforate anus, Hirschsprung disease, celiac disease, bifid scrotum, pelvic anomaly, renal anomaly, neural tube defects, factor VII deficiency, VACTERL association.

ETIOLOGY
This disorder is caused by deletion of part of the long arm of a 13 chromosome. Ring 13 chromosome individuals may have a similar pattern of malformation.

COMMENT
The natural history is dependent on the deleted segment. Patients with proximal deletions not extending into q32 have mild to moderate intellectual disability, variable minor anomalies, and growth retardation. If the q14 region is involved, a significant risk exists for retinoblastoma; intellectual disability; growth deficiency; and major malformations, including microcephaly and central nervous system defects, distal limb anomalies, eye defects, and gastrointestinal malformations. Patients with the most distal deletions, involving q33-q34, have severe intellectual disability but usually lack growth deficiency or gross structural malformations although a case with uncontrolled epilepsy has been described.

Although the majority of patients with deletions of chromosome 13 involving the q14 region develop retinoblastoma, it is estimated that 13% to 20% remain unaffected. Chromosome studies would seem merited in all patients with retinoblastoma.

References

Lele KP, Penrose LS, Stallarf HB: Chromosome deletion in a case of retinoblastoma, *Ann Hum Genet* 27:171, 1963.
Allerdice PW et al: The 13q-deletion syndrome, *Am J Hum Genet* 21:499, 1969.
Taylor AI: Dq-, Dr and retinoblastoma, *Humangenetik* 10:209, 1970.
Yunis JJ, Ramsay N: Retinoblastoma and subband deletion of chromosome 13, *Am J Dis Child* 132:161, 1978.
Riccardi VM, et al: Partial triplication and deletion of 13q: Study of a family presenting with bilateral retinoblastoma, *Clin Genet* 18:332, 1979.
Wilson WG, et al: Deletion (13)(q14.1q14.3) in two generations: Variability of ocular manifestations and definition of the phenotype, *Am J Med Genet* 28:675, 1987.
Brown S, et al: Preliminary definition of a "critical region" of chromosome 13 in q32: Report of 14 cases with 13q deletions and review of the literature, *Am J Med Genet* 45:52, 1993.
Talvik I, et al: Boy with celiac disease, malformations, and ring chromosome 13 with deletion 13q32→qter, *Am J Med Genet* 93:399, 2000.
Walsh LLE, et al: Distal 13q deletion syndrome and the VACTERL association: Case report, literature review, and possible implications, *Am J Med Genet* 98:137, 2001.
Lance EI, et al: Expansion of the deletion 13q syndrome phenotype: A case report, *J Child Neurology* 22:1124, 2007.

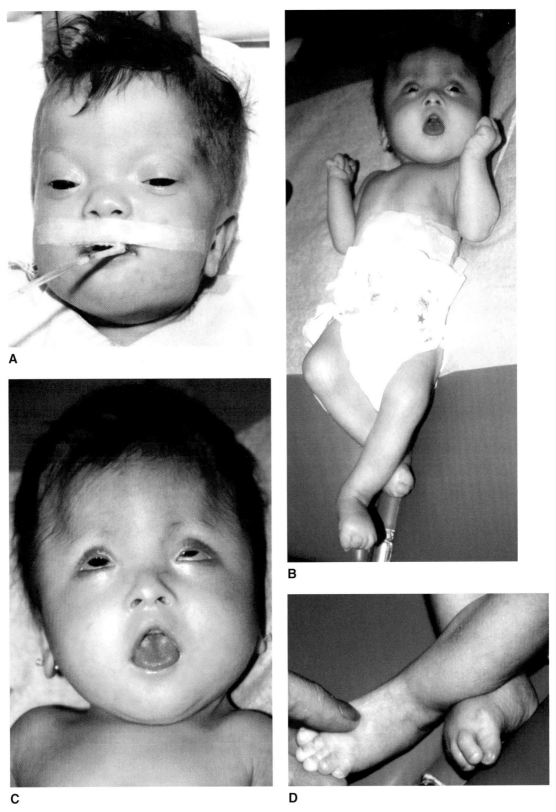

FIGURE 1. Deletion 13q syndrome. **A–D,** Two affected newborns. Note the ptosis, trigonocephaly, metopic ridge, and short big toe. (**A,** Courtesy Dr. Bryan D. Hall, University of Kentucky, Lexington.)

DUPLICATION 15Q SYNDROME
Prominent Nose with Broad Nasal Bridge, Camptodactyly, Cardiac Defects

Initially described by Fujimoto and colleagues, duplication of distal 15q has been described in more than 30 cases. The breakpoints have all been between bands 15q21 and 15q23, except for two families with breakpoints at 15q25 and two families with breakpoints at 15q15. Cases with proximal duplication 15q are more common but have a more variable phenotype.

ABNORMALITIES

Growth. Prenatal growth deficiency (15%), postnatal growth deficiency (60%), tall stature (11%),

Performance. Severe to profound intellectual disability (92%), two patients with duplication of 15q25→qter were only mildly intellectually disabled.

Craniofacial. Microcephaly (37%), sloping forehead (71%), short palpebral fissures (78%), downslanting palpebral fissures (71%), ptosis (56%), prominent nose with broad nasal bridge (96%), long, well-defined philtrum (77%), midline crease in lower lip (86%), micrognathia (88%), puffy cheeks (70%)

Skeletal. Pectus excavatum (46%), scoliosis (60%), short neck with or without vertebral anomalies (68%)

Hands. Arachnodactyly (75%), camptodactyly (100%)

Other. Cardiac defects (69%)

OCCASIONAL ABNORMALITIES

Genital abnormalities, including cryptorchidism and hypoplastic labia majora, preauricular pit.

NATURAL HISTORY

Death primarily related to congenital heart defects, recurrent respiratory infections, and aspiration pneumonia has occurred in one third of patients. A 27-year-old mentally retarded male is the oldest known survivor.

ETIOLOGY

The cause of this disorder is duplication of distal 15q. The majority of cases have resulted from unbalanced translocations, all but one of which were the offspring of a balanced carrier parent. Despite the fact that the second chromosome involved in the reciprocal translocation has varied, the clinical phenotype is consistent.

References

Fujimoto A, et al: Inherited partial duplication of chromosome no. 15, *J Med Genet* 11:287, 1974.

Lacro RV, et al: Duplication of distal 15q: Report of five new cases from two different translocation kindreds, *Am J Med Genet* 26:19, 1987.

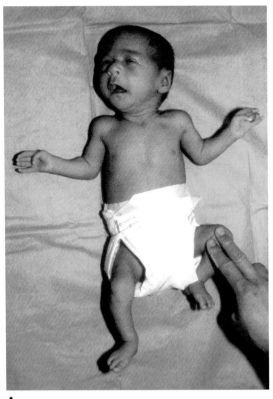

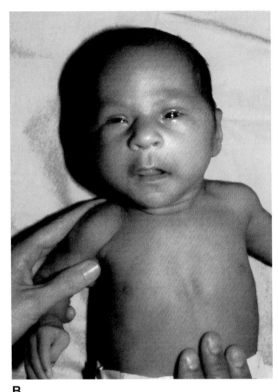

A

B

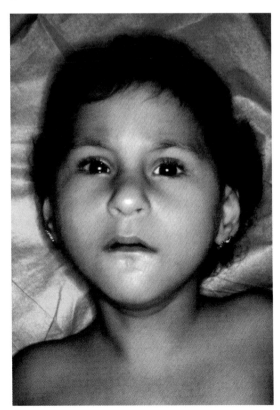

C

FIGURE 1. Duplication 15q syndrome. **A,** Affected newborn female infant. Note the sloping forehead, downslanting palpebral fissures, and prominent nose with broad nasal bridge. Affected girl at birth (**B**) and 41 months (**C**). (**A–C,** From Lacro RV, et al: *Am J Med Genet* 26:719, 1987. Reprinted with permission of Wiley-Liss Inc., a subsidiary of John Wiley & Sons, Inc.)

DELETION 18P SYNDROME (18P- SYNDROME)
Mental and Growth Deficiencies, Ptosis or Epicanthal Folds, Prominent Auricles

Deletion of the short arm of chromosome 18 is one of the most common chromosome deletion syndromes. It was first described by de Grouchy and colleagues in 1963. Since then, more than 150 cases with a terminal deletion have been reported.

ABNORMALITIES

Growth. Mild to moderate growth deficiency.
Central Nervous System. Intellectual disability, tendency toward hypotonia, microcephaly (mild) (29%).
Facial. Ptosis (38%), epicanthal folds (40%), low nasal bridge, hypertelorism (41%), rounded facies, micrognathia (25%), wide mouth, downturning corners of mouth, large protruding ears.
Dental. High frequency of caries (29%).
Limbs. Relatively small hands and feet.
Other. Pectus excavatum.

OCCASIONAL ABNORMALITIES

Immunologic. IgA absence or deficiency, usually asymptomatic.
Central Nervous System and Facial. Holoprosencephaly arrhinencephaly-type defect (12%).
Skin and Hair. Alopecia, hypopigmentation.
Other. Cataract, strabismus (15%), webbed neck, broad chest, cleft palate, kyphoscoliosis, clinodactyly of fifth finger (21%), syndactyly (11%), simian crease, cubitus valgus, pectus excavatum (17%), inguinal hernia, dislocation of hip (9%), talipes equinovarus (13%), genital anomalies (18%), development of rheumatoid arthritis–like signs and symptoms, polymyositis, cardiac defects (10%), ulerythema ophryogenes (i.e., reticular erythema, small horny papules, atrophy, and permanent loss of hairs in outer halves of eyebrows, sometimes extending to adjacent skin, scalp, and cheeks), growth hormone deficiency.

NATURAL HISTORY

There is a mild to severe intellectual disability. IQs range from 25 to 75, with an average of approximately 45 to 50. A correlation between the size of the deletion and the degree of intellectual disability has been suggested. Of seven patients with terminal deletions, all four with a deletion at 18p11.1 were intellectually disabled, while two of the patients with breakpoints at 18p11.21 had normal mental development and one had borderline intellectual disability. There is a dissociation between language ability and practical performance; many do not speak even simple sentences before 7 to 9 years of age. Restlessness, emotional lability, fear of strangers, and lack of ability to concentrate are features of this disorder. The prognosis is poor for those patients with holoprosencephaly-type defect. Otherwise, life expectancy does not seem to be impaired. Alopecia, when a problem, develops during infancy. Adequate adaptation has occurred in some patients, and they are capable of reproduction. Neurologic status of 13 patients between 22 and 62 years of age have been reported. Dystonia has been reported in three of them, pseudo-myotonic deep tendon reflexes in one, speech articulation problems in one, Parkinson-type movements in one, and paranoid schizophrenia in one.

ETIOLOGY

The cause of this disorder is short arm 18 deletion, sometimes as part of the deficiency in a ring 18 chromosome. Parents should undergo chromosome analysis to determine whether either is a balanced translocation carrier or has the unbalanced 18p- deletion.

References

de Grouchy J, et al: Dysmorphie complexe avec oligophrénie: Délétion des bras courts d'un chromosome 17–18, *D R Acad Sci* 256:1028, 1963.
Uchida IA, et al: Familial short arm deficiency of chromosome 18 concomitant with arrhinencephaly and alopecia congenita, *Am J Hum Genet* 17:410, 1965.
Brenk CH, et al: Towards mapping phenotypical traits in 18p- syndrome by array-based comparative genomic hybridization and fluorescent in situ hybridization, *Eur J Hum Genet* 15:35, 2007.
De Ravel TJL, et al: Follow-up of adult males with chromosome 18p deletion, *Eur J Med Genet* 48:189, 2005.
Wester U, et al: Clinical and molecular characterization of individuals with 18p deletion: A genotype-phenotype correlation, *Am J Med Genet* 140A:1164, 2006.

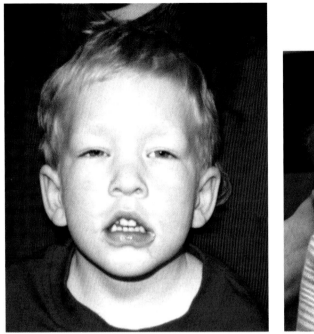

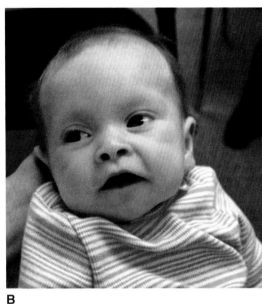

A

B

FIGURE 1.   Deletion 18p syndrome. **A** and **B,** Two affected children. Note the ptosis, hypertelorism, round facies, and wide mouth with downturning corners. (**A,** Courtesy Dr. Bryan D. Hall, University of Kentucky, Lexington; **B,** courtesy Dr. Cynthia Curry, University of California, San Francisco.)

DELETION 18Q SYNDROME
(LONG ARM 18 DELETION SYNDROME, 18Q- SYNDROME)
Midfacial Hypoplasia, Prominent Antihelix, Whorl Digital Pattern

Initially described by de Grouchy and colleagues in 1964, this disorder has been documented in more than 100 cases and occurs in approximately 1 out of 40,000 live births.

ABNORMALITIES

Growth. Postnatal onset of growth deficiency with disproportionate short stature secondary to decreased lower segment.

Performance. Intellectual disability with hypotonia, poor coordination, nystagmus, conductive deafness, seizures.

Craniofacial. Microcephaly, midfacial hypoplasia with deep-set eyes, short palpebral fissures, carp-shaped mouth, narrow palate.

Ears. Prominent antihelix, antitragus, or both; narrow or atretic external canal, with sensorineural or conductive hearing loss.

Limbs. Long hands, tapering fingers, short first metacarpal with proximal thumb, high-frequency whorl digital pattern, distal axial triradius, simian crease, fifth finger clinodactyly, abnormal toe placement, vertical talus with or without talipes equinovarus, short feet.

Genitalia. Female: hypoplastic labia minora; male: cryptorchidism with or without small scrotum and penis, hypospadias.

Other. Skin dimples over acromion and knuckles, cardiac defect.

OCCASIONAL ABNORMALITIES

Eyes. Inner epicanthal folds, slanted palpebral fissures, ocular hypertelorism, microphthalmia, corneal abnormality, iris hypoplasia, coloboma, cataract, retinal defect, abnormal optic disk, myopia, optic atrophy.

Ears. Atretic middle ear, low-set ears, microtia.

Other. Cleft palate (30%), cleft lip, short frenulum, widely spaced nipples, prominent venous pattern on the abdomen, extra rib, horseshoe kidney, celiac disease, lipomata at lateral border of feet, hemihypertrophy, scoliosis, vertebral anomalies, femoral head abnormalities, choreoathetotic movements, eczema, decreased to absent IgA, growth hormone deficiency, atrophy of olfactory and optic nerves, poor myelination of central white matter tracts with relatively normal myelination of corpus callosum, hydrocephalus, porencephaly, cerebellar hypoplasia.

NATURAL HISTORY

Ureteral reflux and urinary tract infection can be a significant problem. Intellectual disability, with IQs from 40 to 85, and growth deficiency, coupled with various visual and hearing problems, may leave these individuals seriously handicapped. Behavioral problems, including difficult or autistic behavior, may be features. However, some patients with this deletion have not been severely affected.

ETIOLOGY

Variable deletions of part of the long arm of chromosome 18 from 18q21.3 or 18q22.2 to qter. In general, the size of the deletion correlates with the severity of the phenotype. Phenotypic variability has been noted even within affected family members.

References

de Grouchy J, et al: Délétion partielle du bras long du chromosome 18, *Pathol Biol (Paris)* 12:579, 1964.
Wertelecki W, Gerald PS: Clinical and chromosomal studies of the 18q- syndrome, *J Pediatr* 78:44, 1971.
Miller G, et al: Neurologic manifestations in 18q- syndrome, *Am J Med Genet* 37:128, 1990.
Kline AD, et al: Molecular analysis of the 18q- syndrome and correlation with phenotype, *Am J Hum Genet* 52:895, 1993.
Cody JD, et al: Congenital anomalies and anthropometry of 42 individuals with deletion of chromosome 18q, *Am J Med Genet* 85:455, 1999.
Margarit E, et al: Familial 4.8 MB deletion on 18q23 associated with growth hormone insufficiency and phenotypic variability, *Am J Med Genet* 158A:611, 2012.

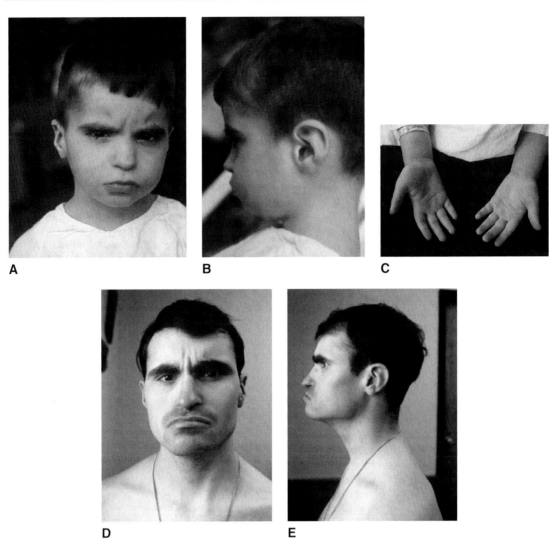

FIGURE 1.   Deletion 18q syndrome. **A–E,** Affected male as child and adult. Note the midface hypoplasia, deep-set eyes, carp-shaped mouth, and prominent antihelix. (Courtesy Dr. Wladimir Wertelecki, University of South Alabama, Birmingham.)

CAT-EYE SYNDROME (COLOBOMA OF IRIS–ANAL ATRESIA SYNDROME)
Coloboma of Iris, Downslanting Palpebral Fissures, Anal Atresia

Anal atresia and colobomata of the iris, initially considered the hallmarks of this disorder, are present in combination in only a minority of affected patients. More than 100 cases have been reported, only 9% of which showed all the major clinical features.

ABNORMALITIES

Performance. Usually mild intellectual disability, some patients have been of normal intelligence but emotionally immature.

Growth. Normal in the majority of cases.

Craniofacial. Mild hypertelorism; downslanting palpebral fissures; inferior coloboma of iris, choroid, and/or retina; micrognathia, preauricular pits, and/or tags.

Cardiac. Cardiac defects in more than one third of cases, including total anomalous pulmonary venous return, persistence of the left superior vena cava, ventricular septal defect, and atrial septal defect.

Anus. Anal atresia with rectovestibular fistula.

Urogenital. Hypospadias, renal agenesis, hydronephrosis, vesicoureteral reflux.

OCCASIONAL ABNORMALITIES

Severe intellectual disability (7%); microcephaly; microphthalmos; ocular motility problems; hearing loss; ventricular dilatation; abnormal EEG; seizures; spasticity; cerebral or cerebellar atrophy; ataxia; facial nerve palsy; low-set, malformed ears with stenotic external canals; biliary atresia; dislocation of hip; radial aplasia; scoliosis; vertebral defects; rib or sternal anomaly; cleft palate; malrotation of gut; agenesis of uterus and fallopian tubes; dysplastic or polycystic kidney; bladder defects; aganglionosis of small and large intestine; ectopic anus; volvulus; Meckel diverticulum.

ETIOLOGY

This syndrome is usually the result of an extra chromosome derived from two identical segments of chromosome 22, consisting of the satellites, the entire short arm, the centromere, and a tiny piece of the long arm (22pter→q11). That segment is thus present in quadruplicate.

The phenotype can also result from an interstitial duplication of the 22q11 region. In this situation, the segment is present in triplicate, which may explain the few reported cases of cat-eye syndrome in which an extra chromosome is not present. Fluorescent in situ hybridization studies have been used successfully to document typical cases, as well as atypical cases in which only a few of the features are present.

References

Schachenmann G, et al: Chromosomes in coloboma and anal atresia, *Lancet* 2:290, 1965.

Darby CW, Hughes DT: Dermatoglyphics and chromosomes in cat-eye syndrome, *Br Med J* 3:47, 1971.

Balci S, et al: The cat-eye syndrome with unusual skeletal malformations, *Acta Paediatr Scand* 63:623, 1974.

Schinzel A, et al: The "cat eye syndrome": Dicentric small marker chromosome probably derived from a No. 22 (tetrasomy 22pter q11) associated with a characteristic phenotype. Report of 11 patients and delineation of the clinical picture, *Hum Genet* 57:148, 1981.

McDermid HE, et al: Characterization of the supernumerary chromosome in cat eye syndrome, *Science* 232:646, 1986.

Liehr T, et al: Typical and partial cat eye syndrome: Identification of the marker chromosome by FISH, *Clin Genet* 42:91, 1992.

Rosias PPR, et al: Phenotypic variability of the cat-eye syndrome, case report and review of the literature, *Genet Counsel* 12:273, 2001.

Rosa RFM, et al: Clinical characteristics of a sample of patients with cat eye syndrome, *Rev Assoc Med Bras* 56:462, 2010.

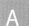

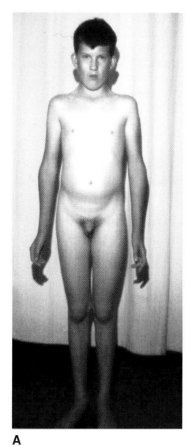

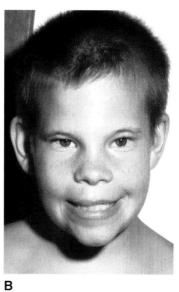

A   **B**

FIGURE 1.   **A** and **B,** Adolescent and preadolescent boys with XXXY syndrome; both are short and of dull mentality. Note the facial dysmorphia, elbow aberrations, and hypogonadism.

XXX AND XXXX SYNDROMES

Initially described by Jacobs and colleagues in 1959 in a woman of normal intelligence who had secondary amenorrhea, the XXX syndrome is recognized to occur in 1 in 1000 newborn females. There is no pattern of malformation associated with this karyotype. Based on studies of unselected newborns with sex chromosome anomalies who have been followed longitudinally, the following can be stated relative to females with a 47,XXX karyotype: Affected individuals are usually tall with average height of 172 cm. Mean occipitofrontal circumference is approximately the 20th percentile. Pubertal development is normal with an average age of menarche of 12 (range, 8 to 12) years. Fertility is probably normal. Delay in achievement of motor milestones, poor coordination, and awkwardness is common. IQ scores cluster in the 85 to 90 range (generally lower than that of their siblings). Problems with verbal learning and expressive language are frequent. Special education classes in high school are required in 60% of these individuals. Behavior problems, including mild depression, conduct disorder, or undersocialization, occur in 30%. Low self-esteem requiring psychological, behavioral, and educational support is common. However, most cope well and adapt as young adults without major problems. Premature ovarian failure is more prevalent than in controls. Cyclothymic and labile personality traits are common. Mortality is increased, with a difference in median survival of 7.7 years.

This is in contrast to the XXXX syndrome, initially described by Carr and colleagues in 1961, in which only 40 cases have been reported. Individuals with the XXXX syndrome have a variable phenotype with the facies suggestive of Down syndrome in several cases.

ABNORMALITIES IN THE XXXX SYNDROME

Except for intellectual disability, all of the other features are variable. The patients are usually of normal to tall stature.

Performance. IQ of 30 to 80, average of 55; speech development is most prominently affected.

Facies. Midfacial hypoplasia, upward slanting palpebral fissures, mild hypertelorism, epicanthal folds, mild micrognathia.

Limbs. Occasional fifth finger clinodactyly, radioulnar synostosis, reduced total finger ridge count.

Other. Tall stature, narrow shoulder girdle, taurodontism, variable amenorrhea, irregular menses.

OCCASIONAL ABNORMALITIES

Seizures, variable EEG abnormalities, mild ventricular enlargement on CT scan, webbed neck.

NATURAL HISTORY

Besides intellectual disability, speech and behavioral problems are frequent in the XXXX syndrome. The patient initially reported by Carr and colleagues, now 56 years old, is in good physical health with no evidence of intellectual deterioration. Her full-scale IQ is 56. Although menstrual disorders are common and fertility is reduced, offspring of these individuals tend to be normal.

ETIOLOGY

The diagnosis is confirmed by chromosomal analysis revealing a XXX or XXXX karyotype. Nondisjunction at maternal meiosis I is the most common cause of 47,XXX. Although not as striking an effect as is seen with trisomy 21, an increased maternal age effect has been seen for 47,XXX females.

References

Jacobs PA, et al: Evidence for the existence of the human "super female", *Lancet* 2:423, 1959.

Carr DH, Barr ML, Plunkett ER: An XXXX sex chromosome complex in two mentally defective females, *Can Med Assoc J* 84:131, 1961.

Berg JM, et al: Twenty-six years later: A woman with tetra-X chromosomes, *J Ment Defic Res* 32:67, 1988.

Robinson A, et al: Sex chromosome aneuploidy: The Denver prospective study, *Birth Defects* 26(4):59, 1991.

Robinson A, et al: Summary of clinical findings in children and young adults with sex chromosome anomalies, *Birth Defects* 26(4):225, 1991.

Liebezeit BU, et al: Tall stature as presenting symptom in a girl with triple X syndrome, *J Pediatr Endocrinol Metab* 16:233, 2003.

Stochholm K, et al: Mortality and incidence in women with 47,XXX and variants, *Am J Med Genet* 152A:367, 2010.

Otter M, et al: Triple X syndrome: A review of the literature, *Eur J Hum Genet* 18:265, 2010.

A

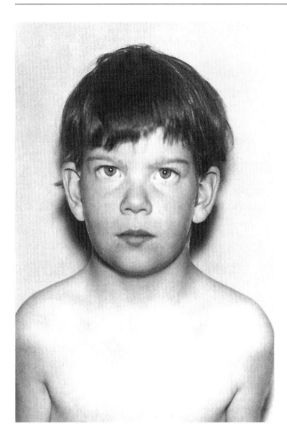

FIGURE 1.   A 6½-year-old girl with XXXX syndrome.

XXXXX SYNDROME (PENTA X SYNDROME)

Upward Slant to Palpebral Fissures, Patent Ductus Arteriosus, Small Hands with Clinodactyly of Fifth Fingers

The first description of an individual with XXXXX was by Kesaree and Wooley in 1963.

ABNORMALITIES

Growth. Prenatal onset of growth deficiency, failure to thrive, short stature; microcephaly.

Performance. Intellectual disability, moderate to severe.

Craniofacial. Mild upward slant to palpebral fissures; low nasal bridge, short neck; hypertelorism; epicanthal folds; low hairline; dental malocclusion; taurodontism and enamel defects, leading to premature loss of deciduous anterior teeth.

Limbs. Small hands with mild clinodactyly of fifth fingers.

Cardiac. Patent ductus arteriosus and ventricular septal defect.

OCCASIONAL ABNORMALITIES

Dandy-Walker malformation; colobomata of iris; low-set ears; preauricular tags; macroglossia; cleft palate; micrognathia; high-frequency, low-arch dermal ridge patterns; simian creases; talipes equinovarus; overlapping toes; multiple joint dislocations, including shoulder, elbow, hips, wrists, and fingers; renal dysplasia; horseshoe kidney; ovarian agenesis.

NATURAL HISTORY

IQ varies from 20 to 75. The oldest known affected individual, a 16-year-old girl, had small nipples, prepubertal external genitalia, and an atrophic vaginal smear. Information on fertility is lacking.

COMMENT AND ETIOLOGY

Of interest is the occurrence in these XXXXX individuals of many of the nonspecific anomalies found in individuals who have Down syndrome, a diagnosis that was initially considered in some of the patients. The diagnosis is confirmed by chromosomal analysis revealing an XXXXX karyotype. Molecular methods have indicated that the X chromosomes are maternally derived.

References

Kesaree N, Wooley PV: A phenotypic female with 49 chromosomes, presumably XXXXX: A case report, *J Pediatr* 63:1099, 1963.

Sergovich F, Uilenberg C, Pozsonyi J: The 49,XXXXX condition, *J Pediatr* 78:285, 1971.

Dryer FR, et al: Pentasomy X with multiple dislocations, *Am J Med Genet* 4:313, 1979.

Funderburk SJ, et al: Pentasomy X: Report of a patient and studies of X-inactivation, *Am J Med Genet* 8:27, 1981.

Deng HX, et al: Parental origin and mechanism of formation of polysomy X: An XXXXX case and four XXXXY cases determined with RFLPs, *Hum Genet* 86:541, 1991.

Myles TD, et al: Dandy-Walker malformation in a fetus with pentasomy X (49,XXXXX) prenatally diagnosed by fluorescent in situ hybridization technique, *Fetal Diagn Ther* 10:333, 1995.

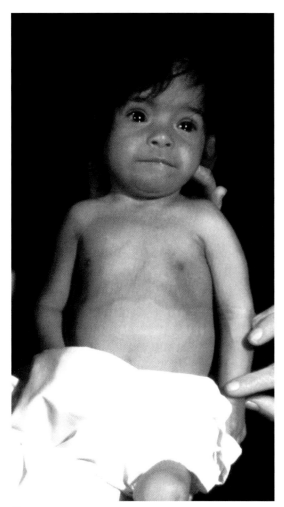

A

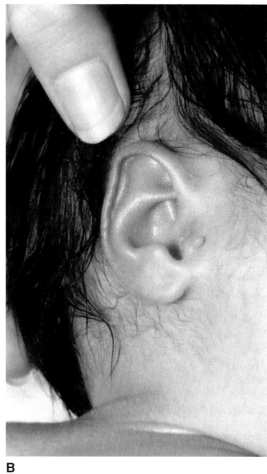

B

C

FIGURE 1. XXXXX syndrome. **A–C,** Note the ocular hypertelorism, preauricular tags, simian crease, and fifth finger clinodactyly.

45X SYNDROME (XO SYNDROME, TURNER SYNDROME)

Short Female, Broad Chest with Wide Spacing of Nipples, Congenital Lymphedema or Its Residua

An association between small stature and defective ovarian development had been noted as early as 1922 by Rossle, who classified the disorder under "sexagen dwarfism." A more expanded syndrome of small stature, sexual infantilism, webbed neck, and cubitus valgus in seven females was described by Turner in 1938. Most 45X conceptuses die early. It is estimated that approximately 1 in 2500 live-born phenotypic females are affected. Health supervision guidelines to assist in caring for affected individuals from birth to adulthood have been established by Bondy et al.

ABNORMALITIES

The following list of abnormalities, with the approximate percentage for each anomaly, includes those of the full monosomic X syndrome. Patients with mosaicism (XX/X mosaics, XY/X mosaics with varying degrees of male-type genitalia) or in whom only a part of one X is missing (X-isochromosome X or X-deleted X) generally have a lesser degree of malformation. The most consistent features for the entire group are small stature and gonadal dysgenesis. Because the latter feature is not evident during childhood, a chromosomal study is indicated in any girl with short stature of unknown cause whose clinical phenotype is not incompatible with the 45X syndrome. In addition, any adolescent with absent breast development by 13 years of age, pubertal arrest, or primary or secondary amenorrhea with elevated follicle-stimulating hormone should undergo karyotype analysis.

Growth. Small stature, often evident by birth; tendency to become obese.

Performance. Mean IQ approximately 90 with performance usually below verbal scores. Although early development is usually normal, delays in motor skills are common, as is poor coordination. Specific neuropsychological deficits are as follows: visual-spatial organization deficits, such as difficulty driving; deficits in social cognition, such as failure to appreciate subtle social cues; problems with nonverbal problem solving, such as math; psychomotor deficits, such as clumsiness; a tendency toward low self-esteem and depression in teenagers and young adults.

Gonads. Ovarian dysgenesis with hypoplasia to absence of germinal elements (>90%).

Lymph Vessels. Congenital lymphedema with residual puffiness over the dorsum of the fingers and toes (>80%). Can be seen at any age; often associated with initiation of growth hormone and/or estrogen therapy.

Thorax. Broad chest with widely spaced nipples that may be hypoplastic, inverted, or both (>80%); often mild pectus excavatum.

Auricles. Anomalous auricles, most commonly prominent (>80%).

Facies. Narrow maxilla (palate) (>80%), relatively small mandible (>70%), inner canthal folds (40%).

Neck. Low posterior hairline, appearance of short neck (>80%), webbed posterior neck (50%).

Extremities. Cubitus valgus or other anomaly of elbow (>70%); knee anomalies, such as medial tibial exostosis (>60%); short fourth metacarpal, metatarsal, or both (>50%).

Other Skeletal. Bone dysplasia with coarse trabecular pattern, most evident at metaphyseal ends of long bones (>50%); dislocation of hip.

Nails. Narrow, hyperconvex, and/or deep-set nails (>70%).

Skin. Excessive pigmented nevi (>50%); distal palmar axial triradii (>40%); loose skin, especially around the neck in infancy; tendency toward keloid formation.

Renal. Most commonly horseshoe kidney, double or cleft renal pelvis, and minor alterations (>60%).

Cardiac. Cardiac defects, the majority of which are bicuspid aortic valve (30%), coarctation of aorta (10%), valvular aortic stenosis, mitral valve prolapse, and aortic dissection later in life.

Central Nervous System. Perceptive hearing impairment (>50%).

OCCASIONAL ABNORMALITIES

Skeletal. Abnormal angulation of radius to carpal bones, Madelung deformity, short midphalanx of fifth finger, short third to fifth metacarpals and/or metatarsals, scoliosis, kyphosis, spina bifida, vertebral fusion, cervical rib, abnormal sella turcica.

Eyes. Ptosis (16%), strabismus, amblyopia, blue sclerae, cataract.

Central Nervous System. Intellectual disability. Agenesis or reduced areas of the genu of the corpus callosum, pons, and lobules VI and VII of the cerebellar vermis and increased area of the fourth ventricle.

Other. Hemangiomata, rarely of the intestine; long hair on arms; idiopathic hypertension; diabetes mellitus; ulcerative colitis; celiac disease; Crohn disease; primary hypothyroidism (10% to 30%); agenesis of corpus callosum (two cases); partial anomalous pulmonary venous return; hypoplastic left heart; persistent left superior vena cava.

NATURAL HISTORY

The congenital lymphedema usually recedes in early infancy, leaving only puffiness of the dorsum of the fingers and toes, although there may be recrudescence of the lymphedema with growth hormone or estrogen replacement therapy. At birth, the skin tends to be loose, especially in the posterior neck where excess skin may persist as the pterygium colli. Small size is often evident at birth, the mean birth weight being 2900 g. From birth up to 3 years of age the growth rate is normal, although there is a delay in bone maturation. Between 3 and 12 years, bone age progression is normal, but height velocity decreases. After 12 years of age, there is a decreased growth rate, deceleration of bone age progression, and relative increase in weight. Mean final height of untreated women with Turner syndrome is 143 cm (4 feet, 8 inches), 20 cm (8 inches) less than the general female population. Regarding treatment for short stature, 99 females with Turner syndrome were enrolled in a U.S. Multicenter Trial of growth hormone and low-dose estrogen. Significant growth hormone–induced improvement in height was demonstrated. Factors that influenced the response to therapy included younger age, lower bone age to chronologic age ratio, lower baseline weight, and greater baseline height at initiation of therapy. Estrogen therapy did not improve gain in near-final height.

Studies of XO abortuses have disclosed near-normal development of the ovaries in early fetal life. Apparently, they usually do not make primary follicles, and the ovary degenerates rather rapidly. In the majority of affected individuals, by adolescence there is seldom any functional ovarian tissue remaining. However, it is important to recognize that 10% to 20% will have spontaneous pubertal development and 2% to 5% will have spontaneous menses, although this is generally transient; at least several 45X individuals have been fertile. Estrogen replacement therapy is indicated, beginning between 12 and 13 years in hypogonadotropic girls.

The actual incidence of early mortality due to congenital heart defects is unknown. An increased risk for dissection of the aorta has been documented in adults. Aortic root dilatation occurs with a prevalence estimated to be between 8% and 42%. Therefore, affected females with normal echocardiograms should be imaged every 5 years, and those with abnormal echocardiograms should be followed yearly. In addition, increased morbidity secondary to diabetes mellitus, hypertension, ischemic heart disease, and stroke has been documented. The types of renal anomalies that occur generally pose no problem to health. However, an increased risk of osteoporosis, autoimmune thyroid disease, and chronic liver disease has been reported with increasing age. Enhancement of physical appearance by plastic surgery for prominent inner canthal folds, protruding auricles, and especially for webbed neck should be given serious consideration before school age. However, there is a markedly increased incidence of keloid formation that must be taken into account.

Approximately 6% of females with Turner syndrome have 45X/46XY mosaicism. In those cases, an exploratory laparotomy in childhood seems indicated to remove any residual gonadal tissue to eliminate the risk for development of gonadoblastoma for which these patients are at increased risk.

If the child has an intellectual disability, a careful search should be made for a chromosome abnormality in addition to that of the sex chromosome. For example, patients with X-autosome translocation are more likely to be mentally deficient. Intellectual disability has also been seen more frequently in individuals with a small ring X chromosome.

ETIOLOGY

Faulty chromosomal distribution leading to 45X individual. The paternal X chromosome is the one more likely to be missing. There has been no significant older maternal age factor for this aneuploidy syndrome. It is generally a sporadic event in a family, although there are, as yet, no adequate data on risk for recurrence. Mosaicism does not ensure survival to term. However, the incidence of sex chromosome mosaicism is higher in live-born than in aborted 45X fetuses.

References

Rossle RI: *Wachstum und Altern*. München, 1922, JF Bergman.

Turner HH: A syndrome of infantilism, congenital webbed neck, and cubitus valgus, *Endocrinology* 23:566, 1938.

Weiss L: Additional evidence of gradual loss of germ cells in the pathogenesis of streak ovaries in Turner's syndrome, *J Med Genet* 8:540, 1971.

Kastrup KW: Oestrogen therapy in Turner's syndrome, *Acta Paediatr Scand Suppl* 343:43, 1988.

Chang HJ, et al: The phenotype of 45X/46XY mosaicism: An analysis of 92 prenatally diagnosed cases, *Am J Hum Genet* 46:156, 1990.

Robinson A, et al: Sex chromosome aneuploidy: The Denver prospective study, *Birth Defects* 26(4):59, 1991.

Hassold T, et al: Molecular studies of parental origin and mosaicism in 45X conceptuses, *Hum Genet* 89:647, 1992.

Gravholt CH, et al: Morbidity in Turner syndrome, *J Clin Epidemiol* 51:147, 1998.

Guarneri MP, et al: Turner's syndrome, *J Pediatr Endocrinol Metab* 14(Suppl 2):959, 2001.

Elsheikh M, et al: Turner's syndrome in adulthood, *Endocr Rev* 23:120, 2002.

Quigley CA, et al: Growth hormone and low dose estrogen in Turner syndrome: Results of a United States multicenter trial to near-final height, *J Clin Endocrinol Metab* 87:2033, 2002.

Pinsker JE: Clinical review:Turner syndrome: updating the paradigm of clinical care, *J Clin Endocrinol Metab* 97:e994, 2012.

Bondy CA, et al: Care of girls and women with Turner syndrome: A guideline of the Turner Syndrome Study Group, *J Clin Endocrinol Metab* 92:10, 2007.

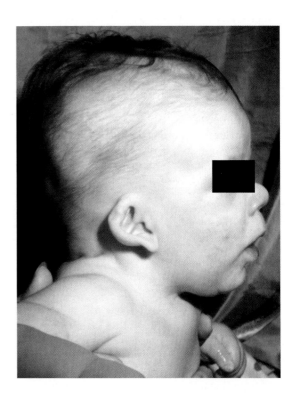

FIGURE 1.   Baby with 45X syndrome. Note the protuberant ears and loose nuchal skin.

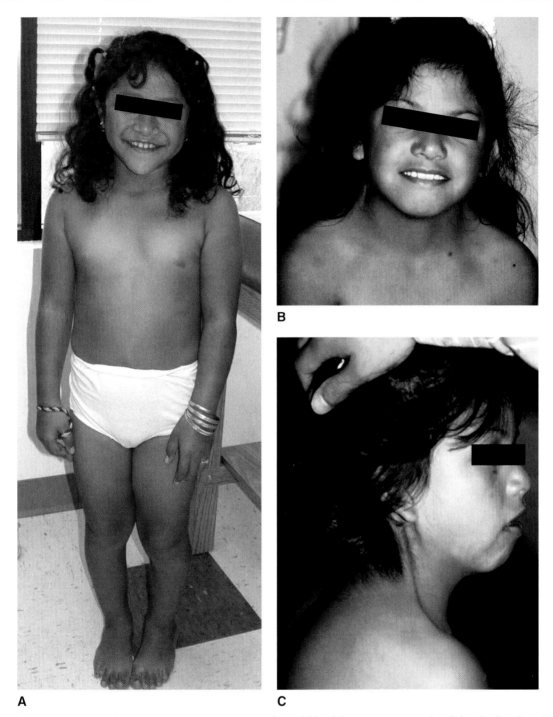

A

B

C

FIGURE 2. Turner syndrome. **A–C,** Note prominent ears, loose folds of skin in posterior neck with low hairline, broad chest with widely spaced nipples. (Courtesy Dr. Lynne M. Bird, Children's Hospital, San Diego.)

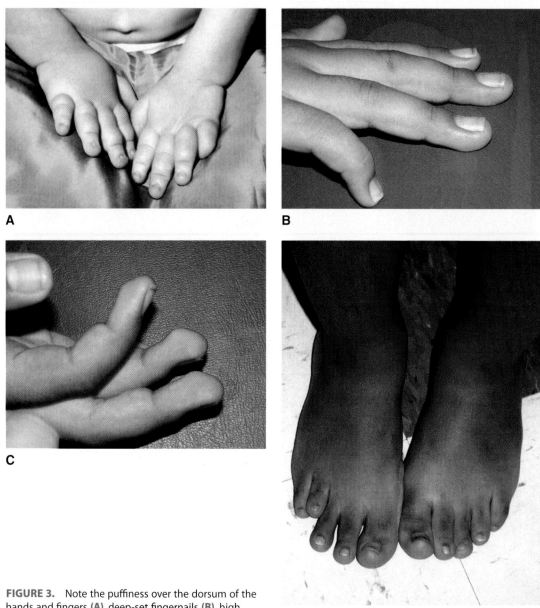

FIGURE 3.   Note the puffiness over the dorsum of the hands and fingers **(A)**, deep-set fingernails **(B)**, high fingertip pads **(C)**, and short fourth metatarsals **(D)**.

A

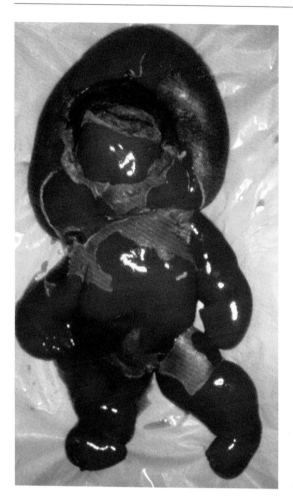

FIGURE 4. Twenty-week fetus with 45X Turner syndrome. Note the massive edema.

B Deletion, Duplication, and Microduplication Syndromes Identifiable Using Molecular Technology

1P36 DELETION SYNDROME (MONOSOMY 1P36 DELETION SYNDROME)
Large Anterior Fontanel, Deep-Set Eyes, Pointed Chin

First delineated in 1997 as a recognizable pattern of malformation, monosomy 1p36 is the most commonly observed terminal deletion in the human population with an estimated prevalence of 1 in 5000.

ABNORMALITIES

Growth. Postnatal onset of growth deficiency, obesity.

Performance. Intellectual disability, severe in the majority of cases although mild in a few; speech more severely affected than motor development. Expressive language absent in the majority of patients. Behavior difficulties, including temper tantrums, self-biting, reduced social interaction, stereotypic behaviors, hyperphagia.

Craniofacial. Microcephaly; brachycephaly; large, late-closing anterior fontanel; straight eyebrows; epicanthal folds; prominent forehead; deep-set eyes; broad nasal root/bridge; midface hypoplasia; low-set, posteriorly rotated ears; thickened ear helices; long philtrum; pointed chin.

Cardiac. Structural defects in 71%, including patent ductus arteriosus, ventricular septal defect (VSD), atrial septal defect (ASD), bicommissural aortic valve, Ebstein anomaly, noncompaction cardiomyopathy, dilated cardiomyopathy in infancy.

Limbs/Skeletal. Brachydactyly, camptodactyly, short feet, bifid/fused/enlarged/missing ribs, scoliosis, delayed bone age.

Neurologic. Hypotonia; seizures with onset between 4 days and 3 years; infantile spasms; electroencephalogram (EEG) abnormalities; central nervous system (CNS) defects including enlarged lateral ventricles, cortical atrophy, enlarged subarachnoid space, diffuse brain atrophy, enlargement of the frontotemporal opercula, and focal pachygyria.

Other. Hypermetropia, hearing loss, renal anomalies, cryptorchidism, hypospadias, scrotal hypoplasia, micropenis, hypoplastic labia minora, clitoral hypertrophy.

OCCASIONAL ABNORMALITIES

Hydrocephalus, visual inattentiveness, strabismus, myopia, nystagmus, sixth nerve palsies, cataracts, colobomas, moderate optic atrophy, cleft lip with or without cleft palate, bifid uvula, facial asymmetry, fifth finger clinodactyly, camptodactyly, hypothyroidism, kyphosis, hip dysplasia, congenital spinal stenosis, metatarsus adductus, polydactyly, shawl scrotum, imperforate anus, anteriorly placed anus, hiatal hernia, pyloric stenosis, abnormal pulmonary lobation, pemphigus vulgaris, sacral/coccygeal dimple.

NATURAL HISTORY

Hypotonia occurs in the majority of neonates. Feeding problems, including poor suck and swallowing, reflux, and vomiting, are common in infancy. Hearing impairment, primarily sensorineural, is common, and visual disturbances have been observed frequently. Full-scale IQ scores are generally less than 60 and IQ less than 20 has been described. Seizures, beginning in infancy, cease in the first few years in some children but persist, requiring long-term therapy, in others. Disturbed behaviors, including temper tantrums, aggressivity, and self-injurious behavior, are common. Survival into adulthood is the rule.

ETIOLOGY

Deletion of the 1p36 chromosome region. The majority of cases are due to a de novo terminal 1p36 deletion. Although in some cases the deletion can be detected by high-resolution karyotype, confirmation by fluorescence in situ hybridization (FISH) analysis or by array comparative genomic hybridization (CGH) is required in most. The size of the deletion does not correlate with the number of characteristic clinical features.

References

Shapira SK, et al: Chromosome 1p36 deletions: The clinical phenotype and molecular characterization of a common newly delineated syndrome, *Am J Hum Genet* 61:642, 1997.

Riegel M, et al: Terminal deletion, del(1)(p36.3), detected through screening for terminal deletions in patients with unclassified malformation syndromes, *Am J Med Genet* 82:249, 1999.

Slavotinek A, et al: Monosomy 1p36, *J Med Genet* 36:657, 1999.

Heilstedt HA, et al: Physical map of 1p36, placement of breakpoints in monosomy 1p36, and clinical characterization of the syndrome, *Am J Hum Genet* 72:1200, 2003.

Gajecka M, et al: Monosomy 1p36 deletions syndrome, *Am J Med Genet C* 145C:346, 2007.

Battaglia A, et al: Further delineation of the deletion 1p36 syndrome in 60 patients: A recognizable phenotype and common cause of developmental delay and mental retardation, *Pediatrics* 121(2):404, 2008.

Rosenfeld A, et al: Refinement of causative genes in monosomy 1p36 through clinical and molecular cytogenetic characterization of small interstitial deletions, *Am J Med Genet A* 152A:1951, 2010.

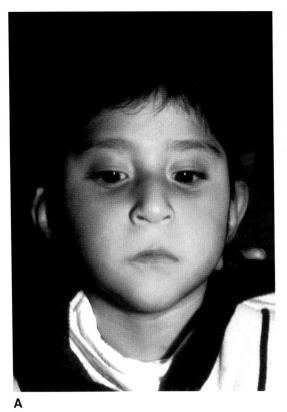

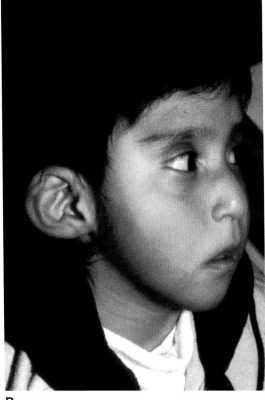

B

A

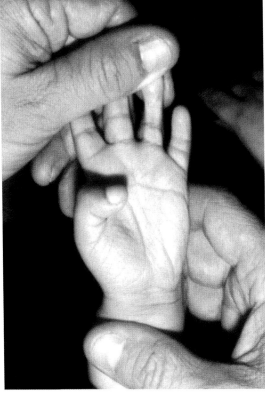

C

FIGURE 1. 1p36 deletion syndrome. **A–C,** Affected child with thickened ear helices, pointed chin, and missing distal crease on fourth finger with contracture (camptodactyly).

1Q41Q42 MICRODELETION SYNDROME
(1Q42 MICRODELETION SYNDROME)
Characteristic Dysmorphic Features, Intellectual Disability, Congenital Diaphragmatic Hernia

Initially reported by Shaffer et al in 2007, more than 15 cases of this syndrome have been reported. The microdeletion appears to be associated with a variable phenotype.

ABNORMALITIES

Growth. Growth retardation (50%).

Performance. Developmental delay, hypotonia, intellectual disability (100%), behavioral problems.

Craniofacial. Microcephaly (40%), bitemporal narrowing, frontal bossing, coarse facies, deep-set eyes, hypertelorism or telecanthus, depressed nasal bridge, bulbous nose with broad nasal tip and anteverted nares, prominent philtrum, full lips, tented upper lip.

Limbs. Short limbs, short fingers, nail hypoplasia, abnormal creases.

Central Nervous System. Seizures, agenesis of corpus callosum, ventriculomegaly, brain atrophy, cortical dysplasia.

Other. Diaphragmatic hernia, congenital heart defects, cleft palate.

OCCASIONAL ABNORMALITIES

Prominent eyebrows, iris anomalies (Brushfield-like spots), cleft palate, supernumerary nipples, talipes equinovarus, short stature, pectus deformities, camptodactyly, male genital anomalies (including micropenis, hypospadias, and cryptorchidism), hypoplasia of labia minora, nail hypoplasia, Pelger-Huët anomaly of granulocytes (abnormal nuclear shape and chromatin organization).

ETIOLOGY

The deletion is nonrecurrent and variable in size ranging from 700 kb to 7 Mb. Initially the smallest region of overlap was 1.17 Mb and included five genes. One of the genes within this common deletion region, *DISP1,* plays a role in the sonic hedgehog signaling pathway, and nonsense mutations have been found in individuals with holoprosencephaly spectrum phenotypes with variable penetrance. However, *DISP1* is not deleted in all patients with the most characteristic dysmorphic phenotype, suggesting that the phenotype cannot be solely attributed to the loss of this gene.

COMMENT

A point mutation in *DISP1* has been found in at least one case of sporadic congenital diaphragmatic hernia (CDH). Deletions and mutations in this gene may be causal for isolated and syndromic CDH.

References

Kantarci S, et al: Findings from aCGH in patients with congenital diaphragmatic hernia (CDH): A possible locus for Fryns syndrome, *Am J Med Genet A* 140:17, 2006.

Rice GM, et al: Microdissection-based high-resolution genomic array analysis of two patients with cytogenetically identical interstitial deletions of chromosome 1q but distinct clinical phenotypes, *Am J Med Genet A* 140:1637, 2006.

Shaffer LG, et al: The discovery of microdeletion syndromes in the post-genomic era: Review of the methodology and characterization of a new 1q41q42 microdeletion syndrome, *Genet Med* 9:607, 2007.

Rosenfeld JA, et al: New cases and refinement of the critical region in the 1q41q42 microdeletion syndrome, *Eur J Med Genet* 54:42, 2011.

B

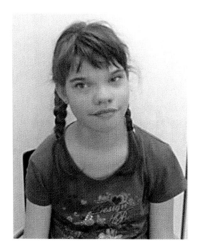
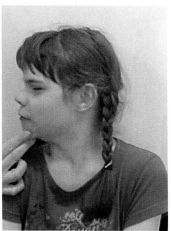

FIGURE 1. Eleven-year-old girl with a 1q41q42 microdeletion. Note coarse facies, deep-set eyes, hypertelorism or telecanthus, depressed nasal bridge, bulbous nose with broad nasal tip and anteverted nares, marked philtrum, full lips, tented upper lip. (Courtesy Dr. Dagmar Wieczorek, Essen, Germany.)

1Q43Q44 MICRODELETION SYNDROME
(1QTER MICRODELETION SYNDROME, SUBTELOMERIC 1Q MICRODELETION)
Microcephaly, Agenesis of Corpus Callosum, Characteristic Facies, Seizures

Since the original report of a terminal 1q43 deletion appeared in 1976 (Mankinen et al), more than 50 individuals with deletions spanning a 25-Mb interval on the subtelomeric region of chromosome 1q (1q42q44) have been reported.

ABNORMALITIES

Growth. Prenatal and/or postnatal growth retardation.

Performance. Moderate to severe intellectual disability with limited or no expressive speech, hypotonia, marked developmental delay. Both friendly and aggressive behaviors have been seen.

Craniofacial. Microcephaly (>50%), rounded face, prominent forehead, deep-set eyes, hypertelorism, epicanthic folds, strabismus, upslanting palpebral fissures, prominent metopic ridge, short nose with a broad or prominent nasal tip, thin bow-shaped upper lip, wide-spaced teeth, low-set malformed large ears, flat nasal bridge, long philtrum, high-arched palate, cleft palate/cleft uvula, microretrognathia, and hearing loss.

Limbs. Tapering fingers, talipes equinovarus, irregular implantation of toes, abnormal palmar creases, joint laxity.

Central Nervous System. Agenesis/hypogenesis of corpus callosum, ventriculomegaly, absence of septum pellucidum, seizures.

OCCASIONAL ABNORMALITIES

Cardiac defects, Dandy-Walker variant, hypoplasia of cerebellar vermis and hemispheres, hypoplasia of brainstem, Rathke cleft cyst, dental anomalies (hypodontia and abnormal size or shape), gastrointestinal reflux, renal and urinary tract anomalies, choroid and retinal coloboma, microphthalmia, blepharophimosis, genital anomalies, hirsutism, scoliosis, café au lait spots, short neck, small hands and feet, congenital hypothyroidism.

NATURAL HISTORY

The shape of the nose and upper lip appear to be the most recognizable features in all patients. Round face and flat nasal bridge are frequently not apparent in older patients, suggesting a change of facial phenotype during life. The degree of intellectual disability is most commonly severe, and seizures can be frequent and resistant to treatment. When adolescents and young adults have been reported, no additional major health problems have occurred.

ETIOLOGY

The critical region identified as the smallest region of overlap for this genotype encompasses a 2-Mb genomic interval between 241.5 Mb and 243.5 Mb from the 1q telomere. Genes within this region include the following: *AKT3* is one of three closely related isoforms of the protein kinase B (PKB/Akt) family. AKT kinases phosphorylate a number of substrates involved in stimulation of cell proliferation, survival, intermediary metabolism and cell growth. *ZNF238* codes for a C2H2-type zinc-finger protein that functions as a transcriptional repressor. *HNRNPU*, the largest component of the heterogeneous ribonucleoprotein complex, which binds to nascent transcripts, is involved in the regulation of embryonic brain development. It appears that deletion of the most proximal portion containing the *AKT3* gene causes microcephaly, deletion of the central portion including *ZNF238* causes agenesis of the corpus callosum, and deletion of the most distal portion containing *HNRNPU* as well as *FAM36A*, *C1ORF199*, may be the critical region for seizures. Cognitive impairment seems to be linked to deletions of all portions of the region. However, these clinical-molecular correlations do not appear to be true for all reported cases.

References

Mankinen CB, Sears JW, Alvarez VR: Terminal (1)(q43) long-arm deletion of chromosome no. 1 in a three-year-old female, *Birth Defects Orig Artic Ser* 12:131, 1976.

Johnson VP, et al: Deletion of the distal long arm of chromosome 1: A definable syndrome, *Am J Med Genet* 22:685, 1985.

van Bever Y, et al: Clinical report of a pure subtelomeric 1qter deletion in a boy with mental retardation and multiple anomalies adds further evidence for a specific phenotype, *Am J Med Genet A* 135:91, 2005.

Boland E, et al: Mapping of deletion and translocation breakpoints in 1q44 implicates the serine/threonine kinase AKT3 in postnatal microcephaly and agenesis of the corpus callosum, *Am J Hum Genet* 81:292, 2007.

van Bon BW, et al: Clinical and molecular characteristics of 1qter microdeletion syndrome: Delineating a critical region for corpus callosum agenesis/hypogenesis, *J Med Genet* 45:346, 2008.

Ballif BC, et al: High-resolution array CGH defines critical regions and candidate genes for microcephaly, abnormalities of the corpus callosum, and seizure phenotypes in patients with microdeletions of 1q43q44, *Hum Genet* 131:145, 2012.

B

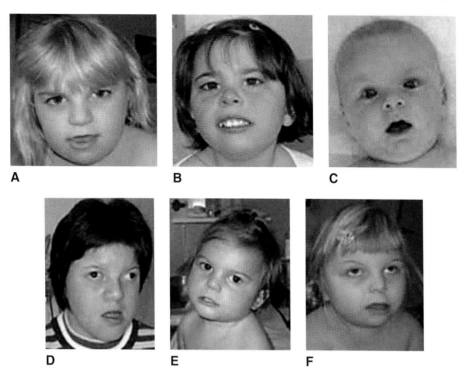

FIGURE 1.   **A–F,** A rounded face is present in almost all patients, a prominent forehead and deep-set eyes in most, hypertelorism in cases **D** and **E,** a short nose with a broad or prominent nasal tip, and a long philtrum in cases **B** and **F.** A thin bow-shaped upper lip is also seen in most patients. The open mouth and protruding tongue reflects significant oral hypotonia. (From Thierry G, et al: *Am J Med Genet A* 158A:1633, 2012.)

2Q31.1 MICRODELETION SYNDROME
Limb Defects, Intellectual Disability, Dysmorphic Features

The clinical phenotype was first delineated by Boles et al. At least 50 patients have been reported. Haploinsufficiency of the *HOXD* cluster has been identified as the cause of the spectrum of limb defects.

ABNORMALITIES

Growth. Pre- and postnatal growth retardation.

Performance. Mild to severe intellectual disability; epilepsy.

Central Nervous System. Large ventricles, delayed myelination, periventricular leukomalacia, partial agenesis of corpus callosum, cortical atrophy.

Craniofacial. Microcephaly, narrow forehead with prominent metopic suture, short downslanting palpebral fissures, deep-set eyes, ptosis, broad eyebrows with lateral flare, small nose with bulbous tip, thin upper lip, thick and everted lower lip, low-set dysplastic ears with thickened helices and lobules, micrognathia, cleft lip with or without cleft palate, cleft palate alone.

Limbs. A wide range of defects. Mild digital abnormalities include camptodactyly, fifth finger clinodactyly with shortening of middle phalanges, partial to complete syndactyly, duplicated halluces, hypoplastic or absent phalanges of third/fourth/fifth fingers, nail hypoplasia, brachymetacarpy, broad first toes, and wide distance between hallux and remaining toes (sandal gap). Severe malformations include multiple fusions of carpal/tarsal and phalangeal bones, split-hand/split-foot, and monodactyly. The lower limbs tend to be more often and more severely affected than the upper limbs.

Ocular. Strabismus, nystagmus, cortical blindness, colobomas, refractive errors.

Cardiac. Septal defects, patent ductus arteriosus.

Genitalia. Hypoplastic male and female genitalia, hypospadias, penoscrotal transposition.

OCCASIONAL ABNORMALITIES

Cataracts, microphthalmia, sex reversal, renal and urinary malformations. Pansynostosis of cranial sutures, myelomeningocele, hydrocephalus, contractures of large joints, hypoplasia or absence of a bone in the forearm or leg, hirsutism.

NATURAL HISTORY

Severe feeding problems and profound developmental delay can occur, and early death from respiratory infection or cardiac defects has occurred in several patients. Patients with smaller deletions can have mild to moderate intellectual disability and a benign course in infancy with near-normal growth.

ETIOLOGY

The deletion of this region is of variable size, ranging from a visible cytogenetic deletion to smaller submicroscopic deletions. Thus the phenotype is variable with more severe growth retardation and developmental delays, as well as multiple major and minor malformations of different systems in larger deletions. However, the deletion of the *HOXD* cluster and its surrounding up/downstream regulatory sequences appear to be responsible for the observed limb anomalies. Deletion of *DLX1* and *DLX2,* two genes in the region affecting limb development in *Drosophila,* do not appear to determine the extent of the limb defects. The critical region covers the interval 1.5 Mb centromeric and 1 Mb telomeric to the *HOXD* genes. The characteristic facial appearance is associated with a 2.4-Mb locus immediately centromeric to the locus for limb anomalies. *HOXD13* mutations and small microdeletions involving *HOXD9-13* and *EVX2* cause a specific synpolydactyly phenotype.

COMMENT

These deletions confirm that a diploid dose of human *HOXD* genes is crucial for normal growth and patterning of the limbs along the anterior-posterior axis.

References

Boles RG, et al: Deletion of chromosome 2q24-q31 causes characteristic digital anomalies: Case report and review, *Am J Med Genet* 55:155, 1995.

Slavotinek A, et al: Two cases with interstitial deletions of chromosome 2 and sex reversal in one, *Am J Med Genet* 86:75, 1999.

Del Campo M, et al: Monodactylous limbs and abnormal genitalia are associated with hemizygosity for the human 2q31 region that includes the HOXD cluster, *Am J Hum Genet* 65:104, 1999.

Veraksa A, Del Campo M, McGinnis W: Developmental patterning genes and their conserved functions: From model organisms to humans, *Mol Genet Metab* 69:85, 2000.

Goodman FR, et al: A 117-kb microdeletion removing *HOXD9-HOXD13* and *EVX2* causes synpolydactyly, *Am J Hum Genet* 70:547, 2002.

Goodman FR: Limb malformations and the human HOX genes, *Am J Med Genet* 112:256, 2002.

Mitter D, et al: Genotype-phenotype correlation in eight new patients with a deletion encompassing 2q31.1, *Am J Med Genet A* 152A:1213, 2010.

Dimitrov B, et al: 2q31.1 microdeletion syndrome: Redefining the associated clinical phenotype, *J Med Genet* 48:98, 2011.

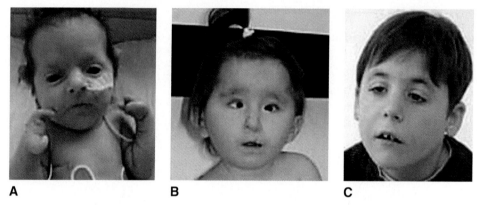

FIGURE 1.   2q31.1 Microdeletion syndrome. Affected children 1 month (**A**), 3 months (**B**), and 11 years (**C**) of age. Note broad eyebrows with lateral flare, short palpebral fissures, ptosis, small nose with bulbous tip and hypoplastic nares, and micrognathia. (From Mitter D, et al: *Am J Med Genet A* 152A:1213, 2010, with permission.)

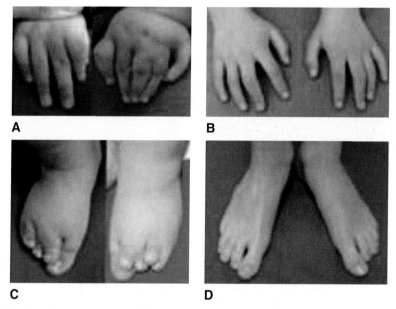

FIGURE 2.   2q31.1 Microdeletion syndrome. **A,** There is camptodactyly of the second and fifth fingers of the right hand and postaxial polydactyly, syndactyly of fingers 3 and 4, and camptodactyly of the second finger of the left hand. **B,** The fingers are tapered, and the thumbs are adducted and proximally placed. Note the bilateral fourth and fifth finger clinodactyly and mild syndactyly of fingers 3 and 4. **C,** Note the syndactyly and overlapping of the second and fourth toes. **D,** There are long halluces, partial cutaneous syndactyly, and short distal phalanges of toes 2 through 5. (From Mitter D, et al: *Am J Med Genet A* 152A:1213, 2010, with permission.)

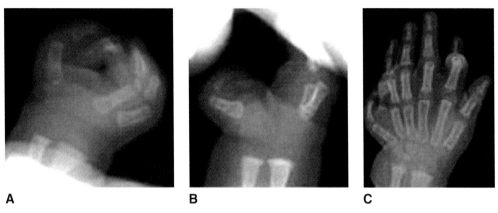

A   B   C

FIGURE 3.   Hand radiographs of patients with a 2q31.1 microdeletion syndrome. **A** and **B,** Newborn radiographs showing aplasia of the second and third fingers. **C,** Radiographs of the left hand of the child, at 1 year of age, whose hand is pictured in Figure 2A. Note dysplastic additional phalanx with an additional metacarpal bone, accelerated bone age, and dysplastic proximal phalanges with low mineralization. (From Mitter D, et al: *Am J Med Genet A* 152A:1213, 2010, with permission.)

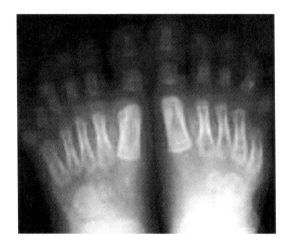

FIGURE 4.   Radiographs of the feet of a 15-month-old with a 2q31.1 microdeletion syndrome. Note the broad halluces, hypoplastic or absent middle or distal phalanges, broad fifth metatarsal bone, and duplication of the proximal fifth phalanx.

2Q37 DELETION SYNDROME
(2QTER SUBTELOMERIC MICRODELETION SYNDROME)

Since the disorder was first reported by Gorski et al in 1989, more than 100 cases of visible or submicroscopic deletions have been described, making this disorder one of the most frequently recognizable subtelomeric deletions.

ABNORMALITIES

Growth. Postnatal onset short stature not manifest until adulthood, obesity.

Performance. Mild to severe intellectual disability, hypotonia, seizures (25%–35%), autism spectrum disorders (25%–35%).

Craniofacial. Sparse hair; sparse, arched eyebrows; frontal bossing; round face with full cheeks; midface hypoplasia; deep-set eyes; epicanthal folds; upslanting palpebral fissures; depressed nasal bridge; short nose; hypoplastic, notched nares; prominent low-set columella; short philtrum; thin upper lip with hypoplastic cupid's bow; high arched palate; microtia.

Limbs. Small hands and feet, short third, fourth and fifth metacarpals (often fourth alone) and metatarsals, brachymetaphalangism, fifth finger clinodactyly, mild cutaneous syndactyly, persistent fetal fingertip pads, abnormal palmar creases.

Cardiac. Defects in 30%, including VSD, ASD, aortic coarctation, hypoplastic aortic arch.

Other. Wide set, distally placed, inverted nipples; supernumerary nipples; pectus carinatum and excavatum; scoliosis; intestinal malrotation; duodenal atresia; anteriorly placed anus; kidney and urinary tract anomalies; joint laxity; inguinal hernias; eczema.

OCCASIONAL ABNORMALITIES

Microcephaly (10%), macrocephaly, hypospadias, cryptorchidism, hypoplastic gonads, bifid uterus, dilated ventricles, hydrocephalus, holoprosencephaly, subependymal cyst, cerebellar anomalies, iris coloboma, diaphragmatic hernia, tracheomalacia, congenital hip dislocation, fused cervical vertebrae, supernumerary ribs, asthma, recurrent infections, Wilms tumor (<5%), alopecia, hypertrichosis, loose skin, cleft palate, hearing loss.

NATURAL HISTORY

Poor feeding and gastroesophageal reflux can lead to failure to thrive. Some patients have early overgrowth with early closure of the epiphyses and adult short stature. Affected women have occasionally given birth, but affected males have not. Screening for Wilms tumor should be considered.

ETIOLOGY

The size of the deletions is variable, ranging from visible deletions in 80% to subtelomeric cryptic deletions in 20%. Several families have shown recurrence for the deletion as a result of a parental balanced translocation (5%). Therefore, as in other subtelomeric deletions, FISH should be performed in all parents. A phenotype reminiscent of Albright Hereditary Osteodystrophy with short stature, obesity, and short fourth and fifth metacarpals and metatarsals seems to occur only in the distal deletions. This phenotype occurs in 50% to 60% of individuals with the 2qter submicroscopic microdeletion syndrome. The interval for autistic behavior is 1.43 Mb in size within the 2q37 region. Wilms tumor has been reported in three patients with breakpoints at or proximal to band 2q37.1.

References

Gorski JL, et al: Terminal deletion of the long arm of chromosome 2 in a mildly dysmorphic hypotonic infant with karyotype 46,XY,del(2)(q37), *Am J Med Genet* 32:350, 1989.

Casas KA, et al: Chromosome 2q terminal deletion: Report of 6 new patients and review of phenotype-breakpoint correlations in 66 individuals, *Am J Med Genet A* 130A:331, 2004.

Lukusa T, et al: Terminal 2q37 deletion and autistic behaviour, *Genet Couns* 16:179, 2005.

Chaabouni M, et al: Molecular cytogenetic analysis of five 2q37 deletions: Refining the brachydactyly candidate region, *Eur J Med Genet* 49:255, 2006.

Falk RE, Casas KA: Chromosome 2q37 deletion: clinical and molecular aspects, *Am J Med Genet C Semin Med Genet* 145C:357, 2007.

B

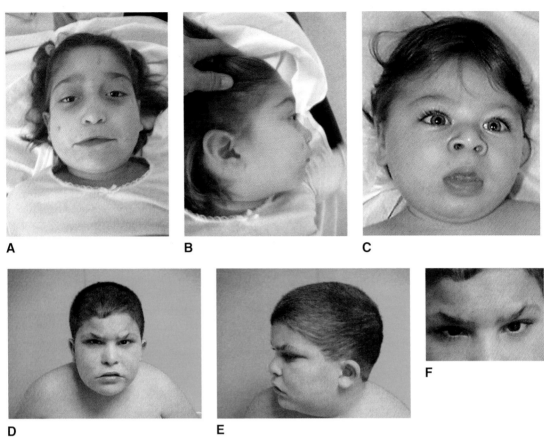

FIGURE 1. 2q37 Microdeletion syndrome. Note the sparse hair, sparse and arched eyebrows, round face with full cheeks, midface hypoplasia, and epicanthal folds (**A–C** and **F**); deep-set eyes, upslanting palpebral fissures (**A, D,** and **F**); depressed nasal bridge, short nose (**B** and **E**); prominent low-set columella, thin upper lip with hypoplastic Cupid's bow (**D** and **E**); and low-set ears (**B** and **E**). (**C,** Courtesy Prof. Bruno Dallapiccola, Ospedale Bambino Gesú, Rome, Italy.)

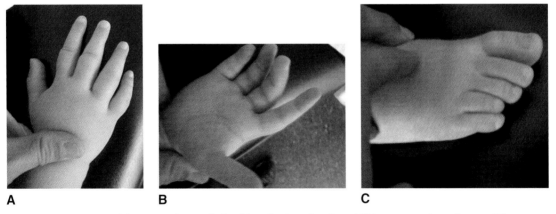

FIGURE 2. 2q37 microdeletion syndrome. **A,** Small hands, short fourth and fifth metacarpals, and tapered fingers. **B,** Altered palmar creases. **C,** Small feet, short fourth and fifth metatarsals.

3Q29 MICRODELETION SYNDROME
Intellectual Disability, Microcephaly, Mild Dysmorphic Features

This recurrent microdeletion syndrome was initially reported in a single case by Rossi et al in 2001. Since then, more than 20 cases have been reported with a consistent, mildly dysmorphic phenotype.

ABNORMALITIES

Growth. Prenatal and postnatal growth are frequently below the 50th percentile, but within the normal range.

Performance. Although normal intelligence has been reported, mild to moderate intellectual disability is the rule. Speech delay, autistic features, ataxic gait, depression, bipolar disorder, and schizophrenia also have been reported.

Craniofacial. Microcephaly (50%), often of postnatal onset; long, narrow face; high nasal bridge; short philtrum; large, low-set, posteriorly rotated ears.

Limbs. Long, tapering fingers.

OCCASIONAL ABNORMALITIES

Macrocephaly, seizures, microphthalmia, cataracts, corneal opacities, high arched palate, cleft lip with or without cleft palate widely spaced teeth, pectus deformities, six lumbar vertebrae, lower limb contractures, ligamentous laxity, abnormal skin pigmentation, anorectal malformation, horseshoe kidney, hypospadias, nasal voice, cerebral sigmoid venous thrombosis, aortic and pulmonic valve stenosis, patent ductus arteriosus.

ETIOLOGY

In most cases, a recurrent deletion of similar size (1.6 Mb) in all patients. The deletion commonly contains 22 genes, many of unknown function. At this stage, it is impossible to attribute the phenotype to any one of the deleted genes, but two genes within the commonly deleted area—*AK2* and *DLG1*—are autosomal homologues of known X-linked mental retardation genes *PAK3* and *DLG3*. Several families have been reported in which most individuals with the 3q29 microdeletion had only mild cognitive disability with no additional health problems, whereas other family members have had major depression, bipolar disease, and schizophrenia. This supports previous linkage of this region to mental disorders. An odds ratio of 17 has been identified for schizophrenia, suggesting this may be a very common adult complication.

COMMENT

The reciprocal microduplication (3q29dup) to the deleted region has been reported in a number of familial and sporadic cases, in which mild intellectual disability, microcephaly, and obesity appear to be the only common features, although major or minor anomalies such as craniosynostosis, high palate, seizures, VSD, excessive hand creases, and pes planus have been reported in more than one case. The fact that the duplication has been found with lower frequency than the deletion suggests many cases with the duplication may have a normal or near-normal phenotype.

References

Rossi E, et al: Cryptic telomeric rearrangements in subjects with mental retardation associated with dysmorphism and congenital malformations, *J Med Genet* 38:417, 2001.

Willatt L, et al: 3q29 microdeletion syndrome: Clinical and molecular characterization of a new syndrome, *Am J Hum Genet* 77:154, 2005.

Baynam G, Goldblatt J, Townshend S: A case of 3q29 microdeletion with novel features and a review of cytogenetically visible terminal 3q deletions, *Clin Dysmorphol* 15:145, 2006.

Ballif BC, et al: Expanding the clinical phenotype of the 3q29 microdeletion syndrome and characterization of the reciprocal microduplication, *Mol Cytogenet* 28:1, 2008.

Li F, et al: 3q29 interstitial microdeletion syndrome: An inherited case associated with cardiac defect and normal cognition, *Eur J Med Genet* 52:349, 2009.

Clayton-Smith J, et al: Familial 3q29 microdeletion syndrome providing further evidence of involvement of the 3q29 region in bipolar disorder, *Clin Dysmorphol* 19:128, 2010.

Mulle JG, et al: Microdeletions of 3q29 confer high risk for schizophrenia, *Am J Hum Genet* 87:229, 2010.

Quintero-Rivera F, Sharifi-Hannauer P, Martinez-Agosto JA: Autistic and psychiatric findings associated with the 3q29 microdeletion syndrome: Case report and review, *Am J Med Genet A* 152A:2459, 2010.

B

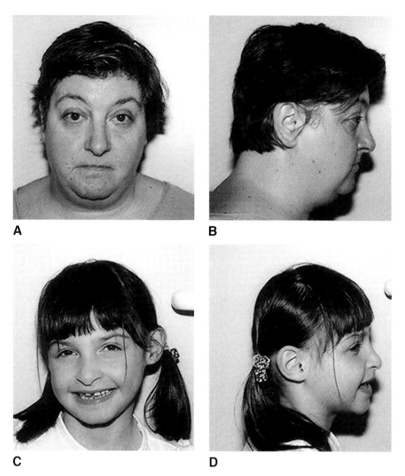

FIGURE 1. Mother (**A** and **B**) and daughter (**C** and **D**), both with the 3q29 microdeletion syndrome. Note the high nasal bridge, short philtrum, and large ears. (Courtesy Prof. Bruno Dallapiccola, Ospedale Bambino Gesú, Rome, Italy.)

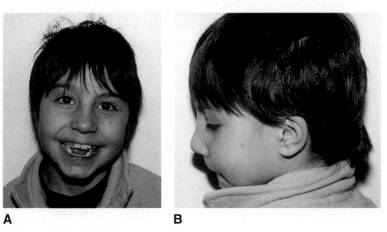

A   **B**

FIGURE 2.   3q29 microdeletion syndrome. **A** and **B,** Note the high nasal bridge. (Courtesy Prof. Bruno Dallapiccola, Ospedale Bambino Gesú, Rome, Italy.)

B

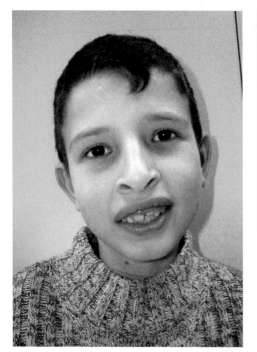 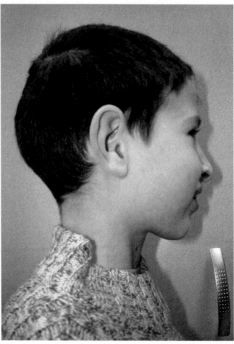

FIGURE 3.   3q29 microdeletion syndrome. Seven-year-old boy with an elongated face, prominent nasal bridge, and large ears. (Courtesy Dr. Jordi Rossell, Hospital Son Espases, Palma de Mallorca, Spain.)

9Q34.3 SUBTELOMERIC DELETION SYNDROME
(KLEEFSTRA SYNDROME)

Initially described as a recognizable pattern of malformation by Dawson et al and by Cormier-Daire et al, the clinical phenotype and the minimal deletion critical region were more fully characterized by Stewart et al and by Kleefstra et al. Mutations and disruptions of the euchromatin histone methyltransferase 1 (*EHMT1*) gene, which is located within the critical region, have recently been identified as being responsible for this phenotype. More than 125 patients have been reported.

ABNORMALITIES

Growth. Prenatal onset overgrowth with respect to weight (9%–20%), short stature (13%–39%), overweight (20%–30%), obesity.

Performance. Developmental delay, mild to severe intellectual disability, hypotonia, speech delay, sleep disturbance. Epilepsy (24%–36%). In older children, outbursts of anger; antisocial, compulsive, and self-stimulating behaviors; and stereotypic movements.

Central Nervous System. Defects in 50% to 61%, including dilated ventricles, white matter anomalies, corpus callosum hypoplasia or agenesis, cerebellar hypoplasia.

Craniofacial. Microcephaly (>50%), brachycephaly, hypertelorism, midface hypoplasia; synophrys, with prominent broad arched eyebrows; short nose with anteverted nares; open mouth with protruding tongue; thin upper lip with downturned corners of mouth; full everted lower lip; prognathism; pointed chin; malformed ears.

Cardiac. Defects in 31% to 44%, including ASD, VSD, patent foramen ovale, tetralogy of Fallot, pulmonary artery stenosis, subaortic/aortic valve stenosis, arrhythmias.

Genital. Abnormalities in 30% to 60%, including cryptorchidism, hypospadias, and micropenis.

OCCASIONAL ABNORMALITIES

Coarse facies, downslanting palpebral fissures, upslanting palpebral fissures, brachydactyly, clinodactyly, syndactyly, tapering fingers, single palmar crease, talipes equinovarus, hydronephrosis, renal cysts, vesicoureteral reflux, hydronephrosis, obesity, natal teeth, widely spaced teeth, joint laxity, tracheomalacia, hernias, anal atresia, sensorineural hearing loss, cortical blindness.

NATURAL HISTORY

Hypotonia results in feeding problems and recurrent aspiration leading to pneumonia as well as motor delay. Intellectual disability is variable in severity. Speech is delayed and can be limited to a few words in severe cases. In general, the severity of the behavioral and motor deficiencies increases over time, and the deficiencies become more apparent after adolescence. Gradual loss of previously learned motor and communication skills, a progressive immobility, and, ultimately, rigid flexion of the arms and hands and a decline in motivational and performance functions occur. The oldest published patient is a 43-year-old woman. Normal pubertal development is common. Four deaths—three that occurred at less than 1 year of age, secondary to respiratory failure or apnea—have been reported.

ETIOLOGY

Submicroscopic deletion of the subtelomere region of chromosome 9q34.3 has been the most frequently identified cause of the phenotype. However, mapping of smaller deletions has shown that haploinsufficiency of the euchromatin histone methyltransferase 1 (*EHMT1*) gene is responsible for this disorder. This was confirmed by the identification of point mutations in the gene in patients who had the typical phenotype but who lacked the microdeletion. *EHMT1* is an epigenetic regulator that affects gene transcription through histone modification leading to chromatin remodeling. Microdeletions have been the cause in 85% of affected individuals and intragenic *EHMT1* mutations in about 15%. Deletions involving the 9q34.3 region do not exceed 3.5 to 4 Mb in size. The virtual lack of detection of larger terminal deletions in live births is thought to reflect lethality. Patients with increased birth weight, obesity, and the "regressive" behavioral phenotype of this disorder are more likely to have point mutations in *EHMT1* than deletions. FISH should always be performed in both parents to rule out a balanced translocation. In addition, three familial cases have been reported in which the deletion was present in the mothers in a mosaic pattern.

COMMENT

Although MRI scanning of the brain in the two eldest patients with a "regressive course" demonstrated multifocal subcortical signal abnormalities, the cause of the apparent neuropsychiatric degeneration is unknown. Recently, memory was restored by *EHMT* re-expression during adulthood in *EHMT*-mutant *Drosophila,* indicating that cognitive defects are reversible in *EHMT* mutants.

References

Dawson AJ, et al: Cryptic chromosome rearrangements detected by subtelomeric assay in patients with mental retardation and dysmorphic features, *Clin Genet* 62:488, 2002.

Cormier-Daire V, et al: Cryptic terminal deletion of chromosome 9q34: A novel cause of syndromic obesity in childhood, *J Med Genet* 40:300, 2003.

Kleefstra T, et al: Disruption of the gene euchromatin histone methyltransferase 1 (*EU-HMTase1*) is associated with the 9q34 subtelomeric deletion syndrome, *J Med Genet* 42:299, 2004.

Kleefstra T, et al: Loss-of-function mutations in euchromatin histone methyl transferase 1 (*EHMT1*) cause the 9q24 subtelomeric deletion syndrome, *Am J Hum Genet* 79:370, 2006.

Stewart DR, et al: Subtelomeric deletion of chromosome 9q: a novel microdeletion syndrome, *Am J Med Genet A* 128:340, 2004.

Stewart DR, Kleefstra T: The chromosome 9q subtelomere deletion syndrome, *Am J Med Genet C* 145C:383, 2007.

Kramer JM, et al: Epigenetic regulation of learning and memory by *Drosophila EHMT/G9a*, *PLoS Biol* 9: e1000569, 2011.

Willemsen M, et al: Familial Kleefstra syndrome due to maternal somatic mosaicism for interstitial 9q34.3 microdeletions, *Clin Genet* 80:31, 2011.

Verhoeven WM, et al: Kleefstra syndrome in three adult patients: Further delineation of the behavioral and neurological phenotype shows aspects of a neurodegenerative course, *Am J Med Genet A* 155A:2409, 2011.

Willemsen MH, et al: Update on Kleefstra syndrome, *Molec Syndromol* 2:201, 2012.

B

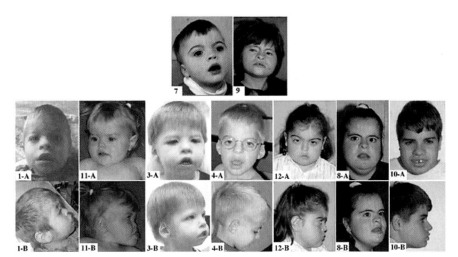

FIGURE 1.   Facial features of nine children with 9q34 microdeletion syndrome from 15 months to 15 years of age. Note the synophrys, arched eyebrows, short anteverted nose, thin tented upper lip, and macroglossia in one case. (From Stewart DW, et al: *Am J Med Genet* 128A:340, 2004.)

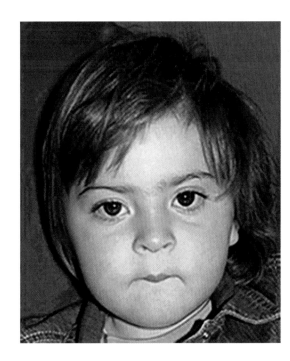

FIGURE 2.   The face of this 3-year-old with a 9q34.3 microdeletion shows synophrys, anteverted nares, and midface hypoplasia. (Courtesy Prof. Bruno Dallapiccola, Ospedale Bambino Gesú, Rome, Italy.)

B

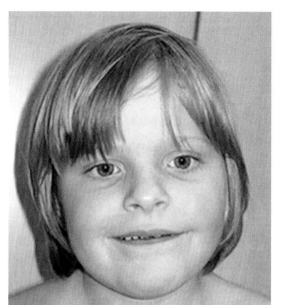 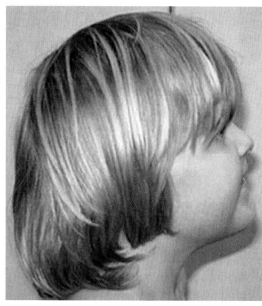

FIGURE 3. Seven-year-old girl with a mutation in *EHMT1*. Midface hypoplasia, short nose with anteverted nares, facial phenotype similar to that of patients with a microdeletion. (Courtesy Dr. Dagmar Wieczorek, Essen, Germany.)

15Q24 MICRODELETION SYNDROME

Although several visible deletions in the region had been reported previously, the first case of this recurrent microdeletion was reported in 2006 by Sharp et al. More than 30 individuals have been reported since then, and the estimated incidence is 1 in 42,000.

ABNORMALITIES

Growth. Prenatal (30%) and postnatal (30%) growth retardation and failure to thrive. Obesity (20%).

Performance. Mild to severe intellectual disability (100%), scarce to absent speech, hypotonia, autistic behavior, food seeking and obsessive compulsive behaviors, poor sleep.

Central Nervous System. Cortical atrophy, neuronal heterotopia, abnormal corpus callosum with cysts, enlarged ventricles, hypoplastic olfactory bulbs, enlarged cisterna magna.

Craniofacial. Microcephaly (20%); long, narrow, triangular face; facial asymmetry; high anterior hairline; high forehead; deep-set eyes; epicanthal folds; hypertelorism; downslanting palpebral fissures; sparse, broad medial eyebrows that taper laterally; low nasal bridge; broad nasal base with notched flaring alae nasi; long, smooth philtrum; full lower lip; small mouth; small pointed chin; abnormal ears (large, protuberant, cup-shaped, thick anteverted lobes).

Ocular. Ocular abnormalities in 60%, especially strabismus and nystagmus but also iris and chorioretinal coloboma, anisocoria, and hypermetropia.

Hearing. Conductive and sensorineural hearing loss (25%).

Hands and Feet. Small hands, short fifth fingers, brachydactyly of fourth and fifth metacarpals, hypoplastic and proximally implanted thumbs, camptodactyly of toes, overriding toes, hypoplastic fifth toes, cutaneous syndactyly of fingers or toes, sandal gap.

Genital. Hypospadias (40%), micropenis, cryptorchidism in males, labial adhesions in females.

Other. Congenital heart defects, joint laxity, scoliosis, kyphosis, hernias, recurrent infections.

OCCASIONAL ABNORMALITIES

Diaphragmatic hernia, bowel atresia, imperforate anus, Pierre Robin sequence, myelomeningocele, café au lait macules, acanthosis nigricans, growth hormone deficiency, hypogonadotropic hypogonadism.

NATURAL HISTORY

Penetrance is 100% for intellectual disability and distinct facial features. Ocular and hearing anomalies are frequent and should be monitored. Connective tissue laxity is evident in many patients, with loose joints, hernias, and scoliosis. Nearly half of the patients have a history of recurrent infections, suggesting some form of immunodeficiency is present, not yet defined. Several adults have been reported, with variable cognitive and behavioral impairment and no major additional health issues. More than 80% of the reported cases have been males.

ETIOLOGY

Most deletions at 15q24 are 1.7 Mb to 6.1 Mb, the smallest region of overlap being a 1.1-Mb region, which includes at least 24 genes. *CYP11A1* encodes an enzyme involved in cholesterol metabolism and may play a role in genital abnormalities. *SEMA7A* and *CPLX3* are highly expressed in brain. Deletion of *STRA6*, the causal gene for the Matthew-Wood syndrome, may cause diaphragmatic hernia, present in several cases. All known cases have been de novo. The actual size and breakpoints of the deletion vary among patients, with most deletions occurring due to nonallelic homologous recombination between segmental duplication blocks (low copy repeats).

COMMENT

The reciprocal duplication of the region 15q24 involving the smallest region of overlap has been reported in several individuals with cognitive deficiency, joint limitations, digital anomalies, and facial features somewhat similar to those present in patients with the deletion. Duplications distal to the deletion critical region also appear to have similar phenotypic consequences, with significant behavioral and cognitive features.

References

Sharp AJ, et al: Discovery of previously unidentified genomic disorders from the duplication architecture of the human genome, *Nat Genet* 38:1038, 2006.

Sharp AJ, et al: Characterization of a recurrent 15q24 microdeletion syndrome, *Hum Mol Genet* 16:567, 2007.

Klopocki E, et al: A further case of the recurrent 15q24 microdeletion syndrome, detected by array CGH, *Eur J Pediatr* 167:903, 2008.

Van Esch H, et al: Congenital diaphragmatic hernia is part of the new 15q24 microdeletion syndrome, *Eur J Med Genet* 52:153, 2009.

Roetzer KM, et al: Further evidence for the pathogenicity of 15q24 microduplications distal to the minimal critical regions, *Am J Med Genet* 152A:3173, 2010.

Mefford HC, et al: Further clinical and molecular delineation of the 15q24 microdeletion syndrome, *J Med Genet* 49:110, 2012.

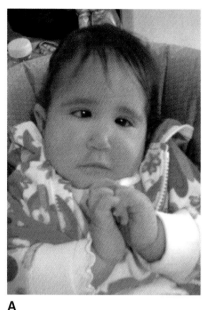
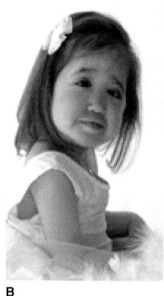
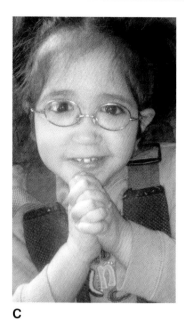

A   B   C

FIGURE 1.   Patient with the 15q24 microdeletion at 9 months **(A),** 2 years **(B),** and 3 years **(C)** of age. Note facial asymmetry, high anterior hairline, high forehead, deep-set eyes, epicanthal folds, hypertelorism, strabismus, downslanting palpebral fissures, low nasal bridge, long prominent philtrum, small pointed chin, and protuberant ears. (Courtesy Prof. HC Mefford, University of Washington.)

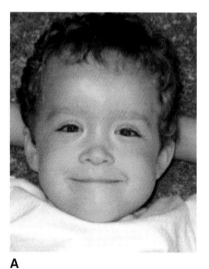
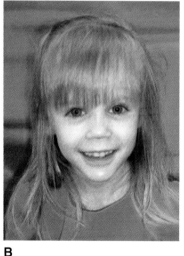

A   B

FIGURE 2.   Two other children with the 15q24 microdeletion. **A,** Note low nasal bridge, mild hypertelorism, sparse medial eyebrows that taper laterally, and broad nasal base with notched alae nasi. **B,** Long, narrow, triangular face with small pointed chin. Both patients show a prominent forehead with a high anterior hairline. (Courtesy Prof. HC Mefford, University of Washington.)

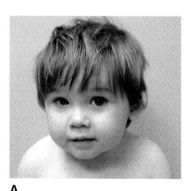
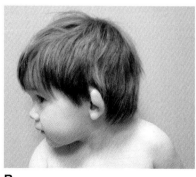

A   B

FIGURE 3.   Frontal **(A)** and lateral **(B)** view of the face of a 2-year-old with the 15q24 microdeletion. Note prominent forehead, mild hypertelorism, strabismus, low nasal bridge, broad nasal base, and small pointed chin. The ears show marked overfolding of the superior helix. (Courtesy Prof. Gail Vance, Indiana University, Indianapolis.)

16P11.2P12.2 MICRODELETION SYNDROME

Although Hernando et al reported the first case of a neonate with del 16p11.2p12.2, Ballif et al initially recognized this disorder as a unique pattern of malformation.

ABNORMALITIES

Growth. Growth has been normal in four patients, below the 3rd percentile in two patients.

Performance. Hypotonia, unsteady gait, intellectual disability, severe expressive language disorder, hyperactivity.

Face. Long, narrow flat face; deep-set eyes; down-slanting palpebral fissures; low-set, malformed, posteriorly rotated ears.

Hands and Feet. Single palmar crease, syndactyly of fingers and/or toes.

Cardiac. Tetralogy of Fallot, pulmonary atresia, bicuspid aortic valve, tricuspid regurgitation.

OCCASIONAL ABNORMALITIES

Craniosynostosis, epicanthal folds, thin upper lip, high arched palate, camptodactyly, long thin fingers, fifth finger clinodactyly, hallux valgus, cutis marmorata, sacral dimple, hemivertebrae.

NATURAL HISTORY

Feeding difficulties and gastroesophageal reflux have occurred in all patients in infancy. Ear infections occur frequently. Moderate intellectual disability is the rule. Speech development is a particular problem, as is hyperactivity with short attention span and impairment of fine motor skills.

ETIOLOGY

Microdeletion involving 16p11.2p12.2, of variable size ranging from 7.1 Mb to 8.2 Mb. The deletions are recurrent and mediated by allelic nonhomologous recombination among blocks of segmental duplications. The telomeric breakpoint appears to be the same in all patients, whereas the proximal breakpoint has been variable. More than 100 genes are involved. The location of the deletions has ranged from 21.4 Mb to 28.5/30.5 Mb from 16pter.

COMMENT

Autism has not been reported in chromosome 16p11.2p12.2 microdeletion syndrome. However, recurrent microdeletion and reciprocal microduplication at a contiguous region on 16p11.2 just centromeric to 16p11.2-p12.2 have been said in some studies to account for approximately 1% of all cases of autism. This frequent deletion is located 29.5 Mb to 30.1 Mb from 16pter.

References

Hernando C, et al: Comparative genomic hybridization shows a partial de novo deletion 16p11.2 in a neonate with multiple congenital malformations, *J Med Genet* 39:E24, 2002.

Ballif BC, et al: Discovery of a previously unrecognized microdeletion syndrome 16p11.2-p12.2, *Nat Genet* 39:1071, 2007.

Weiss LA, et al: Association between microdeletion and microduplication at 16p11.2 and autism, *N Eng J Med* 358:667, 2008.

Battaglia A, et al: Further characterization of the new microdeletion syndrome of 16p11.2-p12.2, *Am J Med Genet A* 149A:1200, 2009.

Hempel M, et al: Microdeletion syndrome 16p11.2-p12.2: Clinical and molecular characterization, *Am J Med Genet A* 149A:2106, 2009.

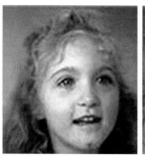
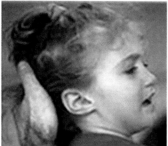

A

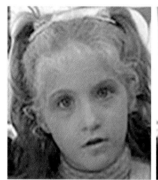
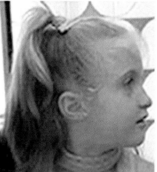

B

FIGURE 1.   A and **B,** Same patient at 3 years of age and at 6 years of age with the 16p11.2p12.2 microdeletion syndrome. Note the deep-set eyes; low-set, posteriorly rotated ears; mildly pointed chin; and thin upper lip. (From Battaglia A, et al: *Am J Med Genet Part A* 149A:1200, 2009, with permission.)

17Q21 MICRODELETION SYNDROME

First reported by Koolen et al and Shaw-Smith et al in 2006, Koolen et al (2008) provided an excellent review of 22 patients with this characteristic phenotype. More than 70 cases have now been reported, with an estimated prevalence of 1 in 16,000. It has recently been shown that haploinsufficiency for a single gene in the interval is the cause of the overall features of this microdeletion.

ABNORMALITIES

Growth. Low birth weight (27%), short stature (18%). Normal growth is most frequent.

Performance. Mild to severe intellectual disability. Marked speech delay and hypotonia occur, epilepsy (>50%). Friendly and cooperative behavior with frequent laughing.

Craniofacial. Present in more than 50%: abnormal hair pigmentation and texture, relative macrocephaly with high/broad forehead, long face, upslanting palpebral fissures, epicanthal folds, tubular or pear-shaped nose, bulbous nasal tip, everted lower lip, high palate, broad chin, large/prominent ears. Less frequent findings are a high nasal bridge, a broad nasal root, a long columella and hypoplastic and/or thick alae nasi, small widely spaced teeth

Ocular. Strabismus, hypermetropia, astigmatism, pale irides, blepharophimosis, ptosis.

Limbs. Slender long fingers (60%), hypoplasia of hand muscles (29%), slender lower limbs (41%), dislocation of the hips (27%), other joint dislocations, and positional deformities of the feet (27%), fetal fingertip pads.

Cardiac. Congenital heart defects (27%), mainly pulmonic stenosis, ASD and VSD, bicuspid aortic valve.

Kidney and Urinary Tract. Anomalies in 32%, including vesicoureteral reflux, hydronephrosis, pyelectasis, duplex renal system, renal dysplasia.

Skeletal. Spine deformities (40%), including scoliosis, lordosis, and kyphosis, pectus excavatum.

Skin. Hyperpigmented nevi, areas of thickened dry skin, deep palmar and plantar creases, hyperelastic skin.

Genital. Cryptorchidism (70%–85% in males).

OCCASIONAL ABNORMALITIES

CNS defects including ventriculomegaly, corpus callosum defects, periventricular leukomalacia, prenatal ischemic infarction, neuronal heterotopia, Chiari malformation type 1. Dilated aortic root, situs inversus, scaphocephaly, metopic synostosis, progressive contractures of distal joints, cleft palate, eczema, ichthyosis, hypodontia, enamel defects, iris and choroid coloboma, conductive and sensorineural deafness, growth hormone deficiency, attention deficit, poor social interaction.

NATURAL HISTORY

Hypotonia, with poor suck and slow feeding, is common. The facial characteristics change with age. In infancy, hypotonia of the face, with an open mouth appearance and a protruding tongue, is characteristic. With increasing age, there is elongation of the face, broadening of the chin, and a more pronounced "tubular" or "pear" shape of the nose. Involvement of ectodermal derivatives—including altered pigmentation of skin and hair, as well as dry thickened skin—are common.

ETIOLOGY

A recurrent heterozygous microdeletion, commonly between 500 kb and 650 kb in size at 17q21.31, is causative. It is most likely mediated by allelic non-homologous recombination of a single copy region flanked by segmental duplications. The smallest region of overlap is 424 kb encompassing at least seven genes, including *KANSL1*. Loss of function mutations of *KANSL1* are responsible for the classic phenotype of the deletion. *KANSL1* is a chromatin modifier gene. It influences gene expression through histone H4 lysine 16 (H4K16) acetylation. All transmitting parents carry a 900-kb inversion polymorphism, which is present in only 20% of the European population and almost absent in Asian and African populations. Therefore, its presence in a parent appears to be a requirement for the occurrence of the deletion in the offspring. Recurrence due to parental mosaicism has been reported.

COMMENT

The reciprocal duplication, microduplication 17Q21 syndrome, has been found in at least six patients with variable developmental delay, microcephaly, facial abnormalities, abnormal digits, and hirsutism, as well as significant behavioral problems including bipolar disorder.

References

Koolen DA, et al: A new chromosome 17q21.31 microdeletion syndrome associated with a common inversion polymorphism, *Nat Genet* 38:999, 2006.

Shaw-Smith C, et al: Microdeletion encompassing MAPT at chromosome 17q21.3 is associated with developmental delay and learning disability, *Nat Genet* 38:1032, 2006.

Kirchhoff M, et al: A 17q21.31 microduplication, reciprocal to the newly described 17q21.31 microdeletion, in a girl with severe psychomotor developmental delay and dysmorphic craniofacial features, *Eur J Med Genet* 50:256, 2007.

Koolen DA, et al: Clinical and molecular delineation of the 17q21.31 microdeletion syndrome, *J Med Genet* 45:710, 2008.

Wright EB, et al: Cutaneous features in 17q21.31 deletion syndrome: A differential diagnosis for cardio-facio-cutaneous syndrome, *Clin Dysmorphol* 20:15, 2011.

Koolen DA, et al: Mutations in the chromatin modifier gene *KANSL1* cause the 17q21.31microdeletion syndrome, *Nat Genet* 44:639, 2012.

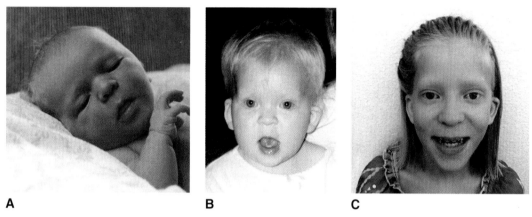

A   **B**   **C**

FIGURE 1. 17q21.31 microdeletion syndrome. Same child at birth **(A)**, 11 months **(B)**, and 12 years **(C)**. In infancy, facial hypotonia and an open mouth posture are noted. Over time, the high forehead, long tubular nasal configuration, and prominent chin are more evident.

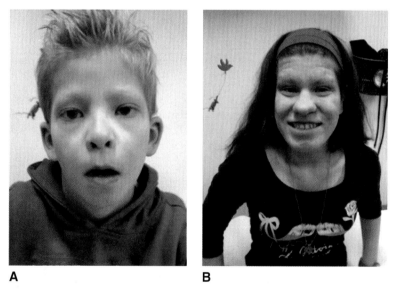

A   **B**

FIGURE 2. 17q21.31 microdeletion syndrome. Two children, ages 9 **(A)** and 17 **(B)**, with the 17q21 deletion. Note the high/broad forehead, long face, upslanting palpebral fissures, epicanthal folds, tubular or pear-shaped nose, bulbous nasal tip, and everted lower lip. (Courtesy Dr. David A. Koolen, Nijmegen, The Netherlands.)

22Q13 DELETION SYNDROME (PHELAN-MCDERMID SYNDROME)

Initially identified as a recognizable pattern of malformation in 1994, this disorder was characterized more completely by Phelan and colleagues in 2001. More than 600 cases have been published. The nonspecificity of the phenotype in newborns suggests that it is far more common than presently recognized.

ABNORMALITIES

Growth. Normal growth is the rule. However, both short and tall stature as well as macrocephaly and microcephaly have been seen more frequently than in the general population.

Performance. Intellectual disability, severe to profound in majority of cases; absent or severely delayed speech; hypotonia; frequent mouthing/chewing of objects; autistic behavior.

Craniofacial. Dolichocephaly; full brow, long eyelashes, and full/puffy eyelids and cheeks; prominent, dysplastic ears; pointed chin.

Limbs. Relatively large, fleshy hands; abnormal, dysplastic toenails.

OCCASIONAL ABNORMALITIES

Bulbous nose, decreased sweating with tendency to overheat, seizures; CNS abnormalities, including ventricular dilatation, delayed myelination, decreased periventricular white matter, and arachnoid cyst; sensorineural hearing loss; ptosis; epicanthal folds; fifth finger clinodactyly; 2-3 toe syndactyly; cardiac defects, primarily patent ductus arteriosus and ventricular septal defects; vesicoureteral reflux and polycystic kidney; puffy, swollen feet; hearing loss; arachnoid cyst; sacral dimple; cyclic vomiting; lymphedema; gastroesophageal reflux; renal anomalies.

NATURAL HISTORY

Hypotonia is common in infancy and is associated with poor oral intake, dehydration, and failure to thrive. Early developmental milestones are often delayed. Although lack of expressive speech is the rule, the ability of affected children to understand language is far more advanced. In one third of cases, a significant regression of skills has been observed. In fact, three adults, ages 40, 41, and 47, had evidence of severe progressive neurologic deterioration.

ETIOLOGY

This disorder is caused by loss of genetic material near the terminal end of the long arm of one chromosome 22 at 22q13. It may result from a simple deletion, an unbalanced translocation, or formation of a ring. Although most cases occur de novo, can be identified with FISH analysis for 22q13, and have no increased risk for recurrence, 10% of cases result from the inheritance of an unbalanced translocation. In those cases, an increased recurrence risk exists. The gene *SHANK3*, which codes for a structural protein found in the postsynaptic density, is thought to be a major factor in the development of the associated neurologic features.

COMMENT

FISH analysis for 22q13 should be considered in all infants presenting with normal growth and hypotonia in the absence of a neurologic cause.

References

Nesslinger NJ, et al: Clinical, cytogenetic, and molecular characterization of seven patients with deletion of chromosome 22q13.3, *Am J Hum Genet* 54:464, 1994.

Phelan MC, et al: 22q13 deletion syndrome, *Am J Med Genet* 101:91, 2001.

Wilson HL, et al: Molecular characterization of the 22q13 deletion syndrome supports the role of haploinsufficiency of SHANK3/PROSAP2 in the major neurological symptoms, *J Med Genet* 40:575, 2003.

Havens JM, et al: 22q13 deletion syndrome: An update and review for the primary pediatrician, *Clin Pediatr* 43:43, 2004.

Phelan K, et al: The 22q13.3 deletion syndrome (Phelan-McDermid syndrome), *Mol Syndromol* 2:186, 2012.

Bonaglia MC, et al: Molecular mechanisms generating and stabilizing terminal 22q13 deletions in 44 subjects with Phelan/McDermid syndrome, *PLoS Genet* 7:e1002173, 2011.

Rollins JD, et al: Growth in Phelan-McDermid syndrome, *Am J Med Genet* 155:2324, 2011.

B

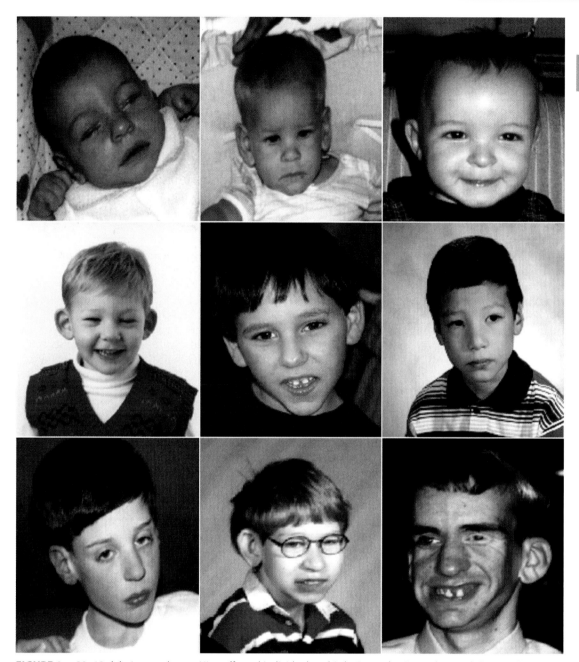

FIGURE 1.   22q13 deletion syndrome. Nine affected individuals at birth, 6 months, 1 year (*top row*); 3 years, 5 years, 7 years (*second row*); 9 years, 13 years, and 24 years (*third row*). (From Phelan MC, et al: *Am J Med Genet* 101:91, 2001, with permission.)

XQ DISTAL DUPLICATION OR DISOMY
(XQ27-Q28 TERMINAL DUPLICATIONS INCLUDING *MECP2* DUPLICATION)
Severe Neurocognitive Deficiency, Autistic Spectrum Disorders, Mild Facial Abnormalities, Recurrent Infections

Duplications of the distal long arm of chromosome X (Xq) include intrachromosomal duplications and partial disomies in males or trisomies in females resulting from unbalanced translocations with an autosome or with a chromosome Y. About 40 cases of Xq functional disomy due to cytogenetically visible rearrangements and more than 100 cases of cryptic duplications have been reported. Clinical manifestations vary depending on the gender and on the gene content of the duplicated segment. The most frequently reported distal duplications involve the Xq28 segment encompassing the *MECP2* gene and yield a specific recognizable phenotype in affected males.

ABNORMALITIES

Growth. Prenatal onset growth retardation. Normocephaly is most common, but microcephaly can occur.

Performance. Severe intellectual disability (99%), absence of speech or severely retarded speech (88%), major axial hypotonia (92%), progressive spasticity (59%) (most prominent in lower limbs), ataxia (54%), epilepsy (52%), autism spectrum disorders (76%), choreiform movements (45%).

Central Nervous System. Hypoplasia of corpus callosum, mild brain atrophy/loss of cerebral volume, external hydrocephalus.

Craniofacial. Premature closure of the fontanels or ridged metopic suture; brachycephaly; facial hypotonia; midface hypoplasia; hypertelorism; epicanthal folds; depressed nasal bridge; upturned nares; small and open mouth; thin tented upper lip; high palate with alveolar ridge hypertrophy; large, low-set, posteriorly rotated ears; other ear anomalies.

Immune System. Recurrent infections, low serum IgA and IgM, elevated serum IgG, poor response to polysaccharide antigen, and poor T-cell response to *Candida*.

Other. Severe constipation (76%), strabismus or amblyopia.

OCCASIONAL ABNORMALITIES
Genital anomalies (hypoplastic genitalia, hypospadias, cryptorchidism), cardiac defects, pectus deformities, scoliosis, small hands and feet, abnormal fingers and toes (syndactyly, clinodactyly, talipes equinovarus). Hearing loss, hypothyroidism, eczema.

NATURAL HISTORY
Severe feeding difficulties with swallowing dysfunction, gastroesophageal reflux, excessive drooling, seizures, and recurrent infections are major challenges from early infancy. Almost 40% of males with *MECP2* duplication reported to date have died before age 25 years. Recurrent infections have decreased with the use of intravenous or subcutaneous immunoglobulins, although the specific immune defect underlying the infections has not been determined in most cases. Up to 72% of patients achieve ambulation. In addition to some individuals who experienced developmental regression, 80% of affected males who initially used words

subsequently regressed and never regained speech. A subset of patients with *MECP2* duplication manifest medication/treatment-refractory epilepsy. Growth retardation, microcephaly and additional malformations (cardiac defects, genital anomalies), or more severe dysmorphic features are characteristic of larger deletions of Xq.

ETIOLOGY

Xq28 duplications can result from unbalanced translocations with an autosome or with a chromosome Y. Most of these cases are de novo, but karyotyping of the parents and FISH should be used to rule out predisposing rearrangements. Most frequently, interstitial duplications ranging from 0.2 Mb to 2.2 Mb are the cause of the phenotype. The smallest region of overlap causing this phenotype contains the gene *MECP2,* which is responsible for the neurologic and dysmorphic phenotype, and the gene *IRAK1,* which encodes the interleukin-1 receptor-associated kinase 1, most likely the cause of the recurring infections. Most Xq duplications observed in males are inherited from their mothers, although a few de novo duplications have been identified. In females, intrachromosomal duplications of the X chromosome are generally associated with a skewed inactivation pattern biased toward the duplicated X chromosome, leading to a normal or near-normal phenotype. However, some carrier females have a variety of neuropsychiatric phenotypes (depression, anxiety, compulsions, autistic features) but normal cognition. Occasionally, females can have short stature, developmental delay, facial dysmorphism, and gonadal dysgenesis. Rarely, a severe phenotype is encountered in females. A copy number effect for *MECP2* has been demonstrated, with several cases of triplication leading to even more severe phenotypes. It has been suggested that duplication of the adjacent *FLNA* gene is responsible for the severe, and often fatal, chronic intestinal pseudo-obstruction and bladder dysfunction phenotype sometimes present in these patients, but constipation is frequent even in those cases without duplication in *FLNA*. Another gene in the interval, *GDI1,* may be responsible for associated microcephaly in larger duplications. Recurrence risk for carrier females is 50% for male offspring.

COMMENT

Deletions or mutations of *MECP2* cause Rett syndrome, a progressive neurodevelopmental disorder primarily affecting girls, with apparently normal psychomotor development during the first 6 to 18 months of life, a short period of developmental stagnation, then rapid regression in language, hand use, and other motor skills, followed by long-term stability. Severe neonatal encephalopathy resulting in death before age 2 years is most frequent in affected males. Dysmorphic features are not usually associated with these phenotypes.

References

Sanlaville D, et al: Functional disomy of the Xq28 chromosome region, *Eur J Hum Genet* 13:579, 2005.

Friez MJ, et al: Recurrent infections, hypotonia, and mental retardation caused by duplication of MECP2 and adjacent region in Xq28, *Pediatrics* 118:e1687, 2006.

del Gaudio D, et al: Increased *MECP2* gene copy number as the result of genomic duplication in neurodevelopmentally delayed males, *Genet Med* 8:784, 2006.

Smyk M, et al: Different-sized duplications of Xq28, including *MECP2,* in three males with mental retardation, absent or delayed speech, and recurrent infections, *Am J Med Genet B Neuropsychiatr Genet* 147B:799, 2008.

Sanlaville D, Schluth-Bolard C, Turleau C: Distal Xq duplication and functional Xq disomy, *Orphanet J Rare Dis* 4:4, 2009.

Ramocki MB, et al: The *MECP2* duplication syndrome, *Am J Med Genet A* 152A:1079, 2010.

Breman AM, et al: *MECP2* duplications in six patients with complex sex chromosome rearrangements, *Eur J Hum Genet* 19:409, 2011.

Honda S, et al: The incidence of hypoplasia of the corpus callosum in patients with dup (X)(q28) involving *MECP2* is associated with the location of distal breakpoints, *Am J Med Genet A* 158A:1292, 2012.

Bijlsma EK, et al: Xq28 duplications including MECP2 in five females: Expanding the phenotype to severe mental retardation, *Eur J Med Genet* 55-540:404, 2012.

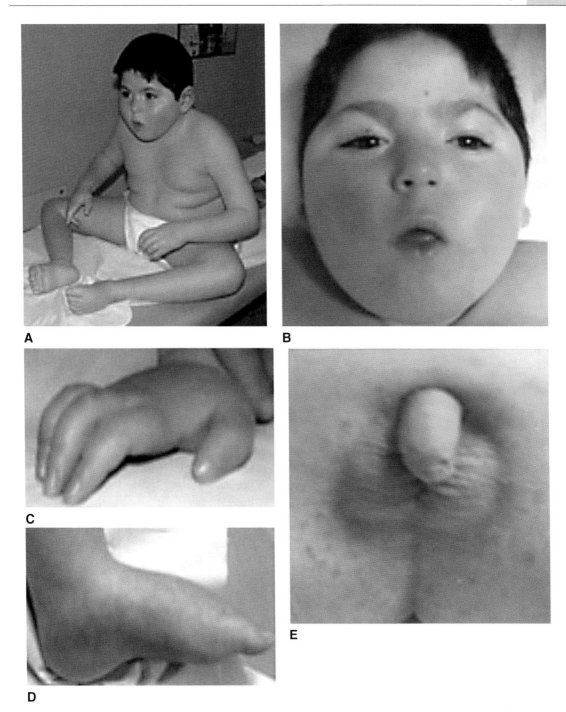

FIGURE 1. Characteristic phenotype of the Xq distal duplication. **A,** Brachycephaly, facial hypotonia, midface hypoplasia. **B,** Hypertelorism, epicanthal folds, depressed nasal bridge, upturned nares, small and open mouth, thin tented upper lip. **C** and **D,** Small hands and small feet. **E,** Cryptorchidism and hypoplastic scrotum. (Courtesy Prof. Bruno Dallapiccola, Ospedale Bambino Gesú, Rome, Italy.)

C Very Small Stature, Not Skeletal Dysplasia

BRACHMANN–DE LANGE SYNDROME
(CORNELIA DE LANGE SYNDROME, DE LANGE SYNDROME)
Synophrys, Thin Downturning Upper Lip, Micromelia

The syndrome was originally reported in 1933 by Cornelia de Lange, although Brachmann described a child with similar features at autopsy in 1916. As the molecular etiology of this condition has been elucidated, both a classical and a milder phenotype are recognized. Percentages of features listed below refer to classical cases.

ABNORMALITIES

Growth. Prenatal onset growth deficiency with length and weight less than 10th percentile. Mean adult height 156 cm (males) and 131 cm (females), Retarded osseous maturation (100%).

Performance. Intellectual disability and sluggish physical activity. Average intelligence quotient (IQ) ranges from below 30 to 86, with an average of 53. Those with higher IQs tend to have a higher birth weight and head circumference and less severe malformations.

Initial hypertonicity	(100%)
Low-pitched, weak, growling cry in infancy	(74%)
High pain tolerance, severe speech and language delays, autism spectrum disorders, seizures	(23%)
Broad-based gait	

Behavior. Hyperactivity, short attention span, aggression, self-injurious behavior, extreme shyness, anxiety, depression, obsessive-compulsive behavior, perseveration, sleep disturbance, circadian rhythm disorders.

Craniofacial. Microbrachycephaly (93%); bushy eyebrows and synophrys (98%), long, thick, curly eyelashes (99%), arched eyebrows (98%); ptosis; high myopia; peripapillary pigmentation; microcornea; tear duct malformation; depressed nasal bridge (83%); anteverted nares (85%); long philtrum, thin upper lip, and downturned angles of mouth (94%); high-arched palate (86%); late eruption of widely spaced teeth (86%); thick dysplastic posteriorly rotated ears; micrognathia (84%); prominent symphysis (66%)

Skin. Hirsutism (78%), cutis marmorata and perioral pale "cyanosis" (56%), hypoplastic nipples and umbilicus (50%), low posterior hairline (92%)

Limbs. Micromelia (93%), phocomelia and oligodactyly (27%), clinodactyly of fifth fingers (74%), single transverse palmar crease (51%), proximal implantation of thumbs (72%), flexion contracture of elbows (64%), syndactyly of second and third toes (86%), cold extremities

Genitalia. Hypoplasia in males (57%), undescended testes (73%), hypospadias (33%), hypoplastic labia majora

Gastrointestinal. Gastroesophageal (GE) reflux (>90%), Barrett esophagus (10%), malrotation with risk for volvulus (>10%)

Imaging. Mandibular spur present up to 3 months of age, dislocated/hypoplastic radial head, hypoplastic first metacarpal and fifth middle phalanx, short sternum with precocious fusion and 13 ribs, enlarged cerebral ventricles, white matter atrophy.

Other. Strabismus, nystagmus, blepharitis; short neck (66%); cleft palate (20%); submucous cleft palate (14%); hearing loss secondary to canal stenosis; ossicular malformation or cochlear anomaly (60%); congenital heart defects (33%); structural renal anomalies; thrombocytopenia, including idiopathic thrombocytopenic purpura

OCCASIONAL ABNORMALITIES

Astigmatism, optic atrophy, coloboma of the optic nerve, cataracts, Coats disease, proptosis, choanal atresia, hypertrophic cardiomyopathy, later-onset dysplastic heart valves, hiatus hernia, diaphragmatic hernia, pyloric stenosis, brachyesophagus, esophageal adenocarcinoma, inguinal hernia, hematometra, split foot, scoliosis, leg length inequality, absent second to third interdigital triradius, thoracic meningocele.

NATURAL HISTORY AND MANAGEMENT

These patients show a marked retardation of growth, evident by the time of birth, and as a rule, they fail to thrive. Feeding difficulties, including regurgitation, projectile vomiting, chewing, and swallowing difficulties, often continue well beyond 6 months. Because of the extremely high rate of GE reflux and intestinal malrotation, search for these features in infancy is critical. Although a high percentage of affected children have severe intellectual disability, a significant number have a much higher potential relative to performance than earlier studies have suggested, particularly among those less classically affected. Hearing loss and visual disturbances are common. Blepharitis improves with age. Chronic sinusitis may be lifelong. Puberty occurs at the normal time although it may be incomplete with irregular menses being common. Adults are small and have a tendency toward obesity. There is some evidence of early aging in adults. Early long-term sequelae of GE reflux, including Barrett esophagus and esophageal adenocarcinoma, have been seen. Episodes of aspiration in infancy, apnea, complications related to bowel obstruction, diaphragmatic hernia, and cardiac defects appear to constitute the major hazards for survival in these patients.

ETIOLOGY

This disorder is a result of mutations in one of three cohesin-associated genes. Mutations in *NIPBL*, located at 5p13, cause 50% of cases, whereas deletions account for 5%. This gene functions in an autosomal dominant fashion. Most cases are sporadic and there is marked variability in expression. Mutations in *SMC1L1*, located at Xp11.22, are responsible for 5% of cases. This gene is inherited in an X-linked manner and accounts for many of the familial, as well as many of the milder, cases observed. One case with a mutation in *SMC3* at 10q25 has been published. Mutations in these genes are fully penetrant. Germline mosaicism is estimated to occur in 3.4% to 5.4% of families. It is expected that mutations in other cohesin-related genes will account for the not quite 50% of cases in which no mutation has yet been identified.

COMMENT

There is preliminary evidence that mutations in cohesin-related genes may impair cellular response to genotoxic treatments.

References

Brachmann W: Ein Fall von symmetrischer Monodaktylie durch ulnadefekt mit symmetrischer Flughautbildung in den Ellenbeugen, sowie anderen Abnormitaten (Zwerghaftigkeit, Halsrippen, Behaarung), *Jahrb Kinderheilk* 84:225–235, 1916.

de Lange C: Sur un type nouveau de dégénération (typus Amstelodamensis), *Arch Med Enfants* 36:713–719, 1933.

Ptacek LJ, et al: The Cornelia de Lange syndrome, *J Pediatr* 63:1000–1020, 1963.

Kline AD, et al: Cornelia de Lange syndrome: clinical review, diagnostic scoring system, and anticipatory guidance, *Am J Med Genet* 143A:1287–1296, 2007.

Krantz ID, et al: Cornelia de Lange syndrome is caused by mutations in NIPBL, the human homolog of the *Drosophila Nipped-B* gene, *Nat Genet* 36:631–635, 2004.

Musio A, et al: X-linked Cornelia de Lange syndrome owing to *SMC1L1* mutations, *Nat Genet* 38:528–530, 2006.

Pehlivan D, et al: NIPBL rearrangements in Cornelia de Lange syndrome: evidence for replicative mechanism and genotype-phenotype correlation, *Genet Med* 14:313–322, 2012.

Oliver C, et al: Cornelia de Lange syndrome: extending the physical and psychological phenotype, *Am J Med Genet* 152A:1127–1135, 2010.

Schrier SA, et al: Causes of death and autopsy findings in a large study cohort of individuals with Cornelia de Lange syndrome and review of the literature, *Am J Med Genet* 155A:3007–3024, 2011.

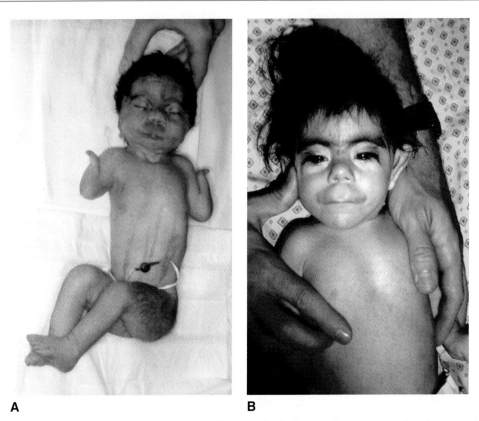

A   **B**

FIGURE 1.   De Lange syndrome. **A–D,** Four different affected individuals. Note the synophrys, thin downturned upper lip, long philtrum, hirsutism, small hands and feet, and severe limb defects.

Continued

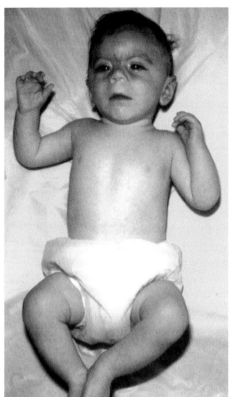

C

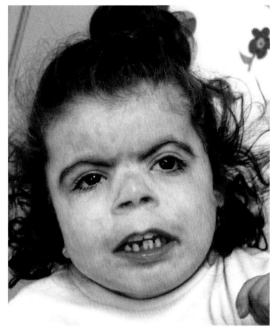

D

FIGURE 1, cont'd

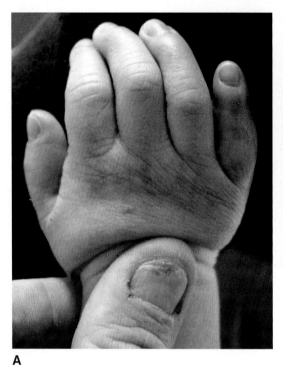

A

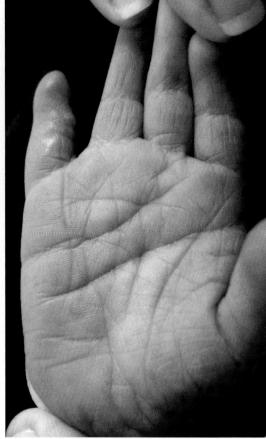

B

FIGURE 2.   **A** and **B,** Note the fifth finger clinodactyly and proximal implantation of the thumb.

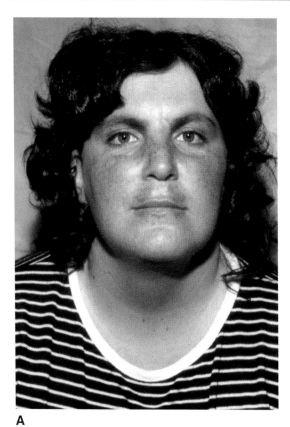

A

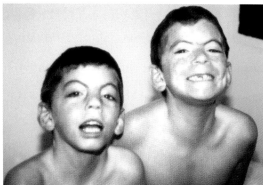

B

FIGURE 3.   **A** and **B,** Mildly affected mother and her severely affected sons.

RUBINSTEIN-TAYBI SYNDROME
Broad Thumbs and Toes, Slanted Palpebral Fissures, Hypoplastic Maxilla

Rubinstein and Taybi set forth this clinical entity in 1963. This disorder is rare, occurring with an estimated frequency of 1 in 100,000 to 1 in 125,000 newborns.

ABNORMALITIES

Growth. Postnatal onset of growth deficiency; in adults, average height of 153 cm in males and 147 cm in females; average weight of 48 kg in males and 55 kg in females. Retarded osseous maturation (74%).

Performance. IQ 30 to 79, with an average of 51; 52% have an IQ less than 50. Speech difficulties (90%), Seizures (23%; however, 57% have an abnormal EEG), Stiff, unsteady gait (85%), Hypotonia (67%), Hyperreflexia (40%).

Behavior. Social and friendly in childhood with short attention span, attention-deficit/hyperactivity disorder, motor stereotypies. In adults, anxiety, depression, mood instability, and aggressive behavior.

Craniofacial. Microcephaly (35%), large anterior fontanel (41%), delayed closure of fontanel (24%), frontal bossing (33%), frontal hair upsweep (20%), low anterior hairline (24%), low posterior hairline (42%), downslanting palpebral fissures (88%; however, only half of children younger than age 5 will manifest this), maxillary hypoplasia with narrow palate (100%), small mouth (56%), prominent or beaked nose with or without nasal septum extending below alae nasi and short columella (90%), deviated nasal septum (71%), micrognathia (49%), low-set and/or malformed ears (84%), heavy eyebrows (76%), highly arched eyebrows (73%), long eyelashes (87%), nasolacrimal duct stenosis (43%), ptosis (36%), epicanthal folds (55%), strabismus (69%), enophthalmos (22%)

Limbs. Broad thumbs with radial angulation (87%), broad great toes (100%), other fingers broad (87%), fifth finger clinodactyly (62%), persistent fetal fingertip pads (31%), deep plantar crease between first and second toes (33%), flat feet (72%)

Other skeletal. Scoliosis (42%), cervical hyperkyphosis (37%)

Imaging. Spina bifida occulta (47%), small flared iliac wings (26%)

Genitourinary. Cryptorchidism (78% of males), renal anomalies (52%)

Skin. Hirsutism (75%), capillary hemangioma (25%), keloid formation (22%)

Cardiac. Defects, most frequent of which are patent ductus arteriosus, ventricular septal defect, and atrial septal defect, occur in approximately one third of cases.

OCCASIONAL ABNORMALITIES
Cataract, glaucoma, ocular coloboma, nystagmus, myopia, Duane retraction syndrome, exophthalmia, talon cusps of teeth, enamel hypoplasia, posterior helical pits, cardiac conduction defects, camptodactyly, polydactyly, syndactyly, simian crease, distal axial triradius, duplicated halluces, patellar dislocation, dislocation of radial head, Perthes disease, bifid uterus, paratubal cystadenoma, pectus excavatum, sternal anomalies, angulated penis, hypospadias, shawl scrotum, Hirschsprung disease, eosinophilic esophagitis, café au lait spots, stereotypic movements, mirror movements, hypohidrosis, obstructive sleep apnea, absence of corpus callosum, large foramen magnum, parietal foramina, Chiari I malformation and syrinx, tethered cord, mediastinal vascular ring, premature thelarche, thyroid hypoplasia, cerebral artery dissection, tumors (neuroblastoma, medulloblastoma, oligodendroglioma, meningioma, pheochromocytoma, thyroid cancer, rhabdomyosarcoma, leiomyosarcoma, seminoma, odontoma, choristoma, pilomatrixomas).

NATURAL HISTORY
Infancy and childhood are complicated by respiratory infections, obstipation, and feeding difficulties. A poor polysaccharide antibody response has been demonstrated in a few patients. Aggressive assessment and treatment of gastroesophageal reflux is warranted. Constipation is very common. Global developmental delay is universal, with most patients testing in the severe to moderate range of intellectual disability. However, performance outside of this range has been reported. Recurrent ear infections with hearing loss and dental problems primarily associated with overcrowding of the teeth occur frequently. Hand and/or foot surgery frequently improves grasp, oppositional function, and comfort. Unusual reactions to anesthesia (respiratory distress and cardiac arrhythmias) have been reported, as well as tracheal collapse after muscle relaxants. Scoliosis may develop in childhood. Management of ingrown toenails and early treatment of paronychia are warranted. More than 90% of affected individuals survive into adulthood and most achieve some independence in self-care and communication. Obesity, eating issues, obstructive sleep apnea,

and keloids are common problems for adults. There is some suggestion that adults may have decreased abilities over time. Affected individuals have an increased risk for a variety of benign and malignant tumors although no screening protocol has been recommended.

ETIOLOGY

The majority of cases (>99%) are sporadic. Mutations in two homologous genes, *CBP* (CREB binding protein) and *EP300,* that encode histone acetyl transferases account for roughly 50% to 75% of cases. The preponderance of affected individuals with a known molecular abnormality have point mutations or small deletions or insertions in *CBP* at 16p13.3. Translocations, inversions, and large deletions involving contiguous genes at 16p13.3 have also been described, and there is some evidence that large deletions are associated with a more severe phenotype and increased mortality. Roughly 3% will have mutations in *EP300*. These cases may have a less severe limb phenotype. A risk for recurrence of 0.5% to 1% for parents of an affected child has been suggested based upon the finding of somatic mosaicism and variable expression in a few families.

COMMENT

Microduplication 16p13.3. Interstitial duplication of 16p13.3, including the gene *CBP,* has been reported in several patients, causing intellectual disability, a recognizable dysmorphic phenotype of midface hypoplasia, a prominent nose with bulbous tip, upslanting short palpebral fissures, thin upper lip, protruding ears, proximally placed short thumbs, camptodactyly of fingers and toes, and talipes equinovarus. Tetralogy of Fallot, atrial septal defect, vertebral fusions, and other anomalies have been noted. Normal growth is common.

References

Rubinstein JH, Taybi H: Broad thumbs and toes and facial abnormalities: a possible mental retardation syndrome, *Am J Dis Child* 105:588–609, 1963.

Rubinstein JH: The broad thumbs syndrome—progress report, 1968, *Birth Defects* 5:25–41, 1969.

Bartholdi D, et al: Genetic heterogeneity in Rubinstein-Taybi syndrome: delineation of the phenotype of the first patients carrying mutations in *EP300, J Med Genet* 44:327–333, 2007.

Breuning MJ, et al: Rubinstein-Taybi syndrome caused by submicroscopic deletions within 16p13.3, *Am J Med Genet* 52:249–254, 1993.

Hennekam RCM: Rubinstein-Taybi syndrome, *Europ J Hum Genet* 14:981–985, 2006.

Petrij F, et al: Rubinstein-Taybi syndrome caused by mutations in the transcriptional co-activator *CBP*, *Nature* 346:348–351, 1995.

Schorry EK, et al: Genotype-phenotype correlations in Rubinstein-Taybi syndrome, *Am J Med Genet A* 146A:2512–2519, 2008.

Stevens CA, Pouncey J, Knowles D: Adults with Rubinstein-Taybi syndrome, *Am J Med Genet Part A* 155:1680–1684, 2011.

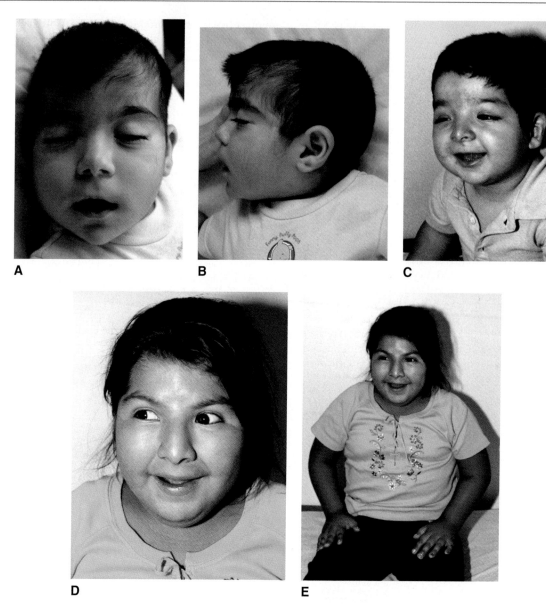

FIGURE 1.   Young infant (**A** and **B**); 21-month-old child (**C**); and 10-year-old child (**D** and **E**) with Rubinstein-Taybi syndrome. Note the hirsutism, downslanting palpebral fissures, maxillary hypoplasia, prominent nose with nasal septum extending below alae nasi, and low posteriorly rotated ears. (**A–E,** Courtesy Dr. Marilyn C. Jones, Children's Hospital, San Diego.)

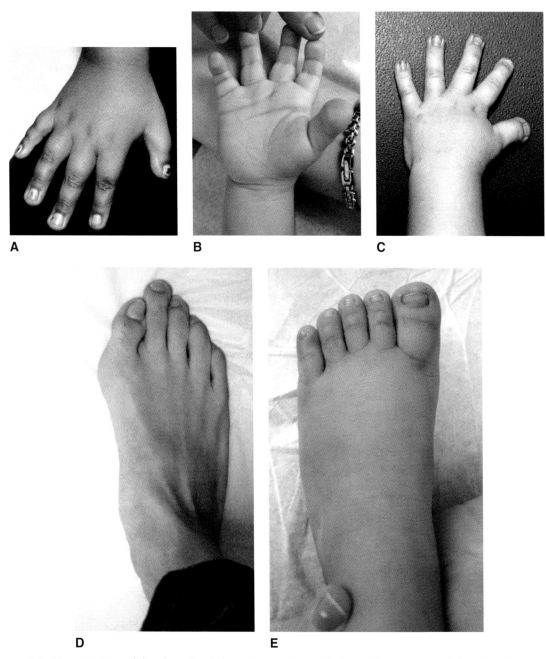

FIGURE 2. **A–C,** Broad thumbs with radial angulation and persistent fingertip pads. **D** and **E,** Broad great toes.

RUSSELL-SILVER SYNDROME
(SILVER SYNDROME, SILVER-RUSSELL SYNDROME)
Short Stature of Prenatal Onset, Skeletal Asymmetry, Small Incurved Fifth Finger

This pattern of malformation was described independently by Silver and colleagues and by Russell in 1953 and 1954. Silver emphasized the skeletal asymmetry as a feature of the disorder. This was a variable finding in the patients described by Russell. Diagnostic criteria for this disorder are inconsistent. Features are most apparent in infancy and early childhood. It is probable that this condition is both under- and overdiagnosed.

ABNORMALITIES

Growth. Small stature, of prenatal onset with length and weight usually equal to –2 SD, minimal postnatal catch-up growth; immature osseous development in infancy and early childhood preservation of head circumference (relative macrocephaly); asymmetry.

Performance. Mild global delay, speech delay.

Craniofacial. Small, triangular facies with frontal prominence, late closure of the anterior fontanel, downturned corners of mouth; facial asymmetry, possible bluish sclerae in early infancy, low-set posteriorly rotated ears, and micrognathia; eye findings include visual refractive errors, strabismus, and tortuous retinal vessels.

Skin. Café au lait spots.

Limbs. Asymmetry, short incurved fifth finger.

Other. Tendency toward excess sweating, especially on the head and upper trunk, during infancy; liability to fasting hypoglycemia from about age 10 months to age 2 to 3 years.

OCCASIONAL ABNORMALITIES

Metopic craniosynostosis, iris coloboma, cleft palate, bifid uvula, velopharyngeal insufficiency, syndactyly of second to third toes, camptodactyly radial hypoplasia, limited elbow supination, absent thumb, scoliosis, Sprengel deformity, hip dysplasia, talipes equinovarus, renal anomaly, posterior urethral valves, hypospadias, cryptorchidism, clitoromegaly, and inguinal hernia; cardiac defects; malignancy, including craniopharyngioma, testicular seminoma, hepatocellular carcinoma, and Wilms tumor; gastrointestinal abnormalities, including gastroesophageal reflux, esophagitis, and food aversion; growth hormone deficiency.

NATURAL HISTORY

Affected children have prenatal onset growth deficiency and typically do not catch up postnatally. Feeding difficulties are seen in 86% and include weak suck, absence of hunger, gastroesophageal reflux, and food aversion. There tends to be a gradual improvement in growth in weight and appearance during childhood and especially during adolescence. Most school-age children eat normally.

As a result, the adult usually appears more normal than the infant with this disorder. Final height attainment can be up to 5 feet. Slow motor development is common. Approximately one third have learning disabilities. Because of the small facies, the upper head may appear large, although head circumference is well within the normal range. This appearance, plus the relatively large fontanels in early infancy, may give rise to a false impression of hydrocephalus, which they do not have. Somewhat frequent feedings and adequate glucose intake during illness should be ensured from age 6 months until age 3 years, the period of enhanced liability to fasting hypoglycemia. Growth hormone (GH) deficiency should be considered if the linear growth rate reaches a plateau. GH treatment has been shown to be of benefit in these patients, even in the absence of GH deficiency.

ETIOLOGY

The majority of cases are sporadic. The condition is genetically heterogeneous. A molecular etiology is identified in up to 60% of patients. Roughly 50% will manifest hypomethylation of the paternal allele of the *H19* gene on chromosome 11p15 associated with imprinting control region 1 (ICR1), which includes *H19* and *IGF2*. Maternal uniparental disomy for chromosome 7 (mat UPD7) accounts for 5% to 10% of cases. UPD7 may be complete or segmental (7p11.2-p13 and 7q31-qter appear to be the critical regions). Other molecular mechanisms include translocations, maternal UPD11, paternal deletions at 7q32, maternal inheritance of duplication within ICR1 and/or ICR2 on 11p15, and multilocus hypomethylation. A small number of patients with submicroscopic deletions or duplications in these imprinted regions have also been described. The remainder are of unknown etiology. Several cases with maternally inherited microduplications or translocations have been familial.

COMMENT

Asymmetry, fifth finger clinodactyly, and congenital anomalies are more obvious in children with ICR1 hypomethylation, who have a more typical presentation. Children with mat UPD7 have less asymmetry, manifest more motor and speech delays, and are at risk for developing myoclonus-dystonia (cervical dystonia, writer's cramp and myoclonic jerks) in later childhood. Myoclonus-dystonia is more commonly due to paternally derived mutations in the imprinted gene e-sarcoglycan (*SGCE*) at 7q21. Russell-Silver syndrome is one of the imprinting disorders that has been associated with the use of assisted reproductive technologies, although the reason for this apparent relationship remains obscure.

References

Silver HK, et al: Syndrome of congenital hemihypertrophy, shortness of stature and elevated urinary gonadotrophins, *Pediatrics* 12:368–376, 1953.

Russell A: A syndrome of "intra-uterine" dwarfism recognizable at birth with craniofacial dysostosis, disproportionately short arms and other anomalies, *Proc R Soc Med* 47:1040–1044, 1954.

Silver HK: Asymmetry, short stature, and variations in sexual development: a syndrome of congenital malformations, *Am J Dis Child* 107:495–515, 1964.

Demars J, et al: New insights into the pathogenesis of Beckwith-Wiedemann and Silver-Russell syndromes: contribution of small copy number variations to 11p15 imprinting defects, *Hum Mut* 32:1171–1182, 2011.

Wakeling EL: Silver-Russell syndrome, *Arch Dis Child* 96:1156–1161, 2011.

Wakeling EL, et al: Epigenotype-phenotype correlations in Silver-Russell syndrome, *J Med Genet* 47:760–768, 2010.

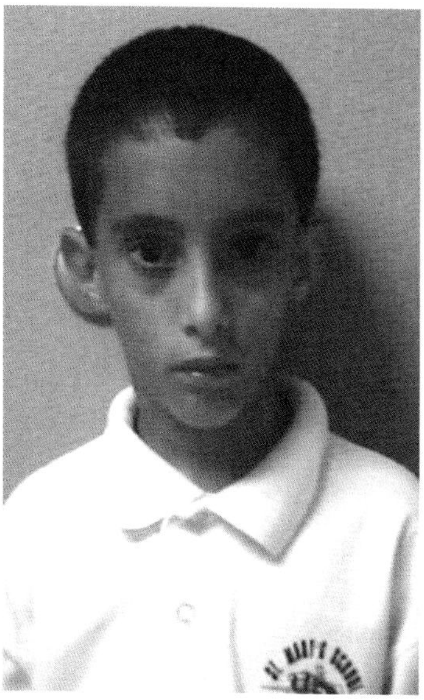

FIGURE 1. Russell-Silver syndrome. **A** and **B,** Note the small triangular face with frontal prominence. **C,** A 3½-year-old boy with his 2-year-old unaffected sister. (**C,** Courtesy Dr. Lynne M. Bird, Children's Hospital, San Diego.) **D** and **E,** A 2-year-old boy. Note the small facies, slimness, and "loose" posture.

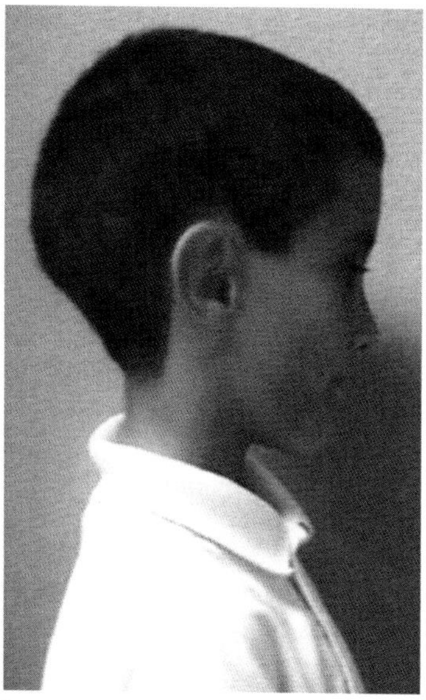

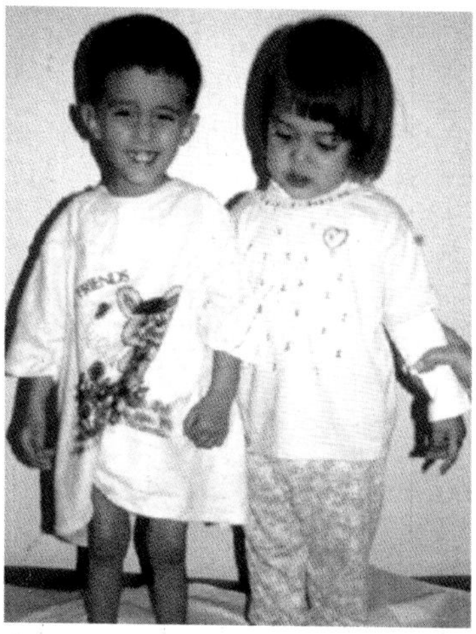

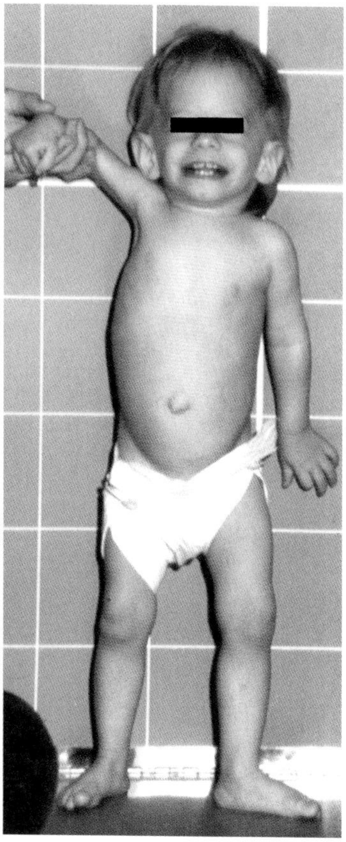

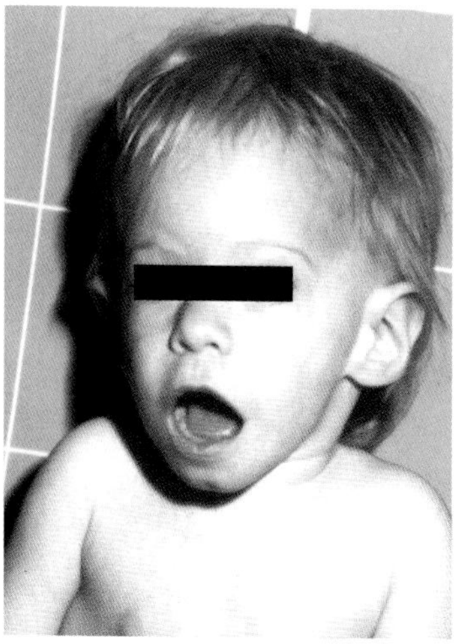

SHORT SYNDROME

First reported in 1975 by Gorlin and colleagues and by Sensenbrenner and colleagues, the acronym SHORT refers to the principal features, which include *s*hort stature, *h*yperextensibility of joints or *h*ernia (inguinal) or both, *o*cular depression, *R*ieger anomaly, and *t*eething delay. Approximately 20 cases have been reported.

ABNORMALITIES

Growth. Mild intrauterine growth restriction (IUGR), postnatal growth deficiency, delayed bone age.

Performance. Delay in speech development with normal mental and motor development.

Craniofacial. "Triangular-shaped" face, prominent ears, broad nasal bridge, telecanthus (lateral displacement of medial canthi), deeply set eyes, Rieger anomaly, hypoplastic ala nasi, micrognathia, delayed dental eruption, prematurely aged appearance.

Limbs. Hyperextensible joints, fifth finger clinodactyly.

Imaging. Large epiphyses, gracile diaphyses, and cone-shaped epiphyses, short metacarpals, Wormian bones.

Other. Inguinal hernia, wrinkled skin.

OCCASIONAL ABNORMALITIES

Sensorineural hearing loss, congenital glaucoma, megalocornea, nystagmus, chin dimple, microcephaly, cardiac defect, lipodystrophy, hip dislocation, anal atresia, late menarche, polycystic ovaries, hypercalcemia, nephrocalcinosis.

NATURAL HISTORY

Although IUGR occurs in the majority of affected children, the growth restriction, involving both height and weight, is most severe postnatally. Illnesses, including chronic vomiting, diarrhea, and feeding problems, are frequent throughout the first 2 years of life, and hospitalization for failure to thrive is common in infancy. Decreased subcutaneous fat in the face has been noted as early as 3 months. Onset of speech has been delayed to 36 months. Diabetes mellitus secondary to insulin resistance has occurred in two patients, at 16 and 13 years of age, respectively, the latter while receiving growth hormone therapy. Nephrocalcinosis (with hypercalcemia, hypercalciuria, and normal levels of vitamin D and parathyroid hormone) has been seen as early as 2 months.

ETIOLOGY

Although autosomal dominant inheritance is most likely, affected siblings born to normal parents have been described. One family, mother and son, has been described with a balanced 1:4 translocation, tt(1;4)(q31.2;q25), which presumably disrupted *PITX2*, the gene responsible for Rieger syndrome. The mother had a Rieger syndrome phenotype with polycystic ovaries, whereas the son had features suggestive of SHORT syndrome. One patient has been documented with a 2.263 Mb deletion on chromosome 14 that includes *BMP4* and 13 other genes. This patient showed normal sequencing and copy number of *PITX2*. Two other patients with SHORT syndrome mentioned in that publication did not have deletions at the chromosome 14 locus. Other patients with larger deletions in the same region have a different phenotype.

References

Gorlin RJ, et al: Rieger anomaly and growth retardation (The SHORT syndrome), *Birth Defects Orig Artic Ser* 11(2):46–48, 1975.

Sensenbrenner JA, Hussels IE, Levin LS: A low birthweight syndrome, Rieger syndrome, *Birth Defects Orig Artic Ser* 11(2):423–426, 1975.

Bankier A, Keith CG, Temple IK: Absent iris stroma, narrow body build and small facial bones: a new association or variant of SHORT syndrome? *Clin Dysmorph* 4:302–304, 1995.

Karadeniz NN, et al: Is SHORT syndrome another phenotypic variation of *PITX2*? *Am J Med Genet A* 130A:406–409, 2004.

Reardon W, Temple IK: Nephrocalcinosis and disordered calcium metabolism in two children with SHORT syndrome, *Am J Med Genet A* 146A:1296–1298, 2008.

Reis LM, et al: *BMP4* loss-of-function mutations in developmental eye disorders including SHORT syndrome, *Hum Genet* 130:495–504, 2011.

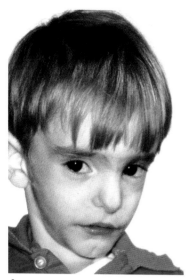

A

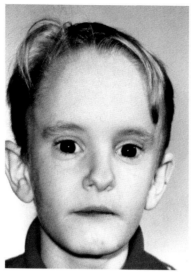

B

FIGURE 1.   SHORT syndrome. **A** and **B,** Brothers with "triangular-shaped" face, deeply set eyes, hypoplastic ala nasi, and micrognathia. (From Gorlin RJ, et al: *Birth Defects* 11:46, 1975.)

3-M SYNDROME
Prenatal and Postnatal Growth Deficiency, Short Neck, Slender Long Bones

Initially described by Fuhrmann and colleagues in 1972, this disorder was designated the 3-M syndrome after the initials of the first three authors of the 1975 paper that delineated the condition (Miller, McKusick, and Malvaux). More than 200 cases have been reported.

ABNORMALITIES

Growth. Prenatal growth deficiency with mean birth length of 40.5 cm and mean birth weight of 2120 g at full term in the absence of maternal or placental pathology, severe postnatal linear growth deficiency with weight below the third percentile for chronological age but increased for height, slightly increased upper/lower segment ratio, delayed bone age, relative macrocephaly.

Craniofacial. Dolichocephaly, frontal bossing, triangular-shaped face, malar hypoplasia, full and pointed chin, fleshy nasal tip, short nose with anteverted nares, long philtrum, full lips, delayed eruption of teeth.

Skeletal. Short neck with prominent trapezius muscles and horizontal clavicles giving appearance of square shoulders, short thorax with pectus (carinatum or excavatum), hyperextensible joints, lumbar hyperlordosis, short fifth fingers, hip dysplasias, prominent heels with fleshy protrusion at the back of the heel.

Imaging. Slender shafts of long bones and ribs, tall vertebral bodies with reduced anterior-posterior diameter particularly in lumbar region, small pelvis, small iliac wings, short femoral necks.

OCCASIONAL ABNORMALITIES

Mild intellectual disability, full eyebrows, prominent dysplastic ears, V-shaped dental arch with anterior crowding and malocclusion, thick patulous lips, dental caries, prominent scapulae, diastasis recti, joint dislocation, decreased elbow extension, congenital hip dislocation, frequent fractures, fifth finger clinodactyly, transverse grooves of anterior chest, pes planus, supernumerary nipple, hypospadias, intracerebral aneurysm, oligohydramnios during pregnancy.

NATURAL HISTORY

Feeding problems are common during the first year. General health is typically good. Although female gonadal function is usually normal with menarche occurring at the usual time, males may have gonadal dysfunction and subfertility or infertility. Final adult height is in the range of 115 to 150 cm (–8 to –4 SD). Developmental milestones and intelligence are normal. Serum growth hormone (GH) levels and insulin-like growth factor 1 (IGF1) levels are typically normal. Growth response to recombinant human GH therapy is variable but typically poor. Evidence suggests resistance in the GH-IGF axis.

ETIOLOGY

This disorder has an autosomal recessive inheritance pattern. Null mutations in several genes that function in the ubiquitin-proteasome pathway targeting proteins for degradation have been identified, including *CUL7* (65%), *OBSL1* (30%), and *CCDC8* (5%).

COMMENT

Several families with clinically diagnosed autosomal recessive Russell-Silver syndrome have been documented to have mutations in one of the genes responsible for 3-M syndrome. The heel abnormalities are most helpful in distinguishing patients with 3-M syndrome from those with Russell-Silver syndrome.

References

Fuhrmann W, et al: Familiärer Minderwuchs mit unproportioniert hohen Wirbeln, *Humangenetik* 16:271–282, 1972.

Miller JD, et al: The 3-M syndrome: a heritable low birth weight dwarfism, *Birth Defects Orig Artic Ser* 11(5):39–47, 1975.

Clayton PE, et al: Exploring the spectrum of 3-M syndrome, a primordial short stature disorder of disrupted ubiquitination, *Clin Endocrinol (Oxf)* 77(3):335–342, 2012. E-pub ahead of print doi:10.1111/j.1365-2265.2012.04428.x.

Huber C, et al: Identification of mutations in *CUL7* in 3-M syndrome, *Nat Genet* 37:1119–1124, 2005.

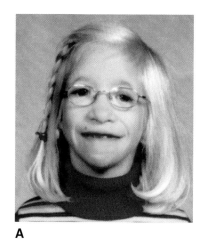

A

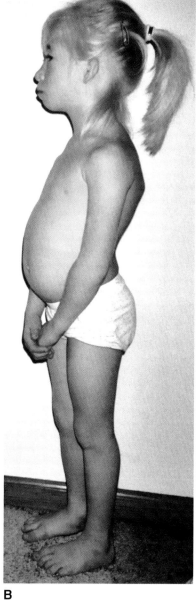

B

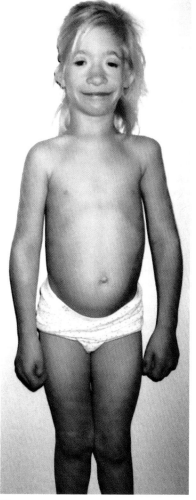

C

FIGURE 1. Dubowitz syndrome.
A–C, Note the short palpebral fissures, asymmetric ptosis, shallow supraorbital ridges, and mild micrognathia. (Courtesy Dr. John M. Opitz, University of Utah, Salt Lake City.)

BLOOM SYNDROME
Short Stature, Malar Hypoplasia, Telangiectatic Erythema of the Face

Since Bloom's original description in 1954, more than 130 patients with this disorder have been reported. The Bloom's Syndrome Registry (*http://weill.cornell.edu/bsr*) contains detailed clinical and natural history information on the most known cases of this disorder.

ABNORMALITIES

Growth. Prenatal onset of growth deficiency mean birth weight of males and females are 1760 and 1754 gm respectively; average adult male height, 149 cm, and adult female height, 138 cm; decreased adipose tissue leads to wasted appearance.

Craniofacial. Mild microcephaly with dolichocephaly; malar hypoplasia, with or without small nose; loss of lower lashes; fissure of lower lip.

Skin. Facial telangiectatic erythema involves the butterfly midface region, is exacerbated by sunlight, and usually develops during the first year. Small and large areas of hyperpigmentation and hypopigmentation.

OCCASIONAL ABNORMALITIES

Mild intellectual disability; short attention span during childhood and learning difficulties, including reading disabilities; telangiectatic erythema of the dorsa of the hands and forearms; high-pitched voice; colloid-body-like spots in Bruch membrane of the eye; lens opacities; optic nerve hypoplasia; absence of upper lateral incisors; prominent ears; ichthyotic skin, hypertrichosis, pilonidal cyst, sacral dimple; syndactyly, polydactyly, clinodactyly of fifth finger, short lower extremity, talipes; café au lait spots; immunoglobulin deficiency, with decreased serum levels of immunoglobulins and an impaired lymphocyte proliferation response to mitogens; compensated hypothyroidism; abnormal lipid profile.

NATURAL HISTORY

These patients show a consistently slow pace of growth not related to growth hormone deficiency or malabsorption. Feeding problems are frequent during infancy, likely secondary to severe gastroesophageal reflux. Susceptibility to infection decreases with age. The facial erythema is very seldom present at birth, usually appearing during infancy following exposure to sunlight; it may excoriate, but improves after childhood. Altered carbohydrate metabolism is present in childhood, with 17.7% developing overt diabetes by adulthood. Some patients have severe chronic lung disease, including bronchiectasis. Although learning disabilities occur, the majority of patients are within the normal range for intelligence. Men are infertile, and women experience early menopause.

Malignancy has been the major known cause of death and develops in 50% of patients. The cancers that develop in Bloom syndrome are similar in type and distribution to those seen in the general population; however, malignancy develops at a much younger age. Multiple cancers may occur in the same individual.

An increased rate of chromosomal breakage and sister chromatid exchange is found in cultured leukocytes and fibroblasts from all patients studied, but not reliably so in the heterozygotes.

ETIOLOGY

The inheritance of this disorder is autosomal recessive. Although reported in all ethnic groups, it is more common in Ashkenazi Jews. The gene, *BLM*, maps to chromosome 15q26.1. The gene product is a member of the highly conserved RecQ family of DNA and RNA helicases, which are responsible for genomic stability. The frequency of the gene carrier in the Ashkenazi Jewish population is estimated at 1:100.

COMMENT

The relation of the in vitro chromosomal breakage and the development of malignancies is not well understood at present. Because of the hypersensitivity of cells in affected individuals to radiation and DNA damaging chemicals, cancer treatment protocols may need modification. Several individuals have developed myelodysplastic disorders following treatment for cancer.

References

Bloom D: Congenital telangiectatic erythema resembling lupus erythematosus in dwarfs, *Am J Dis Child* 88:754–758, 1954.

Bloom D: The syndrome of congenital telangiectatic erythema and stunted growth, *J Pediatr* 68:103–113, 1966.

Diaz A, et al: Evaluation of short stature, carbohydrate metabolism and other endocrinopathies in Bloom's syndrome, *Horm Res* 66:111–117, 2006.

Sawitsky A, Bloom D, German J: Chromosomal breakage and acute leukemia in congenital telangiectatic erythema and stunted growth, *Ann Intern Med* 65:487–495, 1966.

Ellis NA: The Bloom's syndrome gene product is homologous to RecQ helicases, *Cell* 83:655–666, 1995.

C

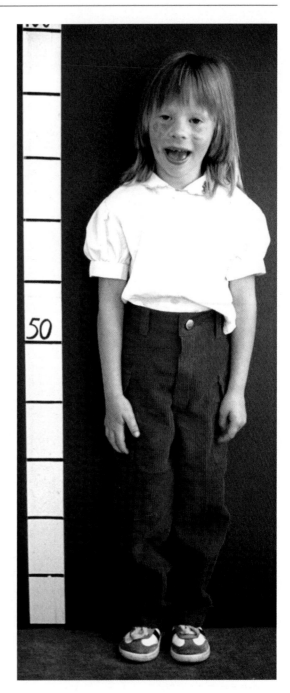

FIGURE 1.   Bloom syndrome. Note the facial telangiectatic erythema involving the butterfly midface region. (From Passarge E: *Color Atlas of Genetics*. New York, 1995, George Thieme Medical Publishers, p 338. Reprinted by permission.)

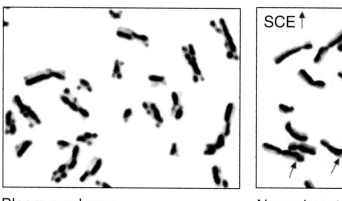
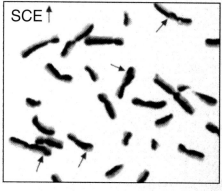

Bloom syndrome   Normal control

FIGURE 2.   Photograph of increased sister chromatin exchange in a child with Bloom syndrome on the left compared to the control on the right. (From Passarge E: *Color Atlas of Genetics.* New York, 1995, George Thieme Medical Publishers, p 338. Reprinted by permission.)

JOHANSON-BLIZZARD SYNDROME
Hypoplastic Alae Nasi, Hypothyroidism, Deafness

In 1971, Johanson and Blizzard reported three cases of this disorder and found one from the previous literature. Fewer than 100 patients have been reported. This syndrome incorporates elements of ectodermal dysplasia with endocrine and exocrine insufficiency plus growth and intellectual disability.

ABNORMALITIES

Growth. Prenatal onset of growth deficiency (60%)

Performance. Intellectual disability, sometimes severe (67%), sensorineural deafness (75%), hypotonia (80%)

Craniofacial. Mild to moderate microcephaly (50%), prominent forehead; frontal upsweep of hair pattern; midline scalp defect most typically posterior but can be anterior or over vertex (87%), variable sparse hair with frontal upsweep (96%), upslanting palpebral fissures; hypoplastic to aplastic alae nasi (100%), nasolacrimal duct cutaneous fistulae (66%), absence of superior or inferior puncta, hypoplastic deciduous teeth, absent permanent teeth (90%).

Anorectal. Imperforate or anteriorly placed anus (40%), rectoureteral or rectovaginal fistula (18%)

Genitourinary. Caliectasis to hydronephrosis; vesicoureteral reflux; defects occurring in 25% include vagina septate or double, cryptorchidism, micropenis, hypospadias, or single urogenital orifice

Endocrine. Hypothyroidism of unknown etiology (30%)

Exocrine. Pancreatic insufficiency with malabsorption (100%)

OCCASIONAL ABNORMALITIES

Severe facial clefting; arrhinencephaly; eyelid colobomas, strabismus, and cataracts; small nipples and absent areolae; radiolucent skull defects; abnormal electroencephalogram; cardiac defects, including septal defects, myxomatous mitral valve, and dilated cardiomyopathy; abdominal and thoracic situs inversus; urethral obstruction sequence; fifth finger clinodactyly; transverse palmar crease; café au lait spots; neonatal cholestasis; Diamond-Blackfan anemia; growth hormone deficiency.

NATURAL HISTORY

Although intellectual disability is frequent, normal intelligence has clearly been documented. Hypothyroidism, only rarely noted in the neonatal period, occurs in approximately one third of cases; it may progress in degree and is unusual in that the cholesterol level is not elevated. This unusual characteristic is possibly related to the concomitant malabsorption. Improvement in growth rate may occur when the patient is treated with thyroid replacement, pancreatic enzymes, and fat-soluble vitamins. Diabetes and loss of glucagon response to hypoglycemia develop in adolescence and adults as a result of ongoing destruction of the pancreas.

ETIOLOGY

The inheritance is autosomal recessive. Homozygous or compound heterozygous mutations in *UBR1* cause this disorder. The protein product is an E3 ubiquitin ligase of the N-end rule pathway, which targets proteins to proteasomal degradation based on the identity of their N-terminal residue. Missense mutations in the gene cause a milder phenotype than those that abolish gene function.

References

Grand RJ, et al: Unusual case of XXY Klinefelter's syndrome with pancreatic insufficiency, hypothyroidism, deafness, chronic lung disease, dwarfism and microcephaly, *Am J Med* 41:478–485, 1966.

Johanson A, Blizzard R: A syndrome of congenital aplasia of the alae nasi, deafness, hypothyroidism, dwarfism, absent permanent teeth, and malabsorption, *J Pediatr* 79:982–987, 1971.

Cheung JC, et al: Ocular manifestations of the Johanson-Blizzard syndrome, *J AAPOS* 13:512–514, 2009.

Rezaei N, et al: Eponym: Johanson-Blizzard syndrome, *Eur J Pediatr* 170:179–183, 2011.

Zenker M, et al: Deficiency of *UBR1*, a ubiquitin ligase of the N-end rule pathway, causes pancreatic dysfunction, malformations and mental retardation (Johanson-Blizzard syndrome), *Nat Genet* 37:1345–1350, 2005.

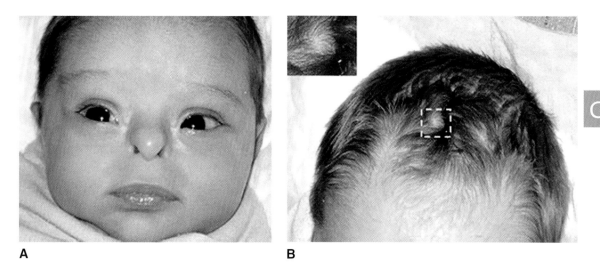

A   **B**

FIGURE 1.   Johanson-Blizzard syndrome. **A,** 2-month-old affected infant with hypoplastic ala nasi and in **B** marked frontal hair upsweep and a mild degree of aplasia cutis noted in insert. (From Al-Dosari MS, et al: *Amer J Med Genet* 146: 1875, 2008. With permission)

MICROCEPHALIC PRIMORDIAL DWARFING SYNDROMES
(MAJEWSKI OSTEODYSPLASTIC PRIMORDIAL DWARFISM [MOPD II], SECKEL SYNDROME, MOPD I)
Severe Short Stature, Microcephaly, Prominent Nose

Since 1960 when Seckel published his monograph reviewing 15 individuals with primordial short stature and microcephaly, the term "Seckel syndrome" has been used broadly to describe what is clearly a heterogeneous group of conditions, each with its own etiology and natural history. The 1982 publications of Majewski did much to delineate specific syndromes among individuals with severe prenatal growth deficiency and microcephaly, the most common of which is not Seckel syndrome but Majewski osteodysplastic primordial dwarfism.

MAJEWSKI OSTEODYSPLASTIC PRIMORDIAL DWARFISM (MOPD II)

Abnormalities

Growth. Severe prenatal growth deficiency with proportionate microcephaly, birth weight ≤ 1500 g, birth length ≤ 40 cm; progressive postnatal microcephaly; progressive disproportion with shortening of middle and distal limbs; final adult height < 100 cm.

Performance. Normal intelligence to mild-moderate intellectual disability; short attention span; hyperactivity; sociable outgoing personality; high, squeaky, nasal voice; sleep disturbance.

Craniofacial. Microcephaly with secondary craniosynostosis; relatively normal forehead; prominent nose; elevated broad nasal root and bridge; hypoplastic ala nasi; micrognathia; prominent cheeks; low-set, simple ears with lack of lobule; relatively large eyes with downslanting palpebral fissures; shallow orbits; strabismus; small teeth; enamel hypoplasia; oligodontia.

Limbs. Short hands in infancy with progressive ligamentous laxity and subluxation, radial and patellar dislocation over time; short broad feet.

Skeletal. Scoliosis.

Genitourinary. Inguinal hernia, renal anomaly. Male: cryptorchidism, hypospadias, small testes. Female: labial hypoplasia.

Skin. Large areola, multiple café au lait spots, freckling, patches of hyper- and hypopigmentation.

Imaging. Gracile long bones, dysharmonic bone maturation with delayed epiphyseal ossification, severe coxa vara, metaphyseal flaring, high narrow ilia, flat acetabular angles, mild platyspondyly, 11 ribs, pseudoepiphyses of metacarpals, small facial bones, large sella, abnormal brain myelination, ventriculomegaly, hypoplasia/cyst of corpus callosum.

OCCASIONAL ABNORMALITIES

Joint dislocation (knee, elbow, hip), glaucoma, mirror movements, subglottic stenosis, vocal cord web, laryngomalacia, anemia.

NATURAL HISTORY

Extremely tiny but proportionate at birth, with disproportion developing over time. The slender body habitus of infancy is replaced by truncal obesity in childhood. Feeding issues are universal in infancy, as are frequent respiratory infections. Farsightedness and sensorineural hearing loss develop over time. Dyslipidemia, cardiomyopathy, and diabetes mellitus type 2 develop at young ages. Vascular tortuosities and aneurysm resembling Moya-moya disease predispose to vascular accidents, stroke, and cognitive decline. Precocious puberty and premature ovarian failure occur in females. Growth hormone treatment has been ineffective.

ETIOLOGY

This disorder has an autosomal recessive inheritance pattern. Loss of function mutations in pericentrin, *PCNT*, are causative.

SECKEL SYNDROME

Abnormalities

Growth. Moderate prenatal onset growth deficiency with severe microcephaly; postnatal growth deficiency with progressive disproportionate microcephaly without skeletal dysplasia or body disproportion.

Performance. Moderate to severe intellectual disability; hyperactive, aggressive behavior; seizures.

Craniofacial. Sloping forehead, upslanting or downslanting palpebral fissures, prominent nose, high nasal bridge, relatively large ears, micrognathia, abnormal teeth.

Imaging. Cerebral atrophy, gyral simplification, subarachnoid dilatation.

OCCASIONAL ABNORMALITIES

Craniosynostosis; iris coloboma; ptosis; pectus carinatum; camptodactyly, syndactyly, polydactyly, and/or clinodactyly; hallux valgus; café au lait macules; white spots; cardiac defect; epiglottic defects; anemia.

NATURAL HISTORY

Growth is less severely affected than in MOPD II, but microcephaly and intellectual disability are more pronounced. Hematologic disorders may develop, and there is some evidence that affected individuals may have increased sensitivity to chemotherapy.

ETIOLOGY

Five distinct genetic loci have been identified for Seckel syndrome (SCKL). Mutations in *ATR* account for SCKL1, *RBBP8* for SCKL2, *CENPJ* for SCKL4, and *SEP152* for SCL5. SCKL3 maps to 14q23q24. All are inherited as autosomal recessive disorders.

All result in impaired signaling of the DNA-damage response protein ATR.

COMMENT

Much of what is written about natural history of "Seckel syndrome" does not account for more recent understanding of genetic heterogeneity.

MOPD I (INCLUDES MOPD III AND PRIMORDIAL DWARFISM, TAYBI-LINDER TYPE)

Abnormalities

Growth. Severe pre- and postnatal growth deficiency with brachymelic body proportions; microcephaly.

Performance. Severe to profound intellectual disability.

Craniofacial. Sloping forehead, prominent nose, micrognathia, sparse eyebrows, alopecia.

Limbs. Preaxial polydactyly, hypoplastic thumbs, dislocated hips and elbows.

Imaging. Platyspondyly; cleft vertebral arches; delayed epiphyseal ossification; low, broad, dysplastic pelvis; poor acetabular formation; short, broad, bowed humeri and femora; unremarkable metaphyses; agenesis of corpus callosum; colpocephaly; marked lissencephaly; heterotopias and other neuromigrational defects; vermis agenesis; arachnoid cyst.

OCCASIONAL ABNORMALITIES

Corneal clouding, cryptorchidism, dysplastic kidney, cardiac defect.

NATURAL HISTORY

Failure to thrive, frequent infections, and very early mortality.

ETIOLOGY

Autosomal recessive. Mutations in *RNU4ATAC*, which encodes a small nuclear RNA component of the U12 spliceosome, cause this condition.

References

Seckel HPG: *Bird-Headed Dwarfs*, Springfield, Ill, 1960, Charles C Thomas.

Majewski F, Goecke T: Studies of microcephalic primordial dwarfism I: approach to a delineation of the Seckel syndrome, *Am J Med Genet* 12:7–21, 1982.

Majewski F, Ranke M, Schinzel A: Studies of microcephalic primordial dwarfism II: the osteodysplastic type II of primordial dwarfism, *Am J Med Genet* 12:23–35, 1982.

Faivre L, et al: Clinical and genetic heterogeneity of Seckel syndrome, *Am J Med Genet* 112:379–383, 2002.

Hall JG, et al: Majewski osteodysplastic primordial dwarfism type II (MOPD II): natural history and clinical findings, *Am J Med Genet A* 130A:55–72, 2004.

Rauch A, et al: Mutations in the pericentrin (*PCTN*) gene cause primordial dwarfism, *Science* 319:816–819, 2008.

Kalay E, et al: CEP152 is a genome maintenance protein disrupted in Seckel syndrome, *Nat Genet* 43:23–26, 2011.

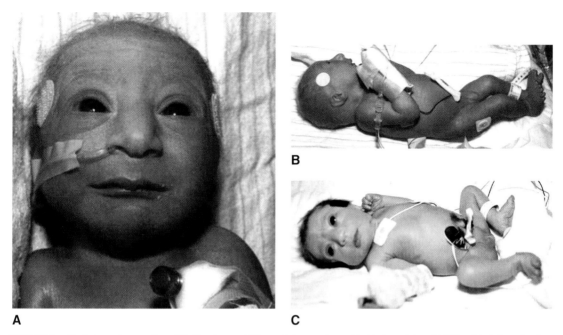

FIGURE 1. Seckel syndrome. **A** and **B,** Newborn at 38 weeks' gestation with birth weight of 1651 g, birth length of 41 cm, and occipitofrontal circumference of 28 cm. **C,** Her sibling. Note the disproportion of nose size to the size of the face and mandible, whereas general body proportions and adiposity are near normal for age. (**A–C,** Courtesy Dr. Marilyn C. Jones, Children's Hospital, San Diego.)

HALLERMANN-STREIFF SYNDROME
(OCULOMANDIBULODYSCEPHALY WITH HYPOTRICHOSIS SYNDROME)
Microphthalmia, Small Pinched Nose, Hypotrichosis

The first report of this disorder was by Audry, who described an incomplete case in 1893. Hallermann, in 1948, and Streiff, in 1950, independently described three cases, recognizing this syndrome as a separate entity. Approximately 150 cases have been reported in the literature.

ABNORMALITIES

Growth. Prematurity, low birth weight, or both in one third of patients; proportionate small stature; postnatal growth deficiency in two thirds of cases, with mean final height of 152 cm in females and 155 to 157 cm in males.

Craniofacial. Brachycephaly with frontal and parietal bossing, thin calvarium, and delayed ossification of the sutures; malar hypoplasia; micrognathia, with hypoplasia of the rami and anterior displacement of the temporomandibular joint; thin, small, pointed nose, with hypoplasia of the cartilage, becoming parrot-like with age; narrow and high-arched palate; hypoplasia or malimplantation of the teeth, neonatal teeth, and partial anodontia; atrophy of the skin, most prominent over the nose and sutural areas of the scalp; thin and light hair with hypotrichosis, especially of the scalp, eyebrows, and eyelashes.

Ocular. Bilateral microphthalmia (80%); cataracts (94%), total or incomplete, which may resorb spontaneously; corneal stromal opacities; nystagmus; strabismus.

Imaging. Large, poorly ossified skull with decreased ossification in sutural areas; Wormian bones; obtuse or straight gonial angle; thin, gracile long bones with widening at the metaphyseal ends; thin ribs; small vertebral bodies; decreased number of sternal ossification centers; thin, gracile metacarpals; delayed bone age.

OCCASIONAL ABNORMALITIES

Scaphocephaly, microcephaly, platybasia, shallow sella turcica, absence of the mandibular condyles, tracheomalacia, double cutaneous chin, microstomia, blue sclerae, downward slant to palpebral fissures, optic disk colobomata, glaucoma, persistence of pupillary membrane, various chorioretinal pigment alterations, retinal detachment, entropion, blepharoptosis, ear anomalies, syndactyly, winging of the scapulae, lordosis, scoliosis, spina bifida, funnel chest, cardiac defects, intellectual disability (15%), hyperactivity, choreoathetosis, generalized tonic-clonic seizures, hypogenitalism and cryptorchidism in the male, renal anomalies, hepatic defects, immunodeficiency, hematopoietic abnormalities, growth hormone deficiency.

NATURAL HISTORY

The patients' narrow upper airway associated with the craniofacial configuration can lead to serious complications, including severe early pulmonary infection, respiratory embarrassment, obstructive sleep apnea, and anesthetic complications. During early infancy, patients with this disorder may have feeding and respiratory problems, sometimes necessitating tracheostomy. Respiratory infections may contribute to the cause of death. Laryngoscopy and endotracheal intubation at the time of anesthesia may be difficult because of the upper airway obstruction. The major handicap is the ocular defect, which usually culminates in blindness despite surgery. Although the majority of the reported patients have been of normal intelligence, motor deficits and intellectual disabilities, even to a severe degree, have been reported. Spontaneous pregnancy has been reported.

ETIOLOGY

All cases have been sporadic occurrences.

References

Audry C: Variété d'alopécia congénitale; alopécie suturale, *Ann Dermatol Syph (Ser. 3)* 4:899, 1893.

Hallermann W: Vogelgesicht und cataracta congenita, *Klin Monatsbl Augenheilkd* 113:315–318, 1948.

Streiff EB: Dysmorphie mandibulo-faciale (tête d'oiseau) et alterations oculaires, *Ophthalmologica* 120:79–83, 1950.

Christian CL, et al: Radiological findings in Hallermann-Streiff syndrome: report of five cases and a review of the literature, *Am J Med Genet* 41:508–514, 1991.

Cohen MM: Hallermann-Streiff syndrome: a review, *Am J Med Genet* 41:488–499, 1991.

Roulez FM, Schuil J, Meire FM: Corneal opacities in the Hallermann-Streiff syndrome, *Ophthalmic Genet* 29:61–66, 2008.

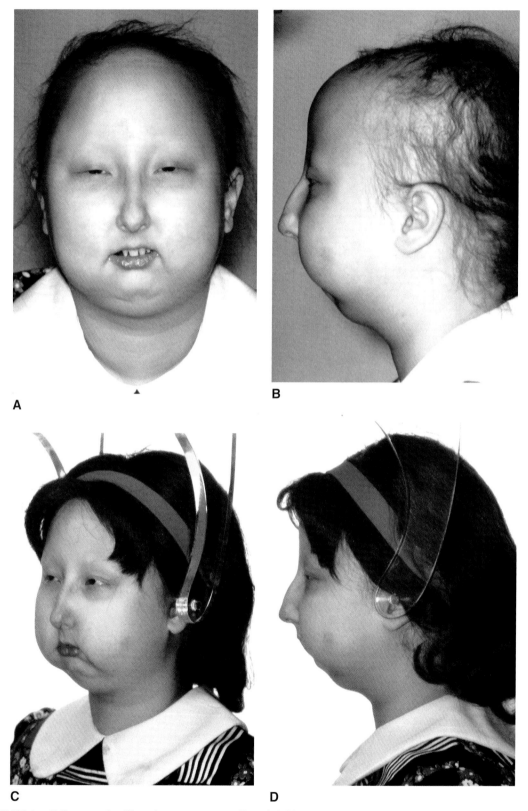

FIGURE 1.   Hallermann-Streiff syndrome. **A–D,** Two affected children. Note the brachycephaly with frontal and parietal bossing, malar hypoplasia, micrognathia, thin nose, microphthalmia, and hypotrichosis. (**A** and **B,** From Cohen MM: *Am J Med Genet* 41:488, 1991, with permission; **C** and **D,** courtesy Dr. Michael Cohen, Dalhousie University, Halifax, Nova Scotia.)

SMITH-LEMLI-OPITZ SYNDROME
Anteverted Nostrils, Ptosis of Eyelids, or Both; Syndactyly of Second and Third Toes; Hypospadias and Cryptorchidism in Male

Four patients with this disorder were described by Smith and colleagues in 1964. Its birth prevalence has been estimated by Opitz to be 1 in 20,000. Tint and colleagues in 1993 identified an abnormality in cholesterol biosynthesis in patients with this disorder that appears to explain much of the clinical phenotype.

ABNORMALITIES

Growth. Moderately small at birth, with subsequent failure to thrive; final height between 143 and 170 cm.

Performance. Moderate to severe intellectual disability, with variable altered muscle tone; approximately 10% of biochemically diagnosed cases have intelligence quotients (IQs) between 50 and 70.

Craniofacial. Microcephaly with narrow frontal area, auricles slanted or low-set, ptosis of eyelids, inner epicanthal folds, strabismus, broad nasal tip with anteverted nostrils, broad maxillary secondary alveolar ridges, micrognathia.

Limb. Simian crease; high frequency of digital whorl dermal ridge patterning; "Y-shaped" syndactyly of second and third toes; short, proximally placed thumb; postaxial polydactyly of hand and, less often, of feet.

Genitourinary. Genital abnormalities (70%), including hypospadias, cryptorchidism, micropenis, hypoplastic scrotum, bifid scrotum, and microurethra; upper tract anomalies (57%), including ureteropelvic junction obstruction, hydronephrosis, renal cystic dysplasia, renal duplication, renal agenesis, and reflux.

Cardiac. Defect in 50%, particularly endocardial cushion defect, hypoplastic left heart, atrial septal defect, patent ductus arteriosus, and membranous ventricular septal defect.

OCCASIONAL ABNORMALITIES
Central and Peripheral Nervous Systems. Seizures; abnormal EEG; demyelination found in cerebral hemispheres, cranial nerves, and peripheral nerves; enlarged ventricles; agenesis of corpus callosum; cerebellar hypoplasia; holoprosencephaly (5%).

Optic. Cataract, sclerosis of lateral geniculate bodies, lack of visual following, opsoclonus, nystagmus, sclerocornea, iris coloboma, heterochromia iridis, posterior synechiae, glaucoma, optic atrophy, microphthalmia.

Limb. Flexed fingers, asymmetrically short finger(s), radial agenesis, clinodactyly, camptodactyly, ectrodactyly, short first toes, metatarsus adductus, vertical talus, dislocation of hip.

Other. Ocular hypertelorism, absent lacrimal puncta, cleft palate, macrostomia, microglossia, bifid tongue, small larynx and vocal cords, sensorineural hearing loss, abnormal pulmonary lobation, hypoplasia of thymus, adrenal enlargement, inguinal hernia, hepatic dysfunction, pancreatic islet cell hyperplasia, deep sacral dimple, rectal atresia, pyloric stenosis, gallbladder aplasia, cholestatic liver disease, intestinal malrotation, diaphragmatic hernia, anal stenosis, Hirschsprung disease, pit anterior to anus, unusually blond hair, short neck.

NATURAL HISTORY
Many of these babies are born in a breech presentation. Stillbirth and early neonatal death are not uncommon. Feeding difficulty and vomiting are frequent problems in early infancy. Oral tactile defensiveness and failure to progress to textured food is common and results in the need for nasogastric tube feeding in 50% of these babies. Gastroesophageal reflux is common because of a small stomach, intestinal dysmotility, and milk or soy protein allergy. Of those who survive, 20% die during the first year. Death appeared to be related to pneumonia in most of them, one of whom had a hemorrhagic necrotizing pneumonia with varicella, suggesting an impaired immune response. Irritable behavior with shrill screaming may pose a problem during infancy. Muscle tone, which may be hypotonic in early infancy, tends to become hypertonic with time. Diminished amount of sleep is common in early infancy. The degree of mental deficiency is usually moderate to severe. However, affected children are sociable, have better receptive than expressive language, and may be mechanically adept. Behavioral characteristics of autism, self-injurious and aggressive behavior, and forceful backward arching are common.

ETIOLOGY

This disorder has an autosomal recessive inheritance pattern. A severe defect in cholesterol biosynthesis has been identified leading to abnormally low plasma cholesterol levels and elevated concentrations of the cholesterol precursor 7-dehydrocholesterol, the result of a deficiency of 7-dehydrocholesterol reductase (DHCR7). The *DHCR7* gene is localized to chromosome 11q12-13. Cholesterol is vitally important in normal development through its contribution to the cell membrane and outer mitochondrial membrane as well as its role in steroid, bile acid, and vitamin D metabolism, and myelination of the nervous system. Its relative deficiency explains many of the variable features of this disorder. Conventional colorimetric techniques to measure cholesterol will not invariably detect the cholesterol abnormalities in this condition. At present, only a chromatographic assay is suitable for measuring 7-dehydrocholesterol.

Prenatal diagnosis has been accomplished successfully on the basis of an elevated 7-dehydrocholesterol in amniotic fluid. One of the earliest signs of an affected fetus is an abnormally low maternal serum level of unconjugated estriol on maternal triple screen. Direct measurement of sterol composition of chorionic villi at 10 weeks' gestation is also reliable.

COMMENT

It is now recognized that the spectrum of defects seen in children with Smith-Lemli-Opitz syndrome is extremely broad. Severely affected patients die in the perinatal period with multiple structural defects, whereas much more mildly affected patients have minor structural anomalies with the characteristic behavioral and learning problems. All patients have a typical craniofacial pattern profile, which includes small skull size, decreased head length and width, narrow forehead, decreased facial depth, flat face, short nose with anteverted nares, and normal width of jaw with retro- or micrognathia. Plasma cholesterol concentration correlates with the degree of severity. Children at the severe end of the spectrum have plasma cholesterol concentrations of less than 2.2 mmol/L, while the less severely affected patients have plasma cholesterol levels equal to or greater than 2.2 mmol/L.

Although dietary cholesterol supplementation has been used frequently to treat children with Smith-Lemli-Opitz syndrome, the only randomized clinical trial of behavioral effects of supplementation showed no difference between treatment and placebo groups.

References

Smith DW, Lemli L, Opitz JM: A newly recognized syndrome of multiple congenital anomalies, *J Pediatr* 64:210, 1964.

Dallaire L, Fraser FC: The syndrome of retardation with urogenital and skeletal anomalies in siblings, *J Pediatr* 69:459, 1966.

Fierro M: Smith-Lemli-Opitz syndrome: Neuropathological and ophthalmological observations, *Dev Med Child Neurol* 19:57, 1977.

Joseph DB, et al: Genitourinary abnormalities associated with the Smith-Lemli-Opitz syndrome, *J Urol* 137:179, 1987.

Irons M, et al: Abnormal cholesterol metabolism in the Smith-Lemli-Opitz syndrome: Report of clinical and biochemical findings in four patients and treatment in one patient, *Am J Med Genet* 50:347, 1994.

Opitz JM: RSH/SLO ("Smith-Lemli-Opitz") syndrome: Historical, genetic and developmental considerations, *Am J Med Genet* 50:344, 1994.

Opitz JM, de La Cruz F: Cholesterol metabolism in the RSH/Smith-Lemli-Opitz syndrome: Summary of an NICHD Conference, *Am J Med Genet* 50:326, 1994.

Tint GS, et al: Defective cholesterol biosynthesis associated with the Smith-Lemli-Opitz syndrome, *N Engl J Med* 330:107, 1994.

Tint GS, et al: Correlation of severity and outcome with plasma sterol levels in variants of the Smith-Lemli-Opitz syndrome, *J Pediatr* 127:82, 1995.

Kelley RI, Hennekam RCM: The Smith-Lemli-Opitz syndrome, *J Med Genet* 37:321, 2000.

Tierney E, et al: Behavior phenotype in the RSH/Smith-Lemli-Opitz syndrome, *Am J Med Genet* 98:191, 2001.

Porter FD. Smith-Lemli-Opitz syndrome: Pathogenesis, diagnosis and management, *Eur J Hum Genet* 16:535, 2008.

Tierney E, et al: Analysis of short term behavioral effects of dietary cholesterol supplementation in Smith-Lemli-Opitz syndrome, *Am J Med Genet A* 152A:91, 2010.

Nowaczyk MJ, et al: Smith-Lemli-Opitz syndrome: Objective assessment of facial phenotype, *Am J Med Genet A* 158A:1020, 2012.

D

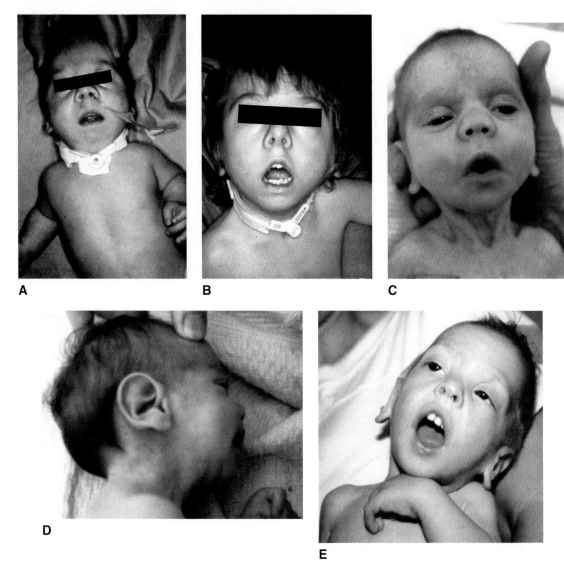

FIGURE 1. Smith-Lemli-Opitz syndrome. **A–E,** Two affected children. Note the narrow frontal area, somewhat prominent glabella, ptosis, broad nasal tip with anteverted nares, and micrognathia.

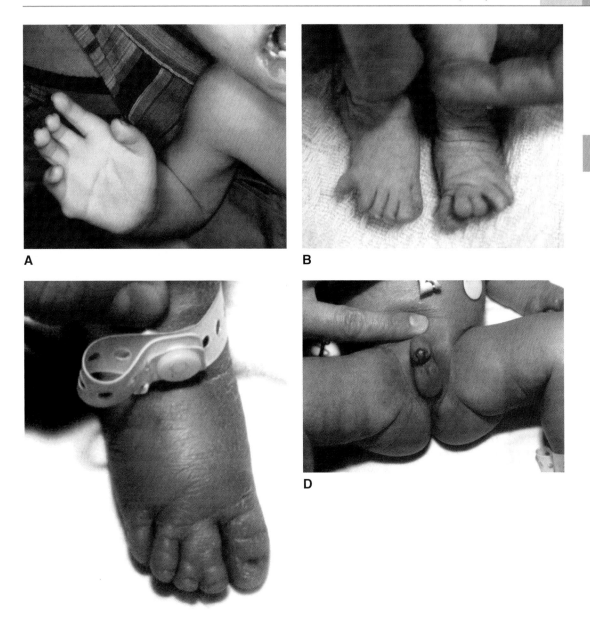

FIGURE 2.   A–D, Note the polydactyly, camptodactyly, 2-3 syndactyly of the toes, and hypospadias.

KABUKI SYNDROME
(KABUKI MAKE-UP SYNDROME, NIIKAWA-KUROKI SYNDROME)
Long Palpebral Fissures, Eversion of Lower Lateral Eyelids, Persistent Fingertip Pads

Initially reported in 1981 by Niikawa and colleagues and by Kuroki and colleagues in 10 unrelated Japanese children, this disorder has now been reported in more than 400 patients, many of them non-Japanese. Because of the facial resemblance of affected individuals to the make-up of actors in *Kabuki*, the traditional Japanese theater, this disorder has been referred to as the Kabuki syndrome.

ABNORMALITIES

Growth. Postnatal growth deficiency, with onset usually occurring in the first year, becomes more marked with increasing age; mean height in children 12 months or older was –2.3 SD.

Performance. Mean developmental quotient in infants and children is 52, and in older patients, mean IQ is 62; severe intellectual disability is uncommon; IQ equal to or greater than 80 in 12%; hypotonia.

Craniofacial. Long palpebral fissures with eversion of the lateral portion of the lower eyelid, ptosis, arced and broad eyebrows with sparse lateral third, blue sclera, strabismus, epicanthal folds, short columella, large protuberant ears, preauricular pit, cleft palate, tooth abnormalities, open mouth with tented upper lip giving myopathic appearance.

Skeletal. Anomalies in 88% including short, incurved fifth finger secondary to short fourth and fifth metacarpals; short middle phalanges; brachydactyly; rib anomalies; vertebral anomaly; hip dislocation; scoliosis, kyphosis, or both.

Cardiac. Defects occur in approximately 50% of patients and include malformations associated with altered hemodynamics such as coarctation of the aorta, bicuspid aortic valve, mitral valve prolapse, membranous ventricular septal defect, pulmonary, aortic, and mitral valve stenosis as well as tetralogy of Fallot, single ventricle with common atrium, double outlet right ventricle, and transposition of great vessels.

Other. Joint hyperextensibility (74%); persistent fetal finger pad (96%); excess digital ulnar loops; renal anomalies, urinary tract anomalies, or both (28%); hearing loss (32%).

OCCASIONAL ABNORMALITIES

Microcephaly; craniosynostosis; polymicrogyria; subarachnoid cyst; hydrocephalus secondary to aqueductal stenosis; autistic behavior; premature graying of hair; vitiligo; cleft lip; lower lip pits; Mondini dysplasias and ossicular anomalies; microtia; short nasal septum; broad nasal root; long eyelashes; preauricular pit; cutaneous syndactyly; nail hypoplasia; cryptorchidism; micropenis; delayed puberty; imperforate anus; umbilical and inguinal hernias; malrotation of colon; premature thelarche; precocious puberty; obesity; seizures; pectus excavatum; diaphragmatic hernia, eventration, or both; biliary atresia; stenosis of bronchial tree; growth hormone deficiency; predisposition to neoplasia.

NATURAL HISTORY

Although many of the characteristic facial features are present in neonates, the features become more obvious with age. Severe feeding problems are common. Susceptibility to infection, particularly otitis media, upper respiratory tract, and pneumonia, is common, and decreased levels of IgA, IgG, and IgM have been documented not infrequently. Obesity often occurs at adolescence. Delays in speech and language acquisition with articulation errors are common.

ETIOLOGY

Approximately 60% of cases are caused by mutations in the the *mixed lineage leukemia 2 gene (MLL2)* gene. *MLL2* encodes proteins involved in histone modification. Nearly all patients with a typical Kabuki syndrome facies have a pathologic *MLL2* mutation. However, three patients, two with classical facial features of Kabuki syndrome and one less characteristic, have been identified with a de novo Xp11.3 microdeletion which included either partial or complete deletions of *KDM6A*. *KDM6A* encodes a histone demethylase that interacts with *MLL2*.

References

Kuroki Y, et al: A new malformation syndrome of long palpebral fissures, large ears, depressed nasal tip, and skeletal anomalies associates with postnatal dwarfism and mental retardation, *J Pediatr* 99:570, 1981.

Niikawa N, et al: Kabuki make-up syndrome: A syndrome of mental retardation, unusual facies, large and protruding ears, and postnatal growth deficiency, *J Pediatr* 99:565, 1981.

Niikawa N, et al: Kabuki make-up (Niikawa-Kuroki) syndrome: A study of 62 patients, *Am J Med Genet* 31:565, 1988.

Philip N, et al: Kabuki make-up (Niikawa-Kuroki) syndrome: A study of 16 non-Japanese cases, *Clin Dysmorph* 1:63, 1992.

Wessels MJ, et al: Kabuki syndrome: A review study of three hundred patients, *Clin Dysmorph* 11:95, 2002.

Matsumoto N, Niikawa N: Kabuki make-up syndrome: A review, *Am J Med Genet C Semin Med Genet* 117C:57, 2003.

Adam M, Hudgins L: Kabuki syndrome: A review, *Clin Genet* 67:209, 2004.

Hoffman JD, et al: Immune abnormalities are a frequent manifestation of Kabuki syndrome, *Am J Med Genet A* 135A:278, 2005.

Ng SB, et al: Exome sequencing identifies MLL2 mutations as a cause of Kabuki syndrome, *Nat Genet* 42:790, 2010.

Hannibal MC, et al: Spectrum of MLL2 (ALR) mutations in 110 cases of Kabuki syndrome, *Amer J Med Genet* 155:1511, 2011.

Banka S, et al: How genetically heterogeneous is Kabuki syndrome? MLL2 testing in 116 patients, review and analyses of mutation and phenotypic spectrum, *Eur J Hum Genet* 20:381, 2012.

Lederer D, et al: Deletion of KDM6A, a histone demethylase interacting with MLL2, in three patients with Kabuki syndrome, *Amer J Human Genet* 90:119, 2012.

D

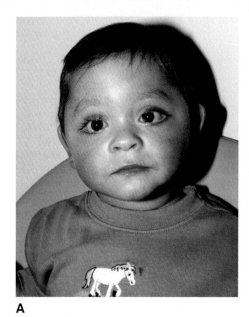

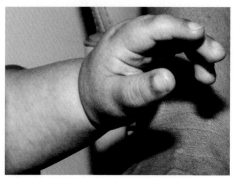

A

B

FIGURE 1.   Kabuki syndrome. **A** and **B,** An 18-month-old boy. Note the long palpebral fissures, eversion of the lateral portion of the lower eyelid, and prominent fingertip pads.

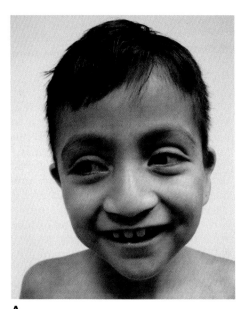

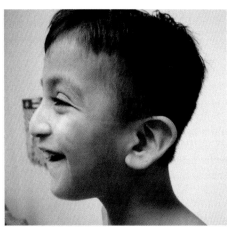

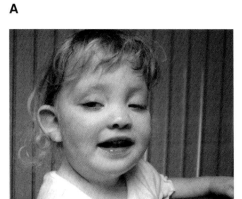

A

B

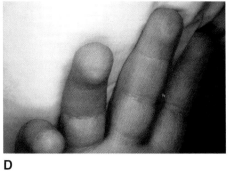

D

C

FIGURE 2.   A–D, A 3-year-old boy and 4-year-old girl. Note the long palpebral fissures, large protruding ears, and prominent fingertip pads.

WILLIAMS SYNDROME (WILLIAMS-BEUREN SYNDROME)
Prominent Lips, Hoarse Voice, Cardiovascular Anomaly

In 1961, Williams and colleagues described this disorder in four unrelated children with mental deficiency, an unusual facies, and supravalvular aortic stenosis. Subsequently, more than 100 cases have been described. Hypercalcemia has been an infrequent finding; cardiovascular anomalies, including supravalvular aortic stenosis, have been variable; and features such as aberrations of growth and performance and the unusual facies are more consistent relative to diagnosis.

ABNORMALITIES

Features vary from among the following:

Growth. Mild prenatal growth deficiency, postnatal growth rate approximately 75% of normal, mild microcephaly.

Performance. Average IQ of approximately 56, with a range from 41 to 80; friendly, loquacious personality; anxious; hoarse voice; hypersensitivity to sound; mild neurologic dysfunction; primarily mild spasticity manifest by tight heel cords and hyperactive deep tendon reflexes and poor coordination; hypotonia; perceptual and motor function more reduced (–3.0 to –3.9 SD) than verbal and memory performance (–2.0 SD); level of general language ability is much greater than general cognitive ability.

Facies. Medial eyebrow flare, short palpebral fissures, depressed nasal bridge, epicanthal folds, periorbital fullness of subcutaneous tissues, blue eyes, stellate pattern in the iris, anteverted nares, long philtrum, prominent lips with open mouth.

Limb. Hypoplastic nails, hallux valgus.

Cardiovascular. Supravalvular aortic stenosis, peripheral pulmonary artery stenosis, pulmonic valvular stenosis, ventricular and atrial septal defect, renal artery stenosis with hypertension, hypoplasia of the aorta, and other arterial anomalies.

Dentition. Partial anodontia, microdontia, enamel hypoplasia, malocclusion.

Musculoskeletal. Joint hypermobility, contractures, lordosis, scoliosis, kyphosis, extra sacral crease.

Urinary. Renal anomalies, including nephrocalcinosis, asymmetry in kidney size, small solitary or pelvic kidney, bladder diverticula, urethral stenosis, vesicoureteral reflux.

Other. Soft lax skin, premature gray hair.

OCCASIONAL ABNORMALITIES

Ocular hypotelorism, amblyopia, strabismus, refractive errors, tortuosity of retinal vessels, high-frequency sensorineural hearing loss, vocal cord paralysis, malar hypoplasia, fifth finger clinodactyly, radioulnar synostosis, small penis, pectus excavatum, inguinal or umbilical hernia, colon diverticula, rectal prolapse, Chiari type I malformation, mucinous cystadenoma of ovary, portal hypertension, celiac disease, hypercalcemia, hypothyroidism, diabetes mellitus, obesity, early onset of puberty.

NATURAL HISTORY

In early infancy, these children tend to be fretful, have feeding problems, vomit frequently, be constipated, and be often colicky. During childhood, they tend to be outgoing and loquacious, easily approach strangers, and have a strong interest in others. Almost two thirds of children older than 3 years of age display more difficult temperament characteristics than controls, including higher activity, lower adaptability, greater intensity, more negative moods, less persistence, greater distractibility, and lower threshold arousal. Most between 4 and 16 years old meet criteria for at least one DSM-IV diagnosis, including Attention-Deficit/Hyperactivity Disorder and Specific Phobia. A diagnosis of Generalized Anxiety Disorder increases with age.

Progressive medical problems are the rule in adults. These include hypertension; progressive joint limitations; recurrent urinary tract infections; and gastrointestinal problems, including obesity, chronic constipation, diverticulosis and cholelithiasis, and hypercalcemia. The vast majority live with their parents, in group homes, or in supervised apartments.

Sudden death has been documented in a number of children with Williams syndrome. Some deaths were associated with the administration of anesthesia. Cardiovascular-associated mortality is 25 to 100 times that of controls. Health supervision guidelines have been established for children with Williams syndrome by the Committee on Genetics of the American Academy of Pediatrics.

ETIOLOGY

Although most individuals with this disorder represent sporadic cases within otherwise normal families, parent-to-child transmission has been documented. Studies using fluorescent in situ hybridization and quantitative Southern analysis indicate that both inherited and sporadic cases of Williams syndrome are caused by a deletion at 7q11.23, a region that includes approximately 17 genes. Hemizygosity for the elastin gene is responsible for supravalvular aortic stenosis as well as other vascular stenosis, and LIM-kinase 1 hemizygosity is a contributing factor to impaired visuospatial construction cognition in this disorder. Many of the other features must be the result of hemizygosity for other genes in the deleted region.

COMMENT

In 2005 Somerville et al described the initial case of 7q11.23 microduplication syndrome. Whereas expressive language fluency is a relative strength in individuals with Williams syndrome, speech is the most affected area in individuals with the reciprocal duplication, and the degree of intellectual disability is less severe. Seizures, autism, subtle dysmorphic features (broad forehead; high, broad nasal bridge; low-set, posteriorly rotated ears; ocular hypertelorism; straight eyebrows; short philtrum; thin upper lip) and occasionally microcephaly and major birth defects (cleft lip and palate, heart defects, vertebral anomalies, cryptorchidism) can occur. The deletion and the duplication are equal in size (commonly 1.56-1.8 Mb containing 26-28 genes) and mediated through nonallelic homologous recombination (NAHR) mediated by flanking segmental duplications.

References

Joseph MC, Parrott D: Severe infantile hypercalcemia with special reference to the facies, *Arch Dis Child* 33:385, 1958.

Williams JCP, Barratt-Boyes BG, Lowe JB: Supravalvular aortic stenosis, *Circulation* 24:1311, 1961.

Jones KL, Smith DW: The Williams elfin facies syndrome: A new perspective, *J Pediatr* 86:718, 1975.

Jensen OA, Marborg M, Dupont A: Ocular pathology in the elfin face syndrome (the Fanconi-Schlesinger type of idiopathic hypercalcaemia of infancy). Histochemical and ultrastructural study of a case, *Opthalmologica* 172:434, 1976.

Morris CA, et al: The natural history of the Williams syndrome: Physical characteristics, *J Pediatr* 113:318, 1988.

Ewart AK, et al: Hemizygosity at the elastin locus in a developmental disorder, Williams syndrome, *Nat Genet* 5:11, 1993.

Pober BR, et al: Renal findings in 40 individuals with Williams syndrome, *Am J Med Genet* 46:271, 1993.

Bird LM, et al: Sudden death in patients with supravalvular aortic stenosis and Williams syndrome, *J Pediatr* 129:926, 1996.

Frangiskakis JM, et al: LIM-kinase 1 hemizygosity implicated in impaired visuospatial constructive cognition, *Cell* 86:59, 1996.

Donnai D, Karmiloff-Smith A: Williams syndrome: From genotype through to the cognitive phenotype, *Am J Med Genet* 97:164, 2000.

Committee on Genetics, American Academy of Pediatrics: Health care supervision for children with Williams syndrome, *Pediatrics* 107:1192, 2001.

Wessel A, et al: Risk of sudden death in the Williams-Beuren syndrome, *Am J Med Genet A* 127A:234, 2004.

Somerville MJ, et al: Severe expressive language delay related to duplication of the Williams-Beuren locus, *N Eng J Med* 353:1694, 2005.

Leyfer OT, et al: Prevalence of psychiatric disorders in 4 to 16-year-olds with Williams syndrome, *Am J Med Genet B Neuropsychiatr Genet* 141B:615, 2006.

Van der Aa N, et al: Fourteen new cases contribute to the characterization of the 7q11.23 microduplication syndrome, *Eur J Med Genet* 52:94, 2009.

Morris CA: The behavioral phenotype of Williams syndrome: A recognizable pattern of neurodevelopment, *Am J Med Genet C Semin Med Genet* 154C:427, 2010.

Pober BR: Williams-Beuren syndrome, *N Engl J Med* 362:239, 2010.

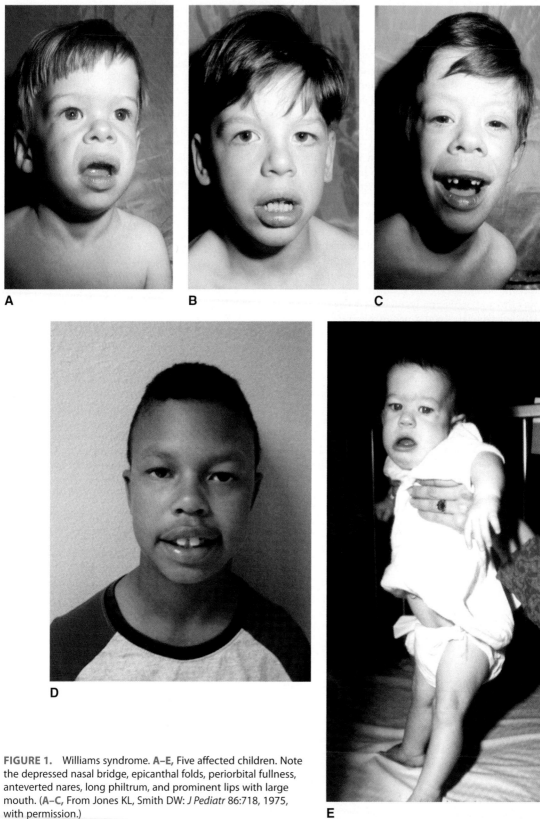

FIGURE 1. Williams syndrome. **A–E,** Five affected children. Note the depressed nasal bridge, epicanthal folds, periorbital fullness, anteverted nares, long philtrum, and prominent lips with large mouth. (**A–C,** From Jones KL, Smith DW: *J Pediatr* 86:718, 1975, with permission.)

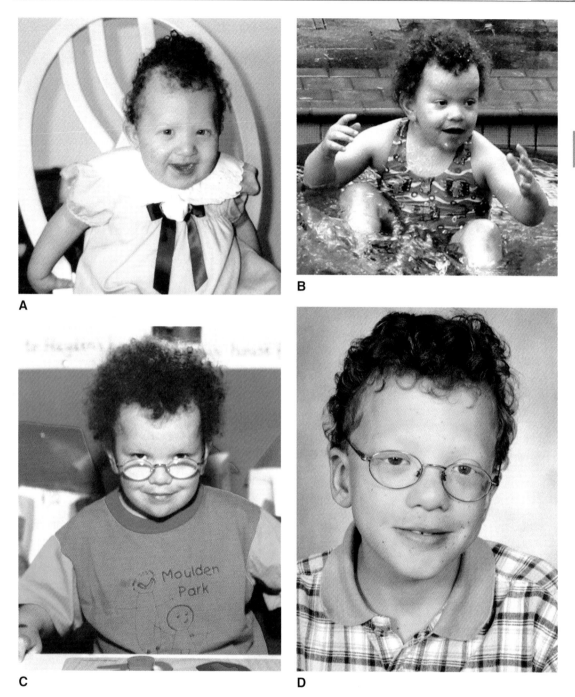

D

FIGURE 2. **A–D,** Note the somewhat sparse curly hair, relative macrocephaly with large prominent forehead, bitemporal narrowing, shallow orbits, and lack of eyebrows and eyelashes. The same girl is depicted in **B** and **C.** The boy in **D** is 11 years old. (Courtesy Dr. John M. Opitz, University of Utah, Salt Lake City.)

AARSKOG SYNDROME
Hypertelorism, Brachydactyly, Shawl Scrotum

Set forth by Aarskog in 1970, there has been increasing recognition of this disorder. It can be misdiagnosed easily as the Noonan syndrome.

ABNORMALITIES

Growth. Slight to moderate short stature, final adult height between 160 and 170 cm, delayed bone age.

Facies. Rounded. Facial edema in children younger than 4 years. Hypertelorism with variable ptosis of eyelids and slight downward slant to palpebral fissures; widow's peak; small nose with anteverted nares, broad philtrum, maxillary hypoplasia, slight crease below the lower lip; upper helices of ears incompletely outfolded; hypodontia, retarded dental eruption, broad central upper incisors (permanent dentition), orthodontic problems.

Limbs. Brachydactyly with clinodactyly of fifth fingers, unusual position of extended fingers with hyperextension of distal interphalangeal (DIP) joints and flexion of proximal interphalangeal (PIP) joints, simian crease, mild interdigital webbing; broad thumbs and great toes.

Radiologic. Short long tubular bones with wide metaphysis; brachyphalangia; hypoplastic middle phalanges of fifth fingers; short, broad first metacarpals and metatarsals; pelvic hypoplasia.

Abdomen. Prominent umbilicus, inguinal hernias.

Genitalia. "Shawl" scrotum in 90%; cryptorchidism.

Other. Short neck with or without webbing; cervical vertebral anomalies, including hypoplasia and synostosis of one or more cervical vertebrae and spina bifida occulta; mild pectus excavatum; protruding umbilicus.

OCCASIONAL ABNORMALITIES

Ocular. Strabismus, amblyopia, hyperopia, astigmatism, latent nystagmus, inferior oblique overaction, blue sclerae, anisometropia, posterior embryotoxon, corneal enlargement.

Skeletal. Scoliosis, cubitus valgus, splayed toes with bulbous tips, metatarsus adductus.

Genitalia. Cleft scrotum, phimosis.

Other. Mild to moderate intellectual disability, scalp defects, anomalous cerebral venous drainage, Hirschsprung disease, midgut malrotation, hypoplastic kidney, dental enamel hypoplasia, delayed eruption of teeth, cleft lip and/or cleft palate, cardiac defects.

NATURAL HISTORY

Growth deficiency may be of prenatal onset. Marked failure to thrive in the first year with feeding difficulties and recurrent respiratory infections in 35% of patients. More commonly, mild growth deficiency is first evident at 1 to 3 years of age and may be associated with slow maturation and a late advent of adolescence. A positive effect of growth hormone treatment on growth and adult height has been suggested. Fertility is normal. Orthodontic correction is often necessary. IQ is normal in the majority of cases. However, hyperactivity and attention deficit disorders are common, particularly in those who are intellectually disabled.

ETIOLOGY

The disorder has an X-linked recessive inheritance pattern, with carrier females often showing some minor manifestations of the disorder, especially in the face and hands. The gene for this disorder, designated *FGD1*, has been mapped to Xp11.21. *FGD1* is a member of the guanine nucleotide exchange factor family, which catalyses the exchange of GDP to GTP and promotes the activity of Rho family GTPases. More than 16 *FGD1* mutations have been reported.

References

Aarskog D: A familial syndrome of short stature associated with facial dysplasia and genital anomalies, *J Pediatr* 77:856, 1970.

Furukawa CT, Hall BD, Smith DW: The Aarskog syndrome, *J Pediatr* 81:1117, 1972.

Brodsky MC, et al: Ocular and systemic findings in the Aarskog (facial-digital-genital) syndrome, *Am J Ophthalmol* 109:450, 1990.

Fryns JP: Aarskog syndrome: The changing phenotype with age, *Am J Med Genet* 43:420, 1992.

Lizcano-Gil LA, et al: The facio-digito-dental syndrome (Aarskog syndrome): A further delineation of the distinct radiological findings, *Genet Couns* 5:387, 1994.

Pasteris NG, et al: Isolation and characterization of the faciogenital dysplasia (Aarskog-Scott syndrome) gene: A putative Rho/Rac guanine nucleotide exchange factor, *Cell* 79:669, 1994.

Logie LG, Porteous MEM: Intelligence and development in Aarskog syndrome, *Arch Dis Child* 79:359, 1998.

Zou W, et al: *MLK3* regulates bone development downstream of the faciogenital dysplasia protein *FGD1* in mice, *J Clin Invest* 121:4383, 2011.

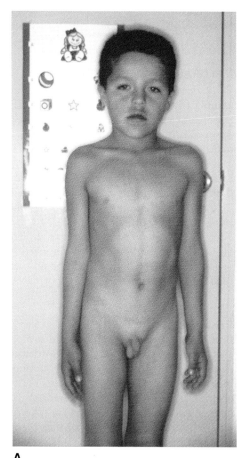

A

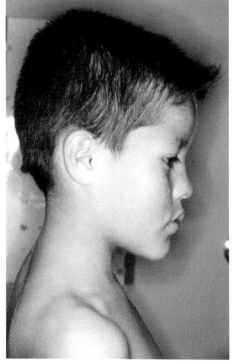

B

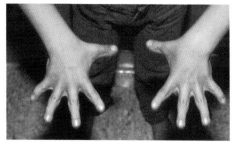

D

D

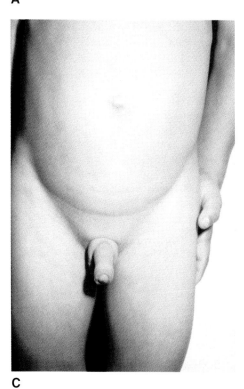

C

FIGURE 1.   Aarskog syndrome. **A** and **B,** Photograph of a 7-year-old boy. Note the round face, hypertelorism, and downslanting palpebral fissures. **C,** "Pouting" umbilicus and "shawl" scrotum in an 8-year-old boy. **D,** Mild brachyclinodactyly with mild syndactyly.

ROBINOW SYNDROME (FETAL FACE SYNDROME)
Flat Facial Profile, Short Forearms, Hypoplastic Genitalia

Initially reported by Robinow and colleagues in 1969, many additional cases of this disorder have been recognized.

ABNORMALITIES

Growth. Slight to moderate shortness of stature of postnatal onset (93%).

Craniofacial. Macrocephaly (44%), large anterior fontanel, frontal bossing (94%), hypertelorism (100%), prominent eyes (86%), downslanting palpebral fissures (80%), small upturned nose (100%), long philtrum (88%), triangular mouth with downturned angles (94%) and micrognathia (87%), hyperplastic alveolar ridges (66%), crowded teeth (96%), posteriorly rotated ears (53%).

Limbs. Short forearms (100%), small hands with clinodactyly (88%), nail dysplasia (48%).

Other Skeletal. Hemivertebrae of thoracic vertebrae (70%), rib anomalies, primarily fusion of or absent ribs (40%), scoliosis (50%).

Genitalia. Small penis, clitoris, labia majora (94%), cryptorchidism (65%).

OCCASIONAL ABNORMALITIES

Oral-Facial. Nevus flammeus (23%), epicanthal folds, macroglossia, high-arched palate, absent or bifid uvula (18%), cleft lip and/or cleft palate (9%), short frenulum of tongue with cleft tongue tip, midline clefting of lower lip.

Limbs. Broad thumbs and toes, bifid terminal phalanges, clinodactyly of fifth finger, hyperextensible fingers, short metacarpals. Madelung-like anomaly of forearm, dislocation of hip, hypoplastic interphalangeal creases, single flexion creases on third and fourth fingers, hypoplastic middle and terminal phalanges of fingers and toes, transverse palmar crease, ectrodactyly.

Other. Seizures; developmental delay and intellectual disability (18%); language deficiency; conductive hearing loss; pectus excavatum (19%); superiorly positioned, broad, and poorly epithelialized umbilicus and inguinal hernia (20%); pilonidal dimple; renal anomalies (29%); vaginal atresia with hematocolpos; cardiac defects, especially right ventricular outlet obstruction (13%).

NATURAL HISTORY

Early death secondary to pulmonary or cardiac complications occurs in 10% of patients. The penile hypoplasia may be sufficient to raise the question of sex of rearing. Although partial primary hypogonadism evidenced by elevated serum follicle-stimulating hormone levels was documented in four affected males, normal pubertal virilization occurred in all three patients older than 16 years. Two adult women are 4 feet 10 inches and 5 feet, respectively, and three adult men are 5 feet 3 inches, 5 feet 7 inches, and 5 feet 10 inches in height. The facial features become less pronounced with age owing to accelerated growth of the nose at adolescence. Performance has been normal in most individuals.

ETIOLOGY

Both an autosomal dominant and a more severe autosomal recessive type of this disorder have been described. The recessive type is distinguished by more severe mesomelic and acromelic dwarfism, multiple rib and vertebral anomalies, radioulnar dislocation, severe hypoplasia of the proximal radius and distal ulna, and a more triangular-shaped mouth. Mutations of *ROR2*, a gene located on chromosome 9q22, which encodes a receptor tyrosine kinase–like orphan receptor 2, are responsible for the recessive type. Mutations of *WNT5A*, which result in amino acid substitutions of highly conserved cysteines, are associated with the dominant form. *ROR4* is a putative *WNT5A* receptor.

COMMENT

Distinguishing features between the two forms are subtle and include the following: Hemivertebrae and scoliosis occur in 75% of the recessive form and in less than 25% of the dominant form. Umbilical hernia (32.3%) and supernumerary teeth (10.3%) occur exclusively in the dominant form.

References

Robinow M, Silverman FN, Smith HD: A newly recognized dwarfing syndrome, *Am J Dis Child* 117:645, 1969.

Wadlington WB, Tucker VL, Schimke RN: Mesomelic dwarfism with hemivertebrae and small genitalia (the Robinow syndrome), *Am J Dis Child* 126:202, 1973.

Bain MD, Winter RM, Burn J: Robinow syndrome without mesomelic brachymelia: A report of five cases, *J Med Genet* 23:350, 1986.

Butler MG, Wadlington WB: Robinow syndrome: Report of two patients and review of the literature, *Clin Genet* 31:77, 1987.

Afzal AR, et al: Recessive Robinow syndrome, allelic to brachydactyly type B, is caused by mutations of *ROR2*, *Nat Genet* 25:419, 2000.

Patton MA, Afzal AR: Robinow syndrome, *J Med Genet* 39:305, 2002.

Mazzeu JF, et al: Clinical characterization of autosomal dominant and recessive variants of Robinow syndrome, *Am J Med Genet A* 143A:320, 2007.

Person AD, et al: *WNT5A* mutations in patients with autosomal dominant Robinow syndrome, *Dev Dyn* 239:327, 2010.

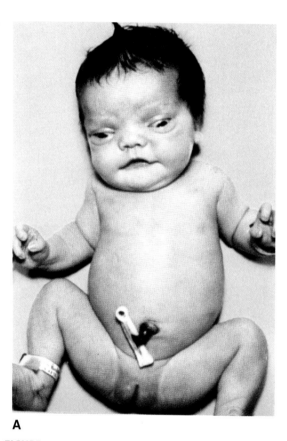
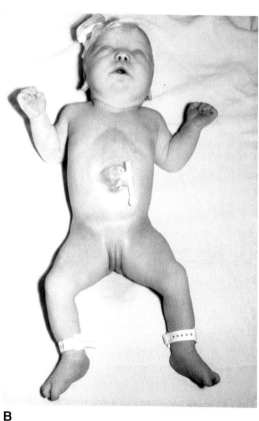

A   **B**

FIGURE 1. Robinow syndrome. **A,** A 2-day-old female with flat facies, hypertelorism, and minute clitoris. (From Robinow M et al: *Am J Dis Child* 117:645, 1969. Copyright 1969, American Medical Association.) **B,** Newborn female with small nose, hypertelorism, and omphalocele.

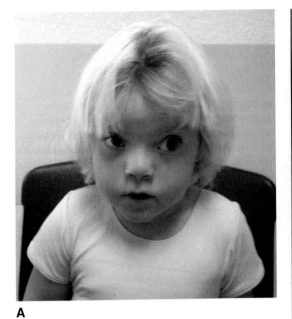

A

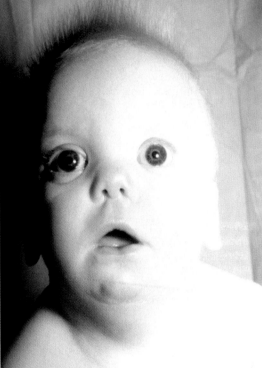

B

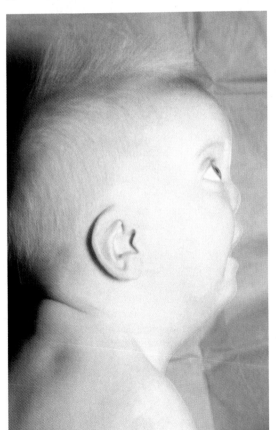

C

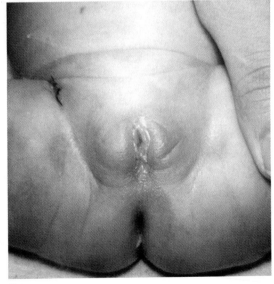

D

FIGURE 2. **A–D,** Note the relative macrocephaly; frontal bossing; hypertelorism; prominent eyes; small, upturned nose; long philtrum; triangular mouth with downturned angles; micrognathia; posteriorly rotated ears; and minute clitoris.

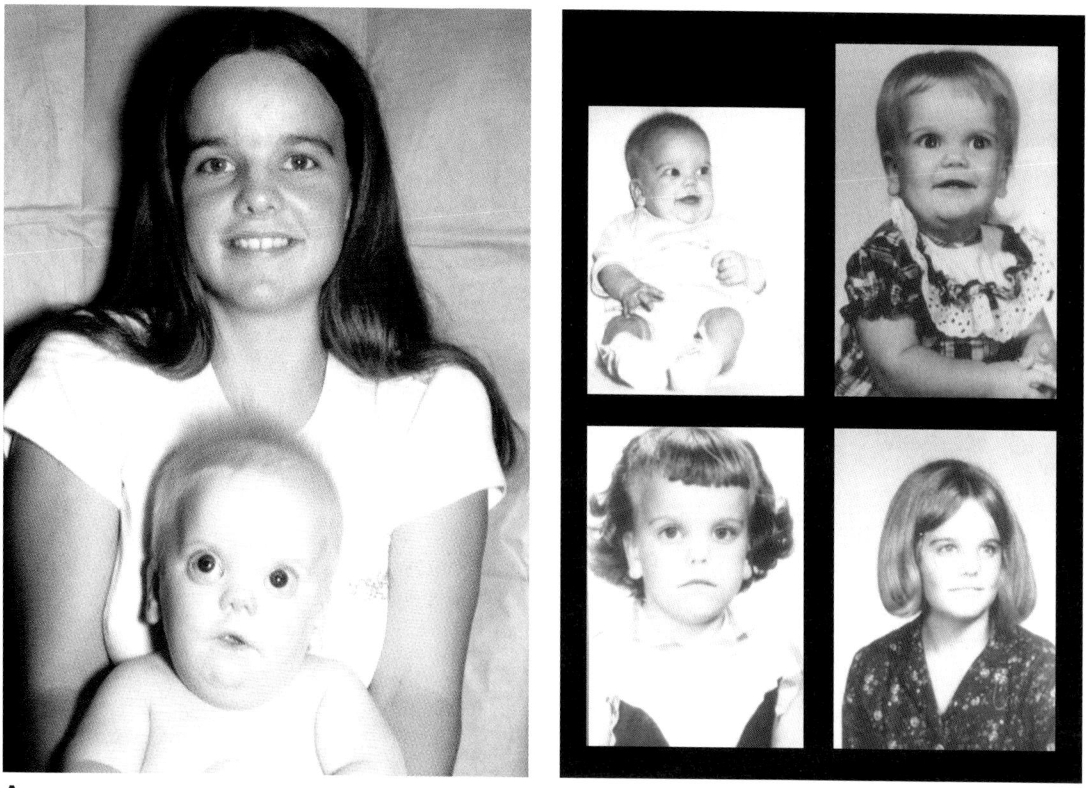

D

FIGURE 3.   **A,** Affected mother and her daughter. **B,** Mother depicted in **A** from birth through 17 years of age shows progression of the phenotype in the autosomal dominant type.

OPITZ G/BBB SYNDROME
(HYPERTELORISM-HYPOSPADIAS SYNDROME, OPITZ-FRIAS SYNDROME, OPITZ OCULO-GENITO-LARYNGEAL SYNDROME)
Hypertelorism, Hypospadias, Swallowing Difficulties

In 1965 and again in 1969, Opitz, Smith, and Summitt reported this condition, previously referred to as the BBB syndrome, in three families in which affected males usually have apparent ocular hypertelorism and hypospadias and affected females have only hypertelorism. In 1969 Opitz and colleagues reported a second disorder referred to as the G syndrome or Opitz-Frias syndrome. It has become clear that these two conditions represent variable manifestations of the same condition, now referred to as the Opitz G/BBB syndrome.

ABNORMALITIES

Performance. Mild to moderate intellectual disability in about two thirds of patients, hypotonia.

Facial. Prominent forehead, ocular hypertelorism, upward or downward slanting of palpebral fissures and epicanthal folds, broad flat nasal bridge with anteverted nostrils, cleft lip with or without cleft palate, short frenulum of tongue, posterior rotation of auricles, micrognathia.

Genital. In males, hypospadias, cryptorchidism, bifid scrotum; in females, splayed labia majora.

Laryngo-Tracheo-Esophageal. Laryngotracheal cleft, malformation of larynx, tracheoesophageal fistula, hypoplastic epiglottis, and high carina.

Other. Hernias.

OCCASIONAL ABNORMALITIES

Cranial asymmetry, widow's peak, strabismus, grooving of nasal tip, flattened elongated philtrum, thin upper lip, bifid uvula, cleft tongue, dental anomalies; brain magnetic resonance imaging findings include agenesis or hypoplasia of corpus callosum, cerebellar vermal hypoplasia, cortical atrophy and ventriculomegaly, macro cisterna magna, pituitary macroadenoma, cranial osteoma, and wide cavum septum pellucidum; malformation of larynx, tracheoesophageal fistula, hypoplastic epiglottis, high carina, pulmonary hypoplasia; renal defect; cardiac defects, most commonly conotruncal lesions; agenesis of gallbladder; duodenal stricture; imperforate anus; hiatal hernia; diastasis recti; increased monozygotic twinning.

NATURAL HISTORY

Swallowing problems with recurrent aspiration, stridulous respirations, intermittent pulmonary difficulty, wheezing, and a weak, hoarse cry should raise concern about a potentially lethal laryngoesophageal defect. In those individuals, mortality is high unless vigorous efforts are made to repair the defect and protect the lungs with gastrostomy or jejunostomy. Although males tend to have more severe and more frequent laryngoesophageal defects, it is important to recognize that this disorder can express itself in both males and females with equal severity. Initial failure to thrive is followed by normal growth in survivors.

ETIOLOGY

Heterogeneity has been demonstrated with an autosomal dominant locus linked to 22q11.2 and an X-linked locus. The gene responsible for the X-linked form, *MID1*, maps to Xp22.3. *MID1* encodes a protein that is highly expressed in tissues that are aberrant in this disorder. Although anteverted nares and posterior pharyngeal clefts have been seen only in the X-linked form, all other manifestations have been seen in both, making it difficult, without molecular testing, to distinguish between the two forms in an affected male who lacks a positive family history.

References

Opitz JM, Smith DW, Summitt RL: Hypertelorism and hypospadias (abst.), *J Pediatr* 67:968, 1965.

Opitz JM, et al: The G syndrome of multiple congenital anomalies, *Birth Defects* 5:95, 1969.

Opitz JM, Summitt RL, Smith DW: The BBB syndrome: Familial telecanthus with associated anomalies. In Bergsma D, editor: *First Conference on Clinical Delineation of Birth Defects*, vol. 5, White Plains, NY, 1969, National Foundation, pp 86–94.

Gonzales CH, Hermann J, Opitz JM: The hypertelorism-hypospadias (BBB) syndrome, *Eur J Pediatr* 12:51, 1977.

Cordero JF, Holmes LB: Phenotypic overlap of the BBB and G syndromes, *Am J Med Genet* 2:145, 1978.

Brooks JK, et al: Opitz (BBB/G) syndrome: Oral manifestations, *Am J Med Genet* 43:595, 1992.

MacDonald MR, et al: Brain magnetic resonance imaging findings in the Opitz/G/BBB syndrome: Extension of the spectrum of midline brain anomalies, *Am J Med Genet* 46:706, 1993.

McDonald-McGinn DM: Autosomal dominant "Opitz" GBBB syndrome due to a 22q11.2 deletion, *Am J Med Genet* 59:103, 1995.

Robin NH, et al: Opitz G/BBB syndrome: Clinical comparisons of families linked to Xp22 and 22q and a review of the literature, *Am J Med Genet* 62:305, 1996.

Quaderi NA, et al: Opitz G/BBB syndrome, a defect of midline development, is due to mutations in a new RING finger gene mapped on Xp22, *Nat Genet* 17:285, 1997.

DeFalco F, et al: X-linked Opitz syndrome: Novel mutations in the *MID1* gene and redefinition of the clinical spectrum, *Am J Med Genet* 120:222, 2003.

D

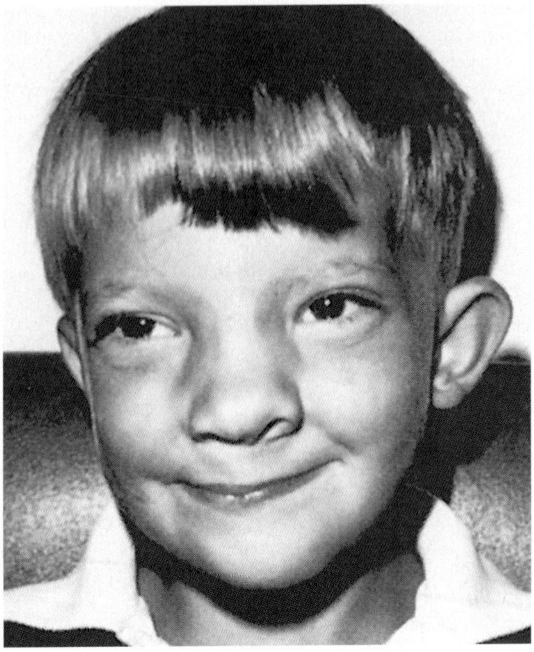

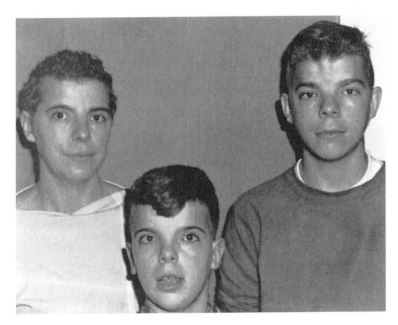

FIGURE 1. A 7-year-old boy with Opitz syndrome. Note hypertelorism, repaired cleft lips, and protruding auricle. Hypospadias was also present. (Courtesy Dr. Robert Fineman.)

FIGURE 2. An affected mother (mild hypertelorism) and two of her affected boys who show hypertelorism and also have hypospadias. (From the B. O. family pedigree of Opitz JM et al: *Birth Defects* 5:86, 1969, with permission.)

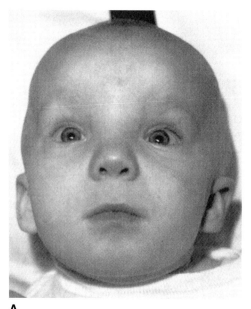

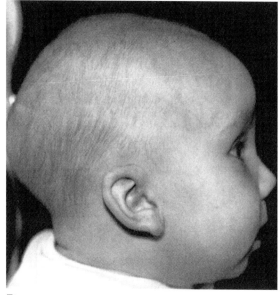

D

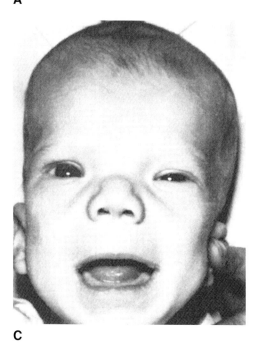

FIGURE 3.   A and B, Photographs of a 1-month-old affected child. C, Photographs of a 7½-month-old affected child. (A–C, From Opitz JM et al: *Birth Defects* 5(2):95, 1969, with permission.)

FLOATING-HARBOR SYNDROME
Postnatal Growth Deficiency, Bulbous Nose, Speech Delay

Pelletier and Feingold described the initial patient with this disorder in 1973. One year later, Leisti and colleagues reported a child with almost identical features and suggested the term "Floating-Harbor syndrome," an amalgam of the names of the hospitals where the initial two patients were evaluated (Boston Floating and Harbor General, Torrance, Calif.). Approximately 50 patients have been reported with this condition.

ABNORMALITIES

Growth. Birth weight and length at third percentile; postnatal growth deficiency, delayed bone age.

Performance. Severe speech and language delay; borderline normal to moderate intellectual disability; behavior problems, including hyperactivity, poor attention span, and aggression.

Craniofacial. Short palpebral fissures with deep-set eyes; triangular shape to nasal tip; wide mouth with downturned corners; low-set posteriorly rotated ears. In midchildhood the nose becomes bulbous with prominent nasal bridge, the columella becomes broad, the philtrum short and smooth, and the vermilion border thin.

Other. Low posterior hairline, short neck, broad chest, fifth finger clinodactyly, brachydactyly, clubbing, broad thumbs, joint laxity.

OCCASIONAL ABNORMALITIES

Microcephaly, trigonocephaly due to metopic suture synostosis, dental problems, abnormal electroencephalograph, pulmonary stenosis, tetralogy of Fallot with atrial septal defect, adult onset hypertension, triangular face, rib anomalies, high-pitched voice, preauricular pit, delayed motor skills, accessory or hypoplastic thumb, subluxated hypoplastic radial head, cone-shaped epiphyses, Perthes disease, clavicular pseudoarthrosis, celiac disease, abdominal distention, constipation, hirsutism, long eyelashes, spinal dysraphism, cerebral aneurysm, postpubertal menorrhagia, precocious puberty, growth hormone deficiency, hypothyroidism.

NATURAL HISTORY

The facial features are most recognizable in midchildhood. During childhood, height and weight tend to parallel the third percentile. The speech difficulties are severe and relate primarily to motor speech production. A slurred quality to the speech is characteristic. Hypernasality is common and often associated with velopharyngeal incompetence. The majority of children are in special education settings. The three adults live in assisted living situations and hold part-time jobs in unskilled positions and have elementary literacy skills.

ETIOLOGY

This disorder presumably has an autosomal dominant inheritance pattern. Mutations in *SRCAP* which encodes SNF2-related CREBB activator protein are responsible. *SRCAP* serves as a coactivator for CREB-binding protein (CREBBP) which is also known as CBP.

COMMENT

CBP is the gene responsible for Rubinstein-Taybi syndrome which has a number of phenotypic similarities to those of Floating-Harbor syndrome.

References

Leisti J, et al: Case report 12, *Syndrome Identification* 2:3, 1973.

Pelletier G, Feingold M: Case report 1, *Syndrome Identification* 1:8, 1973.

Robinson PL, et al: A unique association of short stature, dysmorphic features and speech impairment (Floating-Harbor syndrome), *J Pediatr* 113:703, 1988.

Patton MR, et al: Floating-Harbor syndrome, *J Med Genet* 28:201, 1991.

Houlston RS, et al: Further observations on the Floating-Harbor syndrome, *Clin Dysmorph* 3:143, 1994.

Lacombe D, et al: Floating-Harbor syndrome: Description of a further patient, review of the literature, and suggestion of autosomal dominant inheritance, *Eur J Pediatr* 154:658, 1995.

Hersh JH, et al: Changing phenotype in Floating-Harbor syndrome, *Am J Med Genet* 76:58, 1998.

Paluzzi A, et al: Ruptured cerebral aneurysm in a patient with Floating Harbor syndrome, *Clin Dysmorphol* 17:283, 2008.

White SM, et al: The phenotype of Floating-Harbor syndrome in 10 patients, *Am J Med Genet A* 152A:821, 2010.

Hood RL, et al: Mutations in SRCAP, encoding SNF2-Related CREBBP activator protein, cause floating-harbor syndrome, *Amer J Human Genet* 90:308, 2012.

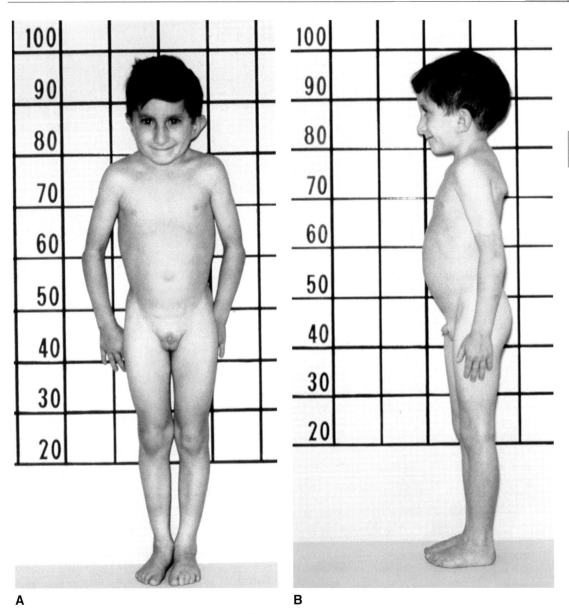

FIGURE 1.   Floating-Harbor syndrome. **A** and **B,** Affected male at 6½ years. Note the proportionate short stature; broad, bulbous nose; and short philtrum. (Courtesy David L. Rimoin, Cedars-Sinai Medical Center, Los Angeles.)

Senile-Like Appearance

PROGERIA SYNDROME (HUTCHINSON-GILFORD SYNDROME)
Alopecia, Atrophy of Subcutaneous Fat, Skeletal Hypoplasia and Dysplasia

The following entry was recorded in the St. James Gazette in 1754: "March 19, 1754 died in Glamorganshire of mere old age and a gradual decay of nature at seventeen years and two months, Hopkins Hopkins, the little Welshman, lately shown in London. He never weighed more than 17 pounds but for three years past no more than twelve." In 1886, Hutchinson described a similar patient. Later, Gilford studied this boy and another patient and termed the condition "progeria," meaning premature aging. DeBusk summarized the findings in 60 cases. Fewer than 50 cases are currently known worldwide.

ABNORMALITIES

Growth. Normal birth size; postnatal growth deficiency becomes evident between 6 and 18 months with subsequent growth rate one third to one half of normal; diminished subcutaneous fat beginning in infancy, last areas of adipose atrophy are cheeks and pubic areas; postnatal microcephaly.

Performance. Normal intelligence, hyperopia, conductive and/or sensorineural hearing loss.

Craniofacial. Facial hypoplasia; prominent eyes; beaked nose; micrognathia; stiff auricular cartilage; small or absent ear lobule; short external auditory canal; delayed eruption of deciduous and permanent dentition; crowding of teeth; ogival palatal arch; anodontia and hypodontia, especially of permanent teeth; discoloration; high incidence of cavities; ankyloglossia; circumoral cyanosis.

Skin. Thin with onset in early to mid-infancy; prominent scalp veins; localized scleroderma-like areas over lower abdomen, upper legs, and buttocks appearing at birth or early infancy; progressive skin hardening; skin dimpling; irregular pigmentary changes over sun-exposed areas that become more prominent with age; alopecia developing in infancy with degeneration of hair follicles; sparse to absent eyelashes and eyebrows.

Nails. Hypoplastic with onset in infancy; nails may be brittle, curved, yellowish.

Limbs. Periarticular fibrosis beginning at 1 to 2 years; stiff or partially flexed prominent joints or both; leads to "horse-riding" stance.

Imaging. Thin calvarium with marked delay in ossification of fontanels; Wormian bones; narrow chest apices; small clavicles; thin ribs; rib fractures; coxa valga; acetabular dysplasia; avascular necrosis of proximal femur, sclerotic changes in the long bones with thinned shafts, reduced corticomedullary ratio, and pathological fractures, particularly of the humerus; progressive loss of bone in clavicle and distal phalanges; delayed bone age; dystrophic calcification. Radiographic findings that become more apparent over time include thinning of ribs, reabsorption of anterior ribs, generalized osteopenia, ulnar minus variant, sagittal suture diastasis, clavicular pseudarthrosis, coxa magna, and enlarged femoral greater trochanter. Cephalometric findings include obtuse angle and steep mandibular plane angle.

OCCASIONAL ABNORMALITIES
Congenital or acquired cataract, microphthalmia, absent breast and nipple, scoliosis, Madelung deformity, bifid rib, ivory epiphyses, dislocated hips, immunologic abnormalities, relatively large thymus, lymphoid and reticular hyperplasia, prolonged prothrombin times, elevated platelet counts, insulin resistance.

NATURAL HISTORY
Although neonatal progeria has been described, the onset of disease manifestations is usually stated as 1 to 2 years. There may be subtle indicators of disease within the first year. The average birth weight for 17 patients is 2.7 kg. The deficit of growth becomes severe after 1 year of age and there is severely delayed sexual maturation. The life span is shortened by the early advent of relentless atherosclerosis associated with hypertension, vascular disease, cardiac valve thickening, transient ischemic attacks, and stroke. The usual cause of death is a cardiovascular event. The average life expectancy is 13 years. Noninvasive measures of vascular dysfunction (carotid-femoral pulse wave velocity and ankle-brachial index) show changes in children as young as 3 years. The tendency to fatigue easily is a factor that limits full participation in childhood activities. Progressive contractures may eventually restrict activities of daily living. Renal ischemia resulting in focal subcortical scars, diffuse glomerulosclerosis, tubular atrophy, and chronic interstitial nephritis occurs in patients surviving into adolescence.

Because intelligence and brain development do not appear to be impaired, children with progeria should be allowed as normal a social life as possible. Low-dose aspirin had been recommended to mitigate vascular events.

ETIOLOGY

Autosomal dominant, new mutation. The classic progeria mutation is a heterozygous c.1824C>T base substitution in *LMNA*, a silent mutation that results in increased usage of a cryptic splice site that deletes 50 amino acids from the lamin A protein, resulting in production and accumulation of progerin, a defective form of lamin A, a constituent of the nuclear membrane. The amino acid deletion renders progerin permanently intercalated into the inner nuclear membrane where it accumulates and exerts progressively more damage to cells as they age. Instances of affected siblings from normal parents are probably the result of gonadal mosaicism.

COMMENT

Three other mutations in *LMNA* have accounted for atypical progeria with either earlier or later ages of onset. There is some clinical overlap with other laminopathies, which has become hard to adjudicate because the diagnosis of progeria is increasingly defined by the presence of the classic mutation.

References

Hutchinson J: Congenital absence of hair and mammary glands with atrophic condition of the skin and its appendages in a boy whose mother had been almost wholly bald from alopecia areata from the age of six, *Trans Med Chir Soc Edinb* 69:473, 1886.

Gilford H: Progeria: A form of senilism, *Practitioner* 73:188, 1904.

Cleveland RH, et al: A prospective study of radiographic manifestations in Hutchinson-Gilford progeria syndrome, *Pediatr Radiol* 42:1089, 2012.

DeBusk FL: The Hutchinson-Gilford progeria syndrome, *J Pediatr* 80:697, 1972.

Eriksson M, et al: Recurrent de novo point mutations in lamin A cause Hutchinson-Gilford syndrome, *Nature* 423:293, 2003.

Merideth MA, et al: Phenotype and course of Hutchinson-Gilford progeria syndrome, *New Eng J Med* 358:592, 2008.

Gerhard-Herman M, et al: Mechanisms of premature vascular aging in children with Hutchinson-Gilford progeria syndrome, *Hypertension* 59:92, 2012.

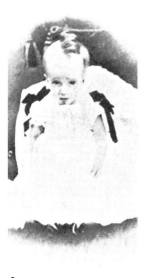 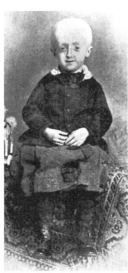 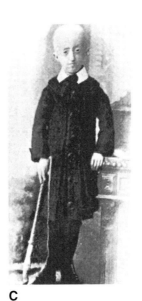 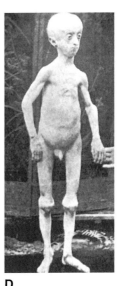

A   **B**   **C**   **D**

FIGURE 1.   Progeria syndrome. **A–D,** Gilford's original patient. (From Gilford H: *Practitioner*, 73:188, 1904, with permission.)

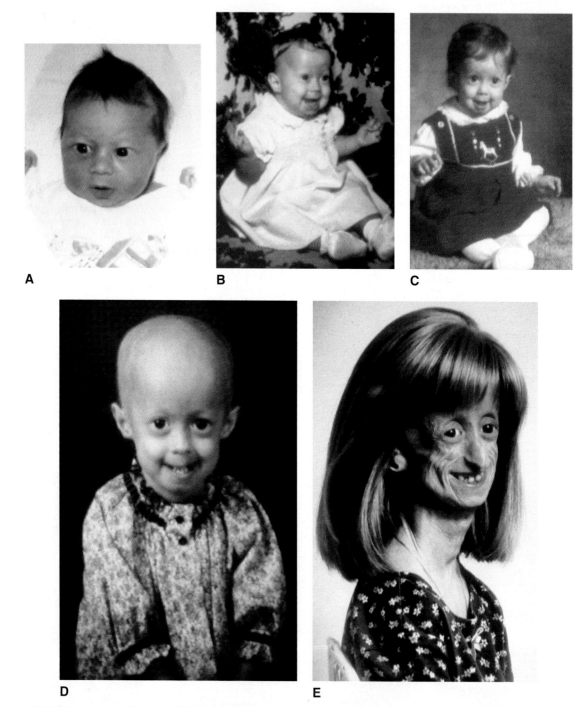

FIGURE 2. **A–E,** An affected child beginning in the neonatal period demonstrates the progression of the phenotype. (From Ackerman J, Gilbert E: *Pediatr Pathol Molec Med* 21:1, 2002, with permission.)

early infancy, and it is not until 2 to 4 years of age that the pattern of anomalies is clearly evident. Personality and behavior tend to correspond to the developmental age, which is delayed. Photosensitivity of the skin may lead to problems with exposure to sunlight. After a variable period of apparent normal growth and development, affected children fail to thrive; decelerate with respect to all growth parameters, eventually becoming cachectic; and develop progressive contractures, kyphosis, hearing loss, and tremors. The most profound intellectual disability is seen in the cases with the earliest onset, smallest heads, and the most severe growth deficiency. The presence of cataracts does not distinguish severity groups. Mean age of mortality in the most severely affected children is 5 years, whereas moderately affected children die at a mean age of 16 years and mildly affected individuals survive into their 30s and have only mild intellectual disability. The most frequent cause of death is pneumonia, followed by kidney failure, seizures, cardiac arrest, liver failure, and stroke.

ETIOLOGY

This disorder has an autosomal recessive inheritance pattern. Mutations in one of two genes, *ERCC6* (65% of cases) and *ERCC8* (35% of cases), cause CS. The protein products of these genes play a critical role in transcription-coupled nucleotide excision repair. This process preferentially targets helix-distorting DNA lesions in actively transcribed genes. Other, as yet unknown functions of these genes likely account for the intellectual disability and growth failure.

COMMENT

In addition to the severe infantile variant of CS, some cases of cerebro-oculo-facio-skeletal (COFS) syndrome are due to mutations in *ERCC6*. COFS presents prenatally with neurogenic congenital contractures, microcephaly, and cataracts. It is a prenatal form of CS. Finally, there exists a Xeroderma Pigmentosum/Cockayne syndrome (XP/CS) complex resulting from mutations in any one of three XP genes. Mutations in two of these genes result in a severe CS phenotype, and mutations in the third result in a mild phenotype. De Sanctis-Cacchione syndrome is a form of XP associated with intellectual disability, profound growth failure, and neurologic deterioration. It is caused by mutations in *ERCC6* and is allelic with CS.

E

References

Cockayne EA: Dwarfism with retinal atrophy and deafness, *Arch Dis Child* 21:52, 1946.

Nance MA, Berry SA: Cockayne syndrome: Review of 140 cases, *Am J Med Genet* 42:68, 1992.

Stefanini M, et al: Genetic analysis of 22 patients with Cockayne syndrome, *Hum Genet* 97:418, 1996.

Troelstra C, et al: *ERCC6*, a member of a subfamily of putative helicases, is involved in Cockayne's syndrome and preferential repair of active genes, *Cell* 71:939, 1992.

Henning KA, et al: The Cockayne syndrome group A gene encodes a WD repeat protein that interacts with CSB protein and a subunit of RNA polymerase II TFIIH, *Cell* 82:555, 1995.

Kraemer KH, et al: Xeroderma pigmentosum, trichothiodystrophy and Cockayne syndrome: A complex genotype-phenotype relationship, *Neuroscience* 145:1388, 2007.

Natale V: A comprehensive description of the severity groups in Cockayne syndrome, *Am J Med Genet A* 155A:1081, 2011.

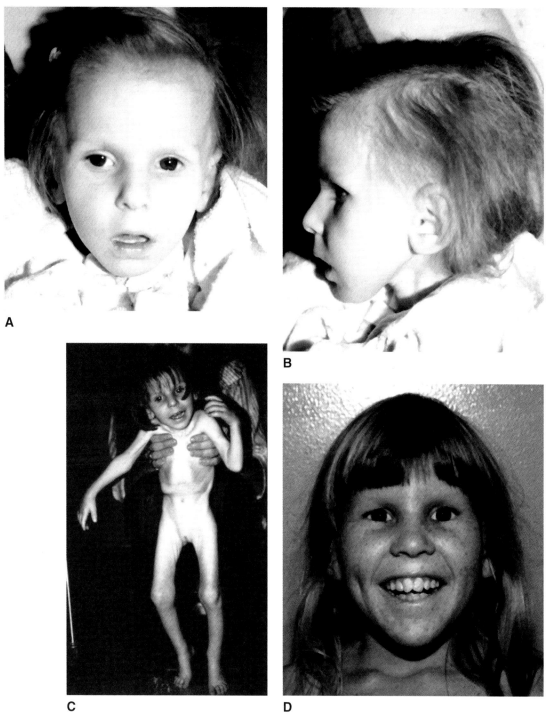

FIGURE 1.   Cockayne syndrome. **A–C,** A 4-year-old girl with severe CS. **D,** A 10-year-old girl with mild CS. Note the loss of facial adipose tissue with slender nose; sunken eyes; thin, dry hair; and evidence of severe neurologic compromise. (**A–D,** Courtesy Dr. Marilyn C. Jones, Children's Hospital, San Diego.)

ROTHMUND-THOMSON SYNDROME
(POIKILODERMA CONGENITALE SYNDROME)
Development of Poikiloderma, Cataract with or without Other Ectodermal Dysplasia

This condition was first described in 1868 by Rothmund, a Munich ophthalmologist who discovered multiple cases among an inbred group of people living in the nearby Alps. More than 300 cases have been reported in the literature.

ABNORMALITIES

Wide variance in expression, the most usual features being the following:

Growth. Small stature of prenatal onset in majority of cases; height and weight at or below 3%; hypogonadism or delayed sexual development (28%).

Craniofacial. Frontal bossing, small saddle nose, prognathism; microdontia and anodontia, ectopic eruption, dental caries (40%), short dental roots, periodontitis.

Eyes. Subcapsular cataract; occasionally corneal dystrophy.

Skin. Irregular erythema progressing to poikiloderma (i.e., telangiectasia, scarring, irregular pigmentation and depigmentation, atrophy); although most marked in sun-exposed areas, skin changes frequently occur on buttocks; hyperkeratotic lesions (33%) may be warty or verrucous; blister formation (20%) occurs before onset of poikiloderma; photosensitivity (35%), hyperkeratosis of palms and soles, cutaneous epithelial neoplasms (5% includes squamous cell carcinoma, basal cell carcinoma, and Bowen disease).

Hair. Sparse, prematurely gray, and occasionally alopecia (80%); thinning of eyebrows and eyelashes occurs initially; scalp, facial, and pubic hair are often only thin.

Nails. Small, dystrophic (32%); pachyonychia.

Skeletal. Small hands and feet (20%), hypoplastic to absent thumbs, syndactyly, forearm reduction defects, absence of patella, clubfeet, osteosarcoma (32%).

Imaging. At least one major radiographic skeletal finding in 75% of cases; abnormal metaphyseal trabeculation; brachymesophalangy; first metacarpal or thumb hypoplasia/agenesis; osteoporosis; radial head dislocation; radial agenesis or hypoplasia; radioulnar synostosis; ulnar hypoplasia or bowing; patella hypoplasia/aplasia; areas of cystic or sclerotic change.

OCCASIONAL ABNORMALITIES

Intellectual disability (3%), microcephaly, hydrocephalus, craniosynostosis, infantile glaucoma, corneal atrophy/scleralization, coloboma, blue sclerae, iris dysgenesis, strabismus, sensorineural hearing loss, cleft palate, hemihypertrophy, hypertension, hypercholesterolemia, hypothyroidism, scoliosis, cryptorchidism, irregular menses, esophageal stenosis, pyloric stenosis, anal stenosis, anteriorly placed anus, annular pancreas, growth hormone deficiency, anhidrosis, skin calcification, bronchiectasis, neutropenia chronic anemia, myelodysplastic to aplastic anemia, leukemia.

NATURAL HISTORY

Feeding or gastrointestinal problems often occur in infancy. Although skin changes were present in six patients at birth, they usually occur between 3 months and 1 year of age. Erythema and blistering develop first on the face and then spread to the buttock and extremities. The progression toward irregular "marbled" hypoplasia, termed "poikiloderma," is mainly noted in the first few years with 89% manifesting poikiloderma by age 2. Cataract most commonly becomes evident between 2 and 7 years of age although cataract is much less frequent than originally suggested. Alopecia progresses and may be complete by the second or third decade. Reduced fertility is frequent, although pregnancy has been reported on several occasions. The major risk to survival is malignancy. Osteosarcoma occurs at a mean age of 14 years. The mean age for skin cancer is 34 years. Regarding management, avoidance of sun exposure and use of sunscreen are mandatory. An annual ophthalologic exam to screen for cataracts is recommended and when initial diagnosis is made, parents should be counseled regarding signs of osteosarcoma, including bone pain, swelling, or an enlarging limb lesion. Radiographs should be performed by 5 years of age, and subsequent radiographs should be taken when merited by clinical signs.

ETIOLOGY

This disorder has an autosomal recessive inheritance pattern. It is genetically heterogeneous. Mutations in the *RECQL4* helicase gene at 8q24.3 account for two thirds of cases. Individuals harboring at least one truncating mutation in *RECQL4* are at increased risk for osteosarcoma and are more likely to have skeletal anomalies. Unlike Bloom syndrome and Werner syndrome, which are also due to mutations in *RECQ* helicase genes and share features of genomic instability and cancer predisposition, no founder mutations have been identified in Rothmund-Thomson syndrome (RTS).

COMMENT

Baller-Gerold syndrome, a craniosynostosis–radial ray reduction disorder is also due to mutations in *RECQL4* and may account for the rare reports of craniosynostosis in RTS. RAPADILINO syndrome, a condition seen primarily in the Finnish population shares with RTS growth deficiency and pigmentary skin abnormalities. It is due to homozygosity for a specific *RECQL4* mutation that is unique to that population. Patients who harbor one of the common truncating mutations in *RECQL4* are always compound heterozygotes.

References

Rothmund A: Ueber Cataracten in Verbindung miteiner eigenthümlichen Hautdegeneration, *Arch Ophthalmol* 14:159, 1868.
Thomson MS: Poikiloderma congenitale, *Brit J Dermatol* 48:221, 1936.

Taylor WB: Rothmund's syndrome–Thomson's syndrome, *Arch Dermatol* 75:236, 1957.

Kitao S: Mutations in *RECQL4* cause a subset of cases of Rothmund-Thomson syndrome, *Nat Genet* 22:82, 1999.

Wang LL, et al: Clinical manifestations in a cohort of 41 Rothmund-Thomson syndrome patients, *Am J Med Genet* 102:11, 2001.

Wang LL, et al: Association between osteosarcoma and deleterious mutations in the *RECQL4* gene in Rothmund-Thomson syndrome, *J Nat Cancer Inst* 95:669, 2003.

Larizza L, et al: Rothmund-Thomson syndrome, *Orphanet J Rare Dis* 5:2, 2010.

Mehollin-Ray AR, et al: Radiographic abnormalities in Rothmund-Thomson syndrome and genotype-phenotype correlation with *RECQL4* mutation status, *AJR Am J Roentgenol* 191:W62, 2008.

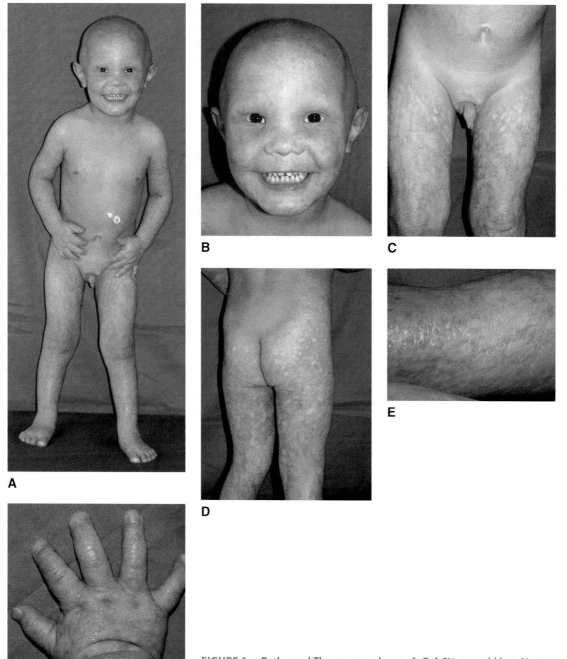

FIGURE 1.   Rothmund-Thomson syndrome. **A–F,** A 2½-year-old boy. Note frontal bossing, absence of lashes, irregular erythema, small hands, and small nails. (Courtesy Dr. Lynne M. Bird, Children's Hospital, San Diego.)

Early Overgrowth with Associated Defects

FRAGILE X SYNDROME (MARTIN-BELL SYNDROME, MARKER X SYNDROME)
Mental Deficiency, Mild Connective Tissue Dysplasia, Macro-Orchidism

In 1943, Martin and Bell published the first pedigree documenting a sex-linked form of mental retardation. Lubs in 1969 showed the presence of a fragile site on the long arm of the X chromosome in affected males and some carrier females in one family. Macro-orchidism without endocrinologic abnormalities was described by Turner and colleagues and Cantu and colleagues in the affected males of a number of families. However, it was not until Sutherland demonstrated that expression of the fragile site was dependent on the nature of the cell culture medium that the association between X-linked mental retardation, macro-orchidism, and the marker X chromosome was made. This subgroup can now be differentiated from other types of X-linked mental retardation.

The disorder appears to be common. An incidence of 1 in 5000 males has been calculated from analysis of newborn blood spots. Among individuals with developmental delay, intellectual disability, and/or autism, between 1% and 3% will have a full mutation. The phenotype is identified most readily in males.

ABNORMALITIES

Growth. Macrocephaly in early childhood; accelerated linear growth in childhood; however, growth velocity slows at adolescence. Obesity with a subset having a Prader-Willi phenotype (hyperphagia and hypogonadism).

Performance. Mild to profound intellectual disability in males with intelligence quotients (IQs) of 30 to 55, but sometimes extending into the mildly retarded to borderline normal range. Hand flapping or biting (60%) and poor eye contact (90%). Cluttered speech in mildly affected males, short bursts of repetitive speech in more severely affected males, and complete lack of speech in severely and profoundly affected males. Strong gaze avoidance, hyperactivity, hyperarousal, anxiety, aggressive outbursts. Sensitivity to stimuli, leading to serious behavior problems in overstimulating situations. Autism spectrum disorder (60%). IQ < 70 in approximately 30% to 50% of females with the full mutation, and IQ < 85 in 50% to 70%. Mean IQ for females 82. Most have shyness and social anxiety.

Craniofacial. Prominent forehead, elongated face, prognathism usually not noted until after puberty, thickening of nasal bridge extending down to the nasal tip, large ears with soft cartilage, pale blue irides, epicanthal folds, high arched palate, dental crowding.

OCCASIONAL ABNORMALITIES
Nystagmus, strabismus, epilepsy, myopia, hypotonia, hyperextensible fingers, mild cutis laxa, soft skin, torticollis, pectus excavatum, kyphoscoliosis, flat feet, cleft palate, mitral valve prolapse, aortic dilation.

NATURAL HISTORY
Life span is normal. Feeding problems and gastroesophageal reflux are common in infancy, as is otitis media. Growth rate is slightly increased in the early years, with delayed motor milestones such that early features may suggest cerebral gigantism. Testicular

size may be increased before puberty, but this increase becomes more obvious postpubertally. Sensory processing disorders are common. Factors such as nurturing home and school environments have been associated with improved performance.

ETIOLOGY

X-linked inheritance. Expansions of a trinucleotide repeat (CGG) in the 5' untranslated region of the *FMR1* gene located at Xq27.3 causes this condition. Normal individuals have from 6 to 54 repeats. Both male and female premutation carriers have 54 to 200 repeats, while affected individuals have greater than 200. Female premutation carriers have a 20% risk for premature ovarian failure and mood and anxiety difficulties. Male premutation carriers also have evidence of anxiety and, with increasing age, may develop deficits in executive function, atypical parkinsonism, cerebellar tremor, and dementia, a constellation of findings referred to as fragile X–associated tremor/ataxia syndrome (FXTAS). Roughly 46% of male and 17% of female premutation carriers develop some signs of FXTAS after age 50. Expansion of premutations to full mutations occurs only in female meiotic transmission and correlates with the size of the premutation. The risk that an individual will be affected clinically is dependent on the position of that individual within the family. Thus the risk that the daughter of a phenotypically normal carrier male will be affected is zero. However, the risk that his daughter's son (his grandson) will be affected is 50%. Most likely based on the phenomenon of X-inactivation, the risk that the daughter of a premutation carrier female will be clinically affected is smaller (approximately 15% to 30% depending on the number of CGG repeats, i.e., the size of the premutation allele). DNA-based molecular analysis allows for identification of both full mutations and permutation carriers.

COMMENT

Expansion of the triplet repeat in *FMR1* leads to DNA methylation and transcriptional silencing. Absence of the gene product, FMRP, a selective m-RNA binding protein, alters translational regulation of its multiple m-RNA partners affecting synaptic plasticity and function in dendrites in the brain. Understanding of the molecular pathogenesis of fragile X is leading to clinical trials of promising therapeutic interventions.

F

References

Lubs HA: A marker X chromosome, *Am J Hum Genet* 21:231, 1969.

Turner G, et al: X-linked mental retardation associated with macro-orchidism, *J Med Genet* 12:367, 1975.

Cantu JM, et al: Inherited congenital normofunctional testicular hyperplasia and mental deficiency, *Hum Genet* 33:23, 1976.

Sutherland GR: Fragile sites on human chromosomes: Demonstration of their independence on the type of tissue culture medium, *Science* 197:265, 1977.

Fu Y, et al: Variation of the CGG repeat at the fragile X site results in genetic instability: Resolution of the Sherman paradox, *Cell* 67:1047, 1991.

Verkerk AJ, et al: Identification of a gene (*FMR-1*) containing a CGG repeat coincident with a breakpoint cluster region exhibiting length variation in fragile X syndrome, *Cell* 67:905, 1991.

Hersh J, et al: Health supervision guidelines for children with fragile X syndrome, *Pediatrics* 127:994, 2011.

Santoro MR, et al: Molecular mechanisms for fragile X syndrome; A twenty-year perspective, *Annu Rev Pathol* 7:219, 2012.

Finucane B, et al: Genetic counseling and testing for *FMR1* gene mutations: Practice guidelines of the National Society of Genetic Counselors, *J Genet Couns* 21:752, 2012.

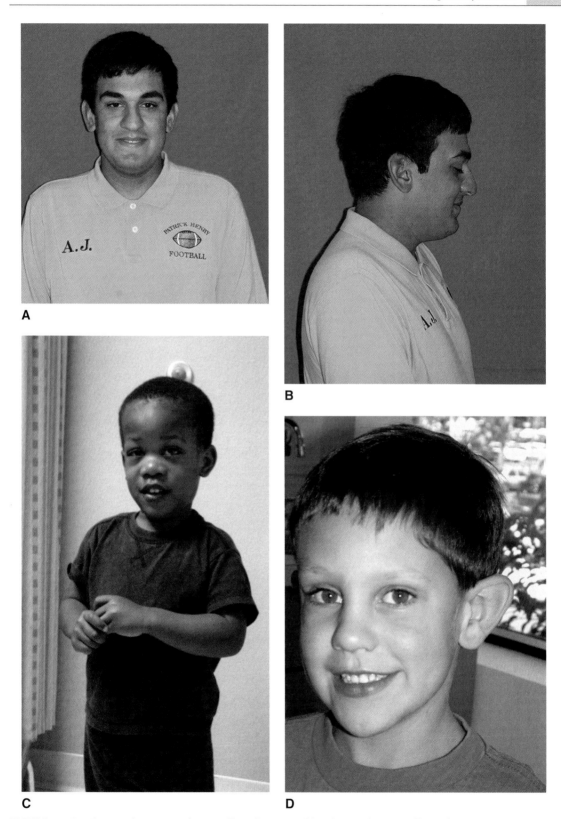

F

FIGURE 1.   Fragile X syndrome. **A** and **B,** An affected 18-year-old male. **C** and **D,** Two affected boys. Note the increased head circumference with prominent forehead, prognathism, and big ears. (**A, B,** and **D,** Courtesy Dr. Lynne M. Bird, Children's Hospital, San Diego.)

SOTOS SYNDROME (CEREBRAL GIGANTISM SYNDROME)
Large Size, Large Hands and Feet, Poor Coordination

Sotos and colleagues described five such patients in 1964, and almost 500 cases have subsequently been reported. The incidence of the condition is estimated at 1 in 10,000 to 1 in 50,000.

ABNORMALITIES

Growth. Prenatal onset of excessive size; at birth, length more likely to be increased than weight; mean full-term birth length 55.2 cm and birth weight 3.9 kg; length increases rapidly, remains at or above 97th percentile throughout childhood and early adolescence, and is more significantly increased than weight; final height often within normal range (average adult height males 182 cm, females 174 cm); relatively large span; large hands and feet (greater than 50th percentile even when plotted for height age); advanced osseous maturation in childhood (84%); macrocephaly of prenatal onset in 50%, by 1 year of age in 100%, persisting into adult life in 86%.

Performance. Variable intellectual disability; IQs of 40 to 129, with a mean of 78; poor coordination; hypotonia; hyperreflexia; delayed gross motor function; significant behavioral abnormalities. In adults, depression, anxiety, social isolation, and hyperactivity.

Craniofacial. Prominent forehead (dolichocephalic); high anterior hairline, sparse hair in frontoparietal region; downslanting palpebral fissures; apparent hypertelorism not always confirmed by measurement; prominent jaw; high, narrow palate with prominent lateral palatine ridges; facial flushing, frequently of nose but also cheeks and perioral region; premature eruption of teeth, dental crowding, hypodontia, deep bite.

Skeletal. Kyphosis, kyphoscoliosis, scoliosis, pes planus, genu valgus.

Imaging. Advanced bone age; abnormalities of the cerebral ventricles, including prominence of the trigone, prominence of the occipital horns, and ventriculomegaly; abnormalities of the corpus callosum with complete or partial agenesis or hypoplasia; increased supratentorial extracerebral fluid spaces; enlarged fluid spaces in the posterior fossa.

Other. Cryptorchidism; thin, brittle fingernails.

OCCASIONAL ABNORMALITIES

Seizures (50% febrile convulsions), electroencephalograph abnormalities, psychosis, strabismus, myopia, nystagmus, optic disc pallor and retinal atrophy, cataracts, iris hypoplasia, glaucoma, cardiac defects (typically atrial septal defect [ASD] and patent ductus arteriosus [PDA]), genitourinary anomalies, diaphragmatic hernia, abnormal glucose tolerance test (14%). Imaging: normal bone age, white matter demyelination, arachnoid cyst.

NATURAL HISTORY

Neonatal problems are frequent, including difficulties with respiration and feeding. An increased incidence of otitis media has been noted, with conductive hearing loss and associated complications. Early developmental milestones are delayed. However, early assessments, which rely heavily on specific motor and verbal skills that are particularly delayed in Sotos syndrome, may well be poor predictors of ultimate intellectual performance. Even in those patients with normal intelligence, delay of expressive language and motor development is characteristically present in infancy. Behavior problems are common. Excessive size, with poor coordination, may lead to problems of social adjustment, often with undue aggressiveness and temper tantrums. Immaturity persisting into adulthood adds to the difficulties with socialization. A variety of psychiatric problems have been noted in some adults. A propensity to fracture with minimal trauma has been documented. A slightly increased risk for malignancy appears to exist (2.2%). Reported tumors include acute leukemia, sacrococcygeal teratoma, neuroblastoma, Wilms tumor, lymphoma, epidermoid carcinoma of vagina, mixed parotid tumor, hepatocarcinoma, hepatoblastoma, blastoma and small cell carcinoma of the lung, yolk sac tumor of the testis, and diffuse gastric carcinoma. Benign tumors include osteochondroma, ganglioglioma, fibromas of the heart and ovary, and presacral ganglioneuroma. Because the sites and types of tumors vary greatly, no routine screening—with the exception of periodic clinical evaluation—seems appropriate.

ETIOLOGY

This disorder has an autosomal dominant inheritance pattern. The majority of cases are sporadic. Mutations in or deletion of *NSD1* (nuclear receptor SET-domain-containing protein) located at 5q35 is responsible for most cases. Gene deletions tend to be associated with greater intellectual disability and more structural anomalies. In the Japanese population, a recurrent 1.9 Mb microdeletion, including *NSD1*, is the most common molecular finding, whereas point mutations are more common in the non-Japanese.

COMMENT

Typical abnormalities have been noted on brain magnetic resonance imaging that can be helpful to diagnosis. Abnormalities of the cerebral ventricles include prominence of the trigone, prominence of the occipital horns, and ventriculomegaly (rarely necessitating shunting). Midline defects include abnormalities of the corpus callosum, with complete or partial agenesis or hypoplasia. The supratentorial extracerebral fluid spaces and the fluid spaces in the posterior fossa are increased in 70% of cases.

References

Sotos JF, et al: Cerebral gigantism in childhood: A syndrome of excessively rapid growth with acromegalic features and a nonprogressive neurologic disorder, *N Engl J Med* 271:109, 1964.

Cole TRP, Hughes HE: Sotos syndrome: A study of the diagnostic criteria and natural history, *J Med Genet* 31:20, 1994.

Douglas J, et al: *NSD1* mutations are the major cause of Sotos syndrome and occur in some cases of Weaver syndrome but are rare in other overgrowth phenotypes, *Am J Hum Genet* 72:132, 2003.

Tatton-Brown K, et al: Genotype-phenotype associations in Sotos syndrome: An analysis of 266 individuals with *NSD1* aberrations, *Am J Hum Genet* 77:193, 2005.

Leventopoulos G, et al: A clinical study of Sotos syndrome patients with review of the literature, *Pediatr Neurol* 40:357, 2009.

Fickie MR, et al: Adults with Sotos syndrome: Review of 21 adults with molecularly confirmed *NSD1* alterations, including a detailed case report of the oldest person, *Am J Med Genet A* 155A:2105, 2011.

F

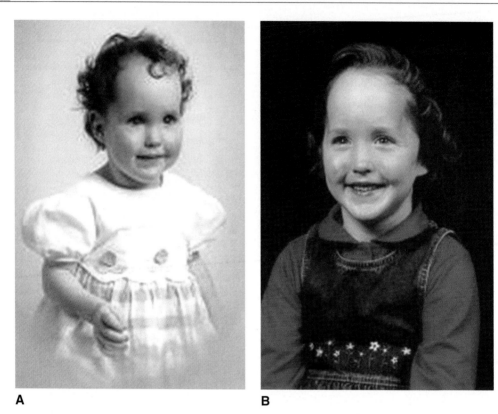

A   **B**

FIGURE 1.   Sotos syndrome. **A–D,** Affected girl from childhood to adolescence. (Courtesy Dr. Angela Lin, Massachusetts General Hospital, Boston.)

Continued

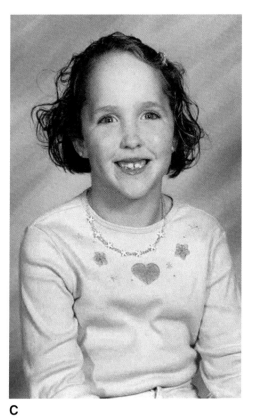

C

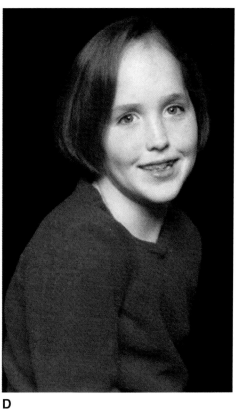

D

F

FIGURE 1, cont'd

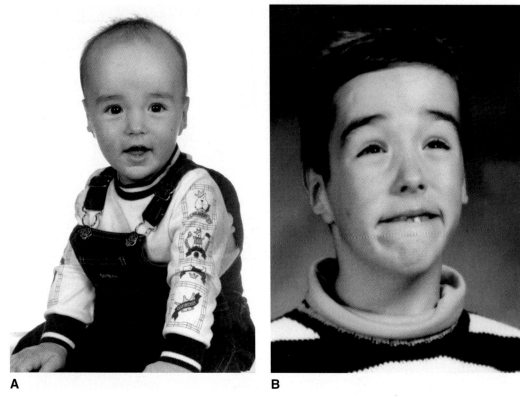

A **B**

FIGURE 2.   A–D, Affected boy from 9 months through 14 years. (Courtesy Dr. Angela Lin, Massachusetts General Hospital, Boston.)

Continued

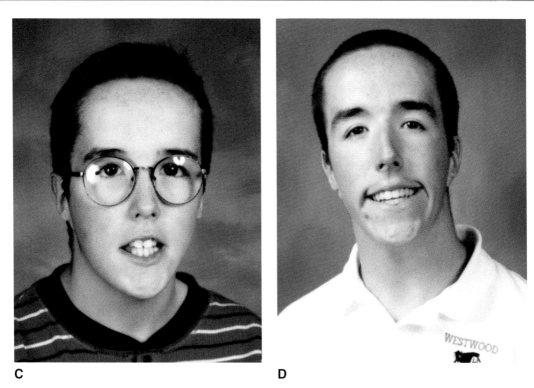

C   D

FIGURE 2, cont'd

F

WEAVER SYNDROME
Macrosomia, Accelerated Skeletal Maturation, Camptodactyly, Unusual Facies

Weaver and colleagues reported two strikingly similar boys with this pattern of overgrowth. Although this condition shares overlapping features with Marshall-Smith and Sotos syndromes, it is clearly a distinct pattern of malformation.

ABNORMALITIES

Growth. Accelerated growth and maturation, of prenatal onset; weight is more significantly increased than height in infancy. However, over time, accelerated skeletal growth is most prominent such that adults are excessively tall. Head circumference, although large, is proportionate to stature.

Performance. Developmental delay or intellectual disability, usually mild (81%); mild hypertonia, coarse low-pitched voice with slurred or dysarthric speech that is delayed in onset; progressive spasticity; poor fine motor coordination and balance.

Craniofacial. Macrocephaly (83%), large bifrontal diameter, flat occiput, ocular hypertelorism, epicanthal folds, depressed nasal bridge, downslanting palpebral fissures, strabismus, large ears, long philtrum, relative micrognathia/retrognathia with a prominent chin crease.

Limbs. Camptodactyly, broad thumbs, thin deep-set nails, prominent fingertip pads, limited elbow and knee extension, clinodactyly leading to overriding of toes, foot deformities including talipes equinovarus, calcaneovalgus, and metatarsus adductus.

Imaging. Accelerated osseous maturation, cervical spine anomalies, ventriculomegaly, delayed myelination, cerebellar hypoplasia, fatty filum terminale, flared metaphyses, especially distal femora and humeri.

Other. Relatively loose skin, pigmented nevi, inverted nipples, thin hair, umbilical hernia, inguinal hernia, cryptorchidism, scoliosis, kyphosis, hypothyroidism, growth hormone deficiency (in adults).

OCCASIONAL ABNORMALITIES

Cardiac defects, cleft palate, atretic ear canal, postaxial polydactyly, hypotonia, instability of the upper cervical spine, seizures, and on imaging diaphragmatic eventration, short ribs, short fourth metatarsals, cyst in the septum pellucidum, cerebral atrophy, enlarged vessels and hypervascularization in the areas of the middle and left posterior cerebral arteries.

NATURAL HISTORY

These children are usually large at birth and show accelerated growth and markedly advanced skeletal maturation during infancy, with carpal centers more advanced than phalangeal centers. In a minority of patients, overgrowth does not develop until a few months of age. Final height 194.2 cm in males and 176.3 cm in females, with occipito-frontal circumference of 61 cm and 59.5 cm in males and females, respectively. Although development is delayed initially, with advancing age, few are described as having clear intellectual disability. Attention deficit and hyperactivity occur occasionally. The lifetime risk for malignancy in Weaver syndrome has been estimated at 11%, although it has been suggested that reporting bias makes this an overestimate. Reported malignancies include leukemia, lymphoma, neuroblastoma, sacrococcygeal teratoma, and endodermal sinus tumor of ovary.

ETIOLOGY

This disorder has an autosomal dominant inheritance pattern. Although the majority of cases are sporadic, Weaver syndrome is genetically heterogeneous. Some cases are due to mutations of *NSD1*, which is the major cause of Sotos syndrome. However, most cases appear to result from de novo mutations in *EZH2*, a histone methyltransferase that acts to repress transcription and has critical roles in stem cell maintenance and cell lineage determination.

COMMENT

Somatic gain-of-function and loss-of-function mutations in EZH2 have been reported in a variety of hematologic malignancies, with activating mutations associated with lymphoma and inactivating mutations associated with myelodysplastic disorders. Since the literature contains no reports of adults older than 30, the actual lifetime risk that an affected individual will develop a malignancy is unknown.

References

Weaver DD, et al: A new overgrowth syndrome with accelerated skeletal maturation, unusual facies, and camptodactyly, *J Pediatr* 84:547, 1974.

Opitz JM, et al: The syndromes of Sotos and Weaver: Reports and review, *Am J Med Genet* 79:294, 1998.

Kelly TE, et al: Cervical spine anomalies and tumors in Weaver syndrome, *Am J Med Genet* 95:492, 2000.

Gibson WT, et al: Mutations in *EZH2* cause Weaver syndrome, *Am J Hum Genet* 90:110, 2012.

Tatton-Brown K, et al: Germline mutations in the oncogene *EZH2* cause Weaver syndrome and increased human height, *Oncotarget* 2:1127, 2011.

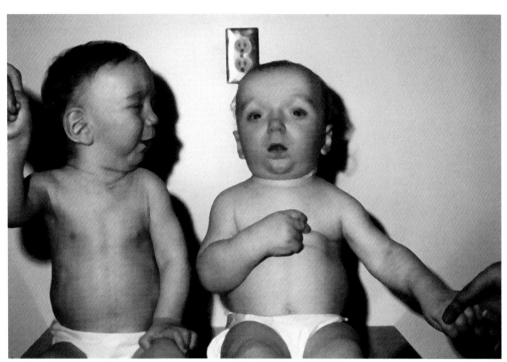

FIGURE 1.   Unrelated affected boys at 18 months and 11 months of age, respectively. (From Weaver DD, et al: *J Pediatr* 84:547, 1974, with permission.)

F

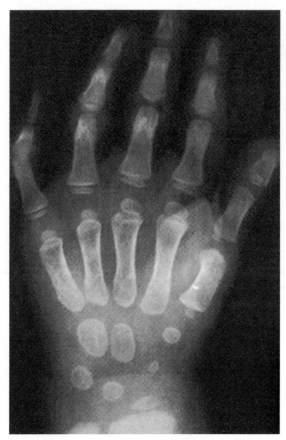

FIGURE 2.   Radiographs showing accelerated osseous maturation and broad distal splaying of femurs. (From Weaver DD, et al: *J Pediatr* 84:547, 1974, with permission.)

Continued

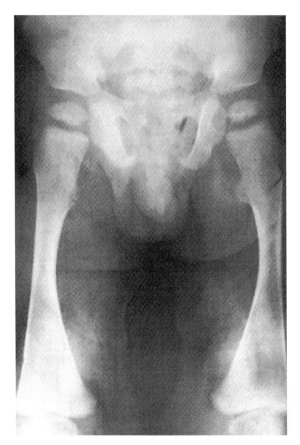

FIGURE 2, cont'd

MARSHALL-SMITH SYNDROME
Accelerated Growth and Maturation, Shallow Orbits, Broad Middle Phalanges

Initially described by Marshall and Smith in 1971, almost 60 patients with this disorder have been reported. Although categorized as an overgrowth syndrome because of large birth size and radiographic evidence of disharmonic advanced skeletal maturation, recent evidence suggests that this disorder involves an intrinsic structural or biochemical defect of cartilage, bone, or connective tissue, rather than generalized or localized cellular hyperplasia.

ABNORMALITIES

Growth. Accelerated linear growth and markedly accelerated skeletal maturation of prenatal onset, underweight for length and failure to thrive in weight. Adults have short stature.

Performance. Moderate to severe intellectual disability, impaired motor development and adaptive functioning, very limited to absent speech, happy demeanor with few maladaptive behaviors.

Craniofacial. Long cranium with prominent forehead; delayed closure of fontanel; shallow orbits with prominent eyes, bluish sclerae, upturned nose, low nasal bridge, small mandibular ramus, micrognathia; large mouth with protruding tongue and full, everted lips over time; progressive coarsening of facies; anterior chamber anomalies; glaucoma.

Skeletal. Kyphoscoliosis, bowed long bones, broad proximal and middle phalanges with narrow distal phalanges; joint laxity and dislocation; nontraumatic fracture; flat feet; calcaneovalgus deformity.

Imaging. Accelerated osseous maturation; long, thin, tubular bones; bullet-shaped middle phalanges; short, narrow, terminal phalanges; osteopenia, sclerotic bones; unusual protrusion of supraoccipital bone and posterior arch of C1, hypoplasia of corpus callosum.

Skin. Hypertrichosis, hyperextensible skin; abnormal scar; ecchymoses.

OCCASIONAL ABNORMALITIES

Choanal atresia, stenosis, or both; abnormal larynx/laryngomalacia; rudimentary epiglottis; dysplastic teeth; craniosynostosis; gingival hyperplasia; deafness and ear anomalies; brain abnormalities, including macrogyria, pachygyria, cerebral atrophy, ventriculomegaly, septo-optic dysplasia; instability of the craniocervical junction with severe spinal stenoses; short sternum; cardiac defect; hypersegmented sacrococcyx; tethered spinal cord; omphalocele; umbilical hernia; pyloric stenosis, diaphragmatic hernia; hydronephrosis; vesicoureteral reflux; cryptorchidism; deep crease between hallux and second toe; immunologic defect, Wilms tumor.

NATURAL HISTORY

Although often large at birth, affected individuals typically fail to thrive, particularly in terms of weight. Life-threatening respiratory problems may occur at any age and include upper airway obstruction (usually at multiple levels: choanal passages, midface, tongue displacement, and airway collapse) and recurrent pneumonia. Although the initially reported cases died by 20 months of age secondary to pneumonia, atelectasis, aspiration, or pulmonary hypertension, aggressive airway management has resulted in long-term survival into adulthood. Many survivors have required tracheostomy. Cervical spine stenosis may result in cord compression requiring decompression. Eyes should be monitored for corneal exposure. Intellectual disability is moderate to severe. Kyphoscoliosis is progressive.

ETIOLOGY

All cases have been sporadic. Heterozygous mutations in *NFIX*, a member of the nuclear factor 1 family of transcription factors, account for some cases of this condition.

COMMENT

Deletions or mutations in *NFIX* that result in haploinsufficiency cause an overgrowth condition resembling Sotos syndrome. The mutations causing Marshall-Smith syndrome appear to produce the disorder through a dominant-negative effect.

References

Marshall RE, et al: Syndrome of accelerated skeletal maturation and relative failure to thrive: A newly recognized clinical growth disorder, *J Pediatr* 78:95, 1971.

Adam MP, et al: Marshall-Smith syndrome: Natural history and evidence of an osteochondrodysplasia with connective tissue abnormalities, *Am J Med Genet A* 137A:117, 2005.

Shaw AC, et al: Phenotype and natural history in Marshall-Smith syndrome, *Am J Med Genet A* 152A:2714, 2010.

Malan V, et al: Distinct effects of allelic NFIX mutations on nonsense-mediated m-RNA decay engender either a Sotos-like or a Marshall-Smith syndrome, *Am J Hum Genet* 87:189, 2010.

Van Balkom IDC, et al: Development and behaviour in Marshall-Smith syndrome: An exploratory study of cognition, phenotype and autism, *J Intellect Disabil Res* 55:973, 2011.

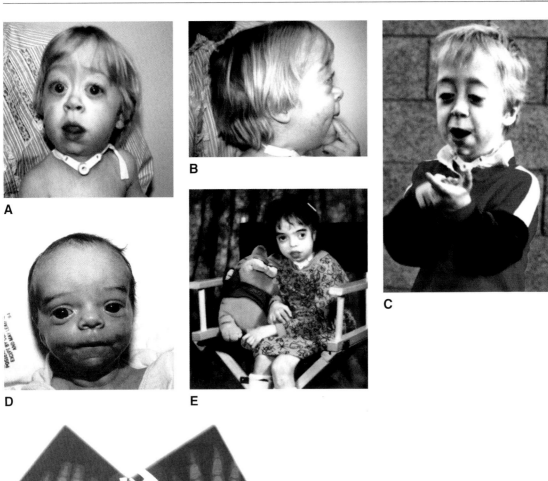

FIGURE 1.   Marshall-Smith syndrome. Affected boy as a neonate and at 7 years (**A–C**) and affected girl as a neonate and at 8 years (**D** and **E**). **A–F,** Note the prominent forehead, shallow orbits with prominent eyes, blue sclera, low nasal bridge, and the hand of one showing an accelerated carpal bone age and broad phalanges. (Courtesy H. Eugene Hoyme, Sanford School of Medicine, University of South Dakota.)

BECKWITH-WIEDEMANN SYNDROME
(EXOMPHALOS-MACROGLOSSIA-GIGANTISM SYNDROME)
Macroglossia, Omphalocele, Macrosomia, Ear Creases

Beckwith and Wiedemann first reported this distinct clinical entity in 1969 and 1964, respectively. The incidence of the condition is reported as 1 in 13,700.

ABNORMALITIES

Growth. Overgrowth beginning in latter half of pregnancy; macrosomia with large muscle mass and thick subcutaneous tissue, hemihyperplasia.

Performance. Development is normal in the absence of chromosome 15p15.5 duplication or serious perinatal complications such as prematurity or refractory hypoglycemia.

Craniofacial. Macroglossia; prominent eyes with relative infraorbital hypoplasia; infraorbital creases; capillary nevus flammeus; central forehead and eyelids; metopic ridge; large fontanels; prominent occiput; malocclusion with tendency toward mandibular prognathism and maxillary underdevelopment; unusual linear fissures in lobule of external ear; indentations on posterior rim of helix.

Internal organs. Large kidneys with renal medullary dysplasia; nephrolithiasis; renal collecting system anomalies; pancreatic hyperplasia, including excess of islets; fetal adrenocortical cytomegaly (a pathognomonic feature); interstitial cell hyperplasia, gonads; pituitary amphophil hyperplasia; cardiomegaly (usually resolves).

Imaging. Accelerated osseous maturation, metaphyseal flaring with overconstriction of diaphyses, diminished tubulation of proximal humerus, nephrocalcinosis.

Other. Neonatal polycythemia, hypoglycemia in early infancy (about one third to one half of cases), omphalocele or other umbilical anomaly, diastasis recti, posterior diaphragmatic eventration, cryptorchidism, cardiovascular defects.

OCCASIONAL ABNORMALITIES

Mild microcephaly, posterior fossa brain anomalies, cleft palate, hepatomegaly, large ovaries/testes, hyperplastic uterus and bladder, bicornuate uterus, hypospadias, clitoromegaly, posterior urethral valves, megaureter, vesicoureteral reflux, immunodeficiency, cardiac hamartoma, cardiomyopathy, hypercalciuria, placentomegaly with excessive extra villous trophoblast, placental mesenchymal dysplasia.

NATURAL HISTORY

Hydramnios and a relatively high incidence of prematurity provide further indication of the rather profound prenatal alterations. Birth weight has averaged 4 kg and length 52.6 cm. Thereafter, length parallels the normal curve at or above the 95th percentile through adolescence. After 9 years of age, mean weight remains between the 75th and 95th percentile. Advanced bone age, most pronounced during the first 4 years, rarely persists until maturity. Spontaneous pubertal development occurs at a normal time. Adults have normal stature. Facial features tend to normalize over time. Severe problems of neonatal adaptation may occur, with apnea, cyanosis, and seizures as symptoms. The large tongue may partially occlude the respiratory tract and lead to feeding difficulties. Infant mortality rate is estimated to be as high as 21%. Detection and treatment of hypoglycemia in any neonate with features of this syndrome are critical. A predisposition for embryonal malignancies exists. Most present by age 8 years although the tumor risk in adults has not been adequately studied. Reported tumors include Wilms tumor, hepatoblastoma, rhabdomyosarcoma, adrenocortical carcinoma, neuroblastoma, gonadoblastoma, pancreatoblastoma, and juvenile fibroadenoma. The risk for tumor is estimated at 7.5% (range 4%–21%). Tumor surveillance screening, including renal ultrasounds and serum alpha-fetoprotein (AFP) every 3 months, has been recommended. The increased risk of malignancy seems to be highest in those children who have hemihypertrophy and nephromegaly. Serum AFP concentration is great in Beckwith-Wiedemann syndrome (BWS) and declines at a slower rate than normal in the first year of life. Affected individuals who survive infancy generally are healthy. Growth may allow adequate oral room for the large tongue. Partial glossectomy has been performed successfully. Evidence suggests the prognathism and dental malocclusion are secondary to the large tongue. Adults may be at risk for hearing loss, aneurismal arterial dilatations (two cases), and male infertility.

ETIOLOGY

Although usually sporadic, autosomal dominant inheritance with preferential maternal transmission has occurred in approximately 10% to 15% of cases. BWS is caused by perturbations of the normal dosage balance of a number of genes clustered at 11p15, a highly imprinted region in the genome. Both genetic (factors that change the structure or copy number of the gene) and epigenetic (factors that influence the function or expression of a gene without changing its structure) play a role. Genetic causes may be heritable, whereas epigenetic causes are not. Genes at 11p15 are organized in two separately controlled imprinted domains.

Domain 1 contains paternally expressed insulin-like growth factor 2 (IGF2) and maternally expressed H19, a noncoding RNA. Mechanisms that increase expression of IGF2—including paternal uniparental disomy (UPD), which also impacts domain 2 (20%); gain of methylation at imprint center 1 (IC1) (5%); and parent-of-origin specific cytogenetic rearrangements and microdeletions in 11p15 (<1%)—all lead to BWS.

Domain 2 contains several imprinted genes, including the growth repressor CDKNIC (10% of sporadic and 40% of familial cases have a mutation of this gene); KCNQ1; and KCNQ1OT1, a paternally expressed transcript that regulates the expression of maternally expressed imprinted genes in domain 2. Loss of methylation at KvDMR (IC2) in the promotor of KCNQ1OT1 accounts for 50% of cases of BWS. Parent-of-origin specific cytogenetic rearrangements and microdeletions also may impact this region. Currently, clinical testing is available for roughly 80% of mechanisms that produce BWS.

COMMENT

BWS has occurred discordantly in a number of monozygotic twins (mostly females with loss of methylation at IC2). BWS secondary to loss of methylation at IC2 is over-represented in pregnancies conceived with assisted reproductive technology, although the absolute risk is low. Individuals with UPD of 11p15.5 or gain of methylation at IC1 have the highest risk for tumor; whereas those with mutations in CDKNIC have the lowest risk. A severe phenotype of BWS usually reflects high levels of paternal UPD for 11p15.5. Some cases of isolated congenital hemihyperplasia represent a forme fruste of BWS.

References

Wiedemann HR: Complexe malformatif familial avec hernie ombilicale et macroglossie—un "syndrome nouveau"? *J Genet Hum* 13:223, 1964.

Beckwith JB: Macroglossia, omphalocele, adrenal cytomegaly, gigantism, and hyperplastic visceromegaly, *Birth Defects* 5(2):188, 1969.

Weksburg R, et al: Disruption of insulin-like growth factor 2 imprinting in Beckwith-Wiedemann syndrome, *Nat Genet* 5:143, 1993.

Tan TY, et al: Tumour surveillance in Beckwith-Wiedemann syndrome and hemihyperplasia: A critical review of the evidence and suggested guidelines for local practice, *J Paediatr Child Health* 42:486, 2006.

Greer KJ, et al: Beckwith-Wiedemann syndrome in adults: Observations from one family and recommendations for care, *Am J Med Genet A* 146A:1707, 2008

Choufani S, et al: Beckwith-Wiedemann syndrome, *Am J Med Genet C* 154C:343, 2010.

Weksberg R, et al: Beckwith-Wiedemann syndrome, *Europ J Hum Genet* 18:8, 2010.

F

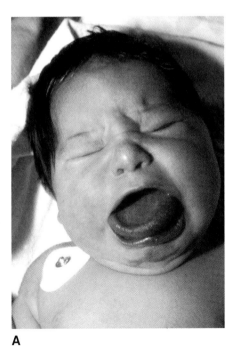
A

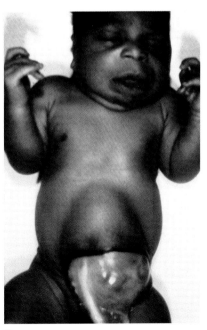
B

FIGURE 1.   Beckwith-Wiedemann syndrome. **A** and **B,** Newborn infants. (Courtesy Dr. Michael Cohen, Dalhousie University, Halifax, Nova Scotia.)

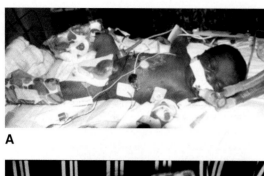

A

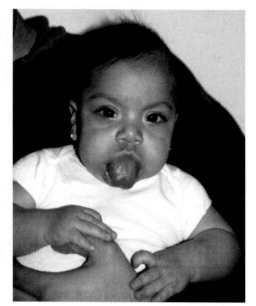

B

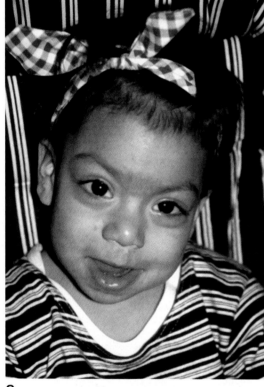

C

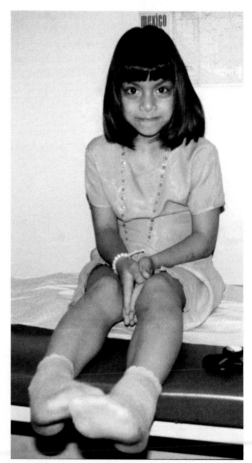

D

FIGURE 2.   A–D, Affected child from birth through 5 years of age. Partial glossectomy was performed at 18 months (see **C**). (Courtesy Dr. Lynne M. Bird, Children's Hospital, San Diego.)

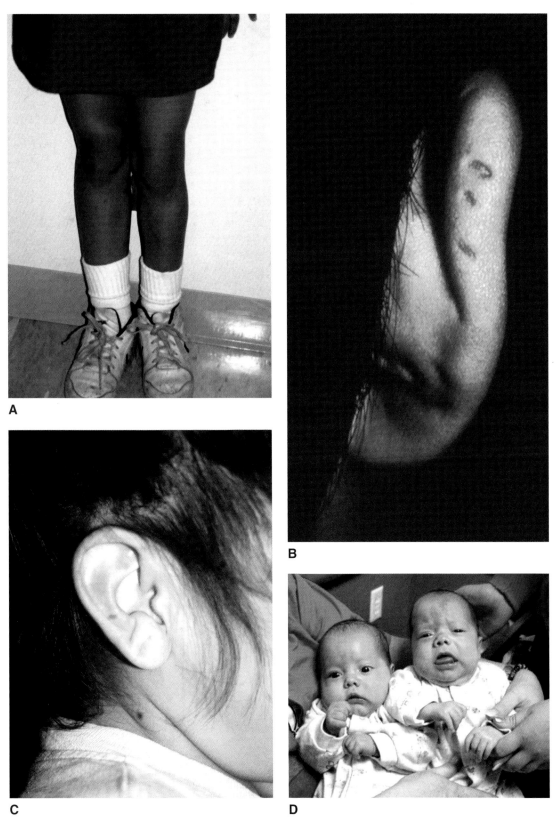

FIGURE 3. **A,** Asymmetry of legs. (Courtesy Dr. Lynne M. Bird, Children's Hospital, San Diego.) **B,** Indentations on the posterior rim of the helix. **C,** Linear crease on the ear lobe. **D,** Newborn monozygotic twins discordant for BWS. (**D,** Courtesy Dr. Cynthia Curry, University of California, San Francisco.)

SIMPSON-GOLABI-BEHMEL SYNDROME

Neri and colleagues and Opitz and colleagues recognized in 1988 that the disorder initially reported by Simpson and colleagues in 1975 was the same as that described in 1984 by both Behmel and colleagues and by Golabi and Rosen. Marked inter- and intrafamilial variability in expression has been documented in this X-linked recessive disorder now referred to as Simpson-Golabi-Behmel syndrome type 1 (SGBS1). Carrier females sometimes have manifestations secondary to skewed X-inactivation. More than 130 patients have been described.

ABNORMALITIES

Performance. Intelligence has varied from severe intellectual disability to normal; average IQ is approximately 1 standard deviation (SD) below the mean; hypotonia.

Growth. Prenatal onset of overgrowth; polyhydramnios; birth weight as high as 5.9 kg; in seven of eight affected adults, height was greater than the 97th percentile and ranged from 188 cm to 210 cm; bone age, initially increased, becomes normal.

Craniofacial. Macrocephaly, present at birth, continues in childhood; coarse facies; downslanting palpebral fissures; ocular hypertelorism; epicanthal folds; furrowed skin over glabella; broad flat nasal bridge with short nose (in infants); macrostomia; macroglossia; midline groove of lower lip; furrowed tongue; broad secondary alveolar ridge; cleft lip and/or submucous cleft palate; bifid uvula; micrognathia (in infants); prognathism (older individuals); low-set posteriorly rotated ears.

Limbs. Postaxial polydactyly of hands, brachydactyly, syndactyly of second and third fingers and toes, nail hypoplasia (particularly of index finger), broad thumbs and great toes.

Imaging. Vertebral segmentation defects, including fusion of posterior elements of C2/C3, cervical ribs, six lumbar vertebrae, and sacral and coccygeal defects; advanced bone age; deep V-shaped sella turcica.

Other. Short webbed neck, cardiac conduction defects, supernumerary nipples, pectus excavatum cryptorchidism, spotty perioral or palatal pigmentation, thickened or dark skin, diastasis recti, umbilical or inguinal hernias.

OCCASIONAL ABNORMALITIES

Indentations on posterior rim of helix; preauricular pits and tags; conductive hearing loss; strabismus, cataracts, coloboma of optic disk; scoliosis; cleft of xiphisternum; preaxial polydactyly of feet; camptodactyly; clinodactyly; scoliosis; cystic hygroma; congenital hip dislocation; clubfeet; short limbs; laryngeal web; subglottal stenosis; gastrointestinal anomalies, including intestinal malrotation, choledochal cyst, diaphragmatic hernia, pyloric ring, polysplenia, hepatosplenomegaly, and increased number of islets of Langerhans; genitourinary anomalies, including large kidneys, cystic kidneys, duplication of renal pelvis, mild hydronephrosis with lobular cystic kidneys, bifid scrotum, and hypospadias; cardiac defects, including ventricular septal defect, pulmonic stenosis, transposition of great vessels, and PDA; central nervous system abnormalities, including agenesis of corpus callosum, hypoplasia of cerebellar vermis, Chiari malformation, and hydrocephalus; seizures; embryonal tumors; diffuse neonatal hemangiomatosis; vascular malformation; carotid artery dissection (adult).

NATURAL HISTORY

Hypoglycemia and airway obstruction from the combined effects of macroglossia and hypotonia may manifest in infancy. Intellectual performance may be normal, but severe intellectual disability has been described. An increased risk exists for development of Wilms tumor, neuroblastoma, hepatoblastoma, hepatocellular carcinoma, and testicular gonadoblastoma.

ETIOLOGY

This disorder has an X-linked recessive inheritance pattern. Most cases have been attributed to mutations or deletion of one or more exons in the glypican-3 gene (*GPC3*) located at Xq26. Glypican 3 is thought to play an important role in growth control in embryonic mesodermal tissue. Duplications in the adjacent gene, *GPC4*, without deletion or mutation in *GPC3* were identified in the original family of Golabi and Rosen.

COMMENT

A severe neonatal form, termed SGBS type 2, has been described in which babies with facial and limb anomalies suggesting SGBS, die in utero or in the neonatal period from cor pulmonale, congenital heart defects or conduction defects, diaphragmatic hernias, overwhelming sepsis, ciliary dysfunction, or hypoglycemia from increased insulin production. The severe form has been mapped to Xp22 and is due to mutation in *CXORF5*, also called *OFD1*, making this condition allelic to oral-facial digital syndrome type 1.

References

Simpson JL, et al: A previously unrecognized X-linked syndrome of dysmorphia, *Birth Defects* 11:18, 1975.

Behmel A, et al: A new X-linked dysplasia gigantism syndrome: Identical with the Simpson dysplasia syndrome? *Hum Genet* 67:409, 1984.

Golabi M, Rosen L: A new X-linked mental retardation-overgrowth syndrome, *Am J Med Genet* 17:345, 1984.

Neri G, et al: Simpson-Golabi-Behmel syndrome: An X-linked encephalo-tropho-schisis syndrome, *Am J Med Genet* 30:287, 1988.

Pilia G, et al: Mutations in *GPC3*, a glypican gene, cause the Simpson-Golabi-Behmel overgrowth syndrome, *Nat Genet* 12:1, 1996.

Budny B, et al: A novel X-linked recessive mental retardation syndrome comprising macrocephaly and ciliary dysfunction is allelic to oral-facial-digital type 1 syndrome, *Hum Genet* 120:171, 2006.

Waterson J, et al: Novel duplication in glypican-4 as an apparent cause of Simpson-Golabi-Behmel syndrome, *Am J Med Genet A* 152A:3179, 2010.

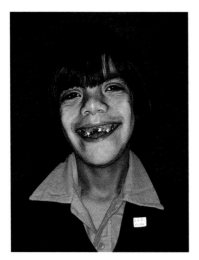
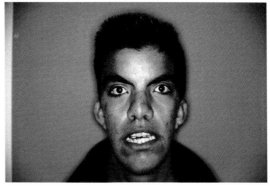
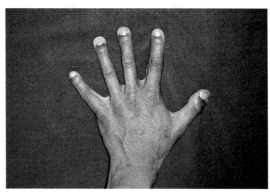

FIGURE 1. Simpson-Golabi-Behmel syndrome. Affected boy at 7 and 16 years of age. Note the ocular hypertelorism, broad flat nose, 2-3 syndactyly, and nail hypoplasia. (From Golabi M, Rosen L: *Am J Med Genet* 17:345, 1984, with permission. Copyright 1984. Reprinted with permission of Wiley-Liss, Inc., a subsidiary of John Wiley & Sons, Inc.)

AMYOPLASIA CONGENITA DISRUPTIVE SEQUENCE

Arms Extended with Flexion of Hands and Wrists, Shoulders Internally Rotated with Decreased Muscle Mass, Bilateral Equinovarus, Variable Contractures of Other Major Joints

ABNORMALITIES

Facies. Round face with micrognathia, small up-turned nose, midline vascular malformation.

Shoulders. Rounded and sloping with decreased muscle mass, internally rotated.

Upper Limbs. Elbows usually in extension with wrists and hands flexed ("policeman tip" position). Severe flexion contractures at metacarpophalangeal joints with mild contractures at interphalangeal joints.

Lower Limbs. Hips, usually flexed, dislocated, adducted, or abducted; knees, flexed or extended; feet, usually equinovarus positioning bilaterally; many combinations of hip and knee positions observed.

Other. Stiff, straight spine.

OCCASIONAL ABNORMALITIES

Cord wrapping of limb, amniotic bands, smashed digits, loss or amputation of digits, cryptorchidism, hypoplastic labia, dimples at contracture sites, torticollis, scoliosis, hernias, gastroschisis, nonduodenal intestinal atresia, defects of muscular layer of trunk and abdominal musculature, Poland sequence, Moebius anomaly, hypoplasia of deltoids and biceps, hemangiomas.

NATURAL HISTORY

There is decreased movement in utero. Seventy percent of pregnancies have first-trimester complications such as bleeding, flu, or fever. Delivery is often difficult and breech presentation is common. Fractures of the limbs secondary to traumatic delivery occur. Intelligence is usually normal unless birth trauma due to stiff joints has occurred. There is decreased bone growth of involved limbs, and there may be increased flexion and pterygium at large joints with time. By 5 years of age, the majority of patients (85%) become ambulatory with good

physical therapy. It is important to begin physical therapy and occupational therapy early to mobilize any muscle tissue present (particularly intrinsic muscles). Splinting and casting are used to maintain and improve range of joint mobility. More than two thirds will require orthopedic surgery, an average of 5.7 procedures per child. All four limbs are involved in the majority of patients; in those with only legs involved, there is an excess of males with bowel atresia and in those with arms alone involved there is an excess of females with gastroschisis. Four percent have three limbs involved: both arms and the right leg or both legs and the left arm. Most will attend regular classrooms at appropriate grade levels and most will be independent in their activities of daily living.

ETIOLOGY

This disorder is sporadic. There is a higher incidence than expected in identical twins, with only one affected. Based on the fact that many of the associated abnormalities have been shown to be caused by an intrauterine vascular accident, it is most likely that hypotension with multiple origins is involved, including placental, maternal, and embryo/fetal factors as well as bleeding, drugs, trauma, and infections. Prenatal diagnosis with use of serial real-time ultrasonography, looking for abnormal movement, could be used to allay parental anxiety.

References

Howard R: A case of congenital defect of the muscular system and its association with congenital talipes equinovarus, *Proc Soc Med* 1:157, 1907.

Hall JG, Reed SD, Driscoll EP: Part I. Amyoplasia: A common sporadic condition with congenital contractures, *Am J Med Genet* 15:571, 1983.

Hall JG, et al: Part II: Amyoplasia: Twinning in amyoplasia—a specific type of arthrogryposis with an apparent excess of discordantly affected identical twins, *Am J Med Genet* 15:591, 1983.

Reid COMV, et al: Association of amyoplasia with gastroschisis, bowel atresia and defects of the muscular layer of the trunk, *Am J Med Genet* 24:701, 1986.

Robertson WL, et al: Further evidence that arthrogryposis multiple congenita in the human sometimes is caused by an intrauterine vascular accident, *Teratology* 45:345, 1992.

Sells JM, et al: Amyoplasia, the most common type of arthrogryposis: The potential for good outcome, *Pediatrics* 97:225, 1996.

Hall JG: Amyoplasia: A problem with angiogenesis? In David W. *Smith Workshop on Malformations and Morphogenesis*, Lake Arrowhead, Calif, 2011.

G

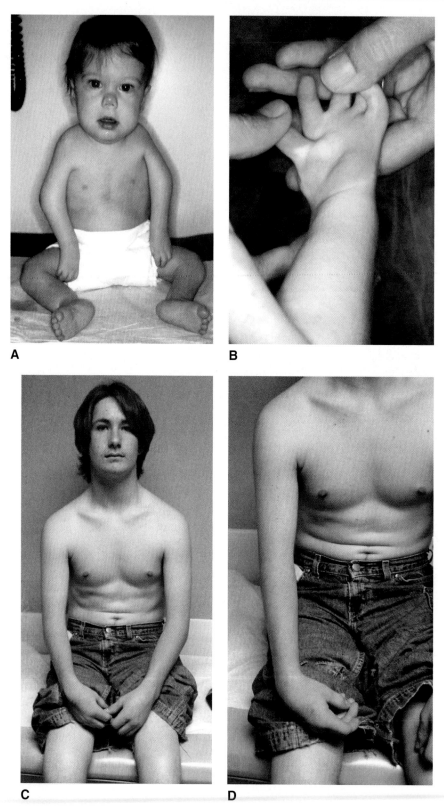

FIGURE 1. Amyoplasia congenita disruption sequence. **A–G,** Note the round face and micrognathia, "policeman tip" position of the arm and hand, the decreased muscle mass and internal rotation of the shoulders, and camptodactyly. (**G,** Courtesy Dr. Lynne M. Bird, Children's Hospital, San Diego.)

Continued

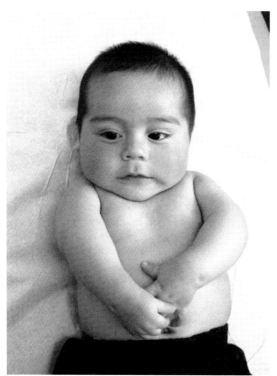

E

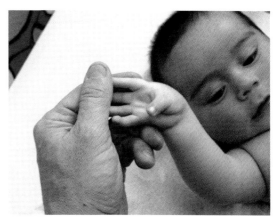

F

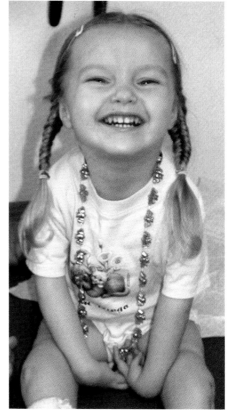

G

FIGURE 1, cont'd

DISTAL ARTHROGRYPOSIS SYNDROME, TYPE 1
Distal Congenital Contractures, Clenched Hands with Medial Overlapping of the Fingers at Birth, Opening of Clenched Hands with Ulnar Deviation

In 1932, Lundblom described a mother and her son with congenital ulnar deviation and flexion of the fingers. In addition, the son had a calcaneovalgus positioning of the feet. Hall recognized this condition as an entity in 1982 in her report of 37 patients with congenital contractures of the distal joints. Two groups of patients were recognized: type I (typical) and type II (atypical), based on the association of other specific anomalies. Bamshad and colleagues have revised and extended the classification to include type 1 (formerly DA type I) through type 10.

ABNORMALITIES

Hands. Neonate's hands are clenched tightly in a fist, with thumb adduction and medially overlapping fingers; hypoplastic/absent flexion creases; ulnar deviation and camptodactyly.
Feet. Position deformities (88%): bilateral calcaneovalgus (33%), bilateral equinovarus (25%), combinations (30%).
Hips. Hip involvement (38%): congenital dislocations, decreased abduction, mild flexion, contracture deformities.
Knees. Mild flexion contractures (30%).
Shoulders. Stiff at birth (17%).

OCCASIONAL ABNORMALITIES
Trismus, mild scoliosis, limited range of motion of proximal joints, small calves, dimples, cryptorchidism, hernias.

NATURAL HISTORY
"Trisomy 18 position" of hand at birth in vast majority. Variable talipes involvement. The hands eventually unclench and may have residual camptodactyly and ulnar deviation. Twenty percent of adults have straight and fully functional fingers. Both neurologic examinations and intelligence are normal. There is remarkably good response to treatment in all joints.

ETIOLOGY
This disorder has an autosomal dominant inheritance pattern with extensive intrafamilial and interfamilial variability. The parent of an affected child might possibly express the gene through mild hand contractures only. Documentation of the genetic basis of DA1 has been elusive. Mutations in 3 contractile genes have been identified in either a single patient or family with DA1. These include *TPM2*, *TNNI2*, and *TNNT3*. In addition, mutations in skeletal muscle slow-twitch myosin binding protein C1 (*MYBPC1*) have been identified in 2 familial cases as well as a mutation in *MYH3*, a gene coding for the heavy chain of myosin, in another family.

COMMENT
Nine additional disorders, all autosomal dominant, have been designated as distal arthrogryposis (DA) syndromes and are listed subsequently.

DA2A. Freeman-Sheldon syndrome (see page 294).
DA2B. Sheldon-Hall syndrome. Less severe than DA2A but more severe than DA1. Affected individuals have vertical talus; ulnar deviation; severe camptodactyly; and a distinctive facies, including a triangular shape, prominent nasolabial folds, downslanting palpebral fissures, small mouth, and a prominent chin. However, no patients have had a pinched mouth or "H-shaped" dimpling of the chin. Inheritance is autosomal dominant. Mutations in one of three skeletal muscle contractile genes—*MYH3*, *TPM2*, *TNNI2,* and *TNNT3*—are responsible. In addition, in one other patient who lacked any of the known DA2B mutations a de novo microdeletion in 8q21 was found.
DA3. Gordon syndrome. Distal arthrogryposis in association with short stature, cleft palate, submucous cleft palate or bifid uvula, ptosis, epicanthal folds, mild facial asymmetry, and short neck (see Hall et al, 1982).
DA4. Distal arthrogryposis in association with scoliosis (see Hall et al, 1982).
DA5. Distal arthrogryposis in association with short stature; unusual stance with short heel cords and pes cavus; short neck; ptosis; immobility of face with or without keratoconus and decreased ocular range of movement; smooth, shiny, tapering fingers with mild camptodactyly; restrictive chest disease (see Hall et al, 1982).
DA6. Distal arthrogryposis in association with sensorineural hearing loss (see Stewart and Bergstrom, 1971).
DA7. Hecht syndrome (see page 308).
DA8. Autosomal dominant multiple pterygium syndrome (see McKowen and Harris, 1982).
DA9. Beals congenital contractural arachnodactyly (see page 618).
DA10. Plantar flexion contractures associated with mild contractures of hips, elbows, wrists, and fingers (see Stevenson et al, 2006).

References

Lundblom A: On congenital ulnar deviation of the fingers of familial occurrence, *Acta Orthop Scand* 8:393, 1932.

Stewart JM, Bergstrom L: Familial hand abnormality and sensorineural deafness: A new syndrome, *J Pediatr* 78:102, 1971.

Hall JG, Reed SD, Greene D: The distal arthrogryposes: Delineation of new entities—review and nosologic discussion, *Am J Med Genet* 11:185, 1982.

McKeown CME, Harris R: An autosomal dominant multiple pterygium syndrome, *J Med Genet* 25:96, 1982.

Bamshad M, et al: A revised and extended classification of the distal arthrogryposis, *Am J Med Genet* 65:277, 1996.

Krakowiak PA: Clinical analysis of a variant of Freeman-Sheldon syndrome (DA2B), *Am J Med Genet* 76:93, 1998.

Sung SS, et al: Mutations in genes encoding fast-twitch contractile proteins cause distal arthrogryposis syndromes, *Am J Hum Genet* 72:681, 2003.

Stevenson DA, et al: A new distal arthrogryposis syndrome characterized by plantar flexion contractures, *Am J Med Genet A* 140A:2797, 2006.

Gurnett CA, et al: Myosin binding protein C1: A novel gene for autosomal dominant distal arthrogryposis type 1, *Hum Mol Genet* 19:1165, 2010.

Alvarado DM, et al: Exome sequencing identifies an *MYH3* mutation in a family with distal arthrogryposis type 1, *J Bone Joint Surg Am* 93:1045, 2011.

Hofmann K, et al: 7 MB de novo deletion within 8q21 in a patient with distal arthrogryposis type 2B (DA2B), *European J of Med Genet* 54:e495–e500, 2011.

G

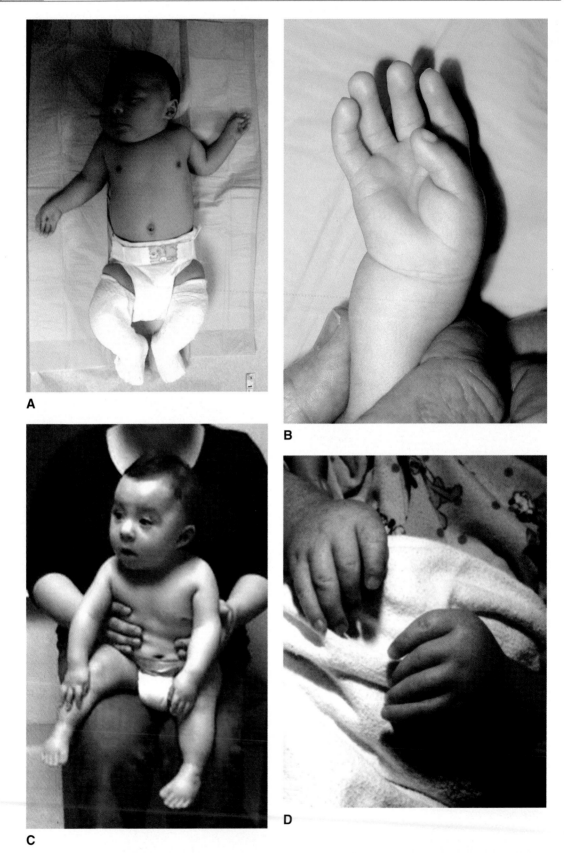

FIGURE 1. Distal arthrogryposis syndrome, type 1. **A–C,** Note the joint contractures involving hands and feet in a child at birth and at 7 months of age. **D,** Camptodactyly in an affected neonate.

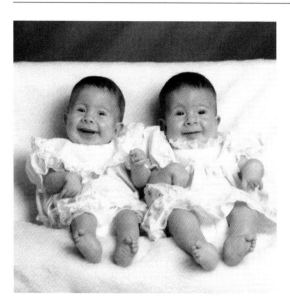

FIGURE 2.   Distal arthrogryposis syndrome, type 2B. Monozygotic twins at 9 months of age. (From Krakowiak PA, et al: *Am J Med Genet* 76:93, 1998, with permission.)

G

PENA-SHOKEIR PHENOTYPE (FETAL AKINESIA/HYPOKINESIA SEQUENCE)
Arthrogryposis, Pulmonary Hypoplasia, Craniofacial Anomalies

In 1974, Pena and Shokeir identified an early lethal disorder involving multiple joint contractures, facial anomalies, and pulmonary hypoplasia with an autosomal recessive mode of inheritance. Subsequently, a number of similar patients have been described. Hall has suggested that this clinical phenotype is secondary to decreased in utero movement, no matter what the cause. As such, it is etiologically heterogeneous and is similar to the fetal akinesia deformation sequence, a pattern of structural defects described by Moessinger in rats that had been curarized in utero. Through an extensive review of published cases, Hall in 2009 delineated 20 distinct familial types.

ABNORMALITIES

Growth. Prenatal onset of growth deficiency; head circumference is frequently spared.

Craniofacial. Rigid expressionless face; prominent eyes; hypertelorism; telecanthus; epicanthal folds; poorly folded, small, and posteriorly angulated ears; depressed nasal tip; small mouth; high-arched palate; micrognathia.

Limbs. Multiple ankylosis (e.g., elbows, knees, hips, and ankles), ulnar deviation of the hands, rocker-bottom feet, talipes equinovarus, camptodactyly, absent or sparse dermal ridges, with frequent absence of the flexion creases on the fingers and palms.

Lungs. Pulmonary hypoplasia.

Genitalia. Cryptorchidism.

Other. Apparent short neck; polyhydramnios, short-gut syndrome with malabsorption, small or abnormal placenta, relatively short umbilical cord.

OCCASIONAL ABNORMALITIES

Cleft palate, cardiac defect.

NATURAL HISTORY

Some of these babies are born prematurely. Those born at term are invariably small for the estimated dates. Approximately 30% are stillborn. Although the majority of those live-born die of the complications of pulmonary hypoplasia within the first month of life, it is important to recognize that the ultimate prognosis for children with this disorder depends on the cause of the decreased fetal movement. The central nervous system and most skeletal muscles are normal with the exception of disuse atrophy.

ETIOLOGY

An autosomal recessive inheritance has been implied in more than one half of the published cases. However, recognition that this phenotype does not have a single etiology makes accurate recurrence risk counseling difficult. A 0% or 25% risk for recurrence seems most appropriate in a sporadic case.

COMMENT

Nineteen additional familial disorders have been recognized, based on differences in natural history and autopsy finding (see Hall 2009). The predominant features of all types are secondary to decreased intrauterine movement. In three of these—referred to as lethal congenital contracture syndrome (LCCS) types 1, 2, and 3—the altered gene has been identified. LCCS-1 is caused by mutations in *GLE* located at 9q34, LCCS-2 is caused by mutations in *ERBB3* located at 12q13, and LCCS-3 is caused by mutations of *PIP5K1C* located at 19p13. All three disorders have an autosomal recessive mode of inheritance.

References

Pena SDJ, Shokeir MHK: Syndrome of camptodactyly, multiple ankyloses, facial anomalies and pulmonary hypoplasia: A lethal condition, *J Pediatr* 85:373, 1974.

Pena SDJ, Shokeir MHK: Syndrome of camptodactyly, multiple ankyloses, facial anomalies and pulmonary hypoplasia: Further delineation and evidence of autosomal recessive inheritance. In Bergsma D, Schimke RM, editors: *Cytogenetics, Environment and Malformation Syndromes*, New York, 1976, Alan R. Liss, pp 201.

Dimmick JE, et al: Syndrome of ankylosis, facial anomalies and pulmonary hypoplasia: A pathologic analysis of one infant. In Bergsma D, Lowry RB, editors: *Embryology and Pathogenesis and Prenatal Diagnosis*, New York, 1977, Alan R. Liss, pp 133.

Chen H, et al: The Pena-Shokeir syndrome: Report of five cases and further delineation of the syndrome, *Am J Med Genet* 16:213, 1983.

Moessinger AL: Fetal akinesia deformation sequence: An animal model, *Pediatrics* 72:857, 1983.

Lindhout D, Hageman G, Beemer FA: The Pena-Shokeir syndrome: Report of nine Dutch cases, *Am J Med Genet* 21:655, 1985.

Hall JG: Invited editorial comment: Analysis of Pena-Shokeir phenotype, *Am J Med Genet* 25:99, 1986.

Lav E, et al: Fetal akinesia deformation sequence (Pena-Shokeir phenotype) associated with acquired intrauterine brain damage, *Neurology* 47:1467, 1991.

Brueton LA, et al: Asymptomatic maternal myasthenia as a cause of the Pena-Shokeir phenotype, *Am J Med Genet* 92:1, 2000.

Hall JG: Pena-Shokeir phenotype (fetal akinesia deformation sequence) revisited, *Birth Defects Res (Part A)* 85:677, 2009.

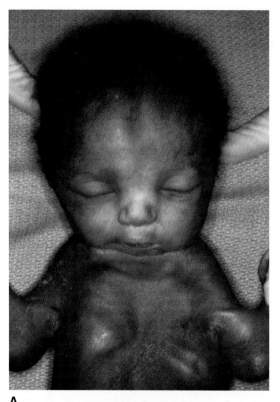

A

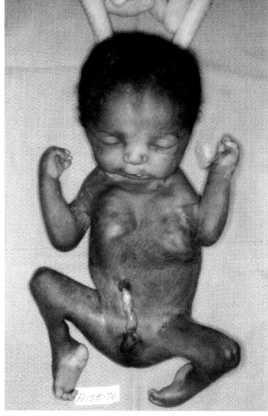

B

G

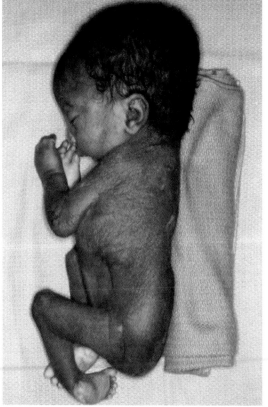

C

FIGURE 1. Lethal multiple pterygium syndrome. **A–C,** Stillborn infant with ocular hypertelorism, epicanthal folds, multiple joint contractures, and pterygia bridging virtually all joints.

NEU-LAXOVA SYNDROME

Microcephaly/Lissencephaly, Canine Facies with Exophthalmos, Syndactyly with Subcutaneous Edema

Neu and colleagues reported three siblings with microcephaly and multiple congenital abnormalities in 1971. An additional family with three affected siblings from a first-cousin mating was reported by Laxova and colleagues in 1972. At least 70 cases have been reported subsequently.

ABNORMALITIES

Growth. Prenatal onset of marked growth deficiency (100%).

Central Nervous System. Microcephaly (84%); lissencephaly (40%); absence of corpus callosum (53%); hypoplasia of cerebellum (53%) and hypoplasia of pons; absence of olfactory bulbs.

Facies. Sloping forehead (100%); ocular hypertelorism (94%); protruding eyes with absent lids (40%); flattened nose; round, gaping mouth and thick everted lips; micrognathia (97%); large ears; short neck.

Skin. Yellow subcutaneous tissue covered by thin, transparent, scaling skin and edema (85%); ichthyosis (50%).

Limbs. Short limbs, syndactyly of fingers and toes (60%), extreme puffiness of hands and feet, overlapping of digits, calcaneovalgus, vertical talus, flexion contractures of major joints with pterygia (79%), poorly mineralized bones.

Other. Cataracts (25%), microphthalmia, persistence of some embryonic structures of eye, absent eyelashes and head hair, muscular atrophy with hypertrophy of fatty tissue, hypoplastic or atelectatic lungs, hypoplastic genitalia (50%), polyhydramnios, short umbilical cord, small placenta.

OCCASIONAL ABNORMALITIES

Hydranencephaly, spina bifida, Dandy-Walker malformation, hypoplastic cerebrum, choroid plexus cysts, hypodontia, patent foramen ovale and ductus arteriosus, atrial septal defect, ventricular septal defect, transposition of great vessels, cleft lip, cleft palate, hepatomegaly, renal agenesis, bifid uterus, cryptorchidism.

NATURAL HISTORY

The majority of patients are stillborn or die in the immediate neonatal period. Three infants survived 7 weeks, 2 months, and 6 months, respectively. The usual cause of death is respiratory failure or sepsis secondary to skin breakdown.

ETIOLOGY

This disorder has an autosomal recessive inheritance pattern.

References

Neu RL, et al: A lethal syndrome of microcephaly with multiple congenital anomalies in three siblings, *Pediatrics* 47:610, 1971.

Laxova R, Ohdra PT, Timothy JAD: A further example of a lethal autosomal recessive condition in siblings, *J Ment Def Res* 16:139, 1972.

Curry CJR: Letter to the editor: Further comments on the Neu-Laxova syndrome, *Am J Med Genet* 13:441, 1982.

Shved IA, Lazjuk GI, Cherstovoy ED: Elaboration of phenotypic changes of the upper limbs in the Neu-Laxova syndrome, *Am J Med Genet* 20:1, 1985.

Ostrovskaya TI, Lazjuk GI: Cerebral abnormalities in the Neu-Laxova syndrome, *Am J Med Genet* 30:747, 1988.

Shapiro I, et al: Neu-Laxova syndrome: Prenatal ultrasonographic diagnosis, clinical and pathological studies, and new manifestations, *Am J Med Genet* 43:602, 1992.

King JAC, et al: Neu-Laxova syndrome: Pathological evaluation of a fetus and review of the literature, *Pediatr Pathol Lab Med* 15:57, 1995.

Manning MA, et al: Neu-Laxova syndrome: Detailed prenatal diagnostic and post-mortem findings and literature review, *Am J Med Genet A* 125A:240, 2004.

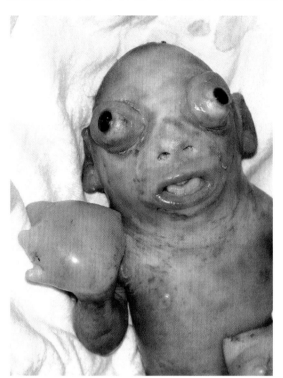

A

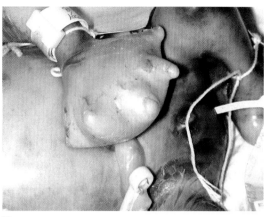

B

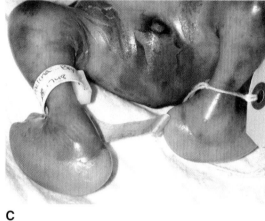

C

FIGURE 1.   Neu-Laxova syndrome. **A–C,** Newborn with microcephaly, sloping forehead, protruding eyes with absent lids, flat nose, gaping mouth and thick lips, scaling skin with edema, extreme puffiness of hands and feet, syndactyly, and joint contractures. (From Manning M, et al: *Am J Med Genet A* 125A:240, 2004, with permission.)

G

RESTRICTIVE DERMOPATHY

Initially described in two infants by Toriello and colleagues in 1983, this disorder has now been reported in approximately 60 patients. Most of the features are constraint-related, the result of restricted in utero movement secondary to the defective skin.

ABNORMALITIES

Growth. Intrauterine growth deficiency.

Craniofacial. Enlarged fontanels, hypertelorism, entropion, small pinched nose, small mouth with ankylosis of the temporomandibular joints, mouth fixed in the "O" position, micrognathia, dysplastic ears.

Skin. Tightly adherent, thin, translucent skin with prominent vessels; erosion may be present; fissures often occur in groin, axilla, and neck; nails may be short or very long; eyelashes, eyebrows, and lanugo are sparse or absent; head hair may be normal; histologically there is hyperkeratosis, delayed maturation of the pilosebaceous and eccrine sweat apparatus, and absence of elastin; the epidermis and subcutaneous fat layer are thickened; the dermis is thin with dense, thin collagen fibers in parallel with the epidermis; there is absence of the rete ridges.

Skeletal. Multiple joint contractures; rocker-bottom feet; bipartite clavicles, ribbon-like ribs, overtubulated long bones of the arms, and a poorly mineralized skull are present on radiographs.

Other. Polyhydramnios, enlarged placenta with short umbilical cord, premature rupture of membranes, absent or small nails, increased anteroposterior diameter of chest, pulmonary hypoplasia.

OCCASIONAL ABNORMALITIES

Natal teeth, microcephaly, short palpebral fissures, eyelid ectropion, choanal atresia, submucous cleft palate, cleft palate, hypospadias, ureteral duplication, dorsal kyphoscoliosis, camptodactyly, adrenal hypoplasia, patent ductus arteriosus, atrial septal defect, dextrocardia.

NATURAL HISTORY

Pregnancy is frequently abnormal with polyhydramnios and decreased fetal activity usually beginning at about 6 months' gestation. Prematurity is common. The majority of affected individuals are stillborn as a result of pulmonary hypoplasia. Intubation is extremely difficult because of the temporomandibular joint ankylosis. Most survivors die within the first week. The longest survival time has been 120 days.

ETIOLOGY

The majority of cases are caused by autosomal recessive *ZMPSTE24* mutations and, less frequently, to de novo dominant mutations in the lamin A gene (*LMNA*). Mutations in both of these genes lead to defective functioning of lamin A, resulting in the characterization of restrictive dermopathy as a laminopathy.

References

Toriello HV, et al: Autosomal recessive aplasia cutis congenita—report of two affected sibs, *Am J Med Genet* 15:153, 1983.

Witt DR, et al: Recessive dermopathy: A newly recognized autosomal recessive skin dysplasia, *Am J Med Genet* 24:631, 1986.

Reed MH, et al: Restrictive dermopathy, *Pediatr Radiol* 23:617, 1992.

Verloes A, et al: Restrictive dermopathy, a lethal form of arthrogryposis multiplex with skin and bone dysplasias: Three new cases and review of the literature, *Am J Med Genet* 43:539, 1992.

Mau U, et al: Restrictive dermopathy: Report and review, *Am J Med Genet* 71:179, 1997.

Wesche WA, et al: Restrictive dermopathy: Report of a case and review of the literature, *J Cutan Pathol* 28:211, 2001.

Smigiel R, et al: Novel frameshift mutations of the *ZMPSTE24* gene in two siblings affected with restrictive dermopathy and review of the mutations described in the literature, *Am J Med Genet A* 152A:447, 2010.

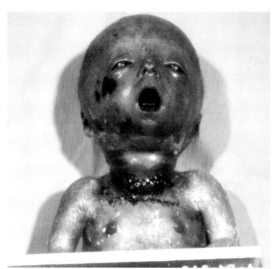

A

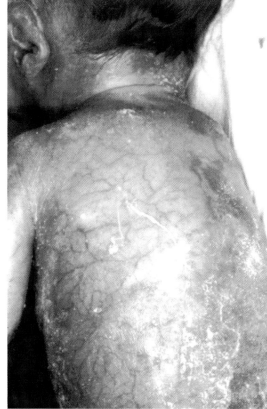

B

G

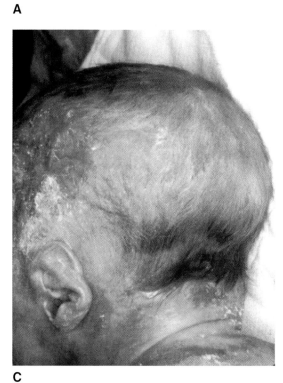

C

FIGURE 1.   Restrictive dermopathy. **A–C,** A newborn infant. Note the small nose, translucent dermis, and flat helix with auricle attached to skin of scalp. (From Toriello HV, et al: *Am J Med Genet* 15:153, 1983. Reprinted with permission of Wiley-Liss, Inc., a subsidiary of John Wiley & Sons, Inc.)

MECKEL-GRUBER SYNDROME (DYSENCEPHALIA SPLANCHNOCYSTICA)

Originally described by Meckel in 1822, later by Gruber, and more recently brought to recognition by Opitz and Howe, more than 200 cases of this severe disorder have been reported. It is now known that Meckel-Gruber syndrome is caused by primary cilia dysfunction and is thus characterized as a ciliopathy.

ABNORMALITIES

Growth. Variable prenatal growth deficiency.
Central Nervous System. Occipital encephalomeningocele; microcephaly with sloping forehead, cerebral and cerebellar hypoplasia; anencephaly; hydrocephaly with or without an Arnold-Chiari malformation; absence of olfactory lobes, olfactory tract, corpus callosum, and septum pellucidum.
Facial. Microphthalmia; cleft palate; micrognathia; ear anomalies, especially slanting type.
Neck. Short.
Limbs. Polydactyly (usually postaxial), talipes.
Kidney. Dysplasia with varying degrees of cyst formation.
Liver. Bile duct proliferation, fibrosis, cysts.
Genitalia. Cryptorchidism, incomplete development of external and/or internal genitalia.

OCCASIONAL ABNORMALITIES

Craniofacial. Craniosynostosis (possibly secondary), coloboma of iris, hypoplastic optic nerve, hypotelorism or hypertelorism, hypoplastic to absent philtrum and/or nasal septum, cleft lip—sometimes midline.
Mouth. Lobulated tongue, cleft epiglottis, neonatal teeth.
Neck. Webbed.
Limbs. Relatively short bowed limbs, syndactyly, simian crease, clinodactyly.
Cardiac. Septal defect, patent ductus arteriosus, coarctation of aorta, pulmonary stenosis.
Lungs. Hypoplasia.
Other. Dandy-Walker malformation, single umbilical artery, patent urachus, omphalocele, intestinal malrotation, enlarged missing and/or accessory spleens, defects in laterality, adrenal hypoplasia, imperforate anus, missing or duplicated ureters, absence or hypoplasia of urinary bladder, enlarged placenta.

NATURAL HISTORY AND MANAGEMENT

These patients seldom survive longer than a few days to a few weeks. Death may be related to the severe central nervous system defects and/or renal defects.

ETIOLOGY

Meckel-Gruber syndrome has an autosomal recessive inheritance pattern, with no recognized expression in the presumed carriers of the gene. Mutations in seven genes—*MKS1, TMEM67, TMEM216, CEP290, CC2D2A, RRPGIP1L,* and *B9D1*—have been reported as responsible. Many of the involved proteins have been localized to the centrosome, the pericentriolar region, or the cilium itself. This disorder is thus referred to as a ciliopathy. A number of other disorders, including Bardet-Biedl syndrome, oral-facial-digital syndrome type I, Alstrom syndrome, hydrolethalus syndrome, and Joubert syndrome, are also due to genes that affect ciliary function and are also referred to as ciliopathies.

COMMENT

Surprising variability of the clinical features exists. In a study of affected siblings of probands, 100% had cystic dysplasia of the kidneys. However, 63% had occipital encephaloceles and only 55% had polydactyly; 18% had no brain anomaly.

References

Meckel JR: Beschreibung zweier durch sehr ähnliche Bildungsabweichung ensteller Geschwister, *Deutsch Arch Physiol* 7:99, 1822.

Gruber GB: Beiträge zur Frage "gekoppelter" missbildungen (Akrocephalosyndactylie und Dysencephalia splanchnocystica), *Beitr Pathol Anat* 93:459, 1934.

Opitz JM, Howe JJ: The Meckel syndrome (dysencephalia splanchnocystica, the Gruber syndrome), *Birth Defects* 5:167, 1969.

Hsia YE, Bratu M, Herbordt A: Genesis of the Meckel syndrome (dysencephalia splanchnocystica), *Pediatrics* 48:237, 1971.

Meckel S, Passarge E: Encephalocele, polycystic kidneys, and polydactyly as an autosomal recessive trait simulating certain other disorders: The Meckel syndrome, *Ann Genet (Paris)* 14:97, 1971.

Fraser FC, Lytwyn A: Spectrum of anomalies in the Meckel syndrome, or "Maybe there is a malformation syndrome with at least one constant anomaly." *Am J Med Genet* 9:67, 1981.

Seppänen U, Herva R: Roentgenologic features of the Meckel syndrome, *Pediatr Radiol* 13:329, 1983.

Salonen R: The Meckel syndrome: Clinicopathological findings in 67 patients, *Am J Med Genet* 18:671, 1984.

Nyberg DA, et al: Meckel-Gruber syndrome. Importance of prenatal diagnosis, *J Ultrasound Med* 9:691, 1990.

Tallila J, et al: Mutation spectrum of Meckel syndrome genes: One group of syndromes or several distinct groups? *Hum Mutat* 30:E813, 2009.

Valente EM, et al: Mutations in *TMEM216* perturb ciliogenesis and cause Joubert, Meckel and related syndromes, *Nat Genet* 42:619, 2010.

Hopp K, et al: *B9D1* is revealed as a novel Meckel syndrome (*MKS*) gene by targeted exon-enriched next-generation sequencing and deletion analysis, *Hum Mol Genet* 20:2524, 2011.

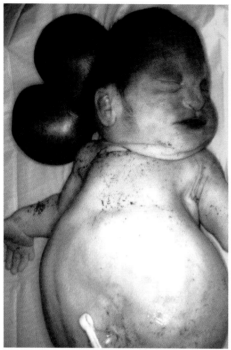

A

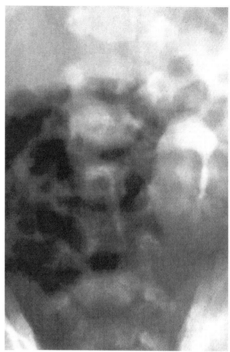

B

G

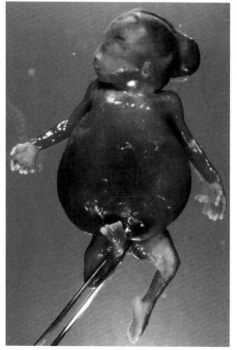

C

FIGURE 1.   Meckel-Gruber syndrome. **A,** A 2-day-old male infant with palpable enlarged kidney who was having frequent seizures and other evidence of central nervous system abnormality. **B,** Intravenous pyelogram showed no visualization on one side and an aberrant calyceal system on the other side. The baby died at 4½ months of age, the oldest known survivor with this syndrome. (**B,** Patient of E. Hutton, Anchorage, Alaska.) **C,** Stillborn infant with posterior encephalocele, postaxial polydactyly, and flank masses caused by massively enlarged cystic kidneys.

PALLISTER-HALL SYNDROME
Hypothalamic Hamartoblastoma, Hypopituitarism, Imperforate Anus, Postaxial Polydactyly

In 1980, Hall and colleagues described six unrelated newborn infants with this pattern of malformation. All died in the neonatal period. However, in subsequent reports, prolonged survival has been documented frequently.

ABNORMALITIES

Growth. Mild intrauterine growth retardation.

Central Nervous System. Hypothalamic hamartoblastoma located on the inferior surface of the cerebrum, extending from the optic chiasma to the interpeduncular fossa, replacing the hypothalamus and other nuclei originating in the embryonic hypothalamic plate; pituitary aplasia/dysplasia; panhypopituitarism.

Craniofacial. Flat nasal bridge and midface with midline capillary hemangioma; short nose; anteverted nares; bathrocephaly; external ear anomalies, including posteriorly rotated, absent external auditory canals, microtia, malformed pinnae, and simple auricles; micrognathia.

Mouth. Multiple frenuli between alveolar ridge and buccal mucosa.

Respiratory. Bifid, hypoplasia, or absence of epiglottis; dysplastic tracheal cartilage; absent lung; abnormal lung lobation.

Limbs. Nail dysplasia, variable degrees of syndactyly and postaxial polydactyly involving both hands and feet; oligodactyly; small, distally placed fourth metacarpal with one or two small fingers associated with it; third metacarpal less frequently affected; fourth metatarsal dysplastic; distal shortening of limbs, particularly the arms.

Anus. Anal defects, including imperforate anus and variable degrees of rectal atresia.

Other. Renal ectopia/dysplasia; congenital heart defects, including endocardial cushion defect, patent ductus arteriosus, ventricular septal defect, mitral and aortic valve defects, and proximal aortic coarctation; pituitary dysplasia/hypopituitarism.

OCCASIONAL ABNORMALITIES

Holoprosencephaly with associated midline cleft lip and palate; arrhinencephaly; Dandy-Walker malformation, polymicrogyria, occipital encephalocele; cleft lip, palate, or uvula; laryngeal cleft; microphthalmia; coloboma; microglossia; natal teeth; narrow cervical vertebrae; hemivertebrae, fused ribs, and multiple manubrial ossification centers; subluxation of the radius; congenital hip dislocation; subluxation of knee; fibular hypoplasia; forearm bowing; blunted metaphyses; acromesomelic limb shortening; simian crease; camptodactyly; hypoplasia of pancreas; underdevelopment of thyroid gland; testicular hypoplasia with micropenis; bifid scrotum, hypospadias; hydrometrocolpos and/or vaginal atresia.

NATURAL HISTORY

Although Pallister-Hall syndrome is not invariably lethal, death before 3 years of age is not uncommon. The major cause of death in the newborn period is hypoadrenalism. Many of the long-term survivors have required L-thyroxine, growth hormone, and corticosteroids from an early age as well as glucose infusions in the neonatal period. The complete spectrum of this disorder is variable. It is now clear that hypothalamic hamartomas and neonatal death are not obligatory features; a number of affected individuals have reproduced, and normal mental capacity has been observed.

ETIOLOGY

This disorder has an autosomal dominant inheritance pattern with variability of expression. A thorough evaluation of the parents of affected children, including brain MRI in some cases, should be performed in order to provide appropriate recurrence risk counseling. Mutations of *GLI3*, which is located on 7p13, are responsible for this disorder. Mutations in the same gene are responsible for the Greig cephalopolysyndactyly syndrome.

References

Hall JG, et al: Congenital hypothalamic hamartoblastoma, hypopituitarism, imperforate anus, and postaxial polydactyly. A new syndrome? Part I: Clinical, causal, and pathogenetic considerations, *Am J Med Genet* 7:47, 1980.

Clarren SK, Alvord EC, Hall JG: Congenital hypothalamic hamartoblastoma, hypopituitarism, imperforate anus, and postaxial polydactyly: A new syndrome? Part II: Neuropathological considerations, *Am J Med Genet* 7:75, 1980.

Culler FL, Jones KL: Hypopituitarism in association with postaxial polydactyly, *J Pediatr* 104:881, 1984.

Iafolla K, et al: Case report and delineation of the congenital hypothalamic hamartoblastoma syndrome (Pallister-Hall syndrome), *Am J Med Genet* 33:489, 1989.

Finnigan DP, et al: Extending the Pallister-Hall syndrome to include other central nervous system malformations, *Am J Med Genet* 40:395, 1991.

Biesecker LG, Graham JM: Pallister-Hall syndrome, *J Med Genet* 33:585, 1996.

Kang S, et al: *GLI3* frameshift mutations cause autosomal dominant Pallister-Hall syndrome, *Nat Genet* 15:266, 1997.

Roscioli T, et al: Pallister-Hall syndrome: Unreported skeletal features of a *GLI3* mutation, *Am J Med Genet A* 136A:390, 2005.

Narumi Y, et al: Genital abnormalities in Pallister-Hall syndrome: Report of two patients and review of the literature, *Am J Med Genet A* 152A:3143, 2010.

G

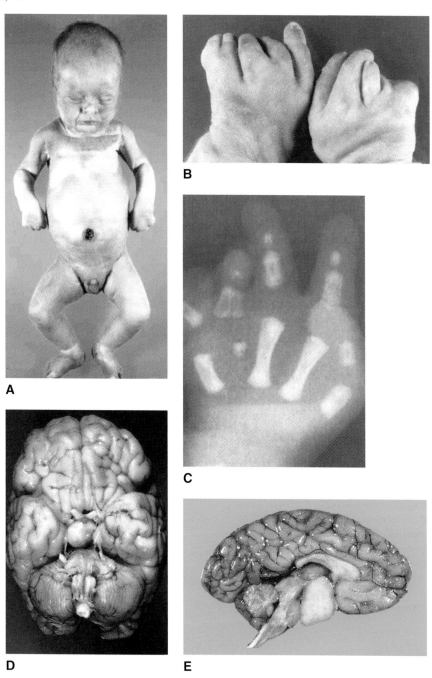

FIGURE 1.   Pallister-Hall syndrome. **A–C,** Male infant who died at 7 days of age. He has camptodactyly, nail dysplasia, postaxial polydactyly, syndactyly, lack of ossification of distal phalanges, and a hypoplastic fourth metacarpal giving rise to two phalanges. **D** and **E,** Note the hamartoblastoma apparent on the inferior cerebral surface and in the sagittal section. (**A–E,** From Hall JG, et al: *Am J Med Genet* 7:47, 1980, with permission. Reprinted with permission of Wiley-Liss, Inc., a subsidiary of John Wiley & Sons, Inc.)

GÓMEZ–LÓPEZ-HERNÁNDEZ SYNDROME
(CEREBELLO-TRIGEMINAL DYSPLASIA, CEREBELLO-TRIGEMINAL-DERMAL DYSPLASIA)
Parieto-Temporal Alopecia, Trigeminal Anesthesia, Rhombencephalosynapsis

Gómez and subsequently López-Hernández described three unrelated children with a similar pattern of malformation, including postnatal growth deficiency, microcephaly, parieto-temporal alopecia, turribrachycephaly with lambdoid synostosis, trigeminal anesthesia. To date, roughly 25 cases have been reported in the literature.

ABNORMALITIES

Growth. Mild prenatal and significant postnatal growth deficiency, microcephaly.

Performance. Mild to moderate cognitive disability. ataxia, jerky movements, head bobbing, central hypotonia with peripheral hypertonia, trigeminal anesthesia, absent corneal reflex, seizures.

Behavior. Self-abusive behavior, attention deficit disorder, bipolar disorder, aggressive behavior, impulsiveness.

Craniofacial. Turribrachycephaly, craniosynostosis (particularly lambdoid sutures), wide anterior fontanel, parieto-temporal alopecia with underdeveloped pili-sebaceous structures and no scarring, corneal opacities, strabismus, ocular hypertelorism, downslanting palpebral fissures, low-set posteriorly rotated or protruding ears, midface hypoplasia, small nose, smooth philtrum, thin upper lip.

Limbs. Hypoplastic/absent thumb. Altered thenar crease. Decreased movement interphalangeal thumb joint, fifth finger clinodactyly, hypoplastic radius and ulna, cubitus valgus, metatarsus adductus.

Genitalia. Hypoplastic labia.

Imaging. Rhombencephalosynapsis (single horseshoe-shaped cerebellar hemisphere, fused cerebellar peduncles, deficient vermis, fused dentate nucleus), ventriculomegaly, arachnoid cyst, absent septum pellucidum, dysgenesis of corpus callosum, brainstem hypoplasia.

OCCASIONAL ABNORMALITIES

Ptosis. nystagmus, retinal detachment, bifid uvula, brisk reflexes, spasticity, dysmetria, dysarthria, growth hormone deficiency, gastroesophageal reflux, single azygous anterior cerebral artery, lipoma of quadrigeminal plate.

NATURAL HISTORY

The majority of affected individuals have significant intellectual disability, although normal cognitive function has also been reported. Trigeminal anesthesia may lead to recurrent facial injuries.

ETIOLOGY

Unknown. All cases to date have been sporadic. Chromosomes have been normal in all patients evaluated. Two patients have had normal comparative genomic hybridization (CGH) arrays.

COMMENT

At least two cases have been identified on prenatal ultrasound imaging, one with ventriculomegaly and a second with cerebellar hypoplasia, later confirmed on MRI to be the result of rhombencephalosynapsis.

References

Fernández-Jaén A, et al: Gomez-Lopez-Hernandez syndrome: Two new cases and review of the literature, *Pediatr Neurol* 40:58–62, 2009.

Gómez MR: Cerebellotrigeminal and focal dermal dysplasia: A newly recognized neurocutaneous syndrome, *Brain Dev* 1:253–256, 1979 (original report).

Gomy I, et al: Two new Brazilian patients with Gómez-López-Hernández syndrome: Reviewing the expanded phenotype with molecular insights, *Am J Med Genet A* 146A:649–657, 2008.

López-Hernández A: Craniosynostosis, ataxia, trigeminal anaesthesia and parietal alopecia with pons-vermis fusion anomaly (atresia of the fourth ventricle). Report of two cases, *Neuropediatrics* 13:99–102, 1982.

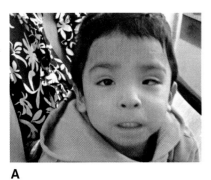
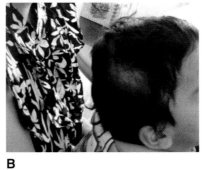
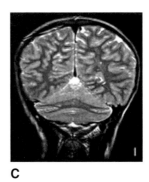

A   B   C

FIGURE 1.   Gómez–López-Hernández. **A** and **B,** Note the parieto-occipital alopecia, strabismus, ocular hypertelorism, smooth philtrum, and thin upper lip. (Courtesy R. Clark, Loma Linda University.) **C,** Rhombencephalosynapsis is noted on the MRI. (From Tully H, et al: *Am J Med Genet* 158:2393, 2012.)

G

X-LINKED HYDROCEPHALUS SPECTRUM
(X-LINKED HYDROCEPHALUS SYNDROME, MASA SYNDROME, L1 SYNDROME)
Hydrocephalus, Short Flexed Thumbs, Mental Deficiency

In 1949, Bickers and Adams first described X-linked recessive hydrocephalus associated with aqueductal stenosis. In 1974, Bianchine and Lewis delineated an X-linked recessive disorder referred to as MASA syndrome, an acronym for mental retardation, adducted thumbs, shuffling gait, and aphasia. Based on the similarities of their clinical phenotype as well as molecular studies that have placed the locus for both disorders, as well as X-linked corpus callosal agenesis and X-linked complicated hereditary spastic paraplegia type 1, at Xq28, it seems clear that the four conditions are phenotypic variations of mutations in the same gene.

ABNORMALITIES

Performance. Mental retardation and spasticity, especially of lower extremities.
Brain. Aqueductal stenosis with hydrocephalus.
Hands. Thumb flexed over palm (cortical thumb) in approximately 50%.

OCCASIONAL ABNORMALITIES
Asymmetry of somewhat coarse facies; brain defects such as absence of the pyramidal tract, fusion of thalamic fornices, agenesis/dysgenesis of corpus callosum, small brainstem, porencephalic cyst.

NATURAL HISTORY
Prenatal hydrocephalus may be severe enough to impede delivery. However, many of the affected males have no hydrocephalus. Such individuals often have a narrow scaphocephalic cranium with an IQ in the range of 30 and tend to have spasticity, a shuffling gait, and aphasia.

ETIOLOGY
This disorder has an X-linked recessive inheritance pattern. A number of different mutations in the gene encoding for the neural cell adhesion molecule, *L1CAM* located at Xq28, have been reported in X-linked hydrocephalus families, in families with MASA syndrome, and in families with X-linked agenesis of the corpus callosum. The carrier female is usually normal but may have dull intelligence and/or adducted thumbs.

COMMENT
Prenatal diagnosis is not always reliable in that ventriculomegaly usually starts after 20 weeks' gestation. Ultrasonographic studies should be performed every 2 to 4 weeks from 16 through 28 weeks' gestation. However, it should be recognized that hydrocephalus might develop postnatally or might never occur.

References

Bickers DS, Adams RD: Hereditary stenosis of the aqueduct of Sylvius as a cause of congenital hydrocephalus, *Brain* 72:246, 1949.
Edwards JH: The syndrome of sex-linked hydrocephalus, *Arch Dis Child* 36:486, 1961.
Holmes LB, et al: X-linked aqueductal stenosis, *Pediatrics* 51:697, 1973.
Bianchine JW, Lewis RC Jr: The MASA syndrome: A new heritable mental retardation syndrome, *Clin Genet* 5:298, 1974.
Fryns JP, et al: X-linked complicated spastic paraplegia, MASA syndrome, and X-linked hydrocephalus owing to congenital stenosis of the aqueduct of Sylvius: Variable expression of the same mutation at Xq28, *J Med Genet* 28:429, 1991.
Van Camp G, et al: A duplication in the *L1CAM* gene associated with X-linked hydrocephalus, *Nat Genet* 4:421, 1993.
Schrander-Stumpel C, et al: The spectrum of complicated spastic paraplegia, MASA syndrome and X-linked hydrocephalus: Contribution of DNA linkage analysis in genetic counseling of individual families, *Genet Couns* 5:1, 1994.
Schrander-Stumpel C, Fryns J-P: Congenital hydrocephalus: Nosology and guidelines for clinical approach and genetic counselling, *Eur J Pediatr* 157:355, 1998.
Weller S, Gartner J: Genetic and clinical aspects of X-linked hydrocephalus (L1 disease): Mutations in the *L1CAM* gene, *Hum Mutat* 18:1, 2001.
Vos YJ, Hofstra RMW: An updated and upgraded *L1CAM* mutation database, *Hum Mutat* 31:E1102, 2010.

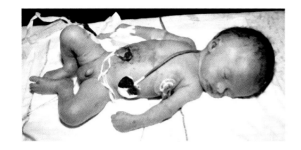

FIGURE 1.   X-linked hydrocephalus spectrum. A male infant, who later died, was shown to have aqueductal stenosis as the cause for hydrocephalus.

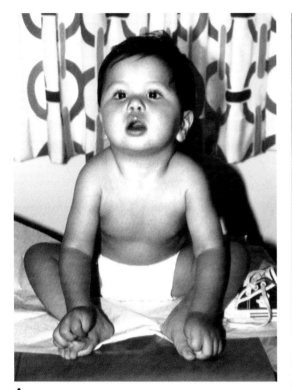

A

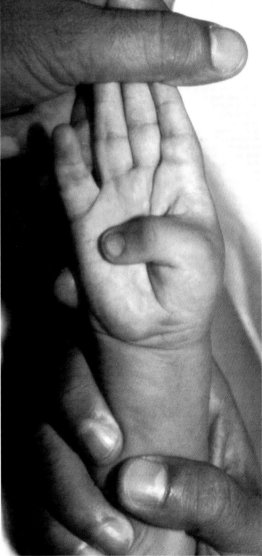

B

FIGURE 2.   **A** and **B,** Boy with MASA syndrome. He has intellectual disability, adducted thumb, shuffling gait, and aphasia.

HYDROLETHALUS SYNDROME
Hydrocephalus, Micrognathia, Polydactyly

This disorder was described initially by Salonen and colleagues in 1981. Hydrolethalus refers to hydramnios, hydrocephalus, and lethality, three of the most common features of this condition. The majority of cases have been from Finland.

ABNORMALITIES

Central Nervous System. Severe prenatal onset of hydrocephalus; absent corpus callosum, septum pellucidum, and olfactory structures; hypoplastic temporal and occipital lobes; hypothalamic hamartoma; hypoplastic brainstem and cerebellum; abnormal gyrations; colobomatous dysplasia and hypoplasia of the optic nerve; cleft in the base of the skull. The foramen magnum and the bony cleft extending posterior from it form a "keyhole-shaped" opening in the base of the skull, which is a constant finding in this disorder.

Craniofacial. Micrognathia, cleft palate, cleft lip that is lateral or midline, broad nose especially at the root, microphthalmia, broad neck relative to the shoulders, malformed low-set ears.

Limbs. Postaxial polydactyly of hands, preaxial polydactyly of feet, clubfeet.

Cardiac. Defects in 50%, most commonly a large ventricular septal defect combined with an atrial septal defect to form an atrioventricular canal.

Respiratory. Defective lung lobation, malformed or hypoplastic larynx, stenotic or rarely dilated trachea and/or bronchi.

Genitourinary. Duplicated uterus, hypospadias, malformations of vagina.

OCCASIONAL ABNORMALITIES

Absent pituitary, arrhinencephaly, hydranencephaly, anencephaly, clefts in the lower lip, bifid nose, agenesis of tongue, hydronephrosis, urethral atresia, short arms, syndactyly, agenesis of the diaphragm, omphalocele.

NATURAL HISTORY

The gestation of most affected patients is complicated by polyhydramnios. Intrauterine growth deficiency is the rule. Seventy percent of cases are stillborn. Live-born infants survive for only a few minutes to a few hours.

ETIOLOGY

Autosomal recessive mutations of two genes involved in ciliogenesis are responsible. *HYLS-1* is required for the apical targeting/anchoring of centrioles at the plasma membrane. Mutations impair *HYLS-1* function in ciliogenesis. Mutations in *KIF7* (the human orthologue of *Drosophila* Costal2, a key component of the hedgehog signaling pathway) also play an important role in human primary cilia, indicating that the Hydrolethalus syndrome is a ciliopathy. Mutations in *KIF7* are also responsible for the acrocallosal syndrome (see page 304).

References

Salonen R, et al: The hydrolethalus syndrome: Delineation of a "new" lethal malformation syndrome based on 28 patients, *Clin Genet* 19:321, 1981.

Toriello H, Bauserman SC: Bilateral pulmonary agenesis: Association with the hydrolethalus syndrome and review of the literature from a developmental field perspective, *Am J Med Genet* 21:93, 1985.

Salonen R, Herva R: Hydrolethalus syndrome, *J Med Genet* 27:756, 1990.

Mee L, et al: Hydrolethalus syndrome is caused by a missense mutation in a novel gene *HYLS1*, *Hum Mol Genet* 14:1475, 2005.

Paetau A, et al: Hydrolethalus syndrome: Neuropathology of 21 cases confirmed by HYLS1 gene mutation analysis, *J Neuropathol Exp Neurol* 67:750, 2008.

Dammermann A, et al: The hydrolethalus syndrome protein HYLS-1 links core centriole structure to cilia formation, *Genes Dev* 23:2046, 2009.

Putoux A, et al: Mutations in *KIF7* cause fetal hydrolethalus and acrocallosal syndromes, *Nat Genet* 43:601, 2011.

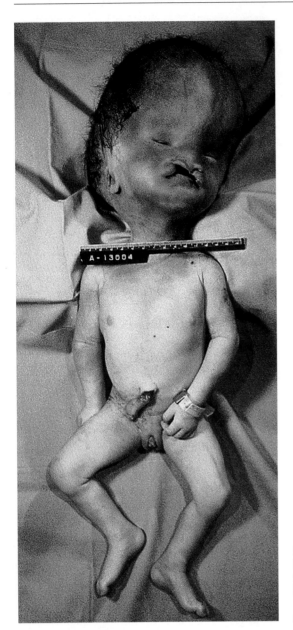

FIGURE 1.   Hydrolethalus syndrome. Newborn infant. Note the broad nasal root, cleft lip, and macrocephaly, which is due to hydrocephalus. (From Toriello HV, Bauserman SC: *Am J Med Genet* 21:93, 1985. Copyright © 1985. Reprinted with permission of Wiley-Liss, Inc., a subsidiary of John Wiley & Sons, Inc.)

G

WALKER-WARBURG SYNDROME
(HARD ± E SYNDROME, WARBURG SYNDROME)
Congenital Muscular Dystrophy, Brain Defects, Anterior Chamber Defects of the Eye

Initially described by Walker in 1942, this disorder was first suggested as a distinct entity by Warburg in 1971. The first familial cases were reported by Chemke and colleagues, and the full spectrum of associated defects was outlined by Pagon and colleagues and by Whitley and colleagues.

ABNORMALITIES

Brain. Type II lissencephaly (100%) manifest by widespread argyria with scattered areas of macrogyria and/or polymicrogyria; abnormally thick cortex with absent white matter interdigitations; absent or hypoplastic septum pellucidum and corpus callosum; cerebellar malformation (100%), including a polymicrogyric or smooth surface and hypoplasia of vermis; occipital encephalocele, which may be small (24%); Dandy-Walker malformation (53%); hydrocephalus, usually from mechanical obstruction in the posterior fossa (53%); ventriculomegaly, even in the absence of increased intracranial pressure (95%).

Eye. Anterior chamber malformation (91%) including cataract, corneal clouding usually secondary to Peters anomaly, and narrow iridocorneal angle with or without glaucoma; retinal malformations (100%), including retrolental masses caused by hyperplastic primary vitreous, coloboma (24%), and retinal detachment secondary to retinal dysplasia; microphthalmia (53%).

Other. Congenital muscular dystrophy (100%), genital anomalies in males (65%).

OCCASIONAL ABNORMALITIES

Cleft lip with or without cleft palate (14%), microcephaly (16%), slit-like ventricles (5%), mild renal dysplasia, imperforate anus, congenital contractures (43%), megalocornea, microtia and absent auditory canals, gonadoblastoid testicular dysplasia.

NATURAL HISTORY

The majority of affected children die within the first year of life secondary to the severe defect in brain development. Patients frequently present as newborns with muscle weakness, hypotonia, or even severe myopathy resulting in fatal respiratory insufficiency. Of those who survive, the majority have profound mental retardation. Five percent to 10%, especially those with less severe intellectual disability, survive longer than 5 years. For those who survive, rolling over and sitting should be expected to commence between 1 and 3 years. Seizures are common with increasing age.

ETIOLOGY

This disorder has an autosomal recessive inheritance pattern. Patients with Walker-Warburg syndrome have mutations in seven genes—*POMT1, POMT2, POMGNT1, FKTN, FKRPL, LARGE,* and *ISPD*—all of which encode proteins involved in the post-translational modification of α-dystroglycan. Mutations in these genes make up 35% to 40% of the genes responsible for this disorder. Mutations in an additional gene, which codes for a major basement membrane protein, collagen IV alpha 1 (COL4A1), implicates a further mechanism for this disorder. Prenatal diagnosis at 20 weeks' gestation has been made on an affected fetus based on the presence of hydrocephalus.

COMMENT

Because of the wide spectrum of brain and eye defects, the diagnosis is frequently not considered. Postmortem examination of the brain and eyes is often necessary. Elevation of the serum creatine kinase and "myopathic" changes on electromyography can be helpful in documenting the presence of congenital muscular dystrophy, which is present in virtually all affected patients.

References

Warburg M: The heterogenicity of microphthalmia in the mentally retarded, *Birth Defects* 7:136, 1971.

Chemke J, et al: A familial syndrome of central nervous system and ocular malformations, *Clin Genet* 7:1, 1975.

Pagon RA, et al: Autosomal recessive eye and brain anomalies: Warburg syndrome, *J Pediatr* 102:542, 1983.

Whitley CB, et al: Warburg syndrome: Lethal neurodysplasia with autosomal recessive inheritance, *J Pediatr* 102:547, 1983.

Dobyns WB, et al: Diagnostic criteria for Walker-Warburg syndrome, *Am J Med Genet* 32:195, 1989.

Monteagudo A, et al: Walker-Warburg syndrome: Case report and review of the literature, *J Ultrasound Med* 20:419, 2001.

Labelle-Dumais C, et al: *COL4A1* mutations cause ocular dysgenesis, neuronal localization defects, and myopathy in mice and Walker-Warburg syndrome in humans, *PLoS Genet* 7:e1002062, 2011. doi:10.1371/journal.pgen.1002062

Willer T, et al: ISPD loss-of-function mutations disrupt dystroglycan O-mannosylation and cause of Walker-Warburg syndrome, *Nat Genet* 44:575, 2012.

Roscioli T, et al: Mutations in ISPD cause Walker-Warburg syndrome and defective glycosylation of α-dystroglycan, *Nat Genet* 44:581, 2012.

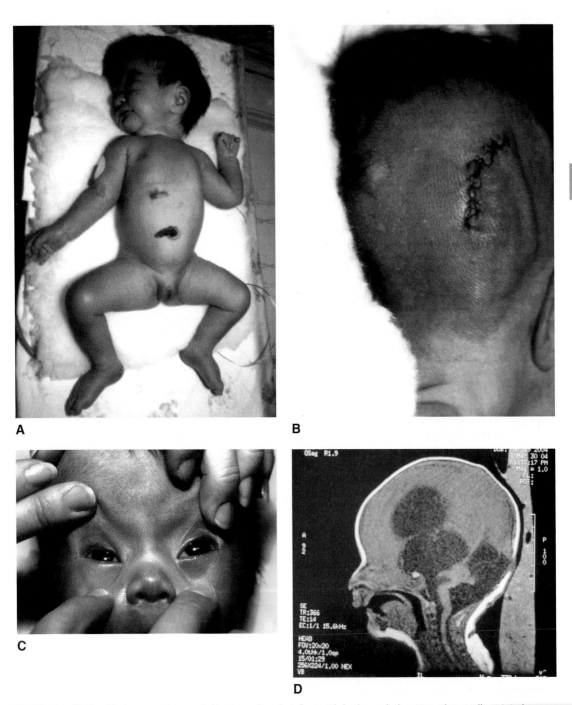

FIGURE 1. Walker-Warburg syndrome. **A,** Newborn female infant with hydrocephalus. Note the small occipital encephalocele (**B**), the unilateral microphthalmic eye (**C**), the encephalocele, and the magnetic resonance image showing an occipital defect (**D**).

MILLER-DIEKER SYNDROME (LISSENCEPHALY SYNDROME)

Miller in 1963 and later Dieker and colleagues described a specific pattern of malformation, one feature of which was lissencephaly (smooth brain). Jones and colleagues expanded the clinical phenotype and introduced the term Miller-Dieker syndrome to distinguish this disorder from other conditions associated with lissencephaly.

ABNORMALITIES

Brain and Performance. Incomplete development of brain, often with a smooth surface, although areas of pachygyria are often seen inferiorly; heterotopias; both frontal and temporal opercula fail to develop, leaving a wide-open Sylvian fossa and a figure-8 appearance on computed tomography; absent or hypoplastic corpus callosum (74%) and large cavum septi pellucidi (77%); small midline calcifications in the region of the third ventricle (45%); brainstem and cerebellum appear grossly normal; severe intellectual disability with initial hypotonia, opisthotonos, spasticity, failure to thrive, seizures, occasionally hypsarrhythmia on electroencephalography.

Craniofacial. Microcephaly with bitemporal narrowing; variable high forehead, vertical ridging and furrowing in central forehead, especially when crying; small nose with anteverted nostrils, upslant to palpebral fissures, protuberant upper lip, thin vermilion border of upper lip, and micrognathia; appearance of "low-set" and/or posteriorly angulated auricles; wide secondary alveolar ridge; late eruption of primary teeth.

Other. Cryptorchidism, pilonidal sinus, fifth finger clinodactyly, transverse palmar crease, polyhydramnios.

OCCASIONAL ABNORMALITIES

Cardiac defect (tetralogy of Fallot, ventricular septal defect, valvular pulmonic stenosis), intrauterine growth retardation, decreased fetal activity, omphalocele, pelvic kidney, cystic dysplasia of kidney, lipomeningocele with tethered cord, sacral tail, cleft palate, cataract.

NATURAL HISTORY

Postnatal failure to thrive; gastrostomy because of feeding problems, poor nutrition, and repeated aspiration pneumonia; brief visual fixation, smiling, and nonspecific motor responses to stimulation are the only developmental skills usually acquired, although a few patients have rolled over occasionally; death usually occurs before 2 years and often within the first 3 months; one child lived to 9 years of age.

ETIOLOGY

A deletion at 17p13.3 has been documented in the majority of patients with this disorder. This defect

has been found in association with ring chromosome 17, terminal deletion 17, unbalanced translocation inherited from a balanced reciprocal translocation carrier, and a recombinant chromosome 17 because of crossover in a pericentric inversion carrier. For de novo abnormalities such as ring 17 or terminal deletions, the recurrence risk is negligible. In families with balanced rearrangements, the recurrence risk might be high. However, prenatal diagnosis is possible. In patients with highly suggestive phenotypes in which high-resolution chromosomal analysis is normal, the diagnosis can sometimes be established with fluorescent in situ hybridization using probes specific for the lissencephaly critical region on 17p. Deletions in 17p13.3 involving the platelet-activating factor acetylhydrolase isoform Ib (*PAFAH1B1*) gene, also known as *LIS-1*, result in lissencephaly. The major facial features of Miller-Dieker syndrome are thought to result from deletion of contiguous genes *YWHAE* and, possibly, *CRK*, in the critical region.

COMMENT

17p13.3 MICRODUPLICATION SYNDROME. Microduplications involving the region deleted in Miller-Dieker syndrome are variable in size and are characterized by autism spectrum disorders, speech delay, intellectual disability, subtle dysmorphic features, and mild hand/foot malformations. Class I duplications involving *YWHAE* but not *PAFAH1B1* are associated with upslanting palpebral fissures, thick eyebrows with synophrys, squared upturned nasal tip, broad nasal bridge, large fleshy ears, prominent cupid bow of upper lip, and prominent chin, whereas class II duplications involving *PAFAH1B1* are associated with a broad midface, low-set ears, frontal bossing, downslanting palpebral fissures, ocular hypertelorism, and broad nasal bridge. Limb anomalies, hallux valgus, large hands with high fetal fingertip pads, and autism are more frequent in class I duplications.

References

Miller JQ: Lissencephaly in two siblings, *Neurology* 13:841, 1963.

Dieker H, et al: The lissencephaly syndrome, *Birth Defects* 5:53, 1969.

Jones KL, et al: The Miller-Dieker syndrome, *Pediatrics* 66:277, 1980.

Dobyns WB, et al: Miller-Dieker syndrome. Lissencephaly and monosomy 17p, *J Pediatr* 102:552, 1983.

Dobyns WB, Stratton RF, Greenberg F: Syndromes with lissencephaly. I: Miller-Dieker and Norman-Roberts syndrome and isolated lissencephaly syndromes, *Am J Med Genet* 22:197, 1984.

Dobyns WB, et al: Clinical and molecular diagnosis of Miller-Dieker syndrome, *Am J Hum Genet* 48:584, 1991.

Hattori M, et al: Miller-Dieker syndrome gene encodes a subunit of brain platelet activating factor, *Nature* 370:216, 1994.

Dobyns WB, et al: Differences in the gyral pattern distinguish chromosome 17-linked and X-linked lissencephaly, *Neurology* 53:270, 1999.

G

Pollin TI, et al: Risk of abnormal pregnancy outcome in carriers of balanced reciprocal translocations involving the Miller-Dieker syndrome (MDS) critical region in chromosome 17p13.3, *Am J Med Genet* 85:369, 1999.

Cardoso C, et al: The location and type of mutation predict malformation severity in isolated lissencephaly caused by abnormalities within the *LIS1* gene, *Hum Mol Genet* 9:3019, 2000.

Sreenath SC, et al: Microdeletions including *YWHAE* in the Miller-Dieker syndrome region on chromosome 17p13.3 result in facial dysmorphisms, growth restriction, and cognitive impairment, *J Med Genet* 46:825, 2009.

Roos L, et al: A new microduplication syndrome encompassing the region of the Miller-Dieker (17p13 deletion) syndrome, *J Med Genet* 46:703, 2009.

Ostergaard JR, et al: Further delineation of 17p13.3 microdeletion involving *CRK*. The effect of growth hormone treatment, *Eur J Med Genet* 55:22, 2012.

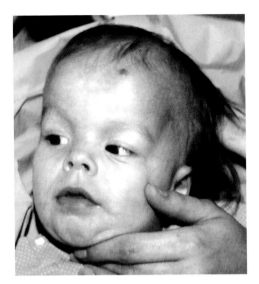

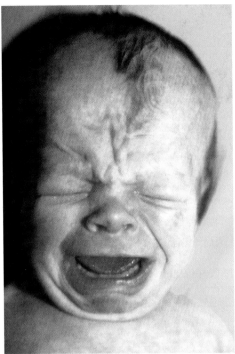

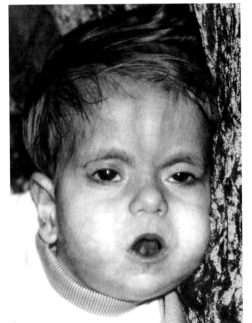

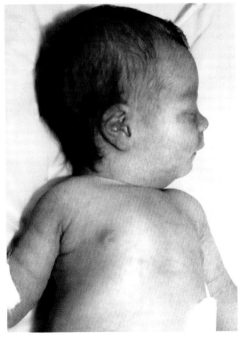

G

FIGURE 1. Facies of an infant with Miller-Dieker syndrome, showing high forehead with vertical soft tissue ridging and furrowing when crying, and small, anteverted nose.

NABLUS MASK-LIKE FACIAL SYNDROME
(MICRODELETION 8Q22.1 SYNDROME)

In 2000, Teebi reported a 4 year old boy with an unusual facial appearance, which he referred to as Nablus mask-like facies syndrome based on having examined the boy in the Palestinian city of Nablus and that the boy appeared as though he was wearing a mask. In 2006, Shieh et al recognized that this syndrome is caused by an 8q21.3-q22.1 microdeletion, which has been present in all cases with the characteristic phenotype. Fewer than 10 patients have been reported.

ABNORMALITIES

Growth. Postnatal growth deficiency.
Performance. Developmental delay and borderline intellectual disability. Happy and social behavior.
Craniofacial. Postnatal onset microcephaly. Almost expressionless long face; tight glistening facial skin, with bluish color especially around the nose; blepharophimosis; lateral displacement of medial canthus (telecanthus); broad flat nasal root, flat and "bulbous" nasal tip with hypoplastic alae and short columella; long prominent philtrum. Small mouth with thin vermillion border, everted lower lip; cheek dimples, maxillary hypoplasia and mild micrognathia; small, posteriorly angulated ears with unfolding of the posterior aspect of the helix, prominent antihelix, prominent antitragus,

and very hypoplastic lobules. Sparse eyebrows, eyelashes, and scalp hair with unusual upsweep of frontal and vertex scalp hair pattern. Short neck.
Extremities. Contractures of the hips, knees, elbows, and wrists; genu valgum; camptodactyly; adducted thumbs; fifth finger clinodactyly; tapering fingers; bilateral single palmar creases; short great toes with wide space between first and second toes; medial deviation and plantar flexion of third and fifth toes.
Other. Curved or indented incisors; laterally displaced hypoplastic nipples; small phallus, cryptorchidism; hypoplastic labia minor and majora.

OCCASIONAL ABNORMALITIES
Prenatal growth deficiency; craniosynostosis; submucous cleft palate; prominent thick tongue, short upper lip frenulum; spigelian hernia.

NATURAL HISTORY
Several patients have undergone surgical intervention to improve their blepharophimosis. Very few data are available regarding natural history.

ETIOLOGY
A microdeletion in the 8q21.3-8q22.1 was detected using array-based comparative genomic hybridization (CGH) in two patients and later confirmed in the original Palestinian patient. The precise

definition of the size of the deletion in several patients has narrowed down a critical region to 2.78 Mb. Several genes in the interval, including cyclin E2, cadherin 17, and *TMEM67,* could contribute to the phenotype. Only sporadic cases have been reported.

COMMENT

Allanson suggested in 2001 that this phenotype was very similar to the blepharo-naso-facial syndrome reported first in 1973 by Pashayan et al. Even though similarities are present, several authors disagree that Nablus mask-like facial syndrome and blepharo-naso-facial syndrome are in fact the same condition. No microdeletion of 8q21 has been described yet in any patient with blepharo-naso-facial syndrome.

References

Teebi AS: Nablus mask-like facial syndrome, *Am J Med Genet* 95:407, 2000.

Allanson J: Nablus mask-like facial syndrome, *Am J Med Genet* 102:212, 2001.

Teebi AS: Differences between Nablus mask-like facial syndrome and blepharonasofacial syndrome, *Am J Med Genet* 102:214, 2001.

Salpietro CD, et al: Confirmation of Nablus mask-like facial syndrome, *Am J Med Genet A* 121A:283, 2003.

Shieh JT, et al: Nablus mask-like facial syndrome is caused by a microdeletion of 8q detected by array-based comparative genomic hybridization, *Am J Med Genet A* 140A:1267, 2006.

Raas-Rothschild A, et al: The 8q22.1 microdeletion syndrome or Nablus mask-like facial syndrome: Report on two patients and review of the literature, *Eur J Med Genet* 52:140, 2009.

G

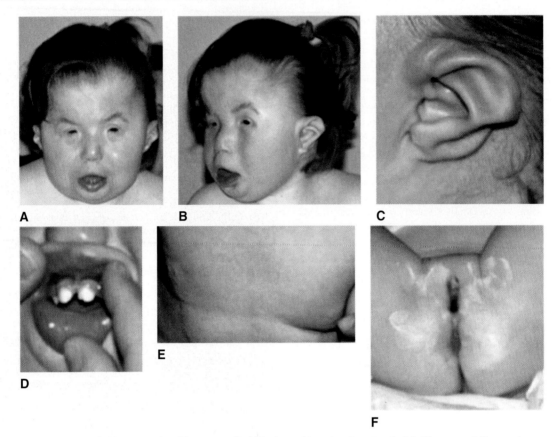

FIGURE 1.   A–C, Child, 21 months old. Note marked blepharophimosis, glistening facial skin, over midface and nose. Hair is sparse and unruly. Small malformed ears with absent lobules. Small mouth with thin vermillion border of the lips. **D,** Small, curved incisors. **E,** Laterally displaced hypoplastic nipples. **F,** Hypoplastic genitalia. (From Salpietro CD, et al: *Am J Med Genet A* 121A:283, 2003, with permission.)

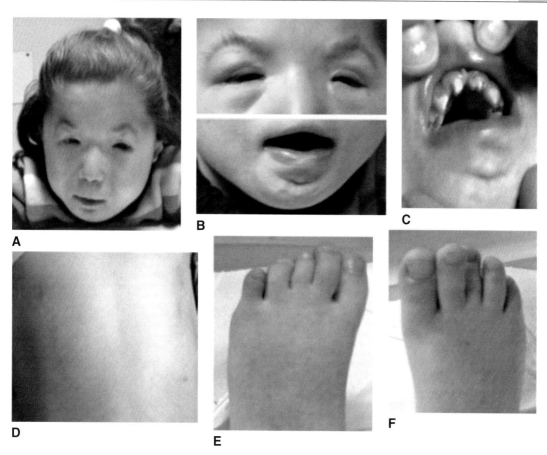

FIGURE 2. **A–C,** Same child as in Figure 1 at 2 years 5 months of age. She has had surgery to correct the blepharophimosis. **D,** Laterally displaced hypoplastic nipples. **E** and **F,** Short first toes with medial deviation and plantar flexion of third and fifth toes. (From Shieh JT, et al: *Am J Med Genet A* 140A:1267, 2006, with permission.)

SMITH-MAGENIS SYNDROME (17P11.2 MICRODELETION SYNDROME)
Broad, Flat Midface with Brachycephaly, Brachydactyly, Speech Delay

Initially described in 1982 by Smith and colleagues, the clinical phenotype, including characteristic behavioral abnormalities, has been more completely delineated by Stratton and colleagues and Greenberg and colleagues. More than 100 cases have been described. The minimum birth prevalence may be as high as 1 in 25,000.

ABNORMALITIES

Growth. Failure to thrive in infancy, postnatal growth deficiency.

Performance. Infantile hypotonia; intelligence quotients range from 20 to 78 with most falling between 40 and 54; speech delay with expressive language more delayed than receptive; working memory is a relative weakness; hoarse, deep voice; self-destructive behavior, including head banging, wrist biting, onychotillomania (pulling out fingernails and toenails), and polyembolokoilamania (insertion of foreign objects into body orifices); sleep disorders; autism spectrum disorders.

Craniofacial. Brachycephaly with flat midface, prominent forehead, broad nasal bridge, synophrys, downturned upper lip with protruding premaxilla, prognathia, low-set ears and/or other ear anomalies.

Limbs. Short broad hands and short fingers (brachydactyly), decreased range of motion at elbows, pes planus/varus.

Other. Cardiac defects; renal anomalies, especially duplication of collecting system; brain anomalies (primarily ventriculomegaly); eye abnormalities, including strabismus, myopia, microcornea, and iris dysplasia; hearing loss (both conductive and sensorineural); scoliosis; insensitivity to pain.

OCCASIONAL ABNORMALITIES

Microcephaly, craniosynostosis, upslanting palpebral fissures, micrognathia (in infancy), Brushfield spots, cleft lip with or without cleft palate, cleft palate, iris coloboma, velopharyngeal incompetence, laryngeal abnormalities (polyps, nodules, edema, and paralysis), bifid rib, hemivertebrae, fifth finger clinodactyly, prominent fingertip pads, lymphedema of hands and feet, short or bowed ulna, cryptorchidism, borderline hypothyroidism, humoral immune dysfunction, jejunal atresia, bladder exstrophy, diaphragmatic hernia.

NATURAL HISTORY

The clinical phenotype is rarely evident before late childhood or early adolescence. With increasing age, the frontal prominence, prognathism, brachydactyly, hoarse deep voice, and coarsening of facial features become apparent. Although onychotillomania, most likely the result of insensitivity to pain, is uncommon in children younger than 5 to 6 years of age, head banging and wrist biting have been documented as early as the second year of life. Severe sleep disturbances are common. Individuals with Smith-Magenis syndrome have a phase shift of their circadian rhythm of melatonin with a paradoxical diurnal secretion of the hormone. It has been hypothesized that some of the hyperactivity and other behavioral problems may occur as the child struggles to remain awake during the day at the time of paradoxical increase in melatonin levels. Treatment with melatonin before bedtime, and repression of its secretion with beta-blocking agents in early morning has been effective. Usual bedtime is early (8:00 or 8:30 PM); one to three arousals throughout the night are common; and affected individuals frequently awaken between 4:00 and 6:00 AM. Exhaustion during morning hours, naps throughout the day, and inability to remain awake during the early evening are associated with tantrums. There is no evidence of general cognitive decline with age.

ETIOLOGY

This disorder is due to an interstitial deletion of chromosome band 17p11.2. Approximately 25 genes, including retinoic acid–induced gene 1 (*RAI1*), which appears to be responsible for most of the features characteristic of Smith-Magenis syndrome, are located within the critical region. *RAI1* regulates, among other things, the transcription of circadian locomotor output cycle kaput (CLOCK), a major component of the mammalian circadian oscillator that transcriptionally regulates many circadian genes.

The deletion can be difficult to detect at resolution levels of less than 500 bands. Although the vast majority of cases have been sporadic, transmission from a mosaic mother has occurred on one occasion, suggesting that parental chromosomes should be examined in all cases.

COMMENT

17p11.2 MICRODUPLICATION (POTOCKI-LUPSKI SYNDROME). Clinical features observed in patients with the Potocki-Lupski syndrome caused by the common dupp11.2p11.2 are distinct from those seen with Smith-Magenis syndrome and include infantile hypotonia, failure to thrive, intellectual disability, autistic features, sleep apnea, and structural and conduction cardiovascular anomalies, aortic root dilatation being most common; several cases of fatal hypoplastic left heart syndrome have also been reported. Hypermetropia, scoliosis, and urinary anomalies can occur. Mild dysmorphic features can be present but do not always allow phenotypic recognition. Shared features include a broad forehead, gentle downslant of the palpebral fissures, wide nasal bridge, epicanthal folds, and relatively long nasal tip. Younger patients have a triangular face with prominence to the angle of the jaw and micrognathia. A more oval-shaped face and larger chin is seen in older individuals. Wide distal phalanges of the hands and an increased gap between the first and second toes have also been seen. More than 50 patients have been reported. The critical region is a 1.3-Mb genomic interval that contains the dosage-sensitive *RAI1* gene. The majority of subjects (60%) harbor the homologous recombination reciprocal product of the common Smith-Magenis syndrome microdeletion (3.7 Mb). Most of the remainder have nonrecurrent duplications ranging in size from 1.3 to 15.2 Mb, always including *RAI1*.

References

Smith ACM, et al: Deletion of the 17 short arm in two patients with facial clefts and congenital heart defects, *Am J Hum Genet A* 34(Suppl):A410, 1982.

Smith ACM, et al: Interstitial deletion of (17)(p11.2p11.2) in nine patients, *Am J Med Genet* 24:383, 1986.

Stratton RF, et al: Interstitial deletion of (17)(p11.2p11.2): Report of six additional patients with a new chromosome deletion syndrome, *Am J Med Genet* 24:421, 1986.

Greenberg F, et al: Molecular analysis of the Smith-Magenis syndrome: A possible contiguous gene syndrome associated with del(17)(p11.2), *Am J Hum Genet* 49:1207, 1991.

Greenberg F, et al: Multi-disciplinary clinical study of Smith-Magenis syndrome (deletion 17p11.2), *Am J Med Genet* 62:247, 1996.

De Leersnyder H, et al: Inversion of the circadian rhythm of melatonin in the Smith-Magenis syndrome, *J Pediatr* 139:111, 2001.

Potocki L, et al: Characterization of Potocki-Lupski syndrome (dup(17)(p11.2p11.2)) and delineation of a dosage-sensitive critical interval that can convey an autism phenotype, *Am J Hum Genet* 80:633, 2007.

Osório A, et al: Cognitive functioning in children and adults with Smith-Magenis syndrome, *Eur J Med Genet* 55:394, 2012. doi:10.1016/eime2012.04.001

Williams SR, et al: Smith-Magenis syndrome results in disruption of CLOCK gene transcription and reveals an integral role for *RAI1* in the maintenance of circadian rhythmicity, *Am J Hum Genet* 90:1, 2012.

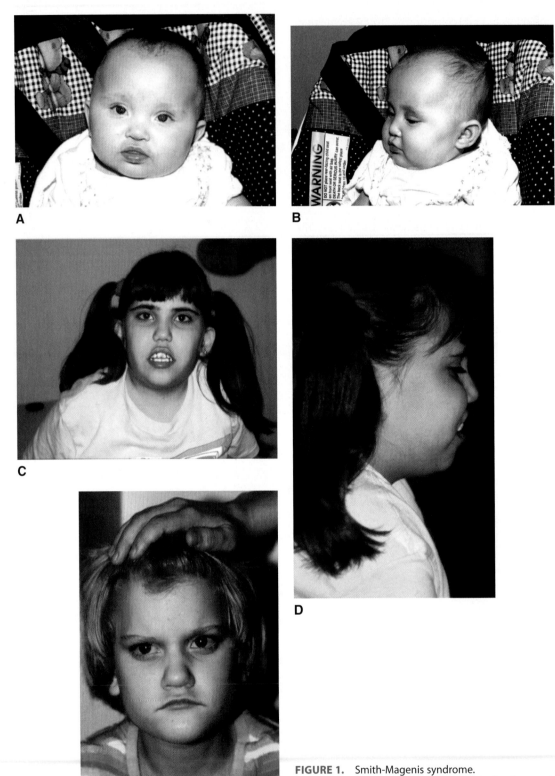

FIGURE 1. Smith-Magenis syndrome.
A and **B,** Neonate showing brachycephaly, flat face, and prominent forehead. Note the similarity of this child's face to that of a child with Down syndrome. **C–E,** Note the downturned upper lip and protruding premaxilla.

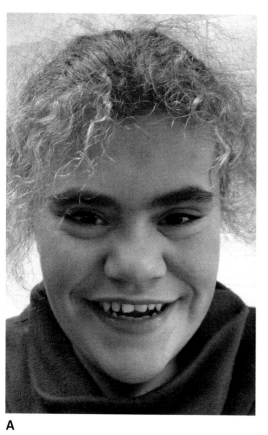

A

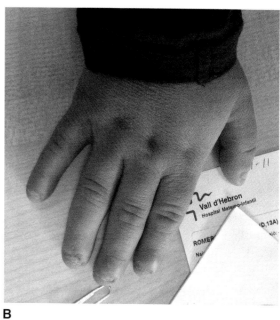

B

G

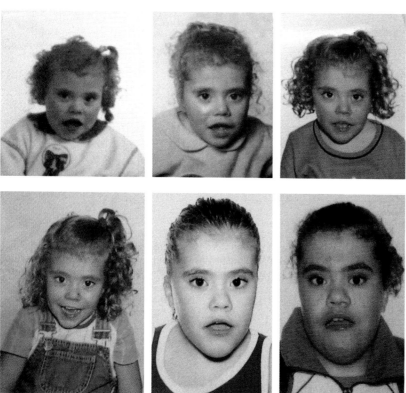

C

FIGURE 2. Sixteen-year-old girl with Smith-Magenis syndrome. **A,** Note upslanting palpebral fissures, midface hypoplasia, and prominent horizontalized philtrum. **B,** The hand shows brachydactyly and evidence of onychotillomania. **C,** The pictures at different ages show a resemblance to Down syndrome in early years, and progressive coarsening.

MENKES SYNDROME (MENKES KINKY HAIR SYNDROME)
Progressive Cerebral Deterioration with Seizures, Twisted and Fractured Hair

Menkes and colleagues described five related male infants with this disease in 1962, and Danks and colleagues subsequently indicated that all features of the disorder are the result of copper deficiency.

ABNORMALITIES

Growth. Deficiency, sometimes small at birth.

Central Nervous System. Severe degenerative process in cerebral cortex with gliosis and atrophy; profound and progressive neurologic deficit beginning at 1 to 2 months of age with hypertonia, irritability, seizures, intracranial hemorrhage, hypothermia, and feeding difficulties.

Facies. Lack of expressive movement, pudgy cheeks.

Hair. Sparse, stubby, and lightly pigmented; shows twisting and partial breakage by magnified inspection.

Skin. Occasionally thick and relatively dry; lax; unequal skin pigmentation at birth, particularly in darkly pigmented patients.

Skeletal. Wormian bones; pectus excavatum; metaphyseal widening, particularly of ribs and femur, with formation of lateral spurs that frequently fracture.

Other. Ocular findings, including very poor visual acuity, myopia, and strabismus; gingival enlargement and delayed eruption of primary teeth; gastric polyps linked to gastrointestinal bleeding; pyloric stenosis; sliding hiatal hernia; umbilical and/or inguinal hernia; bladder diverticula; cardiac defects, widespread arterial elongation and tortuosity noted on arteriograms and at autopsy, most likely caused by deficiency of copper-dependent cross-linking in the internal elastic membrane of the arterial wall.

NATURAL HISTORY

Affected infants appear healthy at birth and develop normally up to 6 to 8 weeks, at which point hypotonia, seizures, and failure to thrive develop. Death occurs usually by 6 years. Hair is normal at birth but by 6 weeks begins to lose pigmentation. Subcutaneous therapy with copper histidine or copper chloride may be an effective treatment in some children if started early. The response to early treatment occurs only in children with mutations that result in some residual copper transport.

ETIOLOGY

This disorder has an X-linked recessive inheritance pattern. The gene (*ATP7A*) responsible for this disorder encodes a copper-transporting ATPase and is located at Xq13.3. Manifestations in the carrier female include hair that is lighter than would be expected for the family, pili torti (180-degree twist of hair shaft), and increased fragility and breakage of hair. Prenatal diagnosis can be made by gene analysis and by demonstrating excessive copper uptake in cultured amniotic fluid cells. The disease results from an abnormality in copper transport so that low levels of serum copper and ceruloplasmin are found in all patients studied. The basic defect at least partially involves reduced ability to incorporate copper into certain enzymes that need it as a cofactor. The clinical phenotype is due to a deficiency of these enzymes; for example, hypopigmentation is caused by tyrosinase deficiency, and vascular tortuosity and bladder diverticula are caused by lysyl oxidase deficiency.

COMMENT

A child with Menkes syndrome presenting with subdural hematomas with a nontraumatic origin has been mistakenly diagnosed as having been the victim of child abuse.

References

Menkes JH, et al: A sex-linked recessive disorder with retardation of growth, peculiar hair, and focal cerebral and cerebellar degeneration, *Pediatrics* 29:764, 1962.

Danks DM, et al: Menkes' kinky hair syndrome. An inherited defect in copper absorption with wide-spread effects, *Pediatrics* 50:188, 1972.

Danks DM, et al: Menkes' kinky hair syndrome, *Lancet* 1:1100, 1972.

Horn N: Menkes X-linked disease: Prenatal diagnosis of hemizygous males and heterozygous females, *Prenat Diagn* 1:121, 1981.

Kaler SG, et al: Gastrointestinal hemorrhage associated with gastric polyps in Menkes disease, *J Pediatr* 122:93, 1993.

Sarkar B, et al: Copper-histidine therapy for Menkes disease, *J Pediatr* 123:828, 1993.

Vulpe C, et al: Isolation of a candidate gene for Menkes disease and evidence that it encodes a copper-transporting ATPase, *Nat Genet* 3:7, 1993.

Bankier A: Menkes disease, *J Med Genet* 32:213, 1995.

Gasch AT, et al: Menkes syndrome: Ophthalmic findings, *Ophthalmology* 109:1477, 2002.

Nassogne MC, et al: Massive subdural haematomas in Menkes disease mimicking shaken baby syndrome, *Childs Nerv Syst* 18:729, 2002.

Kaler SG, et al: Neonatal diagnosis and treatment of Menkes disease, *N Eng J Med* 358:605, 2008.

Hicks JD, et al: Increased frequency of congenital heart defects in Menkes disease, *Clin Dysmorphol* 21:59, 2012.

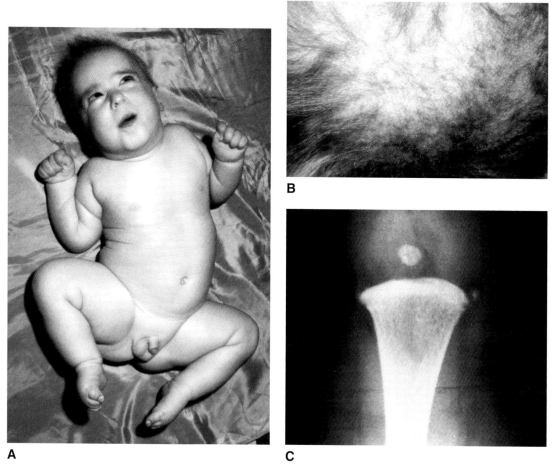

A

B

C

G

FIGURE 1.   Menkes syndrome. **A–C,** Note the sparse, stubby hair and, on radiograph, the metaphyseal widening with lateral spur that has fractured.

PITT-HOPKINS SYNDROME
Intellectual Disability, Wide Mouth, Intermittent Overbreathing

Initially described in 1978 by Pitt and Hopkins in two unrelated patients, more than 60 cases have been described.

ABNORMALITIES

Growth. Postnatal onset microcephaly.

Performance. Severe intellectual disability, absent speech in the majority of cases, hypotonia, motor delay, ataxia/motor incoordination, stereotypic hand movements, hyperventilation/apnea.

Central Nervous System. Aplasia/hypoplasia of corpus callosum, enlarged asymmetric ventricles, bulging caudate nuclei, atrophy of frontal and parietal cortex.

Craniofacial. Bitemporal narrowing, broad mouth with protruding upper lip and everted lower lip, thick lips, widely spaced teeth, upslanting palpebral fissures, deep-set eyes, broad and arched eyebrows that flare medially, prominent nose with pointed tip, wide nasal bridge, flared nares, cup-shaped ears, full cheeks, prognathism.

Eyes. Myopia, astigmatism, strabismus.

Hands. Small with tapering fingers, fifth finger clinodactyly, fetal fingertip pads, single palmar crease, clubbing.

OCCASIONAL ABNORMALITIES

Nystagmus, small optic nerves, pyloric stenosis, supernumerary nipples, short great toes, overlapping fingers, scoliosis, Hirschsprung disease, micropenis, hypospadias, absent clitoris, cryptorchidism.

NATURAL HISTORY

Onset of walking after 5 years of age or not at all is the rule. Speech is almost always absent. Episodes of hyperventilation occur in the majority of cases with onset between first few months and 7 years of age. Episodes start abruptly, last several minutes, and are followed by apnea, cyanosis, and sometimes loss of consciousness. They occur only during wakefulness and are often brought on by emotional outbursts and fatigue. Seizures occur commonly with onset between birth and 5 years of age and are usually controlled with medications. Severe constipation occurs in the majority of cases. Stereotypic hand movements include lateral movements, clapping and flapping, and repeated hand-mouth movements. Facial features coarsen with age and the lower face becomes more protuberant.

ETIOLOGY

Mutations in transcription factor 4 (TCF4), located within the chromosome 18q21.1 interval. TCF4 encodes a class I basic helix-loop-helix transcription factor. Microdeletion of chromosome 18q21.1 has also been responsible for Pitt-Hopkins syndrome.

References

Pitt D, Hopkins I: A syndrome of mental retardation, wide mouth and intermittent overbreathing, *Aust Paediatr J* 14:182, 1978.

Amiel J, et al: Mutations in *TCF4*, encoding a class I basic helix-loop-helix transcription factor, are responsible for Pitt-Hopkins syndrome, a severe epileptic encephalopathy associated with autonomic dysfunction, *Am J Hum Genet* 80:988, 2007.

Zweier C, et al: Haploinsufficiency of *TCF4* causes syndromal mental retardation with intermittent hyperventilation (Pitt-Hopkins syndrome), *Am J Hum Genet* 80:994, 2007.

Zweier C, et al: Further delineation of Pitt-Hopkins syndrome: Phenotype and genotype description of 16 novel patients, *J Med Genet* 45:738, 2008.

Marangi G, et al: The Pitt-Hopkins syndrome: Report of 16 new patients and clinical diagnostic criteria, *Am J Med Genet* 155:1536, 2011.

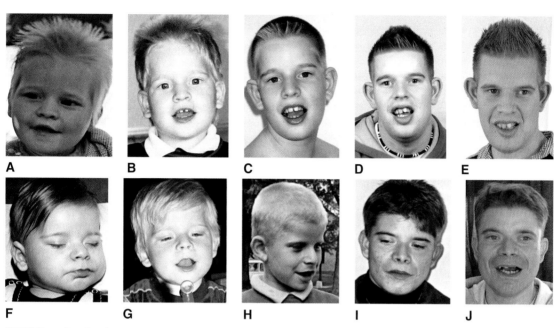

FIGURE 1. Two brothers with Pitt-Hopkins syndrome with mutation in TCF4 born to unaffected parents. Recurrence was due to somatic mosaicism. The younger brother at ages 2 **(A)**, 3 **(B)**, 10 **(C)**, 16 **(D)**, and 24 **(E).** The older brother at ages 2 months **(F)**, 2 years **(G)**, 7 **(H)**, 23 **(I)**, and 30 years **(J).** Note the thick helices, thin medial eyebrows, a broad base to the nose with flared nostrils, as well as a protruding upper lip and full lower lip are present at an early age. Later, there is coarsening of the face, with deep-set eyes, a high nasal bridge, a beaked nose, and prognathism. (Courtesy Prof. Schrander-Stumpel, Maastricht, The Netherlands.)

ANGELMAN SYNDROME (HAPPY PUPPET SYNDROME)
"Puppet-Like" Gait, Paroxysms of Laughter, Characteristic Facies

This disorder, initially described in 1965 by Angelman in three unrelated children with severe mental deficiency, abnormal puppet-like gait, characteristic facies, and frequent paroxysms of laughter, has been more completely delineated by Williams and Frias, who have documented the natural history of this disorder and suggested that the term "happy puppet" is inappropriate.

ABNORMALITIES

Performance. Severe intellectual disability with marked delay in attainment of motor milestones (100%); movement or balance disorder (100%); absent speech or fewer than six words (100%); any combination of frequent laughing/smiling, apparent happy demeanor, easily excitable personality often with uplifted hand-flapping.

Craniofacial. Microbrachycephaly; blond hair (65%); ocular anomalies, including decreased pigmentation of the choroid and iris, the latter resulting in pale blue eyes (88%); maxillary hypoplasia, deep-set eyes, a large mouth with tongue protrusion and widely spaced teeth; prognathia.

Neurologic. Ataxia and jerky arm movements resembling a puppet gait (100%); characteristic position of arms, which are upheld with flexion at wrists and elbows; drooling; excessive chewing/mouthing behavior; seizures varying from major motor to akinetic, beginning usually between 18 and 24 months (86%); electroencephalographic abnormalities consisting of high-amplitude spike and slow waves at 2 to 3 Hz posteriorly, large-amplitude slow waves mixed with spikes facilitated by eye closure, and generalized large-amplitude intermediate slow activity persisting for most of the record (92%); hypotonia and occasionally hyperreflexia; computed tomography shows cerebral atrophy (33%); left hand preference, increased sensitivity to heat, abnormal sleep-wake cycles.

OCCASIONAL ABNORMALITIES

Scoliosis, hypopigmentation (39%), strabismus (42%), myopia and hypermetropia, nystagmus, attraction/fascination with water and with crinkly items such as paper or plastic, obesity in older children, constipation.

NATURAL HISTORY

The intellectual disability, although nonprogressive, is severe. Seizure activity is most severe around 4 years and may stop by 10 years of age. Although the laughter initially was not apparently associated with happiness, it is now felt that it occurs more frequently when the child is involved with adult speech, touch, smiling, laughing, and eye contact. Decreased need for sleep, particularly between 2 and 6 years, has been noted.

Although severe problems exist with speech, the vast majority communicate in other ways, such as sign language. Cognitive skills are stronger than language and motor skills, and receptive language skills are better than expressive. Receptive ability may be sufficient to understand simple commands. Most individuals become toilet-trained by day and some by night. None could live independently.

ETIOLOGY

There are several known genetic mechanisms all involving loss of function of the *UBE3A* gene located on chromosome 15q11-q13, which in the brain is expressed from the maternal chromosome only: a de novo interstitial deletion of maternal 15q11-q13 (70%–75% of cases); paternal uniparental disomy (UPD) of chromosome 15 (3%–7%); an imprinting defect (2%–3%); and a mutation in the E3 ubiquitin protein ligase gene (*UBE3A*) in 10%. No identifiable molecular abnormality has been found in 10% of cases. Whereas the parental origin of the deleted chromosome 15 is paternal in Prader-Willi syndrome, it is always maternal in Angelman syndrome. The fact that the parent of origin of the deleted chromosome impacts the phenotype implies that genes located at 15q11-q13 on the maternally inherited chromosome are expressed differently from those at the same locus on the paternally inherited chromosome, a phenomenon known as genomic imprinting.

The vast majority occur sporadically except in the following situations: a chromosomal rearrangement or unbalanced translocation in which the same rearrangement occurs in the mother, an inherited imprinting center mutation (if present in the mother), and a *UBE3A* mutation (if present in the mother).

Children with deletions are more developmentally delayed than those with nondeletions, with the exception of expressive language.

COMMENT
15q11.1q11.3 DUPLICATIONS AND TRIPLICATIONS. Inv dup(15) is the most frequent supernumerary marker chromosome in humans. They are isodicentric, bisatellited, and consist of two inverted copies of the short (p) arm, the centromere, and variable regions of the proximal long (q) arm, which are fused. Most commonly, a "small" marker, which does not contain the Prader-Willi/Angelman syndrome (PWS/AS) critical region, is found to have no phenotypic effect, making it the most common "benign" chromosomal marker. However, if the PWS/AS region is included in the "large" 15q marker, tetrasomy for this imprinted region will have important phenotypic consequences only when the origin is maternal, including intellectual disability, seizures, and autism spectrum disorders, schizophrenia, strabismus, and subtle dysmorphic features. Interstitial duplications of the PWS/AS regions in the maternally inherited chromosome cause a similar, somewhat milder, phenotype. Overexpression of the maternally expressed gene *UBE3A* is predicted to be the primary cause of the autistic features associated with dup15q.

References

Angelman H: "Puppet" children: A report on three cases, *Dev Med Child Neurol* 7:681, 1965.

Williams CA, Frias JL: The Angelman ("happy puppet") syndrome, *Am J Med Genet* 11:453, 1982.

Boyd SG, et al: The EEG in early diagnosis of the Angelman (happy puppet) syndrome, *Eur J Pediatr* 147:508, 1988.

Clayton-Smith J: Clinical research on Angelman syndrome in the United Kingdom: Observations on 82 affected individuals, *Am J Med Genet* 46:12, 1993.

Knoll JHM, et al: Cytogenetic and molecular studies in the Prader-Willi and Angelman syndromes, *Am J Med Genet* 46:2, 1993.

Nicholls RD: Genomic imprinting and uniparental disomy in Angelman and Prader-Willi syndromes: A review, *Am J Med Genet* 46:16, 1993.

Hall BD: Adjunct diagnostic test for Angelman syndrome: The tuning fork response, *Am J Med Genet* 109:238, 2002.

Clayton-Smith J, Loan L: Angelman syndrome: A review of the clinical and genetic aspects, *J Med Genet* 40:87, 2003.

Battaglia A: The inv dup(15) or idic(15) syndrome: A clinically recognizable neurogenetic disorder, *Brain Dev* 27:365, 2005.

Williams CA, et al: Angelman syndrome 2005: An updated consensus for diagnostic criteria, *Am J Med Genet A* 140A:413, 2006.

Gentile JK, et al: A neurodevelopmental survey of Angelman syndrome with genotype-phenotype correlations, *J Dev Behav Pediatr* 31:592, 2010.

Ramsden SC, et al: Practice guidelines for the molecular analysis of Prader-Willi and Angelman syndromes, *BMC Med Genet* 11:70, 2010.

Adams D, et al: Age related changes in social behavior in children with Angelman syndrome, *Am J Med Genet A* 155A:1290, 2011.

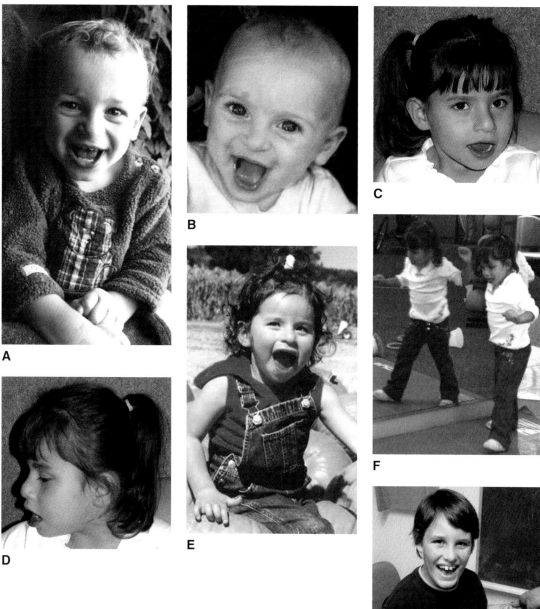

FIGURE 1.   Angelman syndrome. **A–G,** Photographs of affected children with maxillary hypoplasia, deep-set eyes, a large mouth, and prognathism. (**A–F,** Courtesy Dr. Lynne M. Bird, Children's Hospital, San Diego.)

PRADER-WILLI SYNDROME
Hypotonia, Obesity, Small Hands and Feet

Charles Dickens, in *The Pickwick Papers*, described "a fat and red-faced boy in a state of somnolency." The boy was subsequently addressed as "young dropsy," "young opium eater," and "boa constrictor," no doubt in reference to his obesity, somnolence, and excessive appetite, respectively. This may have been the first reported instance of Prader-Willi syndrome.

Prader and colleagues reported this pattern of abnormality in nine children in 1956. The prevalence is estimated to be 1 in 15,000. Health supervision guidelines have been set forth for children with Prader-Willi syndrome.

ABNORMALITIES

Variability in the extent and severity of features based particularly on age.

Growth. Normal birth length with deceleration in the first 2 months of life, steady linear growth rate during childhood, and decrease in adolescence; mean adult height in males is 155 cm and in females is 148 cm.

Obesity. Increased weight beginning at a median age of 2 years.

Craniofacial. Almond-shaped appearance to palpebral fissures, which may be upslanting; narrow bifrontal diameter; strabismus; thin upper lip.

Hair, Eyes, and Skin. Blond to light brown hair with blue eyes and fair skin that is sun-sensitive; picks excessively at sores.

Performance. Intellectual disability is mild (IQ: 60 to 70) in the majority of cases, with 40% having borderline or low normal intelligence and approximately 20% having moderate intellectual disability. Almost three fourths of affected individuals receive special education and function at a sixth-grade level or below in reading and third-grade level or below in math. Strabismus; food-related behavior problems, including excessive appetite, absent sense of satiation, and obsession with eating; speech articulation problems, particularly hypernasal speech; hypotonia, severe in early infancy.

Hands and Feet. Small; slowing in growth of hands and/or feet, usually becoming evident in mid-childhood (one patient wore size 3 shoes at 23 years of age); narrow hands with straight ulnar border.

Genitalia. Small penis and cryptorchidism, hypoplastic labia minora and clitoris, frequent hypogonadism secondary to a combination of hypothalamic and primary gonadal dysfunction.

Other. Scoliosis, osteoporosis, temperature instability, high pain threshold, skill with jigsaw puzzles, decreased vomiting, growth hormone deficiency.

OCCASIONAL ABNORMALITIES

Poor fine and gross motor coordination; upsweep of frontal scalp hair; microcephaly, seizures, clinodactyly, syndactyly, hypoplasia of auricular cartilage; kyphosis; hip dysplasia, early dental caries; diabetes mellitus; early adrenarche; precocious puberty.

NATURAL HISTORY

The mother may have noted feeble fetal activity, and the baby is often born in the breech position. The hypotonia is most severe in early infancy, when there may be respiratory tract and feeding problems, not uncommonly necessitating tube feeding. The degree of mental deficiency may appear to be greater in infancy than at a later age because of the severity of the hypotonia hindering developmental performance. Regarding behavior, these patients have been noted to be cheerful and good-natured. However, behavioral problems, including stubbornness and rage-type responses, tend to become more frequent in later childhood. Verbal perseverance on favorite topics is common. Failure to thrive is frequent in early infancy. Increased weight gain without an increased intake of calories or increased appetite begins at a median age of 2 years. The weight gain becomes associated with an increased interest in food at a median age of onset of 4.5 years. By a median age of 8 years, hyperphagia—with inappropriate food seeking, bizarre and binge eating, and lack of satiation—begins, at which time obesity becomes a major problem. The obesity, which occurs especially over the lower abdomen, buttocks, and thighs, is due to excess intake, reduced activity, and decreased lean body mass. It paradoxically develops at a time when the hypotonia is improving. The presence of a diabetic type of glucose tolerance curve relates to the severity of the obesity, and only an occasional patient develops diabetes mellitus during childhood. Therapy with growth hormone (GH) results in significant improvement of body composition (decreased fat mass, increased muscle mass, and increased linear growth) and physical function (strength and agility). Concern has been raised for a small risk of death in severely obese, respiratory-compromised individuals with

Prader-Willi syndrome within a few months of the start of GH treatment. Hypothyroidism occurs in 25% of patients.

Reduced life expectancy appears to relate to complications of morbid obesity. In addition, the decline of IQ with age is obviated with weight control. Early short-term testosterone therapy has resulted in enlargement of the penis to normal size for age. Any boy who is doing reasonably well at the age of adolescence should be considered for full testosterone replacement therapy, because his testosterone production is usually inadequate. Sixty percent of females have amenorrhea, and the remaining begin to menstruate between 10 and 28 years with an average of 17 years.

Behavior problems occur frequently in patients older than 50 years as do physical problems such as cardiovascular diseases, diabetes, and dermatological and orthopedic problems.

ETIOLOGY

The genetic changes leading to this disorder all result in a loss of expression of the paternally expressed genes on chromosome 15q11.2-q13. Approximately 70% of affected individuals have a deletion of the long arm of chromosome 15 at q11-q13. In all cases studied, the paternally derived chromosome has been deleted. Maternal uniparental disomy (UPD) (i.e., two maternal copies and no paternal copies of 15q) accounts for a further 25% to 30%. The remaining 1% to 3% are due to a mutation of the imprinting center or to a chromosomal translocation involving proximal 15q. Methylation analysis detects all three molecular defects. If the methylation pattern is abnormal, fluorescent in situ hybridization (FISH) can be used to document a deletion, and microsatellite probes can be used to confirm maternal disomy. An abnormal methylation analysis and normal FISH and UPD studies indicate an imprinting defect. Recurrence risk is negligible except for cases involving a chromosome translocation or for those in which there is an imprinting center mutation.

Compared to those with deletion 15q, individuals with UPD 15 are less likely to be hypopigmented or to have the typical facial features, skin picking, skill with jigsaw puzzles, and high pain threshold. However, they are more likely to have psychotic illness and autism spectrum disorders.

COMMENT

15q11.2 MICRODELETION AND MICRODU-PLICATION. Doornbos et al (2009) reported nine patients with a 350-kb microdeletion 15q11.2 between breakpoints 1 (BP1) and 2 (BP2) of the Prader-Willi critical region and suggested an association of the deletion with intellectual disability or variable learning difficulties, behavioral disturbances, dysmorphic features, and an increased risk of congenital malformations. The deletion involves the four highly conserved nonimprinted genes *TUBGCP5*, *NIPA1*, *NIPA2* and *CYFIP1* in all cases. Epilepsy, social withdrawal, and autism spectrum disorders appear frequent. These microdeletions have reduced penetrance and variable expressivity and can be considered a susceptibility disorder. The reciprocal microduplication also appears to have an impact on learning and behavior, and dysmorphic features as well as hypotonia, cardiac problems, and skeletal abnormalities have been seen. In a large study, approximately 87.5% of the patients carrying the deletion and 80% of the patients carrying the duplication had developmental delay or intellectual disability.

The impact of altered dosage of these genes is also reflected in that cases of Prader-Willi syndrome involving this proximal region containing these four genes show a greater tendency toward compulsive behavior, psychological problems, and lower intellectual ability.

References

Prader A, Labhart A, Willi H: Ein Syndrom von Adipositas, Kleinwuchs, Kryptorchismus und Oligophrenie nach myatonieartigem Zustand im Neugeborenenalter, *Schweiz Med Wochenschr* 86:1260, 1956.

Hall BD, Smith DW: Prader-Willi syndrome, *J Pediatr* 81:286, 1972.

Clarren SK, Smith DW: Prader-Willi syndrome, *Am J Dis Child* 131:798, 1977.

Ledbetter DH, et al: Deletion of chromosome 15 as a cause of the Prader-Willi syndrome, *N Engl J Med* 304:325, 1981.

Creel DJ, et al: Abnormalities of the central visual pathways in the Prader-Willi syndrome associated with hypopigmentation, *N Engl J Med* 314:1606, 1986.

Butler MG, et al: Prader-Willi syndrome: Current understanding of cause and diagnosis, *Am J Med Genet* 35:319, 1990.

Donaldson MDC, et al: The Prader-Willi syndrome, *Arch Dis Child* 70:58, 1994.

Cassidy SB, et al: Comparison of phenotype between patients with Prader-Willi syndrome due to deletion 15q and uniparental disomy 15, *Am J Med Genet* 68:433, 1997.

McEntagart ME, et al: Familial Prader-Willi syndrome: Case report and a literature review, *Clin Genet* 58:216, 2000.

Gunay-Aygun M, et al: The changing purpose of Prader-Willi syndrome clinical diagnostic criteria and proposed revised criteria, *Pediatrics* 108(5), 2001. Available at http://www.pediatrics.org/cgi/content/full/108/5/e92.

Boer H, et al: Psychotic illness in people with Prader-Willi syndrome due to chromosome 15 maternal uniparental disomy, *Lancet* 359:135, 2002.

G

Doornbos M, et al: Nine patients with a microdeletion 15q11.2 between breakpoints 1 and 2 of the Prader-Willi critical region, possibly associated with behavioural disturbances, *Eur J Med Genet* 52:108, 2009.

Buiting K, et al: Prader-Willi syndrome and Angelman syndrome, *Am J Med Genet C Semin Med Genet* 154C:365, 2010.

McCandless SE, et al: Clinical report—Health supervision for children with Prader-Willi syndrome, *Pediatrics* 127:195, 2011.

Burnside RD, et al: Microdeletion/microduplication of proximal 15q11.2 between BP1 and BP2: A susceptibility region for neurological dysfunction including developmental and language delay, *Hum Genet* 130:517, 2011.

Sinnema M, et al: Aging in Prader-Willi syndrome: Twelve persons over the age of 50 years, *Am J Med Genet A* 158A:1326, 2012.

Cassidy SB, et al: Prader-Willi syndrome, *Genet Med* 14:10, 2012.

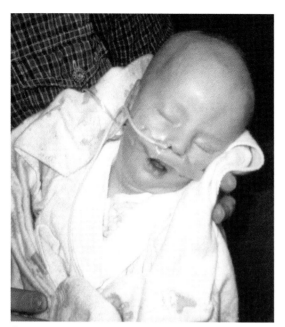

A

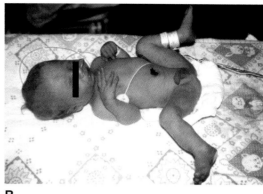

B

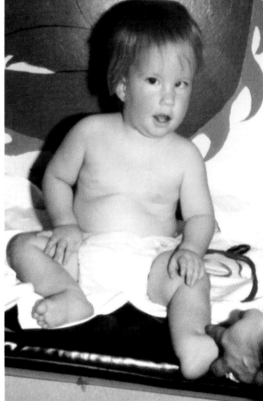

D

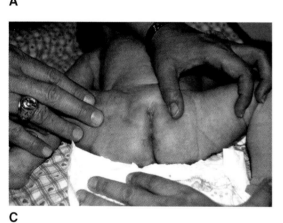

C

G

FIGURE 1. Prader-Willi syndrome. **A–D,** Four children from birth through 14 months. Note the hypotonia, labial hypoplasia, and upslanting palpebral fissures. (**A** and **C,** Courtesy Dr. Suzanne Cassidy, University of California, Irvine; **B,** courtesy Dr. Lynne M. Bird, Children's Hospital, San Diego.)

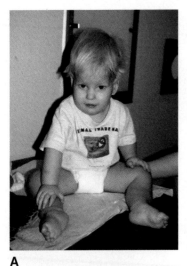

A

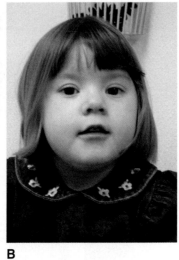

B

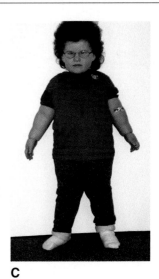

C

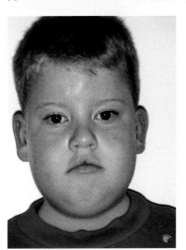

D

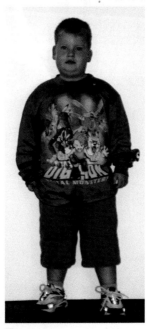

E

FIGURE 2.   **A–E,** Note the almond-shaped eyes, narrow bifrontal diameter, and small hands and feet. (**A** and **B,** Courtesy Dr. Lynne M. Bird, Children's Hospital, San Diego; **C–E,** courtesy Dr. Suzanne Cassidy, University of California, Irvine.)

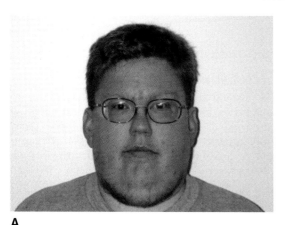

A

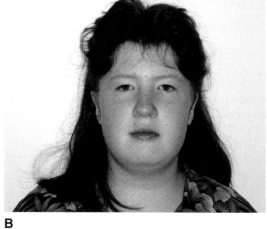

B

G

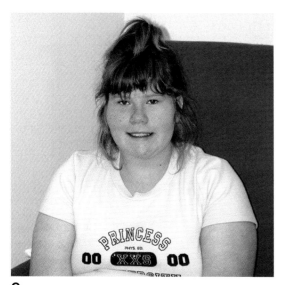

C

FIGURE 3.   A–C, Affected young adults. (Courtesy Dr. Suzanne Cassidy, University of California, Irvine.)

COHEN SYNDROME
Obesity, Progressive Pigmentary Retinopathy, Intermittent Neutropenia

This disorder was recognized in 1973 in two affected siblings and one isolated case by Cohen and colleagues. More than 150 cases, a large percentage from Finland, have been subsequently described. Although the Finnish cases have been clinically homogeneous, cases from outside of Finland have been phenotypically variable. More recently a distinctive clinical phenotype encompassing all populations has been set forth by Chandler et al.

ABNORMALITIES

Growth. Truncal obesity of midchildhood onset, low birth weight, postnatal growth deficiency.

Performance. Persisting hypotonia and weakness, intellectual disability (59% of children older than 8 years in one study had achieved reasonable verbal communication skills. Of the remaining patients, five were using single words only and four were nonverbal), clumsiness. When asked to smile, the patient grimaces.

Craniofacial. Postnatal onset microcephaly, thick head hair, bushy eyebrows and long/thick eyelashes, high nasal bridge and beak-shaped nose, maxillary hypoplasia with mild downslant to palpebral fissures, high-arched or wave-shaped eyelids, short philtrum, open mouth with prominent maxillary central incisors, thin upper lip that does not cover the teeth, high narrow palate, mild micrognathia, large ears.

Eyes. Myopia with onset before 5 years and progression to high myopia by the second decade. strabismus, defective vision in bright light, constricted visual fields, progressive pigmentary retinopathy, with bull's-eye-like maculae, pigmentary deposits, and optic atrophy.

Limbs. Narrow hands and feet with mild shortening of metacarpals and metatarsals, slender fingers that taper, simian creases, hyperextensible joints, camptodactyly, genu valgus, cubitus valgus, pes planovalgus, wide sandal gap.

Spine. Lumbar lordosis with mild scoliosis.

Other. Neutropenia, which is often intermittent. Delayed puberty, cryptorchidism, low hairline.

OCCASIONAL ABNORMALITIES

Cardiac defects, microphthalmia, colobomata, enlarged corpus callosum, cerebellar hypoplasia, mild cutaneous syndactyly, seizures, growth hormone deficiency, ureteropelvic obstruction, tall stature, mitral valve prolapse.

NATURAL HISTORY

Neonatal feeding difficulties; weakness and hypotonia persist beyond infancy, and truncal obesity of moderate degree develops by midchildhood; motor milestones are delayed. Despite their moderate to severe degree of intellectual disability, the majority have a cheerful disposition. Independence levels are poor, but socialization skills are less impaired. Vision begins to deteriorate early but slowly; progressive myopia and progressive retinal dystrophy in all patients older than 5 years.

ETIOLOGY

This disorder has an autosomal recessive inheritance pattern. Mutations in *VPS13B* (previously known as *COH1*), a gene located on chromosome 8q22, are responsible. *VPS13B* encodes a transmembrane protein with a presumed role in vesicle-mediated sorting and intracellular protein transport within the cell. It has recently been established as a Golgi-associated matrix protein required for Golgi integrity.

References

Cohen MM Jr, et al: A new syndrome with hypotonia, obesity, mental deficiency, and facial, oral, ocular, and limb anomalies, *J Pediatr* 83:280, 1973.

Carey JC, Hall BD: Confirmation of the Cohen syndrome, *J Pediatr* 93:239, 1978.

Kousseff BG: Cohen syndrome: Further delineation and inheritance, *Am J Med Genet* 9:25, 1981.

Norio R, Christina R, Lindahl E: Further delineation of the Cohen syndrome: Report on chorioretinal dystrophy, leukopenia, and consanguinity, *Clin Genet* 25:1, 1984.

North C, et al: The clinical features of the Cohen syndrome, *J Med Genet* 22:131, 1985.

Massa G, et al: Growth hormone deficiency in a girl with the Cohen syndrome, *J Med Genet* 28:48, 1991.

Kivitie-Kallio S, et al: Cohen syndrome: Essential features, natural history, and heterogeneity, *Am J Med Genet* 102:125, 2001.

Kolehmainen J, et al: Cohen syndrome is caused by mutations in a novel gene, *COH1*, encoding a transmembrane protein with a presumed role in vesicle-mediated sorting and intracellular protein transport, *Am J Hum Genet* 72:1359, 2003.

Chandler KE, et al: Diagnostic criteria, clinical characteristics, and natural history of Cohen syndrome, *J Med Genet* 40:233, 2003.

Kolehmainen J, et al: Delineation of Cohen syndrome following a large-scale genotype-phenotype screen, *Am J Hum Genet* 75:122, 2004.

Seifert W, et al: Cohen syndrome-associated protein, COH1, is a novel, giant Golgi matrix protein required for Golgi integrity, *J Biol Chem* 286:37665, 2011.

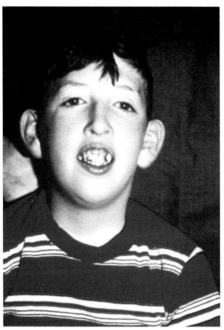

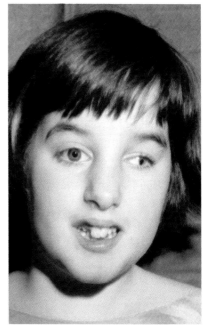

G

A

B

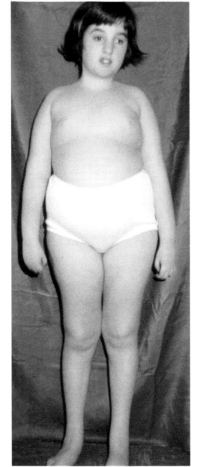

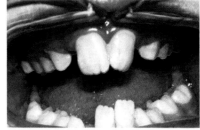

D

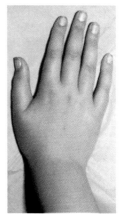

E

FIGURE 1.   Cohen syndrome. **A** and **B,**
Brother and sister at 11 and 14 years of
age, respectively. **C,** An 8-year-old child in
whom obesity developed at 5 to 6 years.
D and **E,** Prominent central incisors and
narrow hands with slim fingers.
(**A–E,** From Cohen MM Jr: *J Pediatr* 83:280,
1973, with permission.)

C

PALLISTER-KILLIAN SYNDROME

(PALLISTER MOSAIC SYNDROME, KILLIAN/TESCHLER-NICOLA SYNDROME, TETRASOMY 12P)

Sparse Anterior Scalp Hair, Long Philtrum with Thin Upper Lip and Distinct Cupid Bow, Streaks of Hypo- and Hyperpigmentation

Teschler-Nicola and Killian described a 3-year-old girl with this disorder in 1981. A second case was reported by Schroer and Stevenson in 1983. It was subsequently recognized that two adults with a similar phenotype and mosaicism for a marker chromosome reported by Pallister and colleagues in 1976 had the same condition. Tetrasomy 12p, either mosaic or total, has been documented in skin fibroblasts from affected individuals but only rarely in peripheral blood.

ABNORMALITIES

Growth. Normal or increased birth length, weight, and head circumference, with postnatal deceleration of length and head circumference; obesity frequently develops.

Performance. Profound intellectual disability with only minimal speech development, seizures, hypotonia with contractures developing with advancing age.

Craniofacial. Sparse anterior scalp hair particularly in temporal areas in infancy, with sparse eyebrows and eyelashes; prominent forehead; coarsening of face over time. Upslanting palpebral fissures; ocular hypertelorism; ptosis; strabismus; epicanthal folds; flat, broad nasal root and short nose with anteverted nostrils; chubby cheeks; long philtrum with thin upper lip and distinct cupid-bow shape; protruding lower lip; delayed dental eruption; large ears with thick protruding lobules; short neck.

Other. Streaks of hyperpigmentation and hypopigmentation, broad hands with short digits, accessory nipples, disproportionate shortening of arms and legs.

OCCASIONAL ABNORMALITIES

Microcephaly; polymicrogyria; cataracts; stenosis of external auditory canal; hearing loss; borderline to normal IQ; hypopigmentation of fundus; macroglossia; prominent lateral palatine ridges; cleft palate; bifid uvula; aortic dilatation; mild skeletal changes, including delayed ossification of vertebrae and pubic bones, flared anterior ribs, and broad metaphyses of long bones, particularly the femur; micrognathia; umbilical and inguinal hernias; hypermobile joints; kyphoscoliosis; hemihypertrophy; fifth finger clinodactyly; distal digital

hypoplasia; postaxial polydactyly of hands and feet; congenital hip dislocation; simian crease; sweating abnormalities; lymphedema; cardiac defect; pericardial agenesis; diaphragmatic hernia; persistence of urogenital sinus/cloaca; intestinal malrotation; imperforate anus; hypospadias; sacral appendage; renal defect; omphalocele.

NATURAL HISTORY

A significant number of affected patients are stillborn or die in the neonatal period. Seizures usually begin in infancy. Survivors are frequently bedridden. Most will never talk. Physical characteristics change with age. Initially sparse, anterior scalp hair grows in by 2 to 5 years; a normal-size tongue becomes macroglossic; initial micrognathia progresses to prognathism, and contractures develop between 5 and 10 years after initial hypotonia. The face of adolescents and adults is coarse with thick lips, an everted lower lip, a broad nasal root, and high forehead. The oldest reported patient is a profoundly retarded, nonambulatory 45-year-old man with multiple joint contractures.

ETIOLOGY

Most cases of this disorder are the result of a supernumerary isochromosome made up of the short arms of chromosome 12 resulting in tetrasomy 12p in skin fibroblasts. Although most patients have had normal karyotypes in peripheral lymphocytes, at least 5 have had lymphocyte mosaicism for the isochromosome 12p. Complete or partial duplication of 12p (trisomy 12p rather than tetrasomy 12p) due to an interstial duplication or unbalanced translocation has also been noted. A minimal critical region at 12p13.31 for the Pallister-Killian phenotype has been identified.

References

Pallister PD, et al: The Pallister mosaic syndrome, *Birth Defects* 13(3B):103, 1976.

Teschler-Nicola M, Killian W: Case report 72: Mental retardation, unusual facial appearance, abnormal hair, *Synd Ident* 7(1):6, 1981.

Buyse ML, Korf BR: Killian syndrome, Pallister mosaic syndrome, or mosaic tetrasomy 12p? An analysis, *J Clin Dysmorphol* 1(3):2, 1983.

Hall BD: Teschler-Nicola/Killian syndrome: A sporadic case in an 11-year-old male, *J Clin Dysmorphol* 1(3):14, 1983.

Schroer RJ, Stevenson RE: Further clinical delineation of the syndrome of unusual facial appearance, abnormal hair and mental retardation reported by Teschler-Nicola and Killian. *Proc Greenwood Genet Cntr* 2:3, 1983.

Reynolds JF, et al: Isochromosome 12p mosaicism (Pallister mosaic aneuploidy or Pallister-Killian syndrome): Report of 11 cases, *Am J Med Genet* 27:257, 1987.

Schinzel A: Tetrasomy 12p (Pallister-Killian syndrome), *J Med Genet* 28:122, 1991.

Bielanska MA, et al: Pallister-Killian syndrome: A mild case diagnosed by fluorescence in situ hybridization: Review of the literature and expansion of the phenotype, *Am J Med Genet* 65:104, 1996.

Stalker HJ, et al: High cognitive functioning and behavioral phenotype in Pallister-Killian syndrome, *Am J Med Genet A* 140A:1950, 2006.

Jamuar S, et al: Clinical and radiological findings in Pallister-Killian syndrome, *Eur J Med Genet* 55:167, 2012.

Izumi K, et al: Duplication12p and Pallister-Killian syndrome: A case report and review of the literature toward defining a Pallister-Killian syndrome minimal critical region, *Am J Med Genet A* 158A:3033, 2012.

G

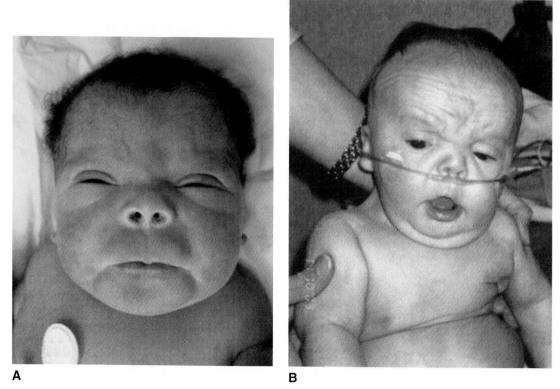

A   **B**

FIGURE 1.   Pallister-Killian syndrome. **A** and **B,** Affected newborn. (**B,** Courtesy Dr. Stephen Braddock, University of Missouri, Columbia.)

ETIOLOGY

This disorder has an autosomal recessive inheritance pattern. Zellweger syndrome is one of a number of peroxisome biogenesis disorders referred to as the Zellweger syndrome spectrum (ZSS) disorders that are manifest by absence or reduced numbers of peroxisomes in tissues as well as multiple enzyme abnormalities. ZSS disorders are caused by a defect in at least 12 PEX genes, which encode peroxins, proteins necessary for peroxisome biosynthesis and import of peroxisomal proteins.

COMMENT

The ZSS disorders include Zellweger syndrome (most severe), neonatal adrenoleukodystrophy (intermediate), and infantile Refsum disease (least severe). In addition to ZSS, peroxisome biogenesis disorders include autosomal recessive chondrodysplasia punctata (see page 504), which is caused by mutations in the *PEX7* gene.

References

Bowen P, et al: A familial syndrome of multiple congenital defects, *Bull Johns Hopkins Hosp* 114:402, 1964.

Smith DW, Opitz JM, Inhorn SL: A syndrome of multiple developmental defects including polycystic kidneys and intrahepatic biliary dysgenesis in two siblings, *J Pediatr* 67:617, 1965.

Opitz JM, et al: The Zellweger syndrome, *Birth Defects* 5:144, 1969.

Goldfischer S, et al: Peroxisomal and mitochondrial defects in the cerebro-hepato-renal syndrome, *Science* 182:62, 1973.

Kelley RI: Review: The cerebrohepatorenal syndrome of Zellweger: Morphologic and metabolic aspects, *Am J Med Genet* 16:503, 1983.

Datta NS, Wilson GN, Hajra AK: Deficiency of enzymes catalyzing the biosynthesis of glycerol ether lipids in Zellweger syndrome, *N Engl J Med* 311:1080, 1984.

Hajra AK, et al: Prenatal diagnosis of Zellweger cerebrohepatorenal syndrome, *N Engl J Med* 312:445, 1985.

G

Solish JI, et al: The prenatal diagnosis of the cerebro-hepato-renal syndrome of Zellweger, *Prenat Diagn* 5:27, 1985.

Wilson GN, et al: Zellweger syndrome: Diagnostic assays, syndrome delineation, and potential therapy, *Am J Med Genet* 24:69, 1986.

Ebberink MS, et al: Genetic classification and mutational spectrum of more than 600 patients with a Zellweger syndrome spectrum disorder, *Hum Mutat* 32:59, 2010.

Moser HW: Genotype-phenotype correlations in disorders of peroxisome biogenesis, *Mol Genet Metab* 68:316, 1999.

Steinberg SJ, et al: Peroxisomal disorders: Clinical and biochemical studies in 15 children and prenatal diagnosis in seven families, *Am J Med Genet* 85:502, 1999.

Suzuki Y, et al: Genetic and molecular bases of peroxisome biogenesis disorders, *Gen Med* 3:372, 2001.

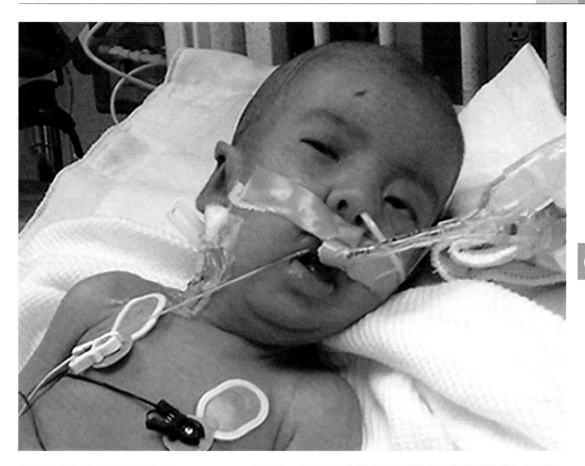

G

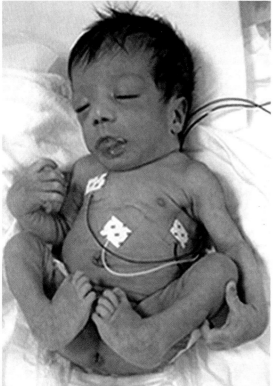

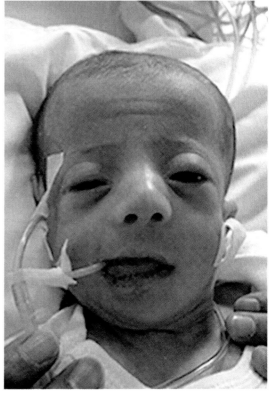

FIGURE 1. Zellweger syndrome. Three affected neonates. Note the hypotonia, high forehead with shallow supraorbital ridges, anteverted nares, and mild micrognathia as well as the talipes equinovarus and contractures at the knees. (From Shaheen, et al: *Clin Genet* 2010, with permission.)

FREEMAN-SHELDON SYNDROME
(WHISTLING FACE SYNDROME, DISTAL ARTHROGRYPOSIS TYPE 2A)
Mask-Like "Whistling" Facies, Hypoplastic Alae Nasi, Talipes Equinovarus

This disorder was described by Freeman and Sheldon in 1938. At least 60 cases have been reported.

ABNORMALITIES

Most of the features are secondary to increased muscle tone.

Facies. Full forehead and mask-like facies with small mouth giving a "whistling" appearance (100%), deep-set eyes, broad nasal bridge, telecanthus, epicanthal folds, strabismus, blepharophimosis, small nose, hypoplastic alae nasi with coloboma, long philtrum, H-shaped cutaneous dimpling on chin, high palate, small tongue, limited palatal movement with nasal speech, dental crowding (100%).

Joints and Skeletal. Ulnar deviation of hands (91%), cortical thumbs, flexion of fingers (88%), thick skin over flexor surface of proximal phalanges, equinovarus with contracted toes (59%), vertical talus, kyphoscoliosis (84%), contracture of hips and/or knees (73%), contractures of shoulders, steeply inclined anterior cranial fossa on radiographs, scoliosis (85%).

Other. Postnatal growth deficiency (62%), strabismus (42%), inguinal hernia (23%), cryptorchidism (42%).

OCCASIONAL ABNORMALITIES

Microcephaly (44%), mental deficiency (31%), seizures (19%), flat face, ptosis, upper airway narrowing, subcutaneous ridge across lower forehead, short neck, low birth weight, dislocation of hip, spina bifida occulta, cerebellar and brainstem atrophy, absent brainstem auditory evoked response, prominent mental protuberance on radiographs of facial bones, frequent fractures (26%), joint dislocations (12%).

NATURAL HISTORY

These patients are not uncommonly born in the breech position, and/or their delivery may be difficult. Feeding difficulties in the neonatal period related in most cases to poor suck. Oro- or nasogastric tube required in 45% and gastrostomy tube in 17%. Vomiting and dysphagia may lead to failure to thrive in infancy. There may be early mortality, often related to aspiration. Difficulties with speech, oral hygiene, and dental treatment secondary to the small mouth can be a problem. Mean age at walking 18 months with a range from 10 to 48 months, and 83% use an ambulatory assist device. Eventual intelligence is in the normal range in the majority of patients. Obstructive sleep apnea/hypopnea exclusively during REM sleep has been described. The average number of surgical procedures is 10.3 per individual. Muscle rigidity following halothane anesthesia has been reported, which gives credence to the theory that this disorder is the result of an underlying myopathy.

ETIOLOGY

This disorder has an autosomal dominant inheritance pattern. Mutations in embryonic myosin heavy chain (*MYH3*) are responsible. The phenotype associated with mutations in *MYH3* includes distal arthrogryposis type 2A (DA2A, also called Freeman-Sheldon syndrome), DA2B (also called Sheldon-Hall syndrome), and DA1 (see page 228).

References

Freeman EA, Sheldon JH: Craniocarpotarsal dystrophy: An undescribed congenital malformation, *Arch Dis Child* 13:277, 1938.

Burian F: The "whistling face" characteristic in a compound cranio-facio-corporal syndrome, *Br J Plast Surg* 16:140, 1963.

Antley RM, et al: Diagnostic criteria for the whistling face syndrome, *Birth Defects* 11:161, 1975.

O'Connell DJ, Hall CM: Cranio-carpotarsal dysplasia: A report of seven cases, *Radiology* 123:719, 1977.

Kousseff BG, McConnachie P, Hadro TA: Autosomal recessive type of whistling face syndrome in twins, *Pediatrics* 69:328, 1982.

Millner MM, et al: Whistling face syndrome: A case report and literature review, *Acta Paediatr Hung* 31:279, 1991.

Jones R, Dolcourt JL: Muscle rigidity following halothane anesthesia in two patients with Freeman-Sheldon syndrome, *Acta Neurol Scand* 102:395, 2000.

Stevenson DA, et al: Clinical characteristics and natural history of Freeman-Sheldon syndrome, *Pediatrics* 117:754, 2006.

Toydemir RM, et al: Mutations in embryonic myosin heavy chain (*MYH3*) cause Freeman-Sheldon syndrome and Sheldon-Hall syndrome, *Nat Genet* 38:561, 2006.

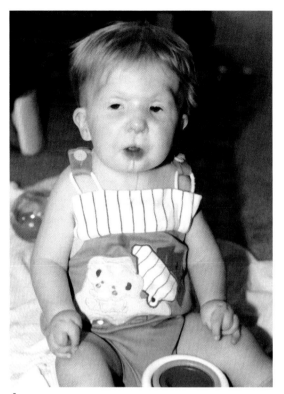

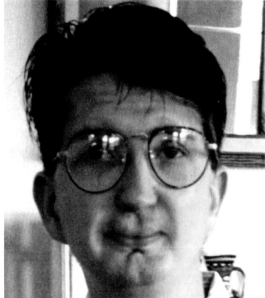

B

G

A

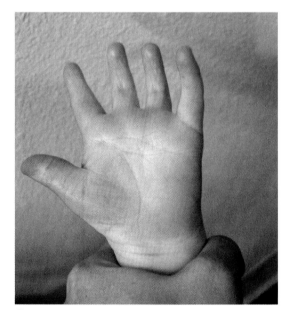

C

FIGURE 1.   Freeman-Sheldon syndrome. **A–C,** Affected boy and his father. Note the crease pattern on chin, deep-set eyes, hypoplastic ala nasi, and camptodactyly. (Courtesy Dr. Michael Bamshad, University of Washington, Seattle, Washington.)

MYOTONIC DYSTROPHY SYNDROME
(MYOTONIC DYSTROPHY TYPE 1, STEINERT SYNDROME, DYSTROPHIA MYOTONICA)
Myotonia with Muscle Atrophy, Cataract, Hypogonadism

The text by Caughey and Myrianthopoulos presents the manifold abnormalities that may occur as features of this single mutant gene. Approximately 1 in 8000 individuals are affected.

ABNORMALITIES

Muscle Degeneration. Myotonia (difficulty in relaxing a contracted muscle), often best appreciated in the hand or jaw or by tapping the tongue; degeneration of swollen muscle cells giving way to thin and atrophic muscle fibers with weakness; ptosis of the eyelids (frequent); myopathic facies.

Eyes. Cataract, often evident only as "myotonic dust" by slit lamp inspection.

Gonadal Insufficiency. Testicular atrophy (80%) in males. Amenorrhea, dysmenorrhea, ovarian cyst in females.

Scalp. Premature frontal hair recession, especially in males.

Cardiac. Conduction defects with arrhythmias.

OCCASIONAL ABNORMALITIES

Hypotonia in infancy, mental deficiency, microcephaly, brain abnormalities (especially the anterior temporal and frontal lobes), talipes, clinodactyly, hernia, cryptorchidism, kyphoscoliosis, hyperostotic cranial bones, atrophic thin skin, macular abnormality, blepharitis, keratitis sicca, goiter, thyroid adenomata, diabetes mellitus.

NATURAL HISTORY

The age of onset is from prenatal life to the sixth or seventh decade, with the average being between 20 and 25 years of age. Lens opacification is usually evident by slit lamp examination in the 20s. Initial signs of the disease are variable. Myotonia may be so mild as to be detected only when specifically tested for. Muscle wasting and weakness, occasionally asymmetric, most often involves the facial and temporal muscles, yielding the expressionless "myopathic facies." The most consistent evident weakness is in the orbicularis oculi muscles. Other involved muscles are the anterior cervical and those of the arms, thighs, and anterior lower leg, with progression from proximal to distal. Ptosis of the eyelids is frequent, and pseudo-hypertrophy is an occasional feature. One of the most sensitive early indicators of muscle dysfunction is the radiologic evidence of partial retention of radiopaque material

in the pharynx after swallowing. Mental deterioration may also be a feature. There is increasing debility, with death, usually by the fifth or sixth decade, as a consequence of pneumonia, cardiac failure, or intercurrent illness.

Congenital myotonic dystrophy is associated with polyhydramnios and decreased fetal activity. Severe hypotonia, difficulty in swallowing and sucking, a tented upper lip, talipes equinovarus (in some cases, multiple joint contractures), cerebral ventricular enlargement, edema, and hematomas of the skin are all frequently present in the newborn period. Myotonia, muscle wasting, and cataracts are not seen initially. An infant mortality rate of approximately 25% has been documented, the majority of deaths occurring in the neonatal period because of respiratory failure. For those who survive, the symptoms diminish. However, at adolescence, typical features of the adult variant develop. Although the vast majority of affected children walk by 3 years of age, psychomotor retardation is present in all survivors. With the exception of five known cases of paternal transmission, congenital myotonic dystrophy has occurred only in the offspring of mothers who have myotonic dystrophy.

ETIOLOGY

This disorder has an autosomal dominant inheritance pattern with variability in expression. The disorder is caused by an unstable trinucleotide repeat expansion containing cytosine-thymidine-guanosine (CTG) in the *DM1* gene located at chromosome region 19q13.3. With transmission of the disorder to family members in subsequent generations, the severity of clinical symptoms increases and their onset occurs earlier. This phenomenon, known as anticipation, is due to expansion of the repeat, which is estimated to have a 93% chance of occurring when the altered allele is passed from parent to child. It is generally thought that the size of the triplet expansion correlates with the severity of the disease and the age of onset. Thus, newborns presenting with congenital myotonic dystrophy have, on average, the largest repeat sizes.

COMMENT

DNA-based testing is indicated for evaluation of neonates with hypotonia and severe feeding problems, for confirmation of a clinical diagnosis, and for evaluation of at-risk asymptomatic individuals with a confirmed family history of myotonic dystrophy.

References

Caughey JE, Myrianthopoulos ND: *Dystrophia Myotonica and Related Disorders*, Springfield, Ill, 1963, Charles C Thomas.

Pruzanski W: Myotonic dystrophy. A multisystem disease. Report of 67 cases and a review of the literature, *Psychiatr Neurol (Basel)* 149:302, 1965.

Calderon R: Myotonic dystrophy: A neglected cause of mental retardation, *J Pediatr* 68:423, 1966.

Pruzanski W: Variants of myotonic dystrophy in preadolescent life (the syndrome of myotonic dysembryoplasia), *Brain* 89:563, 1966.

Bell DB, Smith DW: Myotonic dystrophy in the neonate, *J Pediatr* 81:83, 1972.

Brook JD, et al: Molecular basis of myotonic dystrophy: Expansion of a trinucleotide (CTG) repeat at the 3′ end of a transcript encoding a protein kinase family member, *Cell* 68:799, 1992.

Fu YH, et al: An unstable repeat in a gene related to myotonic dystrophy, *Science* 255:1256, 1992.

Mahadevan M, et al: Myotonic dystrophy mutation: An unstable CTG repeat in the 3′ untranslated region of the gene, *Science* 255:1253, 1992.

Reardon W, et al: The natural history of congenital myotonic dystrophy: Mortality and long-term clinical aspects, *Arch Dis Child* 68:177, 1993.

Wieringa B: Commentary: Myotonic dystrophy reviewed: Back to the future? *Hum Mol Genet* 3:1, 1994.

Keller C, et al: Congenital myotonic dystrophy requiring prolonged endotracheal and noninvasive assisted ventilation: Not a uniformly fatal condition, *Pediatrics* 101:704, 1998.

Meola G: Clinical and genetic heterogeneity in myotonic dystrophies, *Muscle Nerve* 23:1789, 2000.

Zaki M, et al: Congenital myotonic dystrophy: Prenatal ultrasound findings and pregnancy outcome, *Ultrasound Obstet Gynecol* 29:284, 2007.

G

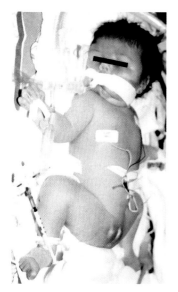

	FETAL-NEONATAL INFANCY	CHILDHOOD	ADULTHOOD
CNS	Mental deficiency – – – – – – – – – – – – – – – – –➤		
OCULAR	Cataracts –➤ Ptosis –➤		
SKELETAL	Clubfeet	Scoliosis/lordosis – – – – – – –➤ Cranial hyperostosis– – – – – – –➤	
RESPIRATORY	Neonatal distress Recurrent infection – – – – – – – – – – – – – – – –		Chronic insufficiency
NEURO – MUSCULAR	Hypotonia/"floppy" Facial diplegia Weakness/atrophy – – – – – – – – – – – – – – – – –➤ Variable myotonia – – – – – – – – – – – – – – – –➤	Dysarthria – – – – – – – – – – –➤	
GI	Poor feeding Impaired deglutition – – – – – – – – – – – – – – – –➤		
GONADAL	Cryptorchidism – – – – – – – – – – – – – – – – –➤		Hypogonadism
CARDIAC		Disturbed conduction – – – – – – –➤	
MISC.		Frontal baldness – – – – – – – –➤ Decreased IgG and IgM – – – – – –➤	

FIGURE 1. *Above left,* Severely affected, almost immobile newborn baby of mother with myotonic dystrophy. (Courtesy David Weaver, Indiana University, Indianapolis.) *Above right,* Correlation of protean features of myotonic dystrophy with age of onset, beginning with earliest age reported.

SCHWARTZ-JAMPEL SYNDROME (CHONDRODYSTROPHIA MYOTONIA)
Myotonia, Blepharophimosis, Joint Limitation

Although Pinto and de Sousa were the first to report this disorder, this fact was only recently appreciated. Schwartz and Jampel described a brother and sister with this condition in 1962, and later Aberfeld and colleagues reported further observations on the same patients. Many, if not most, of the features appear to be secondary to a primary muscle disorder with myotonia. Based on the severity and age of onset of symptoms, two types have been delineated. Type 1A is described subsequently. Type 1B is summarized in the comment section.

ABNORMALITIES

Growth. Small stature, usually of postnatal onset.

Muscle. Myotonia with sad, fixed facies, pursed lips, and narrowed palpebral fissures; small mandible; muscular hypertrophy in one half of patients; hyporeflexia.

Joints. Limitation in hips, wrists, fingers, toes, and spine.

Other Skeletal. Vertical shortness of vertebrae (platyspondyly) with coronal clefts of vertebrae, short neck, kyphoscoliosis, enlarged epiphysis at the knees, progressive dysplasia of femoral heads, diaphyses of leg bones bowed anteriorly, hip dysplasia with acetabular flattening, narrow pelvis, coxa valga/vara, wide metaphyses, osteoporosis, pectus carinatum.

Larynx. Small and high-pitched voice.

Eyes. Blepharophimosis, myopia, medial displacement of outer canthi, long eyelashes in irregular rows.

Other. Low hairline, flat facies, small mouth, low-set ears, small testicles, umbilical and inguinal hernias.

OCCASIONAL ABNORMALITIES

Mental deficiency, intrauterine growth deficiency, delayed bone age, equinovarus foot deformation, hip dislocation, cataract, microcornea.

NATURAL HISTORY

Diagnosis of type 1A is usually made in midchildhood when the myotonic face is recognized. Progressive myotonia, muscle wasting, and orthopedic problems, with slow linear growth occur. Myotonia, which usually reaches a plateau in midchildhood, is almost always recorded on electromyography, even when not present clinically. Light and electron microscopic and histochemical examinations of muscles show inconsistent myopathic abnormalities. Contractures are most severe by midadolescence and then remain static. Anesthesia may constitute a serious risk because of difficulties with intubation and malignant hyperthermia. There is slowing of growth, and there are problems of motor function. Affected patients frequently have a waddling gait and crouched stance. Tiredness results from stiffness of joints. Intelligence is usually considered normal. However, myotonia may result in drooling and indistinct speech. Normal pubertal development occurs. The condition appears to be slowly progressive. Life span is normal.

ETIOLOGY

This disorder has an autosomal recessive inheritance pattern. Mutations of the gene encoding perlecan (HSPG2) located at chromosome 1p34-p36.1 are responsible for types 1A and 1B. Type 2 (the neonatal type) does not map to 1p34-p36.1.

COMMENT

Findings in type 1B are more marked than those in type 1A. Bone dysplasia is present at birth. Long bones are shortened, femurs are dumbbell-shaped in infancy, and epiphyses of long bones are large during childhood. There is flattening of vertebral bodies and coronal clefts. Flared iliac wings, supra-acetabular lateral notches, and a wide ischium are characteristic. A third type, Schwartz-Jampel syndrome type 2 and Stuve-Wiedemann syndrome have now been shown to represent a single disorder due to mutations in the leukemia inhibitory receptor (LIFR) gene, located on chromosome 5p13. That disorder presents in the newborn period, with joint contractures, respiratory and feeding difficulties, and frequent death.

References

Pinto LM, de Sousa JS: Um caso de "doença muscular" de difícil classificação, *Rev Port Pediatr Pueric* 6:1, 1961.

Schwartz O, Jampel RS: Congenital blepharophimosis associated with a unique generalized myopathy, *Arch Ophthalmol* 68:52, 1962.

Aberfeld DC, Hinterbuchner LP, Schneider M: Myotonia, dwarfism, diffuse bone disease and unusual ocular and facial abnormalities (a new syndrome), *Brain* 88:313, 1965.

Horan F, Beighton P: Orthopedic aspects of Schwartz syndrome, *J Bone Joint Surg* 57:542, 1975.

Edward WC, Root AW: Chondrodystrophic myotonia (Schwartz-Jampel syndrome): Report of a new case and follow-up of patients initially reported in 1969, *Am J Med Genet* 13:51, 1982.

Viljoen D, Beighton P: Schwartz-Jampel syndrome (chondrodystrophic myotonia), *J Med Genet* 29:58, 1992.

Al Gazali LI: The Schwartz-Jampel syndrome, *Clin Dysmor-phol* 2:47, 1993.

Giedion A: Heterogeneity in Schwartz-Jampel chondro-dysplasia myotonia, *Eur J Pediatr* 156:214, 1997.

Nicole S, et al: Perlecan, the major proteoglycan of base-ment membranes, is altered in patients with Schwartz-Jampel syndrome (chondrodystrophic myotonia), *Nat Genet* 26:480, 2000.

Dagoneau N, et al: Null leukemia inhibitory factor receptor (LIFR) mutations in Stuve-Wiedemann/Schwartz-Jampel type 2 syndrome *Am J Hum Genet* 74:298, 2004

Nessler M, et al: Multidisciplinary approach to the treat-ment of a patient with chondrodystrophic myotonia (Schwartz-Jampel vel Aberfeld syndrome), *Ann Plast Surg* 67:315, 2011.

G

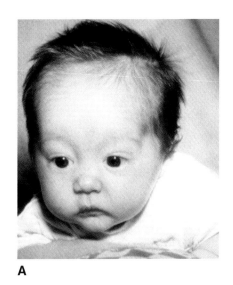

A

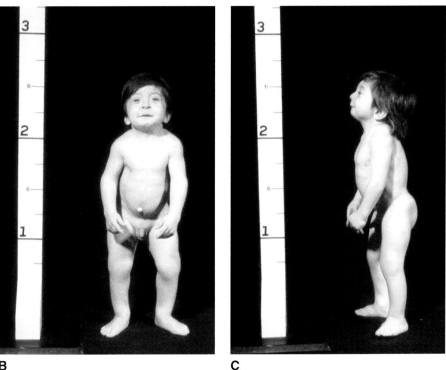

B   C

FIGURE 1. Schwartz-Jampel syndrome. **A–C,** Affected child at 2 months and 12 years. Note the myotonia and sad, fixed face; blepharophimosis; and micrognathia.

MARDEN-WALKER SYNDROME
Blepharophimosis, Joint Contractures, Immobile Facies

This disorder was reported initially in 1966 by Marden and Walker, who described a female infant who died at 3 months of age. Subsequently, approximately 30 affected individuals have been reported.

ABNORMALITIES

Growth. Prenatal (35%) and severe postnatal (88%) growth deficiency.

Performance. Moderate to severe intellectual disability (89%), hypotonia (86%), strabismus (69%).

Craniofacial. Microcephaly (56%), large anterior fontanel, fixed facial expression (100%), blepharophimosis (100%), cleft palate (38%), high-arched palate (88%), micrognathia (100%), small mouth (63%).

Musculoskeletal. Multiple joint contractures present at birth (100%), camptodactyly (69%), arachnodactyly (71%), talipes equinovarus (63%), scoliosis/kyphosis (71%), pectus excavatum/carinatum (75%), decreased muscle mass (92%).

OCCASIONAL ABNORMALITIES

Seizures, electroencephalographic abnormalities, microphthalmia, ventricular dilatation, agenesis of corpus callosum, hypoplasia of cerebellum and inferior vermis, hypoplastic brainstem, Dandy-Walker malformation with vertebral anomalies, short neck, cardiac defect, hypospadias, cryptorchidism, micropenis, microcystic or hypoplastic kidneys, inguinal hernia, radioulnar synostosis, Zollinger-Ellison syndrome, pyloric stenosis and duodenal bands, absent clavicle, hypoplastic lung, patent omphalomesenteric duct.

NATURAL HISTORY

Death has occurred at approximately 3 months of age because of aspiration, sepsis, and/or cardiac failure in 19%. The joint contractures become less severe with age and physical therapy. The vast majority of survivors have been significantly mentally retarded.

ETIOLOGY

This disorder has an autosomal recessive inheritance pattern. The primary abnormality is most likely related to a major defect in central nervous system (CNS) development. Muscle biopsy specimens obtained from some affected individuals have revealed nonspecific changes that are most likely secondary to the primary CNS process.

References

Marden PM, Walker WA: A new generalized connective tissue syndrome, *Am J Dis Child* 112:225, 1966.

Ramer JC, et al: Marden-Walker phenotype: Spectrum of variability in three infants, *Am J Med Genet* 45:285, 1993.

Schrander-Stumple C, et al: Marden-Walker syndrome: Case report, literature review and nosologic discussion, *Clin Genet* 43:303, 1993.

Williams MS, et al: Marden-Walker syndrome: A case report and a critical review of the literature, *Clin Dysmorphol* 2:211, 1993.

Orrico A, et al: Additional case of Marden-Walker syndrome: Support for the autosomal recessive inheritance and refinement of phenotype in a surviving patient, *J Clin Neurol* 16:150, 2001.

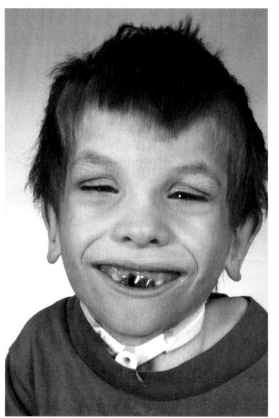

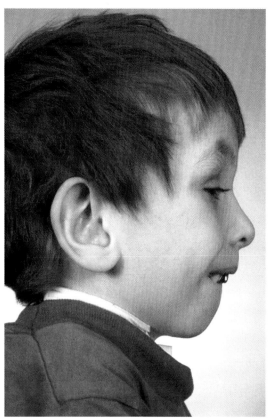

A

B

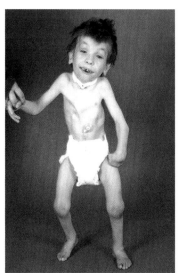

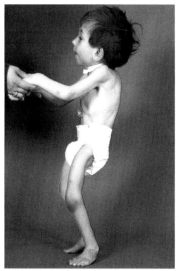

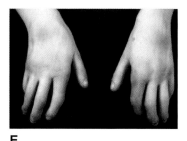

E

C

D

FIGURE 1. Marden-Walker syndrome. **A–E,** A 6-year-old affected boy. (From Williams MS, et al: *Clin Dysmorphol* 2:211, 1993, with permission.)

SCHINZEL-GIEDION SYNDROME
Prominent Forehead, Midface Retraction, Upturned Nose

A brother and sister with this disorder were described in 1978 by Schinzel and Giedion. Slightly less than 50 cases have been reported.

ABNORMALITIES

Growth. Postnatal growth deficiency.

Performance. Profound intellectual deficiency, seizures, opisthotonus, spasticity, hypsarrhythmia, ventriculomegaly secondary to cerebral atrophy and thinning of the corpus callosum.

Craniofacial. Coarse face; widely patent fontanels and sutures (100%) with metopic suture extending anteriorly to nasal root; high, protruding forehead (100%); short nose with low nasal bridge and anteverted nares (83%); shallow orbits with apparent proptosis (100%); deep groove under eyes (100%); ocular hypertelorism (96%); midface hypoplasia (100%); attached helix with protruding lobules of low-set ears (91%).

Limbs. Mesomelic brachymelia, talipes equinovarus or valgus, hyperconvex nails, hypoplastic dermal ridges, simian crease, rocker bottom feet, severe pes planus.

Genital. Anomalies, including hypospadias, short penis, and hypoplastic scrotum in males; deep interlabial sulcus, hypoplasia of labia majora or minora, hymenal atresia, and a short perineum in females.

Renal. Anomalies in 92%, including hydronephrosis, vesicoureteric junction dysplasia, ureteric stenosis, hydroureter, and megacalyces.

Radiologic. Steep short base of skull, sclerotic skull base, wide occipital synchondrosis, multiple wormian bones, hypoplastic first ribs, broad ribs, long or irregular clavicles, hypoplastic/aplastic pubic bones, hypoplastic distal phalanges, short metacarpals of thumbs, broad cortex, and increased density of long bones, widening of distal femurs, tibial bowing.

Other. Short neck with redundant skin, hypoplastic nipples, severe visual impairment, hearing loss.

OCCASIONAL ABNORMALITIES

Macroglossia, wide mouth, bitemporal narrowing, facial hemangiomata (27%), type I Arnold-Chiari malformation, ventriculomegaly, underdeveloped corpus callosum, cortical atrophy, choanal stenosis, alacrima (absence of reflex tearing) and corneal hypoesthesia, hearing loss with tuning-fork malformation of the stapes, visual impairment, postaxial polydactyly, syndactyly, fifth toe overlapping fourth, cardiac defect (30%), short sternum, bicornuate uterus, splenopancreatic fusion, neuroepithelial tumors (17%) including hepatoblastoma, Wilms tumor, extradural ependymoma, malignant sacrococcygeal teratoma.

NATURAL HISTORY

Severe postnatal growth deficiency and profound intellectual disability and seizures as well as visual and hearing problems have occurred in all patients who have survived. Death commonly occurs prior to 2 years of age secondary to respiratory failure or infections. The longest reported survivor was an adolescent. Recurrent pneumonia, feeding intolerance, and refractory seizures are the rule. There is some evidence that this disorder is associated with a severe neurodegenerative process with progressive cerebral and brainstem atrophy.

ETIOLOGY

This disorder has an autosomal dominant mode of inheritance. All cases occur sporadically. Mutations in *SETBP1*, which encodes SET binding protein 1, are responsible. Little is know about the function of the gene. Rare recurrences are most likely the result of gonadal mosaicism.

References

Schinzel A, Giedion A: A syndrome of severe midface retraction, multiple skull anomalies, clubfeet, and cardiac and renal malformations in siblings, *Am J Med Genet* 1:361, 1978.

Donnai D, Harris R: A further case of a new syndrome including midface retraction, hypertrichosis and skeletal anomalies, *J Med Genet* 16:483, 1979.

Kelley RI, Zackai EH, Charney EG: Congenital hydronephrosis, skeletal dysplasia, and severe developmental retardation: The Schinzel-Giedion syndrome, *J Pediatr* 100:943, 1982.

Al-Gazali LI, et al: The Schinzel-Giedion syndrome, *J Med Genet* 27:42, 1990.

Robin NH, et al: New findings of Schinzel-Giedion syndrome: A case with a malignant sacrococcygeal teratoma, *Am J Med Genet* 47:852, 1993.

Labrune P, et al: Three new cases of Schinzel-Giedion syndrome and review of the literature, *Am J Med Genet* 50:90, 1994.

Elliott A, et al: Schinzel-Giedion syndrome: Further delineation of the phenotype, *Clin Dysmorphol* 5:135, 1996.

Shah AM, et al: Schinzel-Giedion syndrome: Evidence for a neurodegenerative process, *Am J Med Genet* 82:344, 1999.

Minn D, et al: Further clinical and sensorial delineation of Schinzel-Giedion syndrome: Report of two cases, *Am J Med Genet* 109:211, 2002.

Lehman AM, et al: Schinzel-Giedion syndrome: Report of splenopancreatic fusion and proposed diagnostic criteria, *Am J Med Genet A* 146A:1299, 2008.

Hoischen A, et al: De novo mutations of *SETBP1* cause Schinzel-Giedion syndrome, *Nat Genet* 42:483, 2010.

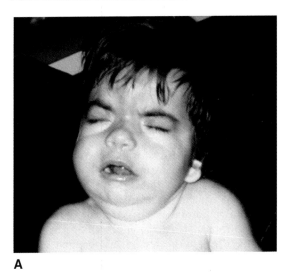

A

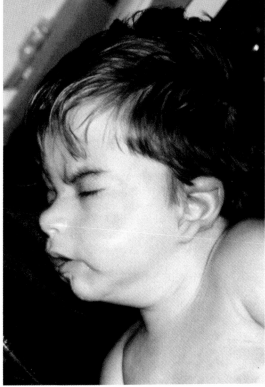

B

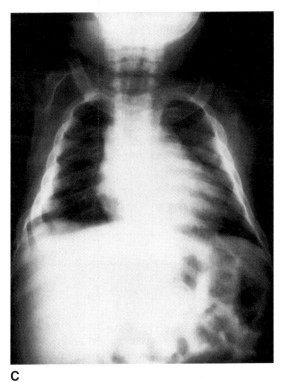

C

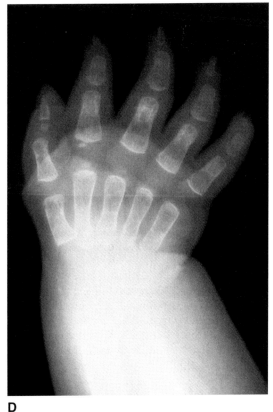

D

G

FIGURE 1. Schinzel-Giedion syndrome. **A–D,** A 13-month-old boy with coarse face, hypertelorism, attached helix with protruding lobule, and (on the radiographs) broad ribs, long clavicles, hypoplastic distal phalanges, and short metacarpals of thumbs. (From Robin NH, et al: *Am J Med Genet* 47:852, 1993. Copyright © 1993. Reprinted with permission of Wiley-Liss, Inc., a subsidiary of John Wiley & Sons, Inc.)

ACROCALLOSAL SYNDROME
Hypoplastic or Absent Corpus Callosum, Postaxial Polydactyly of Hands and Feet, Hallux Duplication

Since the initial description of this disorder by Schinzel in 1979, approximately 26 cases have been reported.

ABNORMALITIES

Neurologic. Hypoplastic or absent corpus callosum; intracranial cysts; other brain anomalies in 20%, including polymicrogyria, cerebral atrophy, hypothalamic dysfunction, hypoplastic pons, medulla oblongata, cerebellar hemispheres, small cerebellum, agenesis or hypoplasia of cerebellar vermis; severe mental retardation (80%); seizures (33%); strabismus; hypotonia.

Craniofacial. Macrocephaly, prominent forehead, large anterior fontanel, hypertelorism, epicanthal folds, downslanting palpebral fissures, small nose with broad nasal bridge and anteverted nares, malformed ears, short philtrum.

Limbs. Postaxial polydactyly of hands and feet, preaxial polydactyly of feet, mild syndactyly of hands and feet, tapered fingers, fifth finger clinodactyly.

Other. Eye findings, including optic atrophy and decreased retinal pigmentation; cardiac defects, primarily septal defects and abnormalities of the pulmonary valves; umbilical hernia.

OCCASIONAL ABNORMALITIES
Mild mental retardation, prominent occiput, hyperreflexia, nystagmus, cerebral atrophy, hypothalamic dysfunction, micropolygyria, hypoplasia of pons, hypoplasia of cerebellar hemispheres, temporal lobe hypoplasia, cleft lip, cleft palate, anterior displaced glottis, laryngomalacia, mixed hearing loss, supernumerary nipples, rib hypoplasia, preaxial polydactyly of hands, syndactyly of feet, simian crease, cryptorchidism, hypospadias, prenatal overgrowth, postnatal growth deficiency, intestinal malrotation.

NATURAL HISTORY
Marked retardation in the attainment of developmental milestones. Neonatal respiratory distress and intercurrent infection leading to early death occur in approximately 15% of patients. Family data documenting an increased incidence of spontaneous abortion suggest an apparent increased lethality of the gene.

ETIOLOGY
This disorder has an autosomal recessive mode of inheritance. Mutations in *KIF7*, the human orthologue of *Drosophila* Costal2, a key component of the hedgehog signaling pathway, are responsible. *KIF7* plays an important role in human primary cilia, indicating that this disorder is a ciliopathy. Mutations in *KIF7* are also responsible for some cases of the hydrolethalus syndrome (see page 250).

COMMENT
Three affected children have had siblings with anencephaly, two of which had polydactyly, suggesting that anencephaly may be the severe end of the spectrum of brain defects in the acrocallosal syndrome.

References

Schinzel A: Postaxial polydactyly, hallux duplication, absence of the corpus callosum, macrencephaly and severe mental retardation: A new syndrome? *Helv Paediatr Acta* 34:141, 1979.

Schinzel A, Schmid W: Hallux duplication, postaxial polydactyly, absence of the corpus callosum, severe mental retardation, and additional anomalies in two unrelated patients: A new syndrome, *Am J Med Genet* 6:241, 1980.

Schinzel A: The acrocallosal syndrome in first cousins: Widening of the spectrum of clinical features and further support for autosomal recessive inheritance, *J Med Genet* 25:332, 1988.

Casamassima AC, et al: Acrocallosal syndrome: Additional manifestations, *Am J Med Genet* 32:311, 1989.

Lurie IW, et al: The acrocallosal syndrome: Expansion of the phenotypic spectrum, *Clin Dysmorphol* 3:31, 1994.

Elson E, et al: De novo *GLI3* mutation in acrocallosal syndrome: Broadening the phenotypic spectrum of *GLI3* defects and overlap with murine models, *J Med Genet* 39:804, 2002.

Koenig R, et al: Spectrum of the acrocallosal syndrome, *Am J Med Genet* 108:7, 2002.

Aykut A, et al: An additional manifestation in acrocallosal syndrome: temporal lobe hypoplasia, *Genet Couns* 19:237, 2008.

Putoux A, et al: Mutations in *KIF7* cause fetal hydrolethalus and acrocallosal syndromes, *Nat Genet* 43:601, 2011.

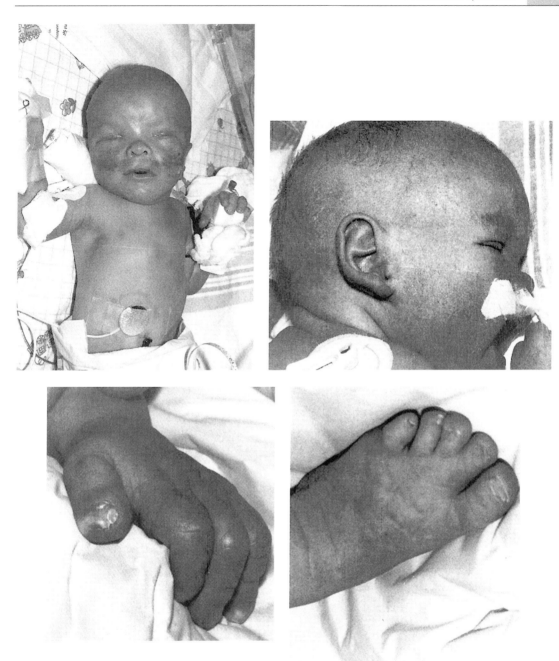

FIGURE 1.   Acrocallosal syndrome. Newborn boy with broad forehead, hypertelorism, broad nose with anteverted nares, abnormal auricles, and redundant nuchal skin. In addition, note the broad thumbs and great toes with partial duplication of the thumb, nail hypoplasia, and syndactyly of the feet. (From Casamassima AC, et al: *Am J Med Genet* 32:311, 1989. Copyright © 1989. Reprinted with permission of Wiley-Liss, Inc., a subsidiary of John Wiley & Sons, Inc.)

G

3C SYNDROME
(RITSCHER-SCHINZEL SYNDROME, CRANIO-CEREBELLO-CARDIAC SYNDROME)
Cerebellar Vermis Hypoplasia, Craniofacial Defects, Cardiac Anomalies

In 1987, Ritscher and colleagues reported two sisters with similar craniofacial anomalies, one of which had a complete common atrioventricular canal and Dandy-Walker variant while the other had a partial atrioventricular canal and a Dandy-Walker malformation. Subsequently Verloes and colleagues reported a third child with this disorder, which they referred to as 3C (craniofacial, cerebellar, cardiac) syndrome.

ABNORMALITIES

Growth. Postnatal growth deficiency with respect to both length and weight.
Performance. Hypotonia, gross motor delay, speech delay.
Craniofacial. Prominent forehead, large anterior fontanel, ocular hypertelorism, depressed nasal bridge, downslanting palpebral fissures.
Central Nervous System. Variable degrees of Dandy-Walker malformation/variant, including cerebellar vermis hypoplasia, enlarged fourth ventricle, enlarged cisterna magna, and hydrocephalus.
Cardiac. Complete/partial atrioventricular canal defects, tetralogy of Fallot, double-outlet right ventricle, atrial septal defect, ventricular septal defect.

OCCASIONAL ABNORMALITIES

Macrocephaly, prominent occiput, mental retardation, coloboma, glaucoma, heterochromatic iris, cleft palate, bifid uvula, micrognathia, hemivertebrae, absent/hypoplastic ribs, short neck, syndactyly, brachydactyly, proximally placed thumb, hypospadias, growth hormone deficiency, bowel malrotation, anal atresia, sensorineural hearing loss, single umbilical artery, scoliosis, hydronephrosis, IgG deficiency.

NATURAL HISTORY

Death before 4 years of age, primarily related to the severity of the cardiovascular malformation, has occurred in one half of reported cases. Feeding difficulties are common. Shunting for hydrocephalus was required infrequently. Limited information is available regarding intellectual performance. A 6-year-old girl performed at the 4½- to 5-year-old level and a 13-year-old child had "mild mental retardation." The initially described case reported by Ritscher et al, now 21 years of age, continues to have short stature but has only mild intellectual disability. The degree to which the growth deficiency is related to growth hormone deficiency is unknown.

ETIOLOGY

This disorder has an autosomal recessive inheritance pattern. Attention has been called to the phenotypic overlap between 3C syndrome and del 6p25 syndrome. It has been suggested that all children diagnosed with 3C syndrome should be tested for del6p25.

References

Ritscher D, et al: Dandy-Walker (like) malformation, atrio-ventricular septal defect and a similar pattern of minor anomalies in two sisters: A new syndrome? *Am J Med Genet* 26:481, 1987.

Verloes H, et al: 3C syndrome: Third occurrence of cranio-cerebello-cardiac dysplasia (Ritscher-Schinzel syndrome), *Clin Genet* 35:205, 1989.

Kosaki K, et al: Ritscher-Schinzel (3C) syndrome: Documentation of the phenotype, *Am J Med Genet* 68:421, 1997.

Leonardi ML, et al: Ritscher-Schinzel cranio-cerebello-cardiac (3C) syndrome: Report of four new cases and review, *Am J Med Genet* 102:237, 2001.

Zanki A, et al: Cranio-cerebello-cardiac syndrome: Follow-up of the original patient, *Am J Med Genet* 118:55, 2003.

Descipio C, et al: Subtelomeric deletions of chromosome 6p: Molecular and cytogenetic characterization of three new cases with phenotypic overlap with Ritscher-Schinzel (3C) syndrome, *Am J Med Genet* 134:3, 2005.

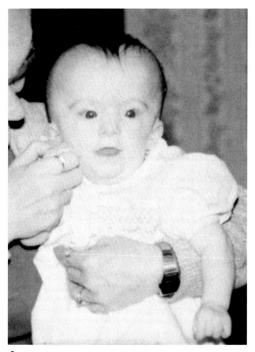

A

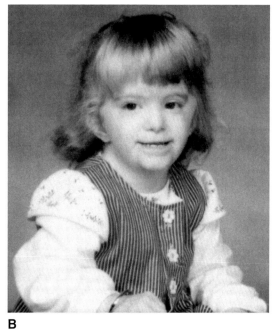

B

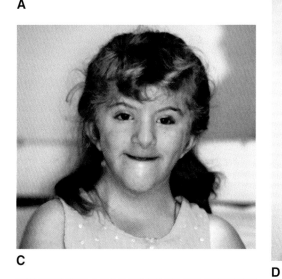

C

D

E

FIGURE 1.   3C syndrome. **A–E,** Affected girl at 8 months, 4 years, and 13 years of age. Note the high forehead, low-set ears, mild maxillary hypoplasia, short fifth fingers, and distal interphalangeal contractures. (From Wheeler PG, et al: *Am J Med Genet* 87:61, 1999, with permission.)

G

HECHT SYNDROME
(TRISMUS PSEUDOCAMPTODACTYLY SYNDROME, DISTAL ARTHROGRYPOSIS TYPE 7, DUTCH-KENTUCKY SYNDROME)
Trismus, Short Flexor Tendons of Hands

This disorder of muscle development and function was first described by Hecht and Beals and by Wilson and colleagues in 1968. Later it was well delineated by Mabry and colleagues in a huge kindred in which the initial U.S. case was a young Dutch girl who arrived in the United States with "crooked hands and a small mouth," thus leading, in some areas, to the designation Dutch-Kentucky syndrome.

ABNORMALITIES

Abnormalities appear to be based on short muscles and especially tendons.

Muscles and Tendons. Limited opening of mouth, sometimes with an enlarged coronoid process; short flexor tendons, so that when the hand is dorsiflexed, the fingers are partially flexed; occasionally short flexor muscles to the feet cause such problems as downturning toes, talipes equinovarus, calcaneovalgus, and metatarsus adductus; short hamstrings and gastrocnemius muscles. Reduced hip flexion occurs occasionally.

NATURAL HISTORY

The newborn baby may have tightly fisted hands and later usually crawls on the knuckles. These patients may have feeding problems because of the small mouth, and they tend to eat slowly. Tonsillectomy and/or intubation may present serious problems. There can be occupational handicaps relative to the military service, typing, or other situations requiring high levels of hand dexterity. Problems with dental hygiene are frequent. Surgical correction of the trismus has been reported in one case.

ETIOLOGY

This disorder has an autosomal dominant inheritance pattern. Mutations in *MYH8* are responsible. *MYH8* encodes the perinatal myosin heavy chain confirming that the known distal arthrogryposes are due to disruption of the contractile complex of fast-twitch myofibers. The rare occurrence of two affected children born to unaffected parents is most likely due to gonadal mosaicism.

References

Hecht F, Beals RK: Inability to open the mouth fully. In Bergsma D, editor: *Birth Defects Original Article Series. Part III: Limb Malformation* (vol V), New York, 1968, National Foundation March of Dimes, pp 96.

Wilson RV, et al: Autosomal dominant inheritance of shortening of flexor profundus muscle tendon. In Bergsma D, editor: *Birth Defects Original Article Series. Part III: Limb Malformation* (vol V), New York, 1968, National Foundation March of Dimes, pp 99.

Mabry CC, et al: Trismus camptomelic syndrome, *J Pediatr* 85:503, 1974.

Lefaivre JF, Aitchison MJ: Surgical correction of trismus in a child with Hecht syndrome, *Ann Plast Surg* 50:310, 2003.

Veugelers M, et al: Mutation of perinatal myosin heavy chain associated with a Carney complex variant, *N Eng J Med* 351:460, 2004.

Toydemir RM, et al: Trismus pseudocamptodactyly is caused by recurrent mutation of *MYH8*, *Am J Med Genet A* 140A:2387, 2006.

Bonapace G, et al: Germline mosaicism for c.2021G>A(p. ARG674GIn) mutation in siblings with trismus pseudocamptodactyly syndrome, *Am J Med Genet A* 152A:2898, 2010.

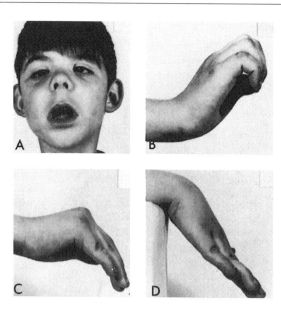

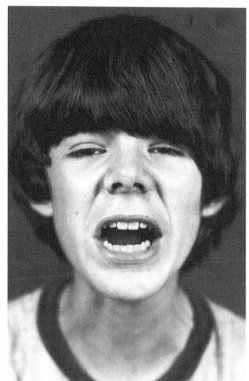

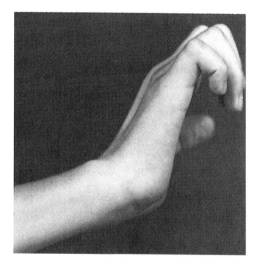

G

FIGURE 1. Hecht syndrome. *Above,* Boy with maximal opening of mouth **(A)**, dorsiflexed hand showing flexion of fingers **(B)**, extended hand with some flexion of fingers **(C)**, but volar flexed hand with no finger flexion **(D)**. *Right,* A 13-year-old boy with maximal mouth opening and flexed fingers following hand flexion. (*Above* and *right,* Courtesy Dr. C. Charlton Mabry, University of Kentucky Medical School, Lexington.)

MOEBIUS SEQUENCE
Sixth and Seventh Nerve Palsy

The basic features of Moebius sequence are mask-like facies with sixth and seventh cranial nerve palsy, usually bilaterally. The necropsy cases implicate at least four modes of developmental pathology in the genesis of the problem. These are (1) hypoplasia to absence of the central brain nuclei, (2) destructive degeneration of the central brain nuclei (most common type), (3) peripheral nerve involvement, and (4) myopathy. Thus, the Moebius sequence is but a sign and is quite nonspecific. Micrognathia, a frequent feature, may be interpreted as secondary to a neuromuscular deficit in early movement of the mandible. It leads to a U-shaped cleft palate or cleft uvula in one third of cases. Some patients have more extensive cranial nerve involvement, including the third, fourth, fifth, ninth, tenth, and twelfth cranial nerves. In cases where there is more extensive cranial nerve involvement, the tongue may be limited in mobility and/or small. There may be ocular ptosis, a protruding auricle, or both. Abnormal tearing, the result of aberrant innervation of the lacrimal gland, and limited involvement of both abduction and adduction are common. Hearing loss, most frequently the result of chronic otitis media, is frequent. Approximately one third of patients have talipes equinovarus, which is most likely the consequence of neurologic deficiency relative to early foot movement. Although autism was once thought to occur in 25% of cases, it is probably much less frequent than that. Although intellectual disability has been estimated to occur in 10% to 15% of cases, performance IQ is more severely affected than verbal IQ. Full-scale IQ using the Wechsler Intelligence Scale for Children, 3rd edition (WISC-III) is not an appropriate test to predict academic performance, which is usually far better than what would be expected using the WISC-III. Feeding difficulties and problems of aspiration often lead to failure to thrive during infancy. The expressionless face and speech impediments create problems in acceptance and social adaptation. Associated non–central nervous system (CNS)-related defects include hypodontia, splenogonadal fusion, bilateral vocal cord paralysis, limb reduction defects, syndactyly, the Poland sequence, and occasionally the Klippel-Feil anomaly.

The Moebius sequence is most commonly a sporadic occurrence in an otherwise normal family. In the majority of those cases, insufficient blood supply to structures supplied by the developing primitive subclavian artery lead to the variable features seen in this disorder. Evidence that a number of affected individuals have been born to women who experienced events during pregnancy that could cause transient ischemic/hypoxic insults to the fetus suggests that this disorder may be due to any event that interferes with the uterine/fetal circulation. Prenatal misoprostol exposure is an example.

The association of seventh cranial nerve palsy with or without sixth cranial nerve palsy but without limb reduction defects may be familial with an autosomal dominant mode of inheritance in some cases.

Facial reanimation procedures are worthwhile to consider in affected children.

References

Moebius PJ: Ueber engeborene doppelseitige Abducens-Facialis-Laehmung, *Munch Med Wochenschr* 35:91, 1888.

Henderson JL: The congenital facial diplegia syndrome: Clinical features, pathology, and aetiology: A review of sixty-one cases, *Brain* 62:381, 1939.

Sugarman GI, Stark HH: Möbius anomaly with Poland's anomaly, *J Med Genet* 10:192, 1973.

Baraitser M: Genetics of Möbius syndrome, *J Med Genet* 14:415, 1977.

Meyerson MD, Foushee DR: Speech, language and hearing in Moebius syndrome, *Dev Med Child Neurol* 20:357, 1978.

Bouwes-Bavinck JN, Weaver DD: Subclavian artery supply disruption sequence: Hypothesis of a vascular etiology for Poland, Klippel-Feil, and Möbius anomalies, *Am J Med Genet* 23:903, 1986.

Lipson AH, et al: Moebius syndrome: Animal model—human correlations and evidence for a brainstem vascular etiology, *Teratology* 40:339, 1989.

St. Charles S, et al: Mobius sequence: Further in vivo support for the subclavian artery supply disruption sequence, *Am J Med Genet* 47:289, 1993.

Vargas FR, et al: Prenatal exposure to misoprostol and vascular disruption defects—a case-control study, *Am J Med Genet* 95:302, 2000.

Strömland K, et al: Mobius sequence—a Swedish multidiscipline study, *Eur J Paediatr Neurol* 6:35, 2002.

Harrison DH, et al: Surgical correction of unilateral and bilateral facial palsy, *Postgrad Med J* 81:562, 2005.

Briegel W, et al: Neuropsychiatric findings of Möbius sequence—a review, *Clin Genet* 70:91, 2006.

Briegel W, et al: Cognitive evaluation in children and adolescents with Möbius sequence, *Child Care Health Dev* 35:650, 2009.

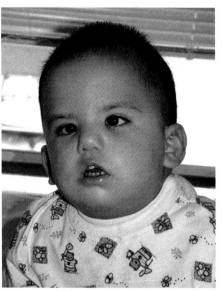

A

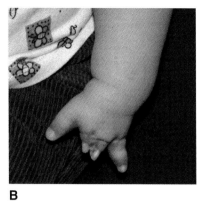

B

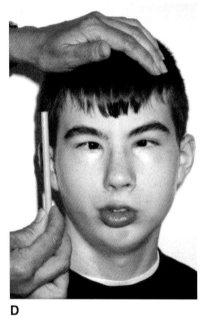

D

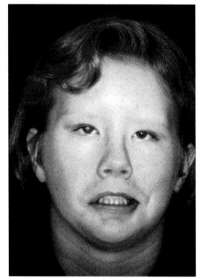

C

E

H

FIGURE 1. Moebius sequence. **A–E,** Affected children at various ages showing high nasal bridge, micrognathia with limited mandibular movement, small mouth with downturned corners, expressionless facies with deficit of lateral gaze, and mild ptosis. (**D** and **E,** From Strömland K, et al: *Eur J Paediatr Neurol* 6:35, 2002.)

BLEPHAROPHIMOSIS-PTOSIS-EPICANTHUS INVERSUS SYNDROME (FAMILIAL BLEPHAROPHIMOSIS SYNDROME)
Inner Canthal Fold, Lateral Displacement of Inner Canthi, Ptosis

Blepharophimosis-ptosis-epicanthus inversus syndrome (BPES), predominantly a dysplasia of the eyelids, was described by Vignes in 1889, and more than 200 families have been reported. The existence of two types has been suggested: type I, associated with infertility in affected females; and type II, transmitted by both males and females.

ABNORMALITIES

Eyes. Inverted inner canthal fold between upper and lower lid, short palpebral fissures with lateral displacement of inner canthi, low nasal bridge and ptosis of eyelids, hypoplasia, fibrosis of the levator palpebrae muscle, strabismus, amblyopia, eyebrows increased in their vertical height and arched.

Ears. Incomplete development, cupping.

Endocrine. Females with type I have menstrual irregularities or amenorrhea, infertility, and elevated gonadotropin levels.

Other. Variable hypotonia in early life.

OCCASIONAL ABNORMALITIES

Intellectual disability; cardiac defect; ocular abnormalities, including microphthalmia, microcornea, hypermetropia, trichiasis, colobomas of the optic disk, trabecular dysgenesis, congenital optic nerve hypoplasia, and nystagmus; endometrial carcinoma; granulosa cell tumor.

NATURAL HISTORY

Plastic surgery is indicated both for cosmetic reasons and for improvement of ocular function. Amblyopia, which occurs in more than 50% of patients, is most frequently associated with asymmetrical ptosis, although it also occurs when the ptosis is bilateral. Although most women with type I have a normal menarche and initially may be fertile, they soon develop ovarian resistance to gonadotropins or true premature ovarian failure. In at least one case, primary ovarian failure has been documented in early childhood.

ETIOLOGY

There is an autosomal dominant inheritance pattern for both type I and type II. Mutations in the forkhead transcription factor gene 2 (*FOXL2*) located at 3q22.3-q23 have been documented in 72% of cases and are responsible for both types. Larger genomic rearrangements, including deletions involving *FOXL2*, account for 10%, and deletions outside the transcription unit of *FOXL2* account for 5% of cases.

Finally, cytogenetically visible apparently balanced translocations or interstitial deletions involving chromosome 3q2 account for approximately 2% of cases. In the majority of these latter cases, non-BPES features such as intellectual disability, microcephaly, and growth delay have been present suggesting that the gene responsible for the additional features is located contiguous to *FOXL2*. It is important to distinguish between the types in order to provide counseling to effected individuals and their families relative to reproductive capabilities and menstrual irregularities, including amenorrhea in females with type I. With the exception of infertility in females, the two types are indistinguishable clinically. Unfortunately, female fertility cannot be definitively predicted based on the *FOXL2* molecular defect. Therefore, separating the two types can be accomplished only through a combination of molecular testing and careful family history. If the affected individual, either male or female, is a member of a family in which the disorder has been transmitted only through males, it is most likely type I, whereas if transmission has occurred through both males and females, it is type II.

References

Vignes A: Epicanthus héréditaire, *Rev Gen Ophthalmol (Paris)* 8:438, 1889.

Sacrez R, et al: Le blépharophimosis compliqué familial: Étude des membres de la famille Blé, *Ann Pediatr (Paris)* 10:493, 1963.

Kohn R, Romano PE: Blepharoptosis, blepharophimosis, epicanthus inversus, and telecanthus—a syndrome with no name, *Am J Ophthalmol* 72:625, 1972.

Zlotogora J, Sagi M, Cohen T: The blepharophimosis, ptosis and epicanthus inversus syndrome: Delineation of two types, *Am J Hum Genet* 35:1020, 1983.

Jones CA, Collin JRD: Blepharophimosis and its association with female infertility, *Br J Ophthalmol* 68:533, 1984.

Oley C, Baraister M: Blepharophimosis, ptosis, epicanthus inversus syndrome (BPES syndrome), *J Med Genet* 25:47, 1988.

Beaconsfield M, et al: Visual development in the blepharophimosis syndrome, *Br J Ophthalmol* 75:746, 1991.

Fokstuen S, et al: FOXL2-mutations in blepharophimosis-ptosis-epicanthus inversus syndrome (BPES): Challenges for genetic counseling in female patients, *Am J Med Genet A* 117A:143, 2003.

De Rue MH, et al: Interstitial deletion of 3q in a patient with blepharophimosis-ptosis-epicanthus inversus syndrome (BPES) and microcephaly, mild mental retardation and growth delay; clinical report and review of the literature, *Am J Med Genet* 137:81, 2005.

Beysen D, et al: FOXL2 mutations and genomic rearrangements in BPES, *Hum Mutat* 30:158, 2009.

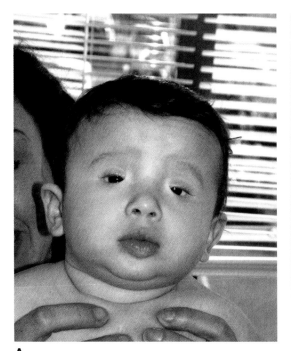

A

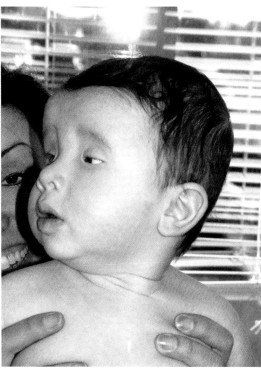

B

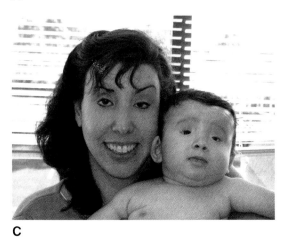

C

FIGURE 1.   Blepharophimosis syndrome. **A-C,** Mother and infant son. (Courtesy Dr. Lynne M. Bird, Children's Hospital, San Diego.)

H

ROBIN SEQUENCE (PIERRE ROBIN SYNDROME)

Micrognathia, Glossoptosis, Cleft Soft Palate; Primary Defect—
Early Mandibular Hypoplasia

The single initiating defect of this disorder may be hypoplasia of the mandibular area before 9 weeks in utero, allowing the tongue to be posteriorly located and thereby impairing the closure of the posterior palatal shelves that must "grow over" the tongue to meet the midline. The mode of pathogenesis is depicted to the right. The rounded contour of the "cleft" palate in some of these patients (see illustration) is compatible with this mode of developmental pathology and differs from the usual inverted V shape of most palatal clefts. The focus of management in the newborn period should be treatment of upper airway obstruction and feeding problems. The tongue-based airway obstruction may require, in order of increasing invasiveness, prone positioning, nasal pharyngeal airway, nasal esophageal intubation, lip-tongue adhesion, mandibular distraction, and tracheostomy. Airway obstruction can lead to hypoxia, cor pulmonale, failure to thrive, and cerebral impairment. Mortality rates as high as 30% have been reported. Significant airway obstruction may develop over the first 2 months of life. Therefore, affected children should be monitored carefully during that period, focusing on the obstruction pathogenesis of the apnea and airway concerns in the condition. In that significant hypoxia may occur without obvious clinical signs of obstruction, serial polysomnography may be helpful over the first month to identify infants at significant risk. Feeding problems requiring nasogastric tube feeding are common and are related in many cases to lower esophageal sphincter hypertonia, failure of lower esophageal sphincter relaxation at deglutition, and esophageal dyskinesis. In 40% of cases, the Robin sequence occurs in otherwise normal individuals, in whom the prognosis is very good if they survive the early period of respiratory obstruction.

However, this disorder commonly occurs as one feature in a multiple malformation syndrome of genetic etiology, the most common of which is Stickler syndrome. The fact that accurate diagnosis of a genetic syndrome is often difficult in the newborn period highlights the need for longitudinal follow-up of affected children. Patients who have Robin sequence as one feature of a multiple malformation syndrome require more aggressive airway and feeding management. The Robin sequence may also be a result of early in utero mechanical constraint, with the chin compressed in such a manner as to limit its growth before palatine closure.

References

Dennison WM: The Pierre Robin syndrome, *Pediatrics* 36:336, 1965.

Latham RA: The pathogenesis of cleft palate associated with the Pierre Robin syndrome, *Br J Plast Surg* 19:205, 1966.

Hanson JW, Smith DW: U-shaped palatal defect in the Robin anomalad: Developmental and clinical relevance, *J Pediatr* 87:30, 1975.

Bull MJ, et al: Improved outcome in Pierre Robin sequence: Effect of multidisciplinary evaluation and management, *Pediatrics* 86:294, 1990.

Baujat G, et al: Oroesophageal motor disorders in Pierre Robin syndrome, *J Pediatr Gastroenterol Nutr* 32:297, 2001.

Evans KN, et al: Robin sequence: From diagnosis to development of an effective treatment plan, *Pediatrics* 127:936, 2011.

Izumi K, et al: Underlying genetic diagnosis of Pierre Robin sequence: Retrospective chart review at two children's hospitals and a systematic literature review, *J Pediatr* 160:645, 2012.

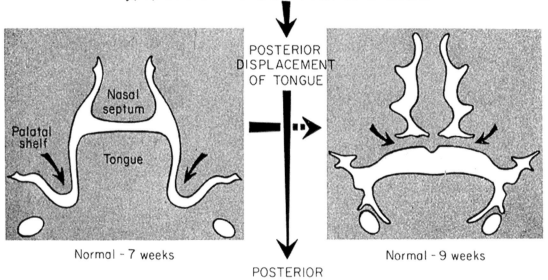

FIGURE 1. **A,** Mode of pathogenesis of the Robin sequence. **B,** Note the severe micrognathia. **C,** Note the unusual rounded shape to palatal "cleft" in a patient with the Robin sequence compatible with the incomplete closure of the palate having been secondary to the posterior displacement of the tongue.

CLEFT LIP SEQUENCE
Primary Defect—Closure of Lip

By 35 days of uterine age, the lip is normally fused, as illustrated in Figure 1. A failure of lip fusion, as shown, may impair the subsequent closure of the palatal shelves, which do not completely fuse until the eighth to ninth week. Thus, cleft palate is a frequent association with cleft lip. Other secondary anomalies include defects of tooth development in the area of the cleft lip and incomplete growth of the ala nasi on the side of the cleft. There may be mild ocular hypertelorism, the precise reason for which is undetermined. Tertiary abnormalities can include poor speech and multiple episodes of otitis media as a consequence of palatal incompetence and conductive hearing loss.

ETIOLOGY AND RECURRENCE RISK COUNSELING

The cause of this disorder is usually unknown. It is more likely to occur in males. The highest birth prevalence is in Asians and Native Americans (1 in 500), followed by Europeans (1 in 1000), and the lowest prevalence is in populations of African descent (1 in 2500). The more severe the defect is, the higher the recurrence risk is for future siblings. For a unilateral defect, the recurrence risk is 2.7%; for bilateral defect, it is 5.4%. The following are the general risk figures: unaffected parents with one affected child, 4% for future siblings; unaffected parents with two affected children, 10% for future siblings. If either the mother or father is affected, the risk for offspring is 4%. An affected parent with one affected child has a 14% risk for future offspring. As many as 15% of infants surviving the newborn period with cleft lip, with or without cleft palate and 42% of those with cleft palate alone have the defect as part of a broader pattern of altered morphogenesis. One should identify such individuals before using the previously mentioned figures for recurrence risk counseling. In addition, the underlying diagnosis may well have an impact on prognosis.

COMMENT

Common alleles in the interferon regulatory factor 6 (*IRF6*) gene and *VAX1* located at chromosome 10q25 are felt to have a role in nonsyndromic cleft lip with or without cleft palate, and a number of other genes are felt to be likely candidates. In addition, prenatal exposure to valproic acid, maternal smoking and alcohol, and mycophenolate mofetil have been identified as environmental factors associated with cleft lip with or without cleft palate.

References

Bixler D: Heritability of clefts of the lip and palate, *J Prosthet Dent* 33:100, 1975.

Carter CO, et al: A three generations family study of cleft lip with or without cleft palate, *J Med Genet* 19:246, 1982.

Shprintzen RJ, et al: Anomalies associated with cleft lip, cleft palate, or both, *Am J Med Genet* 20:585, 1985.

Jones MC: Facial clefting: Etiology and developmental pathogenesis, *Clin Plast Surg* 20:599, 1993.

Dixon MJ, et al: Cleft lip and palate: Understanding genetic and environmental factors, *Nat Rev Genet* 12:167, 2011.

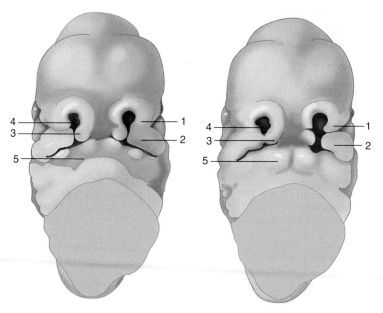

FIGURE 1.   Cleft lip sequence. *Left,* Normal embryo of 35 days. *Right,* Spontaneously aborted 35-day embryo with hypoplasia of the left lateral nasal swelling and, therefore, a cleft lip. *1,* Lateral nasal swelling; *2,* maxillary swelling; *3,* medial nasal swelling; *4,* nares; *5,* mandibular swelling. (*Left* and *right,* Courtesy Prof. G. Töndury, University of Zurich.)

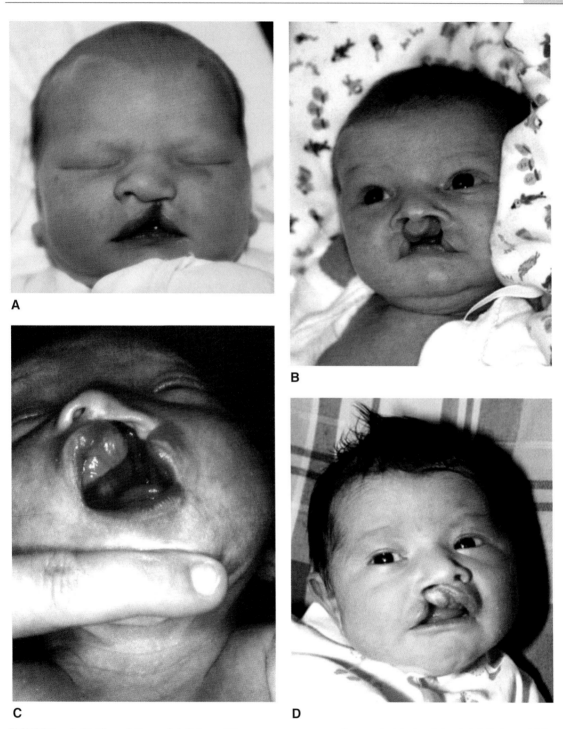

FIGURE 2.   A–D, All gradations of cleft lip and its consequences occur, from an isolated unilateral cleft lip to a widely open cleft with secondary consequences of cleft palate, flared ala nasi, and mild ocular hypertelorism.

VAN DER WOUDE SYNDROME (LIP PIT–CLEFT LIP SYNDROME)

Lower Lip Pit(s), with or without Cleft Lip, with or without Missing Second Premolars

Originally reported by Van der Woude in 1954, this disorder is the most common multiple malformation syndrome associated with cleft lip with or without cleft palate.

ABNORMALITIES

Oral. Lower lip pits (80%); hypodontia, missing central and lateral incisors, canines, or bicuspids; cleft lip with or without cleft palate, cleft palate alone, submucous cleft palate, cleft uvula.

NATURAL HISTORY

Surgical removal of the fistulas, which represent small accessory salivary glands, is recommended because they may produce a watery mucoid discharge that can be embarrassing for the individual. Missing permanent teeth are common.

ETIOLOGY

This disorder has an autosomal dominant inheritance pattern. Mutations in interferon regulatory factor 6 (*IRF6*), which is mapped to chromosome 1q32-41, account for 68% of cases. Microdeletions of *IRF6* account for a very small percentage of cases. Mutations in *IRF6* lead not only to Van der Woude syndrome but also to the popliteal pterygium syndrome. Mutations in Van der Woude syndrome are protein truncation or missense, whereas mutations in popliteal pterygium syndrome are missense. Both disorders have been observed in the same family.

References

Van der Woude A: Fistula labii inferioris congenita and its association with cleft lip and palate, *Am J Hum Genet* 6:244, 1954.

Cervenka J, Gorlin RJ, Anderson VE: The syndrome of pits of the lower lip and cleft lip or cleft palate: Genetic considerations, *Am J Hum Genet* 19:416, 1967.

Janku P, et al: The Van der Woude syndrome in a large kindred: Variability, penetrance, genetic risks, *Am J Med Genet* 5:117, 1980.

Sander A, et al: Evidence for a microdeletion in 1q32-41 involving the gene responsible for Van der Woude syndrome, *Hum Mol Genet* 3:575, 1994.

Kondo S, et al: Mutations in *IRF6* cause Van der Woude and popliteal pterygium syndromes, *Nat Genet* 32:285, 2002.

Muenke M: The pit, the cleft and the web, *Nat Genet* 32:219, 2002.

Oberoi S, Vargervik K: Hypoplasia and hypodontia in Van der Woude syndrome, *Cleft Palate Craniofac J* 42:459, 2005.

De Lima RL, et al: Prevalence and nonrandom distribution of exonic mutations in interferon regulatory factor 6 in 307 families with Van der Woude syndrome and 37 families with popliteal pterygium syndrome, *Genet Med* 11:241, 2009.

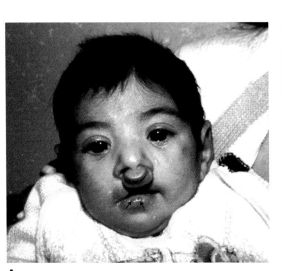

A

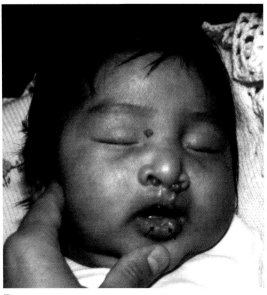

B

FIGURE 1.   Van der Woude syndrome. **A** and **B,** Two affected children. Note the lip pits in both. Bilateral cleft palate has been repaired in **B.**

H

FRONTONASAL DYSPLASIA SEQUENCE
(MEDIAN CLEFT FACE SYNDROME)
Unknown Primary Defect in Midfacial Development with Incomplete Anterior Appositional Alignment of Eyes

DeMyer recognized the transitional gradations in severity of this presumed single primary localized defect in 33 cases and called this pattern of anomaly the median cleft face syndrome. Sedano and colleagues subsequently extended these observations and recommended frontonasal dysplasia as a more appropriate designation for this defect. The accompanying illustration sets forth a crude interpretation of the developmental pathogenesis and gradations of the sequence. A number of additional disorders in which frontonasal dysplasia is one feature have been described (see Comment section).

ABNORMALITIES

The following are defects that may occur in the more severe cases; the milder cases may have only a few of these defects.

Eyes. Ocular hypertelorism, lateral displacement of inner canthi.
Forehead. Widow's peak, deficit in midline frontal bone (cranium bifidum occultum).
Nose. Variability from notched broad nasal tip to completely divided nostrils with hypoplasia to absence of the prolabium and premaxilla with a median cleft lip, variable notching of alae nasi, broad nasal root, lack of formation of nasal tip.

OCCASIONAL ABNORMALITIES
Accessory nasal tags; microphthalmia; preauricular tags, low-set ears, conductive deafness; intellectual disability; frontal cutaneous lipoma or lipoma of corpus callosum; agenesis of the corpus callosum; tetralogy of Fallot.

NATURAL HISTORY
Depending on the severity of the defect, radical cosmetic surgery is usually merited. The majority of affected individuals are of normal intelligence. DeMyer noted that 8% of his patient population (N = 33) had severe intellectual disability and 12% had impairment of intelligence.

ETIOLOGY
The cause of this disorder is unknown.

COMMENT
Six multiple malformation syndromes have been described in which frontonasal dysplasia is one feature. The first three of these disorders are due to autosomal recessive mutations in aristaless-like homeobox genes (*ALX1, ALX3,* and *ALX4*). *ALX* genes encode paired-type homeodomain proteins.

ALX1-*Related Frontonasal Dysplasia.* Features include extreme microphthalmia, bilateral oblique facial clefts, cleft palate, hypertelorism, wide nasal bridge with hypoplasia of ala nasi, and low-set, posteriorly rotated ears. (See Uz et al, 2010.)

Frontorhiny. Features include hypertelorism, wide nasal bridge, short nasal ridge, bifid nasal tip, broad columella, widely separated slit-like nares, long philtrum with prominent vertical ridges, midline notch in upper lip and alveolus. Autosomal recessive mutations in *ALX3.* (See Twigg et al, 2009.)

ALX4-*Related Frontonasal Dysplasia.* Features include alopecia, a large skull defect, coronal craniosynostosis, hypertelorism, depressed nasal bridge, bifid nasal tip, hypogonadism, callosal body agenesis, and intellectual disability. (See Kayserili et al, 2009.)

Frontofacionasal Dysplasia. Features include blepharophimosis, lagophthalmos (inability to completely close eyelids), telecanthus, S-shaped palpebral fissures, facial hypoplasia, eyelid coloboma, widow's peak, cranium bifidum, frontal lipoma, nasal hypoplasia and deformed nostrils, bifid nose cleft lip/palate and premaxilla. Autosomal recessive inheritance. (See Gollop et al, 1984.)

Acromelic Frontonasal Dysplasia. Features include frontonasal dysplasia in association with defects of the CNS and limb anomalies, including tibial hypoplasia/aplasia, talipes equinovarus, and preaxial polydactyly of the feet. Several of the affected children were the offspring of consanguineous marriages, raising the possibility of autosomal recessive inheritance. (See Slaney et al, 1999.)

Frontonasal Dysplasia with Optic Disc Anomalies. Features include frontonasal dysplasia with optic disk anomalies, basal encephalocele, absent corpus callosum, diabetes insipidus, and pituitary deficiency. All cases have been sporadic. (See Lees et al, 1998.)

References

DeMyer W: The median cleft face syndrome: Differential diagnosis of cranium bifidum occultum, hypertelorism, and median cleft nose, lip, and palate, *Neurology [Minn]* 17:961, 1967.

Sedano HO, et al: Frontonasal dysplasia, *J Pediatr* 76:906, 1970.

Gollop TR, et al: Frontofacionasal dysplasia, *Am J Med Genet* 19:301, 1984.

Pascual-Castroviejo I, Pascual-Pascual SI, Pérez-Hiqueras A: Fronto-nasal dysplasia and lipoma of the corpus callosum, *Eur J Pediatr* 144:66, 1985.

Sedano HO, Gorlin RJ: Frontonasal malformation as a field defect and in syndromic associations, *Oral Surg Oral Med Oral Pathol* 65:704, 1988.

Lees MM, et al: Frontonasal dysplasia with optic disc anomalies and other midline craniofacial defects: A report of six cases, *Clin Dysmorphol* 7:157, 1998.

Slaney S, et al: Acromelic frontonasal dysostosis, *Am J Med Genet* 83:109, 1999.

Kayserili H, et al: *AL4* dysfunction disrupts craniofacial and epidermal development, *Hum Mol Genet* 18:4357, 2009.

Twigg SRF, et al: Frontorhiny, a distinctive presentation of frontonasal dysplasia caused by recessive mutations in the *ALX3* homeobox gene, *Am J Hum Genet* 84:698, 2009.

Uz E, et al: Disruption of *ALX1* causes extreme microphthalmia and severe facial clefting: Expanding the spectrum of autosomal-recessive *ALX*-related frontonasal dysplasia, *Am J Hum Genet* 86:789, 2010.

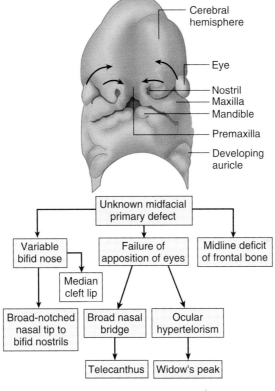

H

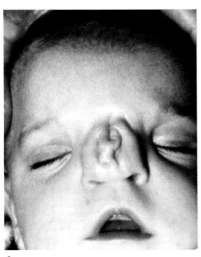
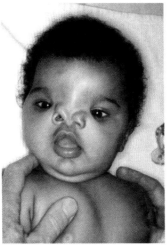
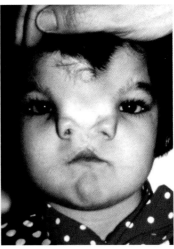

A   B   C

FIGURE 1.   *Top*, Developmental pathogenesis of the frontonasal dysplasia sequence. *Bottom*, Affected individuals.

FRASER SYNDROME (CRYPTOPHTHALMOS SYNDROME)
Cryptophthalmos,* Cutaneous Syndactyly, Genital Anomaly

The association of other malformations in patients with the rare anomaly of cryptophthalmos had been appreciated before 1962, when a rather distinctive syndrome found in two sets of siblings was set forth by Fraser. More than 250 patients have been reported. Because cryptophthalmos is not an obligate feature of this disorder, it is more appropriately termed Fraser syndrome.

ABNORMALITIES

Craniofacial. Cryptophthalmos (85%–93%), usually bilateral and frequently with defect of eye; hair growth on lateral forehead extending to lateral eyebrow, often associated with a depression of underlying frontal bone; hypoplastic notched nares; broad nose with depressed bridge; ear anomalies, most commonly atresia of external auditory canal and cupped ears.

Limbs. Partial cutaneous syndactyly.

Genitalia. Incomplete development: male: hypospadias, cryptorchidism; female: bicornuate uterus, vaginal atresia, clitoromegaly.

Urinary Tract. Renal agenesis/hypoplasia, ureteral agenesis, bladder anomalies.

Other. Laryngeal stenosis or atresia, tracheal abnormalities.

OCCASIONAL ABNORMALITIES

Intellectual disability, microcephaly, hydrocephalus, encephalocele, abnormal gyral pattern, meningoencephalocele, micrognathia, midline groove toward nasal tip, unilateral absence of a nostril, choanal atresia or stenosis, subglottic stenosis, cleft lip with or without cleft palate (4%), cleft palate (3%), tongue tie (6%), dental malocclusion and crowding, bony skull defects, hypertelorism, lacrimal duct defect (9%), coloboma of upper lid (6%), absent eyebrows or eyelashes, microphthalmia, anophthalmia, corneal opacification, partial midfacial cleft, defect of middle ear, fusion of superior helix to scalp, microtia, low-set ears, widely spaced nipples, pulmonary hyperplasia, and hypoplasia, abnormal lung lobation, low-set umbilicus, anal atresia/stenosis, intestinal malrotation, malformation of small bowel, cardiac defects, diaphragmatic hernia, thymic aplasia/hypoplasia, diastasis of symphysis pubis, partial absence of sternum, absent phalanges, hypoplastic or absent thumb, rib anomalies.

NATURAL HISTORY

This disorder should be considered in stillborn babies with renal agenesis. Because the defect of eyelid development is frequently accompanied by ocular anomaly, the likelihood of achieving adequate visual perception is small, although early surgical intervention was of value in one case. Hearing is usually normal. Twenty-five percent of affected individuals are stillborn and an additional 20% die before 1 year of age. Death is related primarily to the renal or laryngeal defects. No affected individual has been reported to have reproduced.

ETIOLOGY

This disorder has an autosomal recessive inheritance pattern. Mutations in *FRAS1, FREM2,* and *GRIP1* are responsible. *FRAS1* and *FREM2* encode extracellular matrix proteins that are important for extracellar-basement membrane adhesion in the mouse. It is assumed that *Grip1, Fras1,* and *Frem2* are critical for the proper localization of the *Fras1/ Frem* protein complex.

References

Fraser CR: Our genetical "load": A review of some aspects of genetical variation, *Ann Hum Genet* 25:387, 1962.

Thomas IT, et al: Isolated and syndromic cryptophthalmos, *Am J Med Genet* 25:85, 1986.

Slavotinek AM, Tifft CJ: Fraser syndrome and cryptophthalmos: Review of the diagnostic criteria and evidence for phenotypic modules in complex malformation syndromes, *J Med Genet* 39:623, 2002.

McGregor L, et al: Fraser syndrome and mouse blebbed phenotype caused by mutations in *FRAS1/Fras1* encoding a putative extracellular matrix protein, *Nat Genet* 34:203, 2003.

Jadeja S, et al: Identification of a new gene mutated in Fraser syndrome and mouse myelencephalic blebs, *Nat Genet* 37:520, 2005.

Van Haelst MM, et al: Fraser syndrome: A clinical study of 59 cases and evaluation of diagnostic criteria, *Am J Med Genet* 143:3194, 2007.

Vogel MJ, et al: Mutations in *GRIP1* cause Fraser syndrome, *J Med Genet* 49:303, 2012.

---

*Cryptophthalmos (hidden eye) fundamentally means absence of the palpebral fissure but usually includes varying absence of eyelashes and eyebrows and defects of the eye, especially the anterior part.

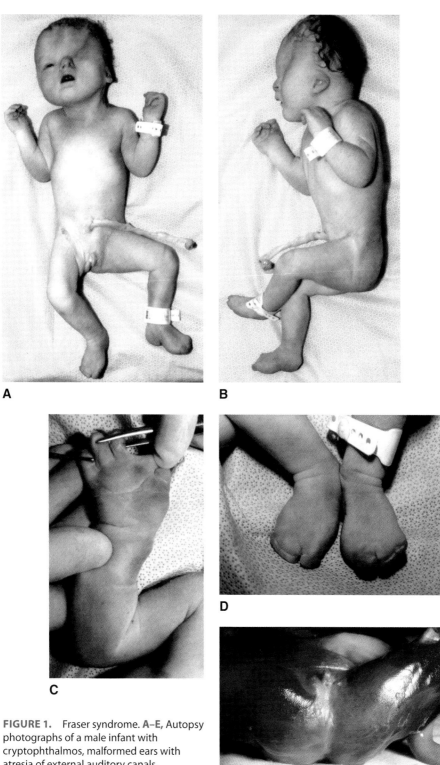

FIGURE 1. Fraser syndrome. **A–E,** Autopsy photographs of a male infant with cryptophthalmos, malformed ears with atresia of external auditory canals, syndactyly, and incomplete development of external genitalia.

H

MELNICK-FRASER SYNDROME (BRANCHIO-OTO-RENAL SYNDROME)
Preauricular Pits, Branchial Fistula/Cysts, Renal Dysplasia

The association of branchial arch anomalies (preauricular pits, branchial fistulas), hearing loss, and renal hypoplasia constitutes the branchio-oto-renal (BOR) syndrome first described by Melnick and colleagues in 1975 and further delineated by Fraser and colleagues. The prevalence is roughly 1 in 40,000. The syndrome occurs in approximately 2% of profoundly deaf children.

ABNORMALITIES

Hearing loss	90%
Preauricular pits	80%
Branchial fistulas or cysts	50%
Anomalous pinna	35%
External auditory canal stenosis	30%
Malformed middle or inner ear	—
Lacrimal duct stenosis/aplasia	10%
Renal dysplasia	65%

OCCASIONAL ABNORMALITIES

Long, narrow face, preauricular tag, congenital cholesteatoma, anomalies of the facial nerve, "constricted palate," deep overbite, microdontia of permanent teeth, cleft palate, bifid uvula, facial paralysis, gustatory lacrimation (the shedding of tears during eating because of misdirected growth of seventh cranial nerve fibers), mitral valve prolapse, congenital hip dislocation, nonrotation of bowel, pancreatic duplication cyst, euthyroid goiter, benign intracranial tumor, temporoparietal linear nevus.

NATURAL HISTORY

The ear pits or branchial clefts may go unnoticed until the hearing loss appears, or they may become infected and require surgery. The hearing loss may be sensorineural (25%), conductive (25%), or mixed (50%) and ranges from mild to severe. Age of onset can be from early childhood to young adulthood, and hearing loss is occasionally precipitous. In some families, it has been progressive. There may be malformations of the middle ear, vestibular system, and cochlea, including displaced, malformed, or fused ossicles and the Mondini malformation of the cochlea. Defects of the external ear range from severe microtia to minor anomalies of the pinna,

which is variously described as cup- or loop-shaped, flattened, or hypoplastic. The external canal can be narrow, slanted upward, or malformed, making otoscopic examination difficult.

The renal anomalies range from minor dysplasia (sharply tapered superior poles, blunting of calyces, duplication of the collecting system) to bilateral renal agenesis with renal failure in approximately 6% of patients.

ETIOLOGY

BOR syndrome is caused by an autosomal dominant gene with variable expression. Mutations in the human homologue of the *Drosophila* eyes absent gene (eya), referred to as *EYA1* and localized to chromosome 8q13.3, are responsible for approximately 50% of cases. Mutations in *SIX1* are also responsible for BOR syndrome but far less frequently. Chromosomal rearrangements of 8q13.3 occur in about 20% of cases. Submicroscopic deletions involving *EYA1* can result in an expanded phenotype that includes variable musculoskeletal defects, speech delay, and developmental delay. This expanded phenotype is most likely due to deletions of contiguous genes.

References

Melnick M, et al: Autosomal dominant branchio-oto-renal dysplasia, *Birth Defects* 11(5):121, 1975.

Melnick M, et al: Familial branchio-oto-renal dysplasia: A new addition to the branchial arch syndromes, *Clin Genet* 9:25, 1976.

Fraser FC, et al: Genetic aspects of the BOR syndrome—branchial fistulas, ear pits, hearing loss, and renal anomalies, *Am J Med Genet* 2:241, 1978.

Fraser FC, Sproule JR, Halal F: Frequency of the branchio-oto-renal (BOR) syndrome in children with profound hearing loss, *Am J Med Genet* 7:341, 1980.

Heimler A, Lieber E: Branchio-oto-renal syndrome: Reduced penetrance and variable expressivity in four generations of a large kindred, *Am J Med Genet* 25:15, 1986.

Vervoort VS, et al: Genomic rearrangements of *EYA1* account for a large fraction of families with BOR syndrome, *Eur J Hum Genet* 10:757, 2002.

Kochhar A, et al: Branchio-oto-renal syndrome, *Am J Med Genet* 143:1671, 2007.

Sanchez-Valle A, et al: HERV-mediated genomic rearrangement of *EYA1* in an individual with branchio-oto-renal syndrome, *Am J Med Genet* 152:2854, 2010.

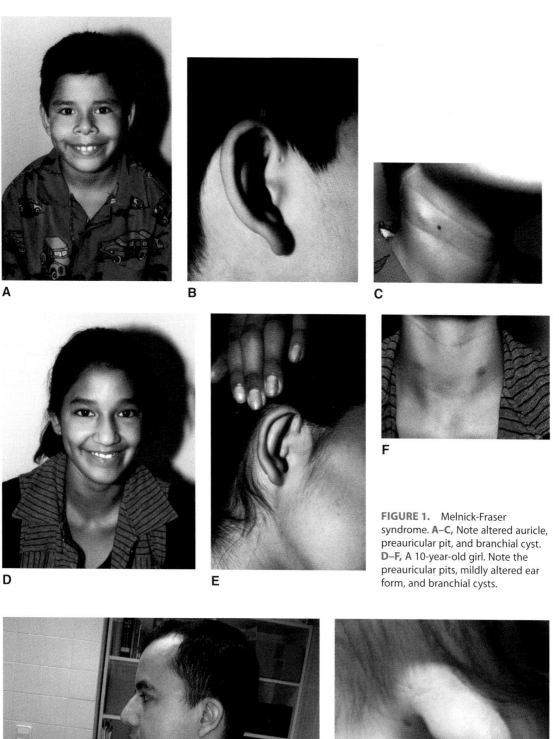

A

B

C

D

E

F

H

FIGURE 1. Melnick-Fraser syndrome. **A–C,** Note altered auricle, preauricular pit, and branchial cyst. **D–F,** A 10-year-old girl. Note the preauricular pits, mildly altered ear form, and branchial cysts.

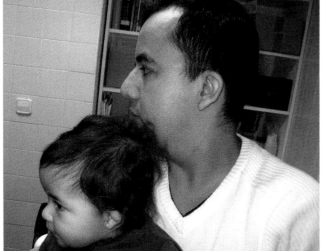

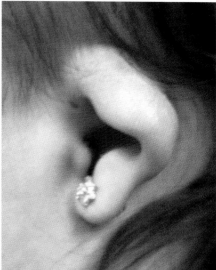

FIGURE 2. A second family with BOR syndrome. Both father and daughter are affected. The father's auricle has normal shape and a preauricular pit, whereas the daughter's auricle is microtic, cup-shaped and also has a pit.

BRANCHIO-OCULO-FACIAL SYNDROME
Branchial Defects, Lacrimal Duct Obstruction, Pseudocleft of Upper Lip

Individuals with this disorder were initially described in 1982 by Lee and colleagues and in 1983 by Hall and colleagues. The designation branchio-oculo-facial syndrome was introduced by Fujimoto and colleagues.

ABNORMALITIES

Performance. Intellectual disability (25%), in most cases mild.

Growth. Prenatal growth deficiency (27%), postnatal growth deficiency (50%).

Branchial. Sinus/fistulous tract (45%), atrophic skin lesion/aplasia cutis congenita/scarring (57%), hemangiomatous lesion (36%).

Ocular. Lacrimal duct obstruction (78%), colobomata (47%), microphthalmia/anophthalmia (44%), upslanting palpebral fissures (48%), telecanthus (58%), myopia (46%).

Auricular. Low-set, posteriorly rotated, over-folded or malformed ears (85%); hypoplastic superior helix (43%); conductive hearing loss (71%); supra-auricular sinuses (15%).

Oral. Abnormal upper lip (90%), which includes pseudocleft (appearance of repaired cleft lip), incomplete or complete cleft lip; dental abnormalities (56%); micrognathia (50%).

Other. Premature graying of hair (67%), renal anomalies (37%).

OCCASIONAL ABNORMALITIES

Microcephaly; temporal bone abnormalities on CT scan, white forelock; ptosis; heterochromic irides, orbital cyst; lacrimal sac fistula; facial nerve paralysis; cataract; strabismus; preauricular pit; posterior auricular pit; microtia; sensorineural hearing loss; cleft palate; upper lip pits; ectopic dermal thymus in cervical region; ectopic dermal parathyroid tissue; thyroglossal duct cyst; iris pigment epithelial cyst; broad or divided nasal tip; subcutaneous cysts of the scalp; renal agenesis; hand anomalies, including polydactyly, clinodactyly, preaxial polydactyly, dysplastic nails, and a single transverse palmar crease; supernumerary nipple; cardiac defects; agenesis of cerebellar vermis; medulloblastoma.

NATURAL HISTORY

Hypernasal speech with conductive hearing loss is common. Premature graying of scalp hair normally begins around 18 years but has been seen as early as 10 years. Intelligence is usually normal. Reduced reproductive fitness in both males and females has been suggested.

ETIOLOGY

This disorder has an autosomal dominant inheritance pattern. Mainly missense mutations in *TFAP2A* are responsible. One case of a complete deletion of the *TFAP2A* gene has been reported. Marked intrafamilial variability has been documented.

References

Lee WK, et al: Bilateral branchial cleft sinuses associated with intrauterine and postnatal growth retardation, premature aging, and unusual facial appearance: A new syndrome with dominant transmission, *Am J Med Genet* 11:345, 1982.

Hall BD, et al: A new syndrome of hemangiomatous branchial clefts, lip pseudoclefts, and unusual facial appearance, *Am J Med Genet* 14:135, 1983.

Fujimoto A, et al: New autosomal dominant branchio-oculo-facial syndrome, *Am J Med Genet* 27:943, 1987.

McCool M, Weaver D: Branchio-oculo-facial syndrome: Broadening the spectrum, *Am J Med Genet* 49:414, 1994.

Milunsky JM, et al: *TFAP2A* mutations result in branchio-oculo-facial syndrome, *Am J Hum Genet* 82:1171, 2008.

Stoetzel C, et al: Confirmation of *TFAP2A* gene involvement in branchio-oculo-facial syndrome (BOFS) and report of temporal bone anomalies, *Am J Med Genet* 149:2141, 2009.

Milunsky JM, et al: Genotype-phenotype analysis of the branchio-oculo-facial syndrome, *Am J Med Genet* 155:22, 2011.

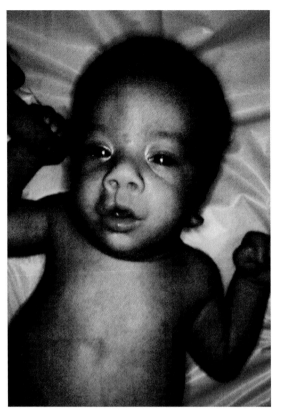

A

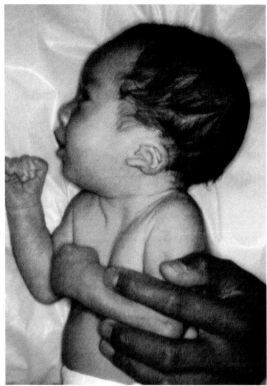

B

H

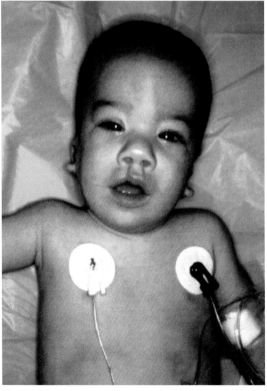

C

FIGURE 1.   Branchio-oculo-facial syndrome. **A–C,** Male infant at 3 days and at 8 months of age. Note the pseudocleft of the lip and the low-set, posteriorly rotated ears with hypoplastic superior helix. (From Fujimoto A, et al: *Am J Med Genet* 27:943, 1987. Copyright © 1987. Reprinted with permission of Wiley-Liss, Inc., a subsidiary of John Wiley & Sons, Inc.)

DONNAI-BARROW SYNDROME
(FACIO-OCULO-ACOUSTIC-RENAL SYNDROME, DBS/FOAR SYNDROME)
Agenesis of Corpus Callosum, Congenital Diaphragmatic Hernia, Ocular Hypertelorism

Donnai and Barrow described siblings with this disorder in 1993 and noted that this condition had significant clinical overlap with a pattern of malformation referred to as facio-oculo-acoustic-renal (FOAR) syndrome reported in 1972 by Holmes and Schepens. Mutations in the gene *LRP2* have been documented in both disorders, indicating that the conditions are allelic. More than 24 cases have been reported.

ABNORMALITIES

Performance. Developmental delay, sensorineural hearing loss.

Craniofacial. Macrocephaly in the newborn period, large anterior fontanel, ocular hypertelorism, prominent eyes, flat nasal bridge, downslanting palpebral fissures, short nose, posteriorly rotated ears.

Ocular. Iris coloboma, high myopia.

Other. Partial or complete agenesis of corpus callosum, congenital diaphragmatic hernia, omphalocele/umbilical hernia, proteinuria.

OCCASIONAL ABNORMALITIES

Increased birth weight; seizures; ocular abnormalities, including megalocornea, microcornea, cataract, rod and cone retinal dysfunction, and retinal pigmentary changes; scoliosis and vertebral anomalies; cardiac defects, including ventricular septal defect, double-outlet right ventricle, and patent ductus arteriosus; bicornuate uterus.

NATURAL HISTORY

Although birth weight is sometimes increased, few data are available regarding final adult weight or height. Developmental delay occurs in the majority of cases. High myopia, which is universal, is a major risk factor for retinal detachment. Severe sensorineural hearing loss occurs in the majority of cases, and patients can benefit from hearing aids.

ETIOLOGY

Autosomal recessive inheritance. This disorder is due to mutations in the gene *LPR2*, located on chromosome 2q23.3-31.1, which encodes the low-density lipoprotein receptor–related protein 2, also called megalin.

COMMENT

Megalin, an endocytic transmembrane receptor, is critical for the reuptake of ligands, including lipoprotein, sterols, vitamin-binding proteins, and hormones. Megalin knockout mice have proteinuria with increased levels of megalin ligands, including retinol-binding (RBP) and vitamin D–binding (DBP) proteins. The proteinuria in the Donnai-Barrow syndrome includes increased spillage of RBP and DBP, which can be used as diagnostic markers of this disorder.

References

Holmes LB, Schepens CL: Syndrome of ocular and facial anomalies, telecanthus, and deafness, *J Pediatr* 81:552, 1972.

Donnai D, Barrow M: Diaphragmatic hernia, exomphalos, absent corpus callosum, hypertelorism, myopia, and sensorineural deafness. A newly recognized autosomal recessive syndrome? *Am J Med Genet* 47:679, 1993.

Kantarci S, et al: Mutations in *LPR2*, which encodes the mutiligand receptor megalin, cause Donnai-Barrow and facio-oculo-acoustico-renal syndromes, *Nat Genet* 39:957, 2007.

Pober BR, et al: A review of Donnai-Barrow and facio-oculo-acoustico-renal (DB/FOAR) syndrome: Clinical features and differential diagnosis, *Birth Defects Res* 85:76, 2009.

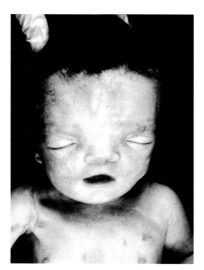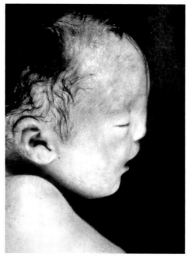

FIGURE 1.   Donnai-Barrow syndrome. Postmortem photograph: note open metopic suture, frontal bossing, downslanting palpebral fissures, ocular hypertelorism, broad nose and vermillion border of upper lip, and on the lateral view, posteriorly angulated ear and flattened facial profile. (From Gripp KW, et al: *Am J Med Genet* 68:441, 1997, with permission.)

CHARGE SYNDROME

This disorder, initially referred to as an association, was first summarized by Hall, and many similar anomalies have been observed in patients ascertained for ocular coloboma. The spectrum was broadened by Pagon and colleagues to include coloboma, heart disease, atresia choanae, retarded growth and development and/or CNS anomalies, genital anomalies and hypogonadism, and ear anomalies and deafness. The genetic etiology was identified by Vissers et al in 2004.

ABNORMALITIES

Performance. Intellectual disability (ranging from mild to profound).
Growth. Deficiency (usually postnatal).
Eyes. Colobomas, including isolated iris coloboma without visual impairment, clinical anophthalmos, and retinal coloboma.
Ears. Structural defects, including small ears, cup-shaped or lop ears, triangular-shaped concha, and hypoplastic semicircular canal. Hearing loss, including either sensorineural or mixed sensorineural, and conductive deafness, ranging from mild to profound.
Heart. Tetralogy of Fallot, patent ductus arteriosus, double-outlet right ventricle with an atrioventricular canal, ventricular septal defect, atrial septal defect, right-sided aortic arch.
Genital. Micropenis and cryptorchidism in males; lack of spontaneous onset of puberty in females.
Other. Atresia choanae (membranous or bony); multiple cranial nerve abnormalities (I, VII, VIII, IX, and/or X); cleft lip ± palate; and/or cleft palate.

OCCASIONAL ABNORMALITIES

Micrognathia, including Robin malformation sequence; feeding difficulties resulting from poor suck and velopharyngeal incompetence; venous malformations of the temporal bone; arrhinencephaly; hypogonadotropic hypogonadism; DiGeorge sequence; renal anomalies; omphalocele; tracheoesophageal fistula; rib anomalies; scoliosis; hemivertebrae; hand anomalies including polydactyly, ectrodactyly, thumb hypoplasia, and altered palmar creases; webbed neck; sloping shoulders; nipple anomalies; ptosis; ocular hypertelorism; microcephaly; anal atresia or stenosis; growth hormone deficiency.

NATURAL HISTORY

In some instances, the severity of these defects has been such that death has occurred during the neonatal period, the result of bilateral choanal atresia, esophageal atresia, severe T-cell deficiency, heart defects, and/or brain anomalies. Death in the post-neonatal period can result from swallowing problems, gastroesophageal reflux, or aspiration and postoperative airway problems that are the result of cranial nerve dysfunction. Although postnatal growth deficiency has been present in some cases, most patients have been appropriate size for gestational age, with linear growth shifting down to or below the 3rd percentile during the first 6 months of life, which in some cases has been due to growth hormone deficiency. Most patients have shown some degree of mental deficiency or CNS defects, and visual or auditory handicaps may further compromise cognitive function. Hypoplasia of the semicircular canals results in balance disturbances and delays in the attainment of motor milestones. Anosmia can be of value in the prediction of hypogonadotrophic hypogonadism. Venous malformations of the temporal bone can lead to serious complications during otologic surgery if not identified.

ETIOLOGY

Mutations in the gene *CHD7*, a member of the chromodomain helicase DNA-binding (CHD) gene family, are responsible. This class of proteins is thought to be important in early embryologic development by affecting chromatin structure and gene expression.

References

Hall BD: Choanal atresia and associated multiple anomalies, *J Pediatr* 95:395, 1979.

Hittner HM, et al: Colobomatous microphthalmia, heart disease, hearing loss, and mental retardation—a syndrome, *J Pediatr Ophthalmol Strabismus* 16:122, 1979.

Pagon RA, et al: Coloboma, congenital heart disease, and choanal atresia with multiple anomalies: CHARGE association, *J Pediatr* 99:223, 1981.

Davenport SLH, et al: The spectrum of clinical features in CHARGE association, *Clin Genet* 29:298, 1986.

Byerly KA, Pauli RM: Cranial nerve abnormalities in CHARGE association, *Am J Med Genet* 45:751, 1993.

Vissers LE, et al: Mutations in a new member of the chromodomain gene family cause CHARGE syndrome, *Nat Genet* 36:955, 2004.

Bergman JEH, et al: Death in CHARGE syndrome after the neonatal period, *Clin Genet* 77:232, 2010.

Bergman JEH, et al: Anosmia predicts hypogonadotrophic hypogonadism in CHARGE syndrome, *J Pediatr* 158:474, 2011.

Bergman JEH, et al: *CDH7* mutations and CHARGE syndrome: The clinical implications of an expanding phenotype, *J Med Genet* 48:334, 2011.

Friedmann DR, et al: Venous malformations of the temporal bone are a common feature in CHARGE syndrome, *Laryngoscope* 122:895, 2012.

H

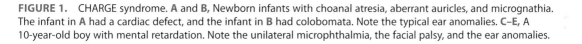

FIGURE 1.   CHARGE syndrome. **A** and **B,** Newborn infants with choanal atresia, aberrant auricles, and micrognathia. The infant in **A** had a cardiac defect, and the infant in **B** had colobomata. Note the typical ear anomalies. **C–E,** A 10-year-old boy with mental retardation. Note the unilateral microphthalmia, the facial palsy, and the ear anomalies.

WAARDENBURG SYNDROME
Lateral Displacement of Medial Canthi, Partial Albinism, Deafness

Waardenburg set forth this pattern of malformation in 1951. He found this syndrome in 1.4% of congenitally deaf children and from these data estimated the incidence to be approximately 1 in 42,000 in Holland. Four types have been described.

ABNORMALITIES

TYPE I
Facies. Lateral displacement of inner canthi with short palpebral fissures and lateral lacrimal dystopia; broad and high nasal bridge with hypoplastic alae nasi; medial flare of bushy eyebrows, which may meet in midline; hypochromic iridis; partial albinism manifested by hypopigmented ocular fundus and white eyelashes, eyebrows, and forelock.

Skin. Hypopigmented skin lesions.

Other. Deafness, aplasia of the posterior semicircular canal, premature graying, broad mandible.

OCCASIONAL ABNORMALITIES
Type I. Patent metopic suture, strabismus, rounded tip of nose, full lips with accentuated "cupid bow" to upper lip, smooth philtrum, cleft lip and palate, anisocoria, cardiac anomaly (ventricular septal defect), imperforate anus, Sprengel anomaly, supernumerary vertebrae and ribs, neural tube closure defect, scoliosis, multicystic dysplastic kidney, absence of vagina and adnexa uteri.

COMMENT
Three additional types designated II, III, and IV have been delineated and are listed subsequently.

Type II. Similar to type I except deafness is more common, lateral displacement of the inner canthi is not present, and all other features occur less frequently than in type I.

Type III. Features of type I with the addition of upper limb defects, including hypoplasia of muscles, flexion contractures, carpal bone fusion, and syndactyly. Camptodactyly occurs occasionally.

Type IV. Features of type II with the addition of Hirschsprung disease.

NATURAL HISTORY
The partial albinism is most commonly expressed as a white forelock and/or isochromic beautiful pale blue eyes with hypoplastic iridic stroma; however, it may be present as heterochromia of the iris, areas of vitiligo on the skin, patches of white hair other than the forelock, and/or mottled peripheral pigmentation of the retina. The white forelock may be present at birth only to become pigmented early in life; the hair may become prematurely gray or white.

Deafness, the most serious feature, is sensorineural, congenital, and usually nonprogressive. It can be unilateral or bilateral and varies from slight to profound, although usually the latter. The defect appears to be in the organ of Corti, with atrophic changes in the spiral ganglion and nerve.

ETIOLOGY
Type I and type III are caused by mutations in the *PAX3* gene encoding the paired box 3 transcription factor and have dominant transmission.

Type II is caused by a number of genes with various patterns of inheritance. In 15% of cases, mutations in *MITF* (dominant transmission) are responsible. Mutations in *SOX10* occur in 15% of cases (dominant transmission). Mutations in the endothelin-B receptor gene (*EDNRB*) and the gene for its ligand endothelin-3 (*EDN3*) (dominant transmission) and in *SNA12* (recessive transmission) are responsible for a small percentage of cases of type II.

Type IV is caused by *SOX10* mutations in 50% of cases (dominant transmission) and in 20% to 30% of cases to *EDN3* and *EDNRB* mutations (not fully recessive, not fully dominant inheritance).

Some patients with Types II and IV due to a SOX10 mutation are associated with neurologic features including peripheral demyelinating neuropathy or central neuropathy.

References

Waardenburg PJ: A new syndrome combining developmental anomalies of the eyelids, eyebrows and nose root with pigmentary defects of the iris and head hair and with congenital deafness, *Am J Hum Genet* 3:195, 1951.

DiGeorge AM, Olmsted RW, Harley RD: Waardenburg's syndrome, *J Pediatr* 57:649, 1960.

Hageman MJ, Delleman JW: Heterogeneity in Waardenburg syndrome, *Am J Hum Genet* 29:468, 1977.

Klein D: Historical background and evidence for dominant inheritance of the Klein-Waardenburg syndrome (type III), *Am J Med Genet* 14:231, 1983.

Tassabehji M, et al: Waardenburg's syndrome patients have mutations in the human homologue of the *PAX-3* paired box gene, *Nature* 355:635, 1992.

Hoth CF, et al: Mutations in the paired domain of the human PAX3 gene cause Klein-Waardenburg syndrome (WS-III) as well as Waardenburg syndrome type I (WS-I), *Am J Hum Genet* 52:455, 1993.

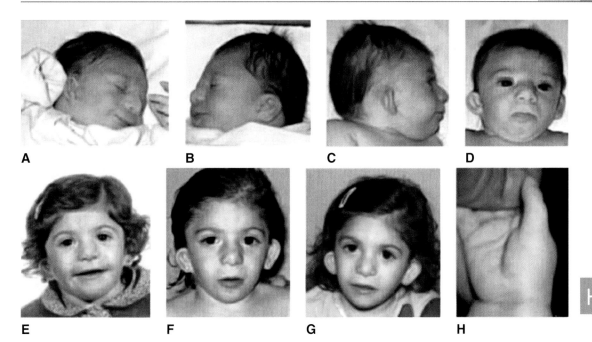

FIGURE 1. Affected child as a newborn (**A** and **B**), at age 3 months (**C** and **D**), at age 10 months (**E**), at age 3 years (**F**), and at age 7 years (**G**). Note the prominent nasal bridge, dysplastic ears, malar hypoplasia, microretrognathia, and hypoplastic thumb (**H**). (From Wieczorek D, et al: *Am J Med Genet A* 149A:837, 2009, with permission.)

MARSHALL SYNDROME

In 1958, Marshall described seven family members in three generations with a disorder characterized by cataracts, sensorineural deafness, and an extremely short nose with a flat bridge.

ABNORMALITIES

Growth. Short stature.

Facies. Short depressed nose with flat nasal bridge and anteverted nares; appearance of large eyes; flat midface; prominent, protruding upper incisors; thick lips.

Eyes. Ocular hypertelorism, myopia, cataracts, esotropia.

Hearing. Sensorineural or mixed loss, primarily affecting high frequencies and usually progressive.

Skeletal. Calvarial thickening; absent frontal sinuses; falx, tentorial, and meningeal calcifications; spondyloepiphyseal abnormalities, including mild platyspondyly, slightly small and irregular distal femoral and proximal tibial epiphyses, outward bowing of radius and ulna, and wide tufts of distal phalanges.

Other. Brachycephaly; sparse scalp hair, eyebrows, and eyelashes.

OCCASIONAL ABNORMALITIES

Mental retardation, glaucoma, retinal detachment, spontaneous rupture of lens capsule, type 1 vitreous anomaly, cleft palate, asymptomatic dysfunction of central and peripheral vestibular system, cryptorchidism, fifth finger clinodactyly.

NATURAL HISTORY

The cataracts may spontaneously resorb. Hearing loss has been noted in early childhood and often progresses to moderate or severe by adulthood.

ETIOLOGY

This disorder has an autosomal dominant inheritance pattern. Mutations in the gene encoding the a1 chain of type XI collagen (*COL11A1*), mapped to chromosome 1p21, are responsible. Some cases of Stickler syndrome are also due to mutations in *COL11A1*.

References

Marshall D: Ectodermal dysplasia: Report of a kindred with ocular abnormalities and hearing defect, *Am J Ophthalmol* 45:143, 1958.

Zellweger H, Smith JK, Grützner P: The Marshall syndrome: Report of a new family, *J Pediatr* 84:868, 1974.

O'Donnell JJ, Sirkin S, Hall BD: Generalized osseous abnormalities in the Marshall syndrome, *Birth Defects* 12(5):299, 1976.

Aymé S, Preus M: The Marshall and Stickler syndromes: Objective rejection of lumping, *J Med Genet* 21:34, 1984.

Shanske AL, et al: The Marshall syndrome: Report of a new family and review of the literature, *Am J Med Genet* 70:52, 1997.

Griffith AJ, et al: Marshall syndrome associated with a splicing defect at the *COL11A1* locus, *Am J Hum Genet* 62:816, 1998.

Griffith AJ, et al: Audiovestibular phenotype associated with a *COL11A1* mutation in Marshall syndrome, *Arch Otolaryngol Head Neck Surg* 126:891, 2000.

Majava M, et al: A report on 10 new patients with heterozygous mutations in the *COL11A1* gene and a review of genotype-phenotype correlations in type XI collagenopathies, *Am J Med Genet* 143:258, 2007.

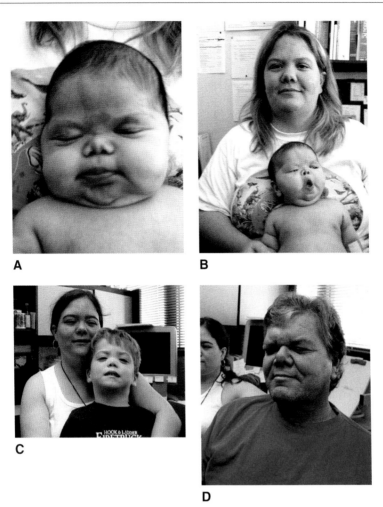

FIGURE 1. Marshall syndrome. **A–D,** Three-generation family, including a father, his two daughters, and two of his grandchildren. Note the short depressed nose, flat nasal bridge, anteverted nares, and appearance of large eyes.

H

CERVICO-OCULO-ACOUSTIC SYNDROME (WILDERVANCK SYNDROME)
Klippel-Feil Anomaly, Abducens Paralysis with Retracted Globes, Sensorineural Deafness

Initially described by Wildervanck in 1952, this disorder was further characterized by the same investigator, who summarized the clinical features of 62 affected patients in 1978.

ABNORMALITIES

Craniofacial. Asymmetry with a short neck and low hairline, preauricular skin tags, and pits.

Eyes. Duane anomaly (abducens paralysis with retraction of the globe and narrowing of the palpebral fissure of the affected eye on adduction), epibulbar dermoids.

Hearing. Sensorineural, conductive, or mixed loss; a malformed vestibular labyrinth is usually present; the cochlea is sometimes altered.

Skeletal. Klippel-Feil anomaly (fusion of two or more cervical and sometimes thoracic vertebrae), torticollis, scoliosis, Sprengel deformity.

OCCASIONAL ABNORMALITIES

Intellectual disability; growth deficiency; occipital meningocele; cerebellar and brainstem hypoplasia, primarily involving the pons and medulla; cervical diastematomyelia; pseudopapilledema; tearing during oral feeding; hydrocephalus; cleft palate; ear anomalies; cardiac defects; cervical ribs; absent kidney; cholelithiasis.

NATURAL HISTORY

Severe deformations of the craniofacial area can progress in cases with significant degrees of torticollis. Intelligence in the vast majority of cases is normal. Computed tomography should be performed to document any abnormality of the inner ear. Magnetic resonance imaging for craniospinal abnormalities should be considered.

ETIOLOGY

The cause of this disorder is unknown; all cases have been sporadic. The majority of affected individuals have been females. One affected child was born to consanguineous parents.

References

Wildervanck LS: The cervico-oculo-acusticus syndrome. In Vinken PJ, Bruyn GW, editors: *Handbook of Clinical Neurology: Congenital Malformations of the Spine and Spinal Cord (vol 32)*, Amsterdam, NY, 1978, Elsevier/North-Holland Biomedical.

West PDB, et al: Wildervanck's syndrome: Unilateral Mondini dysplasia identified by computed tomography, *J Laryngol Otol* 103:408, 1989.

Gupte G, et al: Wildervanck syndrome (cervico-oculo-acoustic syndrome), *J Postgrad Med* 38:180, 1992.

Brodsky MC, et al: Brainstem hypoplasia in the Wildervanck (cervico-oculo-acoustic) syndrome, *Arch Ophthalmol* 116:383, 1998.

Balci S, et al: Cervical diastematomyelia in the cervico-oculo-acoustic (Wildervanck) syndrome: MRI findings, *Clin Dysmorphol* 11:125, 2002.

Di Maio L, et al: Cervico-oculo-acoustic syndrome in a male with consanguineous parents, *Can J Neurol Sci* 33:237, 2006.

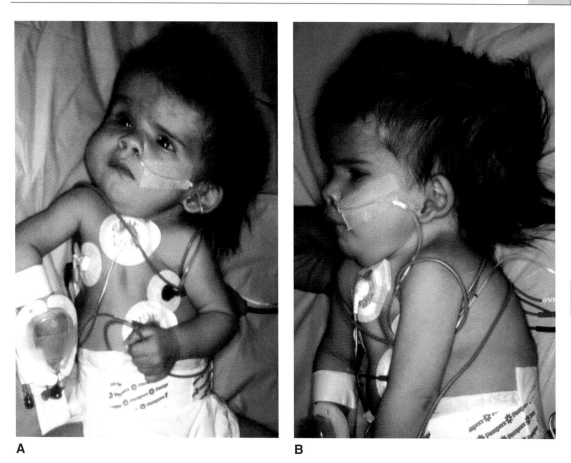

A   **B**

FIGURE 1.   Cervico-oculo-acoustic syndrome. **A** and **B,** Note the short neck with low hairline, preauricular skin tag, and ear anomalies.

H

Facial-Limb Defects as Major Feature

MILLER SYNDROME (POSTAXIAL ACROFACIAL DYSOSTOSIS SYNDROME)
Treacher Collins–Like Facies; Limb Deficiency, Especially Postaxial

In 1979, Miller and colleagues brought together six cases, four of which were from the literature, and recognized this disorder as a concise entity. The facial appearance is similar to that of Treacher Collins syndrome and, in combination with limb defects, resembles Nager syndrome. The severity of the postaxial deficiencies distinguishes it from the latter syndrome.

ABNORMALITIES

Craniofacial. Malar hypoplasia, sometimes with radiologic evidence of a vertical bony cleft, with downslanting palpebral fissures; colobomata of eyelids and ectropion; micrognathia; cleft lip and/or cleft palate; hypoplastic, cup-shaped ears.

Limbs. Absence of fifth digits of all four limbs with or without shortening and incurving of forearms with ulnar and radial hypoplasia; syndactyly.

Other. Accessory nipple(s).

OCCASIONAL ABNORMALITIES

Postnatal growth deficiency, choanal atresia, conductive hearing loss, thumb hypoplasia, low-arch dermal pattern, pectus excavatum, radioulnar synostosis, supernumerary vertebrae, rib defects, congenital hip dislocation, heart defects, absence of hemidiaphragm, pyloric stenosis, renal anomalies, cryptorchidism, midgut malrotation.

NATURAL HISTORY

These individuals are usually of normal intelligence. Hearing evaluation is indicated in all cases. The craniofacial appearance sometimes changes with increasing age with a progressively greater degree of ectropion and facial asymmetry as well as a more triangular facial appearance with thin lips.

ETIOLOGY

This disorder has an autosomal recessive inheritance pattern. Mutations of *DHODH,* which encodes the enzyme dihydroorotate dehydrogenase, are responsible. Dihydroorotate dehydrogenase plays an important role in de novo biosynthesis of pyrimidines. Identification of this gene represents the first successful use of exome sequencing to discover the cause of a Mendelian disorder.

References

Genée E: Une forme extensive de dysostose mandibulofaciale, *J Genet Hum* 17:45, 1969.

Smith DW, Pashayan H, Wildervanck LS: Case report 28, *Synd Ident* 3(1):7, 1975.

Miller M, Fineman R, Smith DW: Postaxial acrofacial dysostosis syndrome, *J Pediatr* 95:970, 1979.

Ogilvy-Stuart AL, Parsons AC: Miller syndrome (postaxial acrofacial dysostosis): Further evidence for autosomal recessive inheritance and expansion of the phenotype, *J Med Genet* 28:695, 1991.

Chrzanowska K, Fryns JP: Miller postaxial acrofacial dysostosis: The phenotypic changes with age, *Genet Couns* 4:131, 1993.

Ng SB, et al: Exome sequencing identifies the cause of a Mendelian disorder, *Nat Genet* 42:30, 2010.

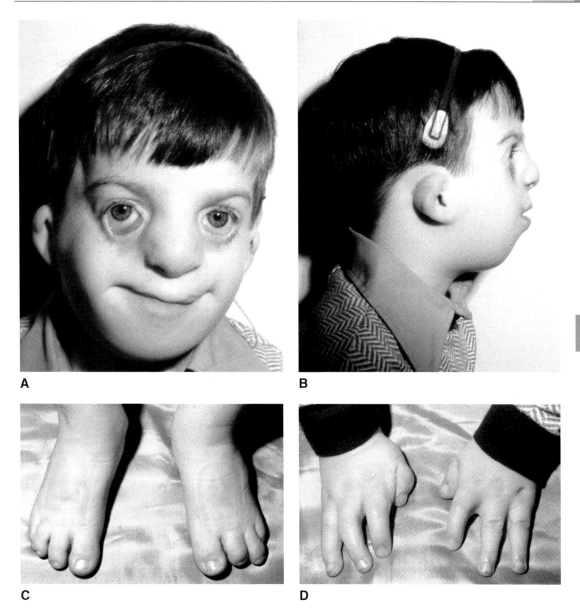

A

B

C

D

FIGURE 1.   Miller syndrome. **A–D,** Affected individual showing striking malar and maxillary hypoplasia and lower lid defects. Note the hearing aid, required for middle ear deafness. The deficiency in the hands and feet is complete for the fifth ray and incomplete for the other digits. (From Miller M et al: *J Pediatr* 95:970, 1979, with permission.)

NAGER SYNDROME (NAGER ACROFACIAL DYSOSTOSIS SYNDROME)
Radial Limb Hypoplasia, Malar Hypoplasia, Ear Defects

Nager and de Reynier described a Treacher Collins syndrome–like patient with radial limb defects in 1948, and subsequently more than 90 cases have been reported.

ABNORMALITIES

Performance. Intelligence normal; conductive deafness, usually bilateral; problems with articulation.

Craniofacial. Malar hypoplasia with downslanting palpebral fissures; high nasal bridge; micrognathia; partial to total absence of lower eyelashes; low-set, posteriorly rotated ears; preauricular tags; atresia of external ear canal; cleft palate.

Limbs. Hypoplasia to aplasia of thumb, with or without radius; proximal radioulnar synostosis and limitation of elbow extension; short forearms.

OCCASIONAL ABNORMALITIES

Intellectual disability; microcephaly; hydrocephalus secondary to aqueductal stenosis; polymicrogyria; postnatal growth deficiency; lower lid coloboma; projection of scalp hair onto lateral cheek; cleft lip; velopharyngeal insufficiency; hypoplasia of larynx or epiglottis; temporomandibular joint fibrosis and ankylosis; syndactyly, clinodactyly, or camptodactyly of hands; duplicated and triphalangeal thumbs; missing or hypoplastic toes; overlapping toes; syndactyly of toes; posteriorly placed hypoplastic halluces, hallux valgus, broad hallux; absent distal flexion creases on toes; limb reduction defects; hip dislocation; clubfeet; hypoplastic first rib; scoliosis; cervical vertebral and spine anomalies; cardiac defects; genitourinary anomalies; Hirschsprung disease; urticaria pigmentosa.

NATURAL HISTORY

The recommendations for early detection of deafness, hearing aid augmentation, and plastic surgery are similar to those for Treacher Collins syndrome. Anesthetic complications should be considered seriously. Delays in speech and language development are related to hearing loss. Early respiratory and feeding problems frequently occur. Gastrostomy or gavage feeding is often necessary. The incidence of prematurity is high. Perinatal mortality is approximately 20% and is related to respiratory distress secondary to micrognathia and palatal anomalies. Management should be the same as that for the Robin sequence.

ETIOLOGY

This disorder has an autosomal dominant pattern of inheritance. About 60% of cases are due to mutations of SF3B4, which encodes SAP49, a spliceosomal protein. Spliceosomes are involved in intron splicing as well as alternative splicing and thus play an important role in gene-expression pathways. Most cases have been sporadic.

References

Nager FR, de Reynier JP: Das Gehörorgan bei den angeborenen Kopfmissbildungen, *Pract Otorhinolaryngol (Basal)* 10(Suppl 2):1, 1948.

Bowen P, Harley F: Mandibulofacial dysostosis with limb malformations (Nager's acrofacial dysostosis), *Birth Defects* 10(5):109, 1974.

Meyerson MD, et al: Nager acrofacial dysostosis: Early invention and long-term planning, *Cleft Palate J* 14:35, 1977.

Halal F, et al: Differential diagnosis of Nager acrofacial dysostosis syndrome: Report of four patients with Nager syndrome and discussion of other related syndromes, *Am J Med Genet* 14:209, 1983.

Aylsworth AL, et al: Nager acrofacial dysostosis: Male-to-male transmission in 2 families, *Am J Med Genet* 41:83, 1991.

McDonald MT, Gorski JL: Nager acrofacial dysostosis, *J Med Genet* 30:779, 1993.

Groeper K, et al: Anaesthetic implications of Nager syndrome, *Paediatr Anaesth* 12:365, 2002.

Bernier FP, et al: Haploinsufficiency of SF3B4, a component of the pre-mRNA spliceosomal complex, causes Nager syndrome, *Am J Hum Genet* 90:925, 2012.

Schlieve T, et al: Temporomandibular joint replacement for ankylosis correction in Nager syndrome: Case report and review of the literature, *J Oral Maxillofac Surg* 70:616, 2012.

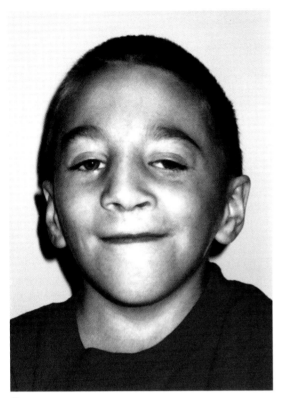 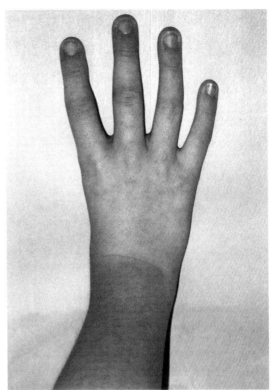

A   **B**

FIGURE 1. Nager syndrome. **A** and **B,** Note the malar hypoplasia, downslanting palpebral fissures, high nasal bridge, micrognathia, and thumb aplasia. (Courtesy of Dr. Stephen Braddock, University of Missouri, Columbia.)

TOWNES-BROCKS SYNDROME
Thumb Anomalies, Auricular Anomalies, Anal Anomalies

Townes and Brocks first described this disorder in 1972, and at least 65 affected individuals have been reported.

ABNORMALITIES

Craniofacial. Auricular anomalies, including overfolding of the superior helix and small, sometimes cupped ears; variable features of hemifacial microsomia, especially preauricular tags.

Hearing. Sensorineural loss, ranging from mild to profound; a small conductive component is often present.

Limbs. Hand anomalies, including broad, bifid, hypoplastic, or triphalangeal thumb; hypoplastic thenar eminence; preaxial polydactyly; distal ulnar deviation of thumb; pseudoepiphysis of second metacarpals; fusion of triquetrum and hamate; absence of triquetrum and navicular bones; fusion or short metatarsals; prominence of distal ends of lateral metatarsals; absent or hypoplastic third toe; clinodactyly of fifth toe.

Anus. Imperforate anus, anterior placement, and stenosis; rectovaginal or rectoperineal fistula.

Genitourinary. Unilateral or bilateral hypoplastic or dysplastic kidneys, renal agenesis, multicystic kidney, posterior urethral valves, vesicoureteral reflux, meatal stenosis.

OCCASIONAL ABNORMALITIES

Intellectual disability; microcephaly; microtia; preauricular pit; structural middle ear anomalies; cataracts; microphthalmia; optic nerve atrophy; coloboma; epibulbar dermoids; mandibular hypoplasia; cardiac defect; duodenal atresia; cystic ovary; prominent perineal raphe; bifid scrotum; hypospadias; second and third, and third and fourth, syndactyly of fingers; abnormalities of toes, including fifth toe clinodactyly, absence or hypoplasia of third toe, third and fourth syndactyly of toes, overlapping second, third, and fourth toes; scoliosis.

NATURAL HISTORY

Hearing loss can be progressive and is worse in the high frequencies. Renal failure or impaired renal function occurs in some cases. Lifelong monitoring of renal function is indicated.

ETIOLOGY

This disorder has an autosomal dominant inheritance pattern with marked variability in the severity of expression for each feature. Mutations in *SALL1*, which is expressed in all organs affected in this disorder and is located at 16q12.1, are responsible in 64% to 83% of cases. Deletions of 16q12.1, which include the *SALL1* gene, have been responsible for a few cases.

COMMENT

This single-gene disorder encompasses many of the features of both the VATER association and the facio-auriculo-vertebral malformation sequence.

References

Townes PL, Brocks ER: Hereditary syndrome of imperforate anus with hand, foot and ear anomalies, *J Pediatr* 81:321, 1972.

Reid IS, Turner G: Familial anal abnormality, *J Pediatr* 88:992, 1976.

Kurnit DM, et al: Autosomal dominant transmission of a syndrome of anal, ear, renal and radial congenital malformations, *J Pediatr* 93:270, 1978.

Walpole IR, Hockey A: Syndrome of imperforate anus, abnormalities of hands and feet, satyr ears, and sensorineural deafness, *J Pediatr* 100:250, 1982.

Monteiro de Pino-Neto J: Phenotypic variability in Townes-Brocks syndrome, *Am J Med Genet* 18:147, 1984.

O'Callaghan M, Young ID: The Townes-Brocks syndrome, *J Med Genet* 27:457, 1990.

Cameron TH, et al: Townes-Brocks syndrome in two mentally retarded youngsters, *Am J Med Genet* 41:1, 1991.

Kohlhase J, et al: Molecular analysis of *SALL1* mutations in Townes-Brocks syndrome, *Am J Hum Genet* 64:435, 1999.

Powell CM, Michaelis RC: Townes-Brocks syndrome, *J Med Genet* 36:89, 1999.

Kosaki R, et al: Wide phenotypic variations within a family with *SALL1* mutations: Isolated external ear abnormalities to Goldenhar syndrome, *Am J Med Genet* 143:1087, 2007.

Miller EM, et al: Implications for genotype-phenotype predictions in Townes-Brocks syndrome: Case report of a novel *SALL1* deletion and review of the literature, *Am J Med Genet* 158:533, 2012.

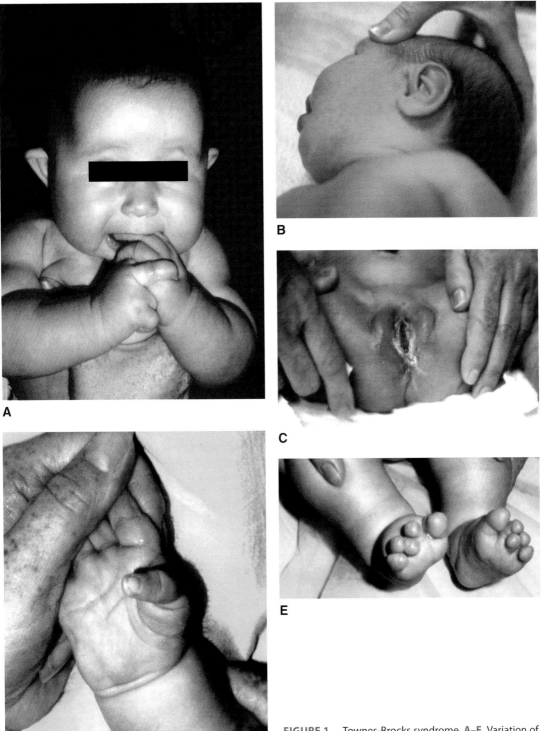

FIGURE 1. Townes-Brocks syndrome. **A–E,** Variation of facial morphogenesis with large protruding ears, preauricular tags, and features resembling facio-auriculo-vertebral sequence (hemifacial microsomia, Goldenhar syndrome). Note the imperforate anus, hypoplastic thenar eminence and thumb, and hypoplastic third toe.

LAURIN-SANDROW SYNDROME
Cup-Shaped Hands, Mirror Image Feet, Flat Nose with Grooved Columella

Laurin and colleagues described, in 1964, a newborn boy with complete polysyndactyly of hands, mirror polysyndactyly of feet, bilateral ulnar and fibular dimelia, and absent tibia and radii. Sandrow and colleagues described a similarly affected father and daughter who had, in addition, anomalies of the ala nasi and columella. Martínez-Frías et al referred to this disorder as Laurin-Sandrow syndrome.

ABNORMALITIES

Growth. Normal pre- and postnatal growth with short stature due to limb anomalies.
Performance. Normal cognitive function, motor challenges secondary to limb anomalies.
Nose. Deep groove running the length of a short columella, flat nasal bridge, bulbous nasal tip, unfused nares, hypoplastic alar and columellar cartilage.
Upper Limbs. Complete polysyndactyly; cup-appearing, rosebud, or mitten hands; phalanges of differing sizes and shapes; disorganized interphalangeal joints; abnormal carpal bones.
Lower Limbs. Polydactyly with variable syndactyly, mirror image feet, talipes equinovarus, abnormal tarsal bones, absent/hypoplastic tibia.
Imaging. Large mandibular condyles; duplication of ulna; malformed scaphoid and lunate bones; absence of the trapezia, triquetrum, and pisiform bones; synostosis/malformation of tarsals; synostosis of talus, calcaneus, cuboid, and navicular bones; supernumerary metacarpals and metatarsals; asymmetric shortening of metacarpals; bony syndactyly of phalanges; radioulnar synostosis; absent/hypoplastic patella.

OCCASIONAL ABNORMALITIES

Frontal prominence, hydrocephalus, agenesis of corpus callosum, neuronal migration defects, developmental delay, hypotonia, absent radius, decreased pronation/supination at elbows, restricted extension at wrist, short fibula, fibular duplication, cryptorchidism.

NATURAL HISTORY

Although one affected 33-week premature infant with agenesis of the corpus callosum and dilatation of the lateral ventricles died of unknown etiology in the newborn period, life expectancy appears to be normal. An affected 54-year-old male with mild intellectual disability who appeared older than his age was described as cheerful and apparently healthy.

ETIOLOGY

Based on one instance of male-to-male transmission, autosomal dominant is the most likely mode of inheritance. The causative gene has not been identified

References

Laurin CA, et al: Bilateral absence of the radius and tibia with bilateral reduplication of the ulna and fibula, *J Bone Joint Surg Am* 46:137, 1964.

Sandrow RE, et al: Hereditary ulnar and fibular dimelia with peculiar facies, *J Bone Joint Surg Am* 52:367, 1970.

Martínez-Frías ML, et al: Laurin-Sandrow syndrome (mirror hands and feet and nasal defects): Description of a new case, *J Med Genet* 31:410, 1994.

Mariño-Enríquez A, et al: Laurin-Sandrow syndrome: Review and redefinition, *Am J Med Genet A* 146A:2557, 2008.

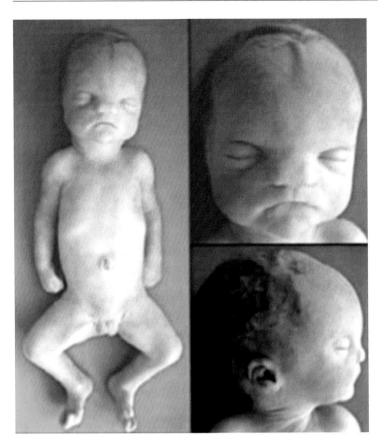

FIGURE 1. Laurin-Sandrow syndrome. Note frontal bossing, hypertelorism, broad nasal bridge, flat midface and nose with a deep longitudinal groove on the tip of the nose and the columella, downturned corners of mouth. (From Mariño-Enríquez A et al: *Am J Med Genet A* 146A:2557, 2008, with permission.)

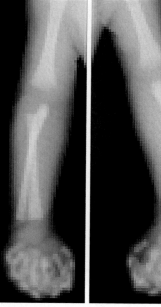

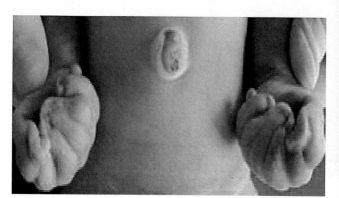

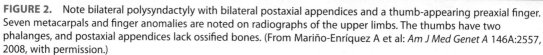

FIGURE 2.   Note bilateral polysyndactyly with bilateral postaxial appendices and a thumb-appearing preaxial finger. Seven metacarpals and finger anomalies are noted on radiographs of the upper limbs. The thumbs have two phalanges, and postaxial appendices lack ossified bones. (From Mariño-Enríquez A et al: *Am J Med Genet A* 146A:2557, 2008, with permission.)

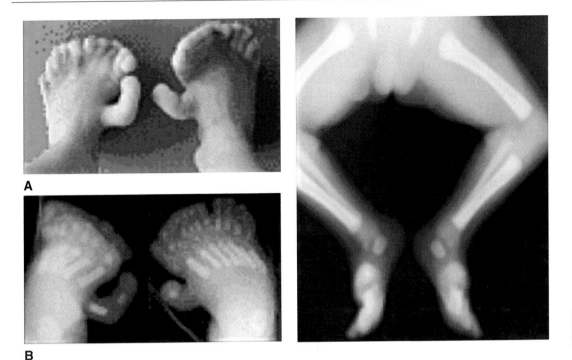

FIGURE 3. Feet of affected child. **A,** Bilateral polysyndactyly with prominent preaxial accessory digit. **B,** Radiographic appearance showing four lateral toes with three identically shaped phalanges, and other phalanges showing variable shapes and sizes. Preaxial accessory digit has three bones on the left side and two on the right. There are seven metatarsals and a single anomalous tarsal bone. On the radiograph of the lower limbs, note the hypoplastic tibiae, which are shorter than the fibula. (From Mariño-Enríquez A et al: *Am J Med Genet A* 146A:2557, 2008, with permission.)

ORAL-FACIAL-DIGITAL SYNDROME (OFD SYNDROME, TYPE I)
Oral Frenula and Clefts, Hypoplasia of Alae Nasi, Digital Asymmetry

Papillon-Léage and Psaume set forth this condition as a clinical entity in 1954. More than 160 cases have been reported. Thirteen different oral-facial-digital syndromes have been delineated. Only types I and II have been set forth in detail in this text.

ABNORMALITIES

Performance. Variable degrees of intellectual disability in approximately 57%, with average IQ of 70.

Oral. Multiple and/or hyperplastic frenuli between the buccal mucous membrane and alveolar ridge, median cleft lip, lobated/bifid tongue with nodules, cleft of alveolar ridge (at area of lateral incisors, which may be missing), cleft palate, dental caries, and anomalous anterior teeth.

Facial. Hypoplasia of alar cartilages, lateral placement of inner canthi; milia of ears and upper face in infancy.

Digital. Asymmetric shortening of digits with clinodactyly, syndactyly, or brachydactyly of hands and preaxial polydactyly of feet.

Scalp. Dry, rough, sparse hair; dry scalp.

Renal. Adult polycystic kidney disease; histologically, there is a predominance of glomerular cysts.

Imaging. Increased naso-sella-basion angle at base of cranium; absence of corpus callosum; intracerebral cyst; porencephaly; hydrocephalus; vermis hypoplasia; focal polymicrogyria; cortical, periventricular, subarachnoid heterotopia; and Dandy-Walker malformation.

OCCASIONAL ABNORMALITIES

Enamel hypoplasia, supernumerary teeth, hamartoma of tongue, fistula in lower lip, choanal atresia, frontal bossing, hypoplastic mandibular ramus and zygoma, nonprogressive metaphyseal rarefaction, alopecia, granular seborrheic skin, pre- and postaxial polydactyly of hands.

NATURAL HISTORY

Patients may do poorly in early infancy; as many as one third die during this period. Management is directed toward plastic surgical correction of oral clefts and dental care, including dentures when indicated. Psychometric evaluation is merited because about one half of the reported patients have intellectual disability. Polycystic renal disease is progressive, with onset of hypertension and renal insufficiency after 18 years of age. Fibrocystic disease of liver and pancreas becomes a problem in adulthood.

ETIOLOGY

This disorder has an X-linked dominant inheritance pattern with lethality in the vast majority of affected males. Mutations in *OFD1* (formerly named Cxorf5), which has an important effect on ciliary function, are responsible for type I. Thus, oral-facial-digital syndrome type I (OFD I) is regarded as a ciliopathy.

COMMENT

Gurrieri et al have set forth the major features that distinguish types III through XIII. With the exception of type V, all have similar oral, facial, and digital abnormalities. Significant overlap exists between the 13 types, making it difficult to provide appropriate counseling relative to prognosis. Furthermore, only the gene for OFD I has been identified.

Type III (Sugarman syndrome), an autosomal recessive disorder, is distinguished clinically by postaxial polydactyly, a bulbous nose, extra and small teeth, and macular red spots associated with see-saw winking of eyelids, myoclonic jerks, or both. Affected siblings have been reported.

Type IV (Baraitser-Burn syndrome), an autosomal recessive disorder, is distinguished by severe tibial dysplasia, occipitoschisis, brain malformations, ocular colobomas, intrahepatic and renal cysts, anal atresia, and joint dislocations.

Type V (Thurston syndrome), an autosomal recessive condition, includes midline cleft lip, duplicated frenulum, and postaxial polydactyly of hands and feet.

Type VI (Varadi-Papp syndrome), an autosomal recessive condition, is distinguished by preaxial polysyndactyly of toes and postaxial polydactyly of fingers, Y-shaped metacarpal with central polydactyly, and cerebellar anomalies (vermis hypoplasia/aplasia or Dandy-Walker anomaly). Occasional features include growth hormone deficiency, hypogonadotrophic hypogonadism, and a hypothalamic hamartoma. The latter findings are features of Pallister-Hall syndrome and raise the possibility that these two disorders are the same.

Type VII (Whelan syndrome) has been reported in a mother-daughter pair. Features that distinguish this condition include congenital hydronephrosis, coarse hair, facial asymmetry, facial weakness, and preauricular tags. It is not clear if this disorder is separate from OFD I.

Type VIII (Edwards syndrome) is an X-linked recessive disorder distinguished from type I by pre- and postaxial polydactyly of hands and bilateral duplication of halluces, shortness of long bones, abnormal tibiae, short stature, laryngeal anomalies, absent or abnormal central incisors, broad or bifid nasal tip, and metacarpal forking. It overlaps with type II.

Type IX (Gurrieri syndrome) is an autosomal recessive disorder. Features that distinguish this condition are retinal coloboma and hallucal duplication.

Type X (Figuera syndrome) has the distinguishing features of mesomelic limb shortening due to radial hypoplasia and fibular agenesis. The digital defects include oligodactyly and preaxial polydactyly.

Type XI (Gabrielli syndrome) is distinguished by craniovertebral anomalies, including fusion of vertebral arches of C1, C2 and C3 and clefts in vertebral bodies, midline cleft of the palate, vomer, ethmoid and crista galli, and apophysis.

Type XII (Moran-Barroso syndrome) has distinguishing features, including myelomeningocele, stenosis of aqueduct of Sylvius, and cardiac anomalies.

Type XIII (Degner syndrome) has distinguishing features that include major depression, epilepsy, and MRI findings of the brain such as patched loss of white matter of unknown origin.

References

Papillon-Léage E, Psaume J: Une malformation héréditaire de la muqueuse buccale: Brides et freins anormaux, *Rev Stomatol (Paris)* 55:209, 1954.

Gorlin RJ, Psaume J: Orodigitofacial dysostosis—a new syndrome, *J Pediatr* 61:520, 1962.

Doege TC, et al: Studies of a family with the oral-facial-digital syndrome, *N Engl J Med* 271:1073, 1964.

Majewski F, et al: Das oro-facio-digitale Syndrom: Symptome und Prognose, *Z Kinderheilkd* 112:89, 1972.

Donnai D, et al: Familial orofaciodigital syndrome type I presenting as adult polycystic kidney disease, *J Med Genet* 24:84, 1987.

Toriello HV: Oral-facial-digital syndromes, 1992, *Clin Dysmorphol* 2:95, 1993.

Toriello HV, et al: Six patients with oral-facial-digital syndrome IV: The case for heterogeneity, *Am J Med Genet* 69:250, 1997.

Doss BJ, et al: Neuropathologic findings in a case of OFDS type VI (Varadi syndrome), *Am J Med Genet* 77:38, 1998.

Ferrante MI, et al: Identification of the gene for oral-facial-digital type I syndrome, *Am J Hum Genet* 68:569, 2001.

Gurrieri F, et al: Oral-facial-digital syndromes: Review and diagnostic guidelines, *Am J Med Genet* 143:3314, 2007.

Chetty-John S, et al: Fibrocystic disease of liver and pancreas; under-recognized features of the X-linked ciliopathy oral-facial digital syndrome type I (OFD I), *Am J Med Genet* 152:2640, 2010.

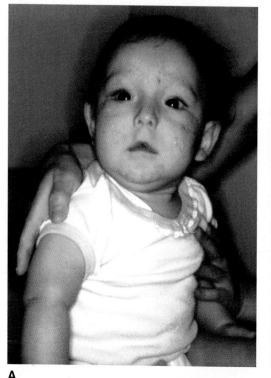

A

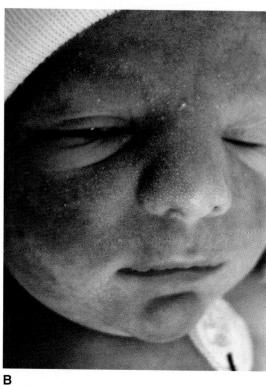

B

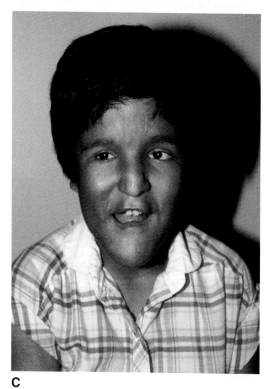

C

FIGURE 1.   Oral-facial-digital syndrome, type I.
A–C, Note the milia of the ears and upper face in infancy,
the median cleft lip, and the hypoplastic ala nasi.

Continued

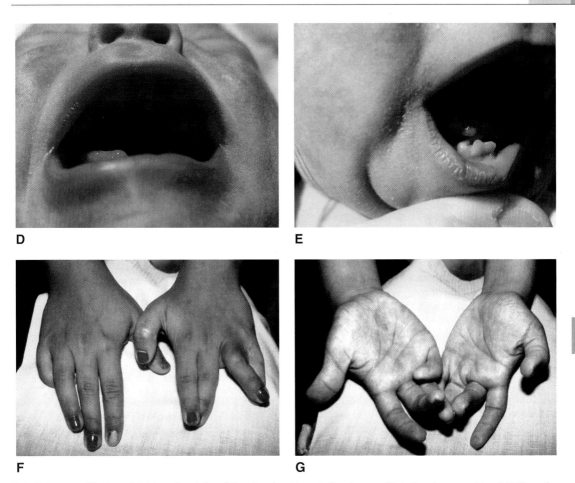

FIGURE 1, cont'd   **D** and **E,** Note the clefts of the alveolar ridge, cleft palate, and lobulated tongue. **F** and **G,** Note the asymmetric shortening of digits with syndactyly and clinodactyly.

MOHR SYNDROME (OFD SYNDROME, TYPE II)
Cleft Tongue, Conductive Deafness, Partial Reduplication of Hallux

Mohr described this pattern in several male siblings in 1941. More than 30 cases have been reported.

ABNORMALITIES

Growth and Performance. Mild shortness of stature, conductive deafness apparently due to defect of incus.

Craniofacial. Low nasal bridge with lateral displacement of inner canthi; broad nasal tip, sometimes slightly bifid; midline partial cleft of lip; hypertrophy of usual frenula; midline cleft of tongue, nodules on tongue; flare to alveolar ridge; hypoplasia of zygomatic arch, maxilla, and body of mandible.

Limbs. Partial reduplication of hallux and first metatarsal, cuneiform, and cuboid bones; relatively short hands with clinodactyly of fifth finger; bilateral postaxial polydactyly of hands; bilateral preaxial polysyndactyly of feet (occasionally only unilateral); metaphyseal flaring and irregularity.

OCCASIONAL ABNORMALITIES

Wormian cranial bones, missing central incisors, cleft palate, multiple frenula, pectus excavatum, scoliosis.

NATURAL HISTORY

These patients apparently have normal intelligence, and plastic surgery is indicated for the clefts, frenula, and partial reduplication of the hallux.

ETIOLOGY

This disorder has an autosomal recessive inheritance pattern.

References

Mohr OL: A hereditary sublethal syndrome in man, *Skr Norske Vidensk Akad I Mat Naturv Klasse* 14:3, 1941.

Rimoin DL, Edgerton MT: Genetic and clinical heterogeneity in the oral-facial-digital syndromes, *J Pediatr* 71:94, 1967.

Pfeiffer RA, Majewski F, Mannkopf H: Das syndrome von Mohr und Classen, *Klin Paediatr* 184:224, 1972.

Levy EP, Fletcher BD, Fraser FC: Mohr syndrome with subclinical expression of the bifid great toe, *Am J Dis Child* 128:531, 1974.

Baraitser M: The orofacial digital (OFD) syndromes, *J Med Genet* 23:116, 1986.

Hosalkar HS, et al: Mohr syndrome: A rare case and distinction from orofacial digital syndrome I, *J Postgrad Med* 45:123, 1999.

Sakai N, et al: Oral-facial-digital syndrome type II (Mohr syndrome): Clinical and genetic manifestations, *J Craniofac Surg* 13:321, 2002.

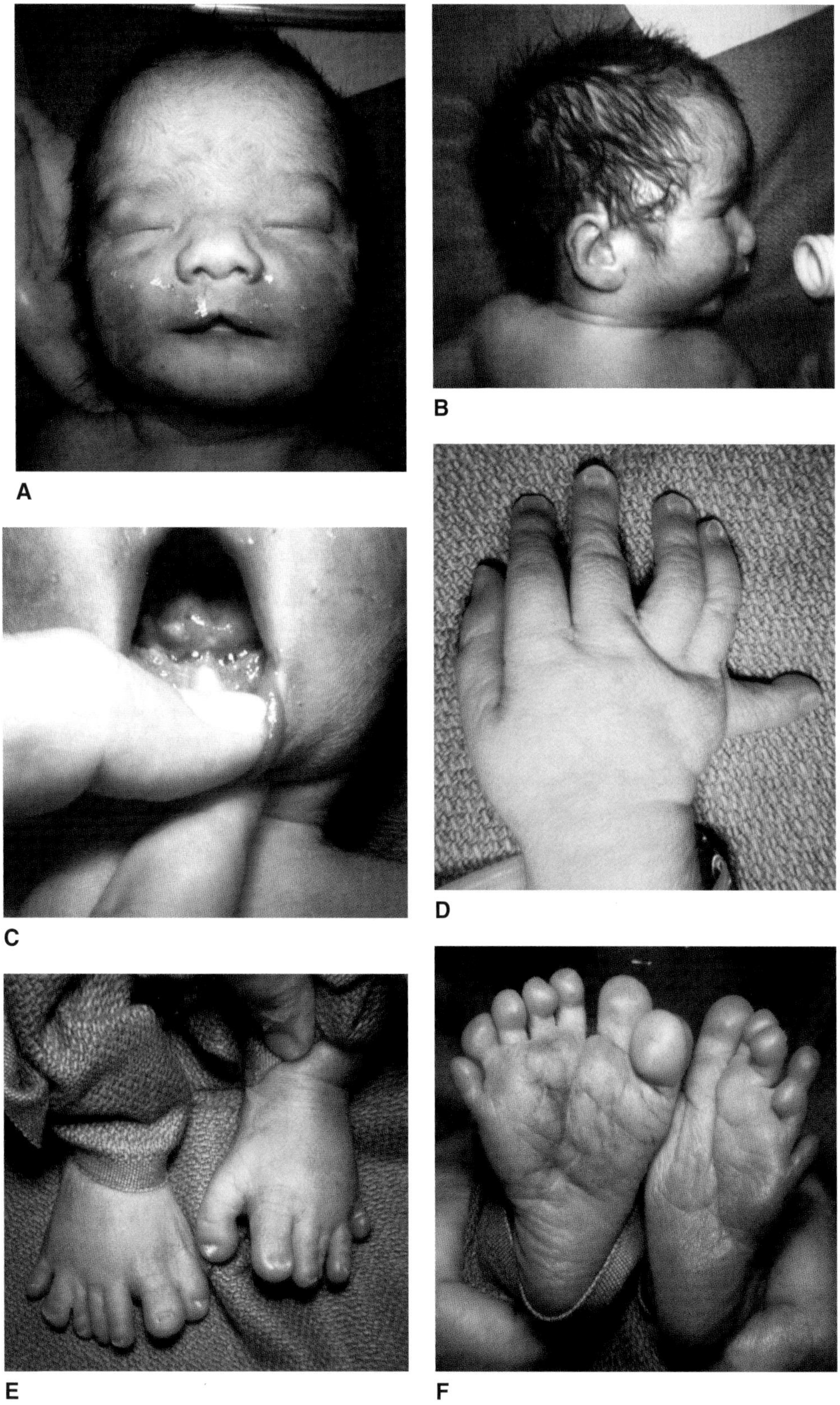

FIGURE 1.   Mohr syndrome. **A–C,** Note the midline cleft of the upper lip, lateral displacement of the medial canthi, broad nasal tip, and tongue nodules. **D–F,** Note the postaxial polydactyly of hands and feet and preaxial polydactyly of feet.

22Q11.2 MICRODELETION SYNDROME
(VELO-CARDIO-FACIAL SYNDROME, DIGEORGE SYNDROME, SHPRINTZEN SYNDROME)

In 1965, DiGeorge described a patient with hypoparathyroidism and cellular immune deficiency secondary to thymic hypoplasia. The pattern of malformation expanded rapidly to include other defects of the third and fourth branchial arches as well as dysmorphic facial features. In 1978, Shprintzen and colleagues reported a group of children with cleft palate or velopharyngeal incompetence, cardiac defects, and a prominent nose (velo-cardio-facial syndrome). It was subsequently determined that individuals with velo-cardio-facial syndrome and the majority of those with the condition described by DiGeorge have a deletion of chromosome 22q11.2. It is now known that the two disorders represent different manifestations of the same genetic defect.

ABNORMALITIES

Performance. Normal development or mild learning problems (62%); moderate or severe learning problems (18%); IQ generally ranges from 70 to 90, with some slightly higher; psychiatric disorders in approximately 10% of cases. Decreased motor tone and axial instability. Motor milestones delayed. Walking occurs at 16 to 24 months.

Growth. Postnatal onset of short stature (36%).

Ears and Hearing. Conductive hearing loss secondary to cleft palate; minor auricular anomalies.

Craniofacial. Cleft of the secondary palate, either overt or submucous; velopharyngeal incompetence; small or absent adenoids; prominent nose with squared nasal root and narrow alar base; narrow palpebral fissures; abundant scalp hair; deficient malar area; vertical maxillary excess with long face; retruded mandible with chin deficiency; microcephaly (40%–50%).

Limbs. Slender and hypotonic with hyperextensible hands and fingers (63%).

Cardiac. Defects present in 85%, the most common being ventricular septal defect (62%); right aortic arch (52%); tetralogy of Fallot (21%); aberrant left subclavian artery.

OCCASIONAL ABNORMALITIES

Robin malformation sequence; cleft lip; asymmetric crying facies; facial nerve palsy; nasal dimple; enlargement, medial displacement, tortuosity, or other abnormalities of internal carotid arteries (25%); umbilical or inguinal hernias; structural brain defects, including cerebral atrophy, cerebellar hypoplasia, cerebral vascular defect, septum pellucidum cyst, hydrocephalus, hypoplastic corpus callosum, polymicrogyria, and enlarged ventricles; absent, dysplastic, or multicystic kidneys; obstructive uropathy; vesicoureteral reflux; cryptorchidism; hypospadias; uterine didelphys, anal anomalies; laryngeal web; tortuosity of retinal vessels (30%); small optic disks; ocular coloboma; cataracts; holoprosencephaly; neural tube closure defect; hypothyroidism; Graves disease; abnormal T-cell function and absent thymic tissue; pre- and postaxial polydactyly; talipes equinovarus; scoliosis; abnormal vertebrae; arthritis.

NATURAL HISTORY

Death, due almost exclusively to cardiac defects, has occurred in 8% of cases, over one half in the first month of life and the majority before 6 months. Hypotonia in infancy is frequent (70%–80%). Transient neonatal hypocalcemia occurs in 60% of cases. Seizures (21%) are usually the result of hypocalcemia. Speech development is often delayed, and language is impaired. Speech is almost always hypernasal, with the pharyngeal musculature being hypotonic. Socialization skills may surpass intellectual skills. Personality may tend toward perseverative behavior, with concrete thinking secondary to intellectual impairment or learning disorders. Approximately 10% of affected individuals have developed psychiatric disorders, primarily chronic schizophrenia and paranoid delusions, with onset varying between 10 and 21 years of age. Obstructive sleep apnea has been noted following pharyngeal surgery to improve speech in several patients. The abnormalities of the internal carotid arteries can be diagnosed by the demonstration of visible pulsations in the posterior pharyngeal wall musculature using fiberoptic nasopharyngoscopy and with magnetic resonance imaging (MRI) of the pharynx. Clinically significant immunologic problems are not common.

ETIOLOGY

This disorder has an autosomal dominant inheritance pattern. Affected individuals have an interstitial deletion of chromosome 22q11.2, which is detectable using fluorescent in situ hybridization (FISH). At least 30 genes have been mapped to the deletion region. Much of the clinical phenotype appears related to haploinsufficiency of one of those genes, *TBX1*. *TBX1* encodes a T-box transcription factor, which plays an important role in early vertebrate development. Strong evidence for its role in the deletion 22q11.2 syndrome is based on the fact that individuals with *TBX1* mutations who lack del22q11.2 have clinical features consistent with the deletion 22q11.2 syndrome and that *Tbx1*-null mouse mutants express all the features of the deletion 22q11.2 syndrome. Because of the marked variability of expression, both parents of an affected child should be tested to determine if they carry the deletion.

COMMENT
22Q11.2 Microduplication

Reciprocal duplications of the 22q11.2 common deletions (a large 3-Mb duplication or a 1.5-Mb proximal nested duplication) have been reported in more than 50 patients with a highly variable but generally mild phenotype, ranging from normal to learning difficulties/intellectual disability, autistic features, growth retardation, hypotonia, and shared structural abnormalities with the 22q11.2 deletion syndromes (DiGeorge/velo-cardio-facial syndrome [DG/VCFS]), although with a much lower frequency, including heart defects, urogenital abnormalities, and velopharyngeal insufficiency with or without cleft palate. The subtle and variable dysmorphic features do not allow clinical recognition. Most individuals (70%) have inherited the duplication, most commonly from a normal or near-normal parent, whereas deletions occur de novo in 90% of cases. *TBX1* gain-of-function mutations have also been observed, resulting in the same phenotypic spectrum, confirming that *TBX1* overexpression might be responsible for the dup22q11.2 syndrome.

Atypical and Distal 22q11.2 Microdeletions and Microduplications

Deletions located distally to the ~1.5 Mb proximal deletion region in DG/VCFS are phenotypically different from deletions in the common interval (3 Mb) or the smaller proximal interval (1.5 Mb) containing *TBX1* as a major causal gene. A history of prematurity, prenatal and postnatal growth delay, developmental delay, intellectual disability, behavioral problems, and mild skeletal abnormalities was prevalent. Cardiovascular malformations, particularly truncus arteriosus, as well as cardiac defects atypical for VCFS can occur, but they are less frequent than in common 22q11.2 deletions. A single patient had a cleft palate. Characteristic facial dysmorphic features are subtle and include arched eyebrows, deep-set eyes, a smooth philtrum, a thin upper lip, hypoplastic alae nasi, and a small, pointed chin. Choanal atresia and features of the oculo-auriculo-vertebral spectrum have also been seen. *CRKL* and *ERK2/MAPK1* have been proposed to cause the heart defects. *Ueb2l3* causes severe growth retardation in mice and could account for growth retardation in these patients. Distal duplications show low penetrance and marked variable expression for developmental delay.

References

Shprintzen RJ, et al: A new syndrome involving cleft palate, cardiac anomalies, typical facies, and learning disabilities: Velo-cardio-facial syndrome, *Cleft Palate J* 15:56, 1978.

Young D, Shprintzen RJ, Goldberg RB: Cardiac malformations in the velo-cardio-facial syndrome, *Am J Cardiol* 46:643, 1980.

Shprintzen RJ, et al: The velo-cardio-facial syndrome: A clinical and genetic analysis, *Pediatrics* 67:167, 1981.

Williams MA, Shprintzen RJ, Goldberg RB: Male-to-male transmission of the velo-cardio-facial syndrome: A case report and review of 60 cases, *J Craniofac Genet Dev Biol* 5:175, 1985.

Driscoll DA, et al: Deletions and microdeletions of 22q11.2 in velo-cardio-facial syndrome, *Am J Med Genet* 44:261, 1992.

Scrambler PJ, et al: The velo-cardio-facial syndrome is associated with chromosome 22 deletions which encompass the DiGeorge syndrome locus, *Lancet* 339:1138, 1992.

Goldberg R, et al: Velo-cardio-facial: A review of 120 patients, *Am J Med Genet* 45:313, 1993.

Ryan AK, et al: Spectrum of clinical features associated with interstitial chromosome 22q11 deletions: A European collaborative study, *J Med Genet* 34:798, 1997.

Wooden M, et al: Neuropsychological profile of children and adolescents with the 22q11.2 microdeletion, *Genet Med* 3:34, 2001.

Yagi H, et al: Role of *TBX1* in human del22q11.2 syndrome, *Lancet* 362:1366, 2003.

Liao J, et al: Full spectrum of malformations in velo-cardio-facial syndrome/DiGeorge syndrome mouse models by altering *Tbx1* dosage, *Hum Mol Genet* 13:1577, 2004.

Scheuerle A: Teenager with uterine didelphys, absent kidney and 22q11.2 deletion, *Am J Med Genet* 146:800, 2008.

Wentzel C, et al: Clinical variability of the 22q11.2 duplication syndrome, *Eur J Med Genet* 51:501, 2008.

Gerkes EH, et al: Bilateral polymicrogyria as the indicative feature in a child with a 22q11.2 deletion, *Eur J Med Genet* 53:344, 2010.

Verhagen JM, et al: Phenotypic variability of atypical 22q11.2 deletions not including *TBX1*, *Am J Med Genet A* 2012 Aug 14. (Epub ahead of print)

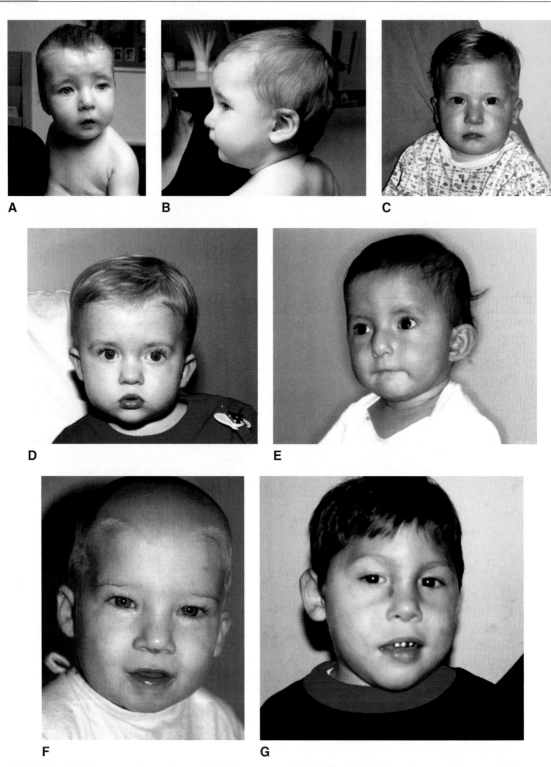

FIGURE 1.   Deletion 22q11.2 syndrome. **A–G,** Phenotype in children from 8 months to 3 years of age. Note the narrow nose with squared nasal root and narrow ala nasi; the short palpebral fissures; and the somewhat smooth philtrum. (**C, F,** and **G,** Courtesy Dr. Lynne M. Bird, Rady Children's Hospital, San Diego.)

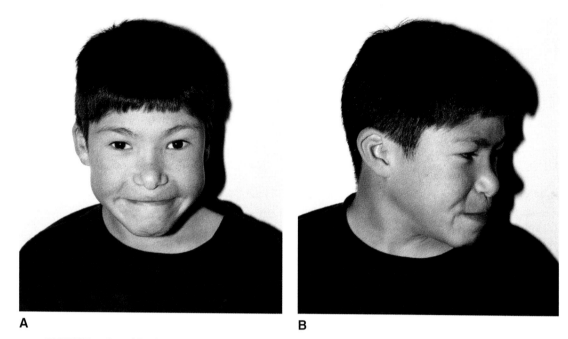

A B

FIGURE 2. **A** and **B,** Photograph of 12-year-old boy. Facial features emphasizing the nasal configuration.

OCULODENTODIGITAL SYNDROME (OCULODENTODIGITAL DYSPLASIA)
Microphthalmos, Enamel Hypoplasia, Camptodactyly of Fifth Fingers

Originally described in 1920 by Lohmann, this pattern was more fully characterized by Gorlin, Meskin, and St. Geme in 1963. More than 200 cases have been reported.

ABNORMALITIES

Eyes. Microphthalmos, microcornea, fine porous iris; short palpebral fissures and epicanthal folds.
Nose. Thin, hypoplastic alae nasi with small nares.
Teeth. Enamel hypoplasia.
Hands and Feet. Syndactyly of fourth and fifth fingers, third and fourth toes; camptodactyly of fifth fingers; midphalangeal hypoplasia or aplasia of one or more fingers or toes.
Hair. Fine, dry, or sparse and slow growing.
Neurologic. Dysarthria, neurogenic bladder, spastic paraparesis, ataxia, nystagmus, anterior tibial muscle weakness, paresthesias, and seizures.
Other Skeletal. Broad tubular bones and mandible with wide alveolar ridge.

OCCASIONAL ABNORMALITIES

Intellectual disability, microcephaly, glaucoma, cataract, atrophy of optic disc, hearing loss, bony orbital hypotelorism with normal inner canthal distance, partial anodontia, microdontia, premature loss of teeth, cleft lip and palate, conductive hearing impairment, cubitus valgus, hip dislocation, osteopetrosis, poor posture, skull and vertebral hyperostosis, abnormal central nervous system white matter on MRI, calcification of basal ganglia.

NATURAL HISTORY

Intellectual performance is usually normal. Progressive neurologic dysfunction is frequent, usually presenting with spastic bladder or gait disturbances, often by the second decade. Demonstration on MRI of diffuse bilateral abnormalities in the subcortical cerebral white matter can be indicative of a slowly progressive leukodystrophy. Facial features become more obvious after the first 3 to 4 years of life. Because open-angle glaucoma has been reported as a late complication, periodic ophthalmic evaluation is recommended.

ETIOLOGY

This disorder has an autosomal dominant inheritance pattern with variable expression. Many cases represent fresh mutations. Mutations in the gap junction alpha 1 (*GJA1*) gene encoding the connexin-43 protein are responsible for this disorder. Autosomal recessive inheritance has been documented in one consanguineous family in which two daughters had a homozygous nonsense mutation in the first transmembrane domain of connexin 43. Both parents were heterozygous for the mutation.

References

Lohmann W: Beitrag zur Kenntnis des reinen Mikrophthalmus, *Arch Augenh* 86:136, 1920.

Gorlin RJ, Meskin LH, St. Geme JW: Oculodentodigital dysplasia, *J Pediatr* 63:69, 1963.

Eidelman E, Chosack A, Wagner ML: Orodigitofacial dysostosis and oculodentodigital dysplasia: Two distinct syndromes with some similarities, *Oral Surg* 23:311, 1967.

Judisch GF, et al: Oculodentodigital dysplasia, *Arch Ophthalmol* 97:878, 1979.

Loddenkemper T, et al: Neurological manifestations of the oculodentodigital dysplasia syndrome, *J Neurol* 249:584, 2002.

Paznekas WA, et al: Connexin 43 (*GJA1*) mutations cause the pleiotropic phenotype of oculodentodigital dysplasia, *Am J Hum Genet* 72:408, 2003.

Richardson RJ, et al: A nonsense mutation in the first transmembrane of connexin 43 underlies autosomal recessive oculodentodigital syndrome, *J Med Genet* 43:e37, 2006.

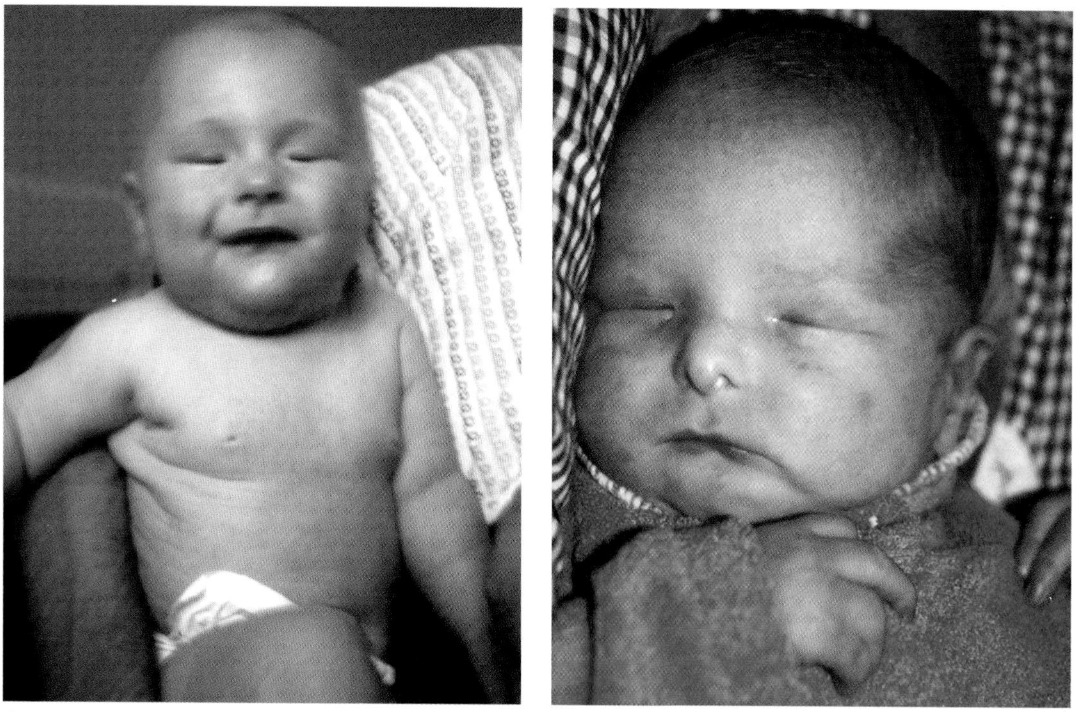

FIGURE 1.   **A** and **B,** Infants with oculodentodigital syndrome. Note the small alae nasi, small mandible, and cutaneous syndactyly of fourth and fifth fingers.

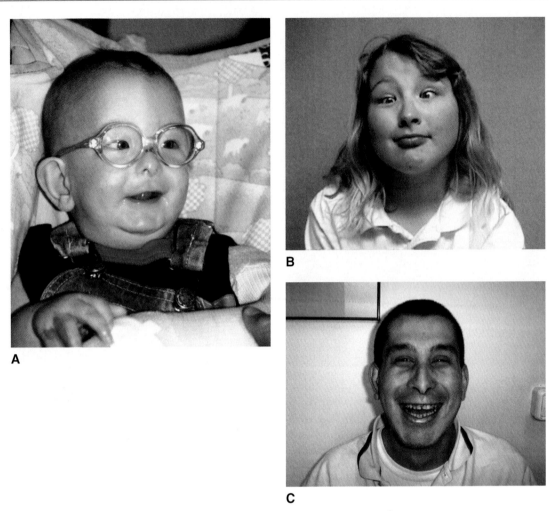

FIGURE 2.   A–C, Note the microcornea; short palpebral fissures; thin, hypoplastic alae nasi; and enamel hypoplasia. (**C,** Courtesy Dr. Blanca Gener Querol, Universitat Pompeu Fabra, Barcelona.)

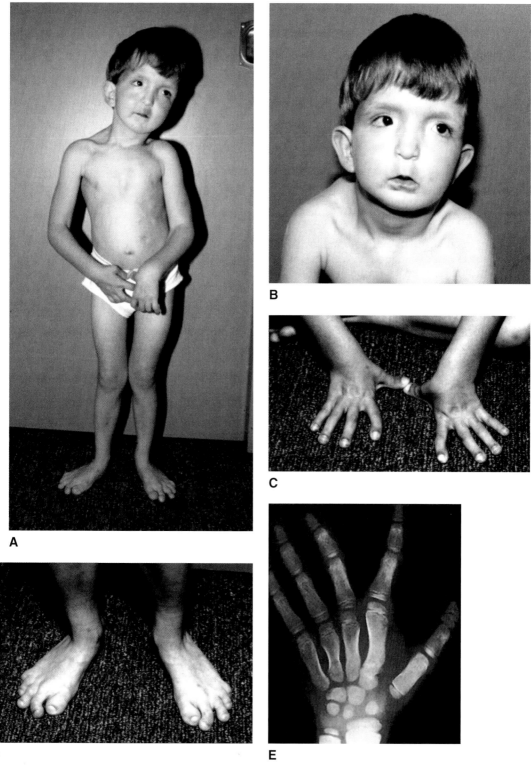

FIGURE 1.   Oto-palato-digital syndrome, type I. **A–E,** Note the frontal prominence of the skull; small trunk and pectus excavatum; limited elbow extension; and irregular length and form of distal phalanges, especially thumb and great toe. (**E,** Radiograph from Dudding BA, Gorlin RJ, Langer LO: *Am J Dis Child* 113:214, 1967, with permission. Copyright 1967, American Medical Association.)

OTO-PALATO-DIGITAL SYNDROME, TYPE II

Fitch and colleagues and, later, Kozlowski and colleagues each described this pattern of malformation in two half brothers. More than 20 cases have been reported.

ABNORMALITIES

Growth. Postnatal growth deficiency in survivors.

Craniofacial. Late closure of large anterior fontanel; wide sutures; prominent forehead; low-set malformed ears; ocular hypertelorism; downslant to palpebral fissures; flat nasal bridge; small mouth; micrognathia; cleft palate; radiographic evidence of dense fontanels, supraorbital ridge, and skull base with undermineralization of cranial vault; small mandible with obtuse angle.

Limbs. Flexed, overlapping fingers; short broad thumbs and great toes; polydactyly; variable syndactyly of hands and feet; clinodactyly of second finger; bowing of radius, ulna, femur, and tibia; small to absent fibula; hypoplastic, irregular metacarpals; nonossified fifth metatarsal; short, absent, or poorly ossified phalanges of fingers and toes; subluxed elbows, wrists, and knees; congenital hip dislocation; rocker-bottom feet.

Other. Intellectual disability, microcephaly, conductive hearing loss, pectus excavatum, a narrow chest with thin wavy clavicles and ribs, flattened vertebral bodies, hypoplastic ilia, widened lumbosacral canal, obstructive uropathy, cardiac defects, posterior fossa brain anomalies.

OCCASIONAL ABNORMALITIES

Hydrocephalus, congenital cataracts, corneal clouding, congenital glaucoma, dental abnormalities, bifid tongue, transverse capitate bone, clinodactyly of second finger, retarded carpal bone age and advanced phalangeal bone age, absent halluces, omphalocele, cryptorchidism, hypospadias, absent adrenal glands.

NATURAL HISTORY

The majority of affected individuals have been stillborn or died before 5 months of age, in most cases, because of respiratory difficulties. The incidence of cognitive impairment in survivors is unknown. Although significant developmental delay has been documented, one 18-month-old and one 6-year-old affected boy are developmentally normal. The facial appearance and the bone curvatures tend to normalize with age. Both membranous ossification and bone remodeling appear to be defective.

ETIOLOGY

This disorder has an X-linked transmission pattern with intermediate expression in females and complete expression in males. Mutations in *FLNA*—a gene that encodes filamin A, which is a protein that regulates reorganization of the cytoskeleton—are responsible. Manifestations such as broad face, downslant of palpebral fissures, and cleft palate or bifid uvula occur in heterozygote females. *FLNA* has been mapped to Xq28.

COMMENT

Oto-palato-digital syndrome types I and II, frontometaphyseal dysplasia, and Melnick-Needles syndrome are allelic conditions, all caused by mutations in *FLNA*.

References

Fitch N, Jequier S, Papageorgiou A: A familial syndrome of cranial, facial, oral and limb anomalies, *Clin Genet* 10:226, 1976.

Kozlowski K, et al: Oto-palato-digital syndrome with severe x-ray changes in two half brothers, *Pediatr Radiol* 6:97, 1977.

Fitch N, Jequier S, Gorlin R: The oto-palato-digital syndrome, proposed type II, *Am J Med Genet* 15:655, 1983.

Brewster TG, et al: Oto-palato-digital syndrome, type II—an X-linked skeletal dysplasia, *Am J Med Genet* 20:249, 1985.

Blanchet P, et al: Multiple congenital anomalies associated with an oto-palatal-digital syndrome type II, *Genet Couns* 4:289, 1993.

Holder SE, Winter RM: Otopalatodigital syndrome type II, *J Med Genet* 30:310, 1993.

Preis S, et al: Oto-palato-digital syndrome type II in two unrelated boys, *Clin Genet* 45:154, 1994.

Savarirayan R, et al: Oto-palato-digital syndrome, type II: Report of three cases with further delineation of the chondro-osseous morphology, *Am J Med Genet* 95:193, 2000.

Robertson SP, et al: Localized mutations in the gene encoding the cytoskeletal protein filamin A cause diverse malformations in humans, *Nat Genet* 33:487, 2003.

Robertson SP. Otopalatodigital syndrome spectrum disorders: Otopalatodigital syndromes type 1 and 2, frontometaphyseal dysplasia and Melnick-Needles syndrome, *Eur J Hum Genet* 15:3, 2007.

Murphy-Ryan M, et al: Bifid tongue, corneal clouding, and Dandy-Walker malformation in a male infant with otopalatodigital syndrome type 2, *Am J Med Genet* 155:855, 2011.

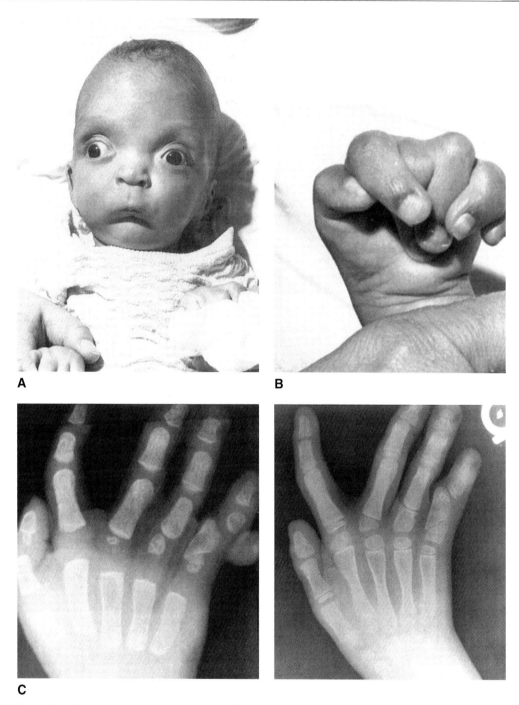

FIGURE 1. **A** and **B,** Neonate with oto-palato-digital syndrome, type II. Note the prominent forehead, ocular hypertelorism, flat nasal bridge, small mouth, micrognathia, and the flexed overlapping fingers. **C,** Radiographs of the hand at 1 and 5 years of age reveal hypoplastic irregular metacarpals, abnormal epiphyses of proximal phalanges 4 and 5, and postaxial polydactyly. (**A–C,** From Fitch N et al: *Am J Med Genet* 15:655, 1983, with permission.)

COFFIN-LOWRY SYNDROME
Downslanting Palpebral Fissures, Bulbous Nose, Tapering Fingers

Coffin and colleagues in 1966 and Lowry and colleagues in 1971 independently described a mental retardation syndrome associated with coarse facies, short stature, and thick, soft hands with tapering fingers. Temtamy et al recognized the similarity between the two and referred to the disorder as Coffin-Lowry syndrome. The facies may appear similar to that of Williams syndrome.

ABNORMALITIES

Growth. Mild to moderate growth deficiency, apparently of postnatal onset; delayed bone age.

Performance. Intellectual disability, usually severe; relative weakness; hypotonia.

Facies. Coarse appearance, with downslanting palpebral fissures and maxillary hypoplasia, mild hypertelorism, prominent brow, and short, broad nose with thick alae nasi and septum, and anteverted nares; large open mouth with thick, everted lower lip; prominent ears.

Dental. Hypodontia, malocclusion, widely spaced teeth, and large medial incisors.

Thorax. Short bifid sternum with pectus carinatum, and excavatum (80%).

Spine. Anterior superior marginal vertebral defects, thoracolumbar scoliosis, and kyphosis.

Limbs. Broad, soft hands with stubby, tapering, limp fingers that are wide at the base and narrow distally; tufted drumstick appearance to distal phalanges on roentgenogram; small fingernails; accessory transverse hypothenar crease; fullness of the forearms due to increased subcutaneous fat; flat feet; lax ligaments.

OCCASIONAL ABNORMALITIES

Microcephaly; thick calvarium; dilated lateral ventricles; seizures (5%); cardiomyopathy; mitral valve prolapse (15%); radiographically, there are hypoplastic sinuses and mastoids, delayed closure of anterior fontanel, narrowing of the foramen magnum, and in the thoracolumbar vertebrae, narrowing of the intervertebral spaces, irregular endplates, and anterior wedging; simian crease; inguinal hernia; rectal prolapse; uterine prolapse; mitral valve insufficiency; left ventricular noncompaction cardiomyopathy; sensorineural hearing loss (30%); spasticity; recurrent drop episodes; cataracts; retinal changes; premature loss of primary teeth.

NATURAL HISTORY

In males, the intellectual disability is usually of severe degree, leaving the patient without speech.

Fullness of the brows and lips become more exaggerated with advancing age. The vertebral dysplasia and kyphoscoliosis generally do not develop until after 6 years and are often progressive, requiring surgery. Stooped posture is common. Late eruption and premature loss of teeth are common. Psychotic behavior with onset around 20 years sometimes occurs in affected females, whereas males are usually cheerful, easygoing, and friendly. Drop attacks triggered by unexpected tactile or auditory stimuli or by excitement, in which the patient experiences episodes of falling backward, begin in midchildhood or the teenage years. Life expectancy may be reduced in affected males, related primarily to cardiac, respiratory, neurologic, and kyphoscoliosis-related causes.

ETIOLOGY

This disorder has an X-linked inheritance pattern with striking similarity between the severely affected hemizygous males. Clinical findings in affected females include slight to moderate intellectual disability, mild facial changes, tapered fingers, obesity and short stature, although some patients are completely normal. Mutations in the *RSK2* gene, which encodes the ribosomal protein S6 kinase-2, are responsible. *RSK2* has been mapped to Xp22.2.

References

Coffin GS, Siris E, Wegienka LC: Mental retardation with osteocartilaginous anomalies, *Am J Dis Child* 112:205, 1966.

Lowry B, Miller JR, Fraser FC: A new dominant gene mental retardation syndrome, *Am J Dis Child* 121:496, 1971.

Temtamy SA, et al: The Coffin-Lowry syndrome: A simply inherited trait comprising mental retardation, facio-digital anomalies and skeletal anomalies, *Birth Defects* 11(6):133, 1975.

Hunter AGW, Partington MW, Evans JA: The Coffin-Lowry syndrome: Experience from four centres, *Clin Genet* 21:321, 1982.

Vles JSH, et al: Early signs in Coffin-Lowry syndrome, *Clin Genet* 26:448, 1984.

Gilgenkrautz S, et al: Coffin-Lowry syndrome: A multicenter study, *Clin Genet* 34:230, 1988.

Hartsfield JK, et al: Pleiotropy in Coffin-Lowry syndrome: Sensorineural hearing deficit and premature tooth loss as early manifestations, *Am J Med Genet* 45:552, 1993.

Hanauer A, Young ID: Coffin-Lowry syndrome: Clinical and molecular features, *J Med Genet* 39:705, 2002.

Hunter AGW: Coffin-Lowry syndrome: A 20-year follow-up and review of long-term outcomes, *Am J Med Genet* 111:345, 2002.

Herrera-Soto JA, et al: The musculoskeletal manifestations of the Coffin-Lowry syndrome, *J Pediatr Orthop* 27:85, 2007.

Pereira PM, et al: Coffin-Lowry syndrome, *Eur J Hum Genet* 18:627, 2010.

Martinez HR, et al: Coffin-Lowry syndrome and left ventricular noncompaction cardiomyopathy with a restrictive pattern, *Am J Med Genet* 155:3030, 2011.

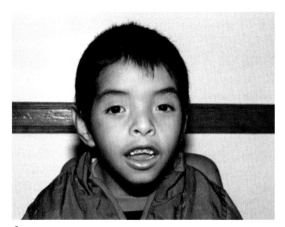

A

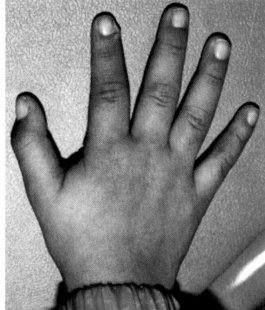

B

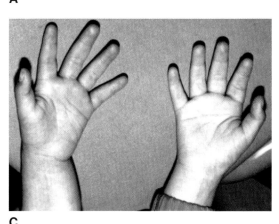

C

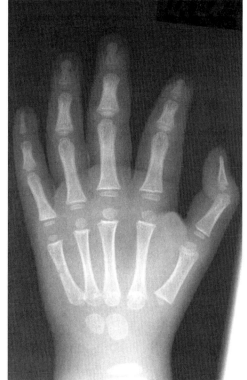

FIGURE 1.   Coffin-Lowry syndrome. **A–D,** Note the downslanting palpebral fissures; maxillary hypoplasia; prominent brow; large, open mouth with everted lower lip; prominent ears; dental malocclusion; tapering fingers; and tufted drumstick appearance to terminal phalanges on radiograph.

D

X-LINKED α-THALASSEMIA/MENTAL RETARDATION SYNDROME (ATR-X SYNDROME)
Severe Intellectual Disability, Characteristic Face, Genital Abnormalities

First described in 1990 by Wilkie and colleagues, this disorder was further characterized by Gibbons and colleagues in 1991. More than 200 affected individuals have been identified.

ABNORMALITIES

Performance. Severe intellectual disability, initial hypotonia frequently followed by spasticity, seizures, self-biting/hitting, extreme emotion.

Growth. Postnatal growth deficiency sometimes not evident until adolescence, delayed bone age.

Craniofacial. Microcephaly; telecanthus; epicanthal folds; low nasal bridge; small, triangular nose with anteverted nares; midface hypoplasia; large "carp-like" mouth that is frequently held open; full lips; large, protruding tongue; wide-spaced incisors; small, simple, deformed, low-set, or posteriorly rotated ears; preauricular pit.

Limbs. Tapering fingers; fifth-finger clinodactyly; overlapping fingers and toes; foot deformities including talipes equinovarus, pes planus, and talipes calcaneovalgus.

Genitalia. Cryptorchidism, testicular dysgenesis, shawl and/or hypoplastic scrotum, small penis, hypospadias.

Hematologic. Mild hypochromic microcytic anemia; mild form of hemoglobin H disease (a type of α-thalassemia) can be detected by hemoglobin electrophoresis or by the presence of hemoglobin H inclusions on 1% brilliant cresyl blue (BCB) stained peripheral smears.

OCCASIONAL ABNORMALITIES

Mild intellectual disability, cerebral atrophy, cleft palate, kyphoscoliosis, hemivertebra, missing rib, ovoid vertebral bodies, short sternum, small or drumstick-like terminal phalanges on radiographs, absent frontal sinuses, flexion deformity of index finger, single palmar crease, umbilical hernia, cardiac defects, renal agenesis, hydronephrosis, male pseudohermaphroditism, asplenia, colonic hypoganglionosis, gastric pseudovolvulus.

NATURAL HISTORY

Severe intellectual disability with lack of expressive speech, limited comprehension, and the development of only partial bladder and bowel control is the rule. Some patients do not walk independently until their late teens, and some do not walk at all. Apneic and cyanotic episodes as well as cold and/or blue extremities occur frequently. Regurgitation of food often is induced by putting fingers down the throat. Excessive salivation, gastroesophageal reflux, and constipation also occur. Death in early childhood from aspiration of vomitus and subsequent pneumonia has been reported. Recurrent urinary tract and chest infections as well as blepharitis and conjunctivitis are common.

ETIOLOGY

This disorder has an X-linked recessive inheritance pattern. Mutations in the X-linked α-thalassemia/mental retardation (*ATRX*) gene, which maps to Xq13.3, are responsible for this disorder. More than 70 mutations of the gene have been reported. The ATRX protein is most likely important in chromatin remodeling. Mutations in the helicase domain are associated with milder phenotypes than mutations in the plant homeodomain-like domain. The function of the X-linked α-thalassemia/mental retardation protein is not yet completely understood. The most sensitive diagnostic test is the demonstration of hemoglobin H inclusions in red blood cells after incubation with BCB. The inability to demonstrate hemoglobin H electrophoretically should not exclude the diagnosis. Carrier females frequently have rare cells containing hemoglobin H in their peripheral blood after incubation with 1% BCB. A faint band of hemoglobin H is sometimes visible on electrophoresis.

References

Wilkie AO, et al: Clinical features and molecular analysis of the alpha thalassemia/mental retardation syndromes. I. Cases due to deletions involving chromosome band 16p13.3, *Am J Hum Genet* 46:1112, 1990.

Wilkie AO, et al: Clinical features and molecular analysis of the alpha thalassemia/mental retardation syndromes. II. Cases without detectable abnormality of the alpha globin complex, *Am J Hum Genet* 46:1127, 1990.

Gibbons RJ, et al: A newly defined X linked mental retardation syndrome with alpha thalassemia, *J Med Genet* 28:729, 1991.

Gibbons RJ, et al: X linked alpha-thalassemia/mental retardation (ATR-X) syndrome: Localization to Xq12-q21.31 by X inactivation and linkage analysis, *Am J Hum Genet* 51:1136, 1992.

Gibbons RJ, et al: Clinical and hematological aspects of the X-linked alpha-thalassemia/mental retardation syndrome (ATR-X), *Am J Med Genet* 55:288, 1995.

Gibbons RJ, et al: Mutations in a putative global transcriptional regulator cause X-linked mental retardation with alpha-thalassemia (ATR-X syndrome), *Cell* 80:837, 1995.

McPherson EW, et al: X-linked alpha-thalassemia/mental retardation (ATR-X) syndrome: A new kindred with severe genital anomalies and mild hematological expression, *Am J Med Genet* 55:302, 1995.

Yntema HG, et al: Expanding the phenotype of XNP mutations: Mild to moderate mental retardation, *Am J Med Genet* 110:243, 2002.

Leahy RT, et al: Asplenia in ATR-X syndrome: A second report, *Am J Med Genet* 139:37, 2005.

Badens C, et al: Mutations in PHD-like domain of the *ATRX* gene correlate with severe psychomotor impairment and severe urogenital abnormalities in patients with ATRX syndrome, *Clin Genet* 70:57, 2006.

Martucciello G, et al: Gastrointestinal phenotype of ATR-X syndrome, *Am J Med Genet* 140:1172, 2006.

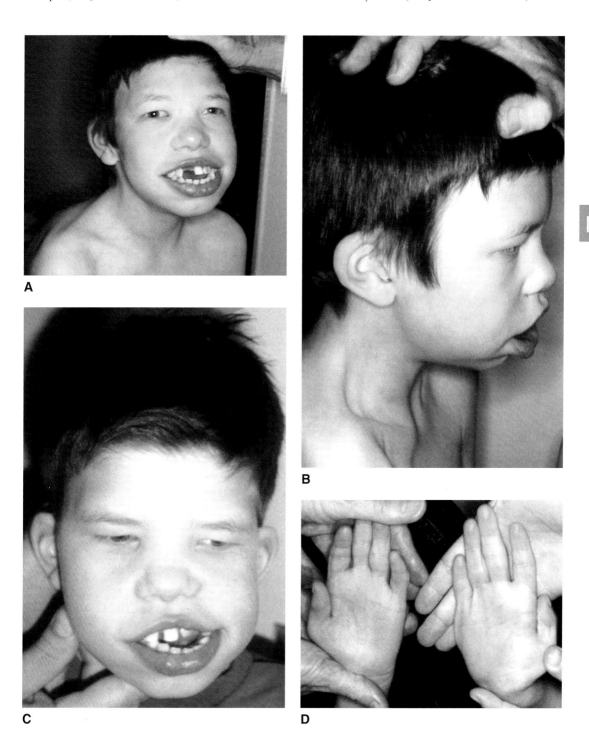

FIGURE 1. X-Linked α-thalassemia/mental retardation syndrome. **A** and **B,** Affected boy at 12 years of age. **C,** Same patient at 15 years of age. Note the telecanthus, epicanthal folds, low nasal bridge, and large mouth with thick lips. **D,** Note the tapering fingers and fifth-finger clinodactyly.

FG SYNDROME (OPITZ-KAVEGGIA SYNDROME)
Imperforate Anus, Hypotonia, Prominent Forehead

Initially described by Opitz and Kaveggia in three brothers and two of their male first cousins. Many cases of this X-linked recessive disorder have been documented.

ABNORMALITIES

Performance. Intellectual disability (97%); delayed motor development or hypotonia (90%); electroencephalographic disturbances with seizures (70%); strabismus (52%); hyperactive behavior with short attention span (70%); affable, extroverted personality with occasional temper tantrums in response to frustration (54%).

Growth. Postnatal onset of short stature.

Craniofacial. Postnatal onset of macrocephaly (74%); large anterior fontanel (77%); narrow, tall head and forehead (95%); frontal hair upsweep (91%); long, narrow face; ocular hypertelorism (83%); puffy eyelids; open mouth; prominent lower lip (44%); small ears with simple structure (66%); facial skin wrinkling; fine, sparse hair (66%); epicanthal folds; short downslanting palpebral fissures (85%); narrow palate; large-appearing cornea (75%).

Gastrointestinal. Anal anomalies, including stenosis, imperforate anus, and anteriorly placed anus (38%); constipation (69%).

Skeletal. Broad thumbs and great toes (81%), clinodactyly (53%), camptodactyly (55%), multiple joint contractures, syndactyly (54%), simian crease (60%), minor vertebral defects (64%), abnormal sternum (69%).

Other. Complete or partial agenesis of the corpus callosum, sacral dimple, tethered spinal cord, cryptorchidism (36%), low total dermal ridge count, persistent fetal fingertip pads (50%).

OCCASIONAL ABNORMALITIES

Craniosynostosis, cleft palate, cleft lip, choanal atresia, hydrocephalus, stenotic ear canal, short neck, defects of neuronal migration, malrotation of cecum, absence of mesentery, pyloric stenosis, dilatation of urinary tract, hypospadias, cardiac defect, ectrodactyly, sensorineural deafness, high-pitched voice.

NATURAL HISTORY

Death due to pulmonary complications may occur in the first 2 years of life. Constipation, common in infancy, usually resolves in midchildhood. The initial hypotonia with lax joints tends to evolve into spasticity with joint contractures and unsteady gait in adulthood. Performance is characterized by variable intellectual disability with relative strengths in socialization and daily living skills. Anxiety and attentional issues are common and persist into adulthood. Beginning at puberty, aggressive or self-abusing behaviors sometimes develop.

ETIOLOGY

This disorder has an X-linked recessive inheritance pattern. A p.R961W mutation in the *MED12* gene located at Xq13 is responsible. *MED12* encodes a thyroid hormone receptor-associated protein.

References

Opitz JM, Kaveggia EG: Studies of malformation syndromes of man XXXIII: The FG syndrome. An X-linked recessive syndrome of multiple congenital anomalies and mental retardation, *Z Kinderheilkd* 117:1, 1974.

Romano C, et al: A clinical follow-up of British patients with FG syndrome, *Clin Dysmorphol* 3:104, 1994.

Graham JM, et al: FG syndrome: Report of three new families with linkage to Xq12-q22.1, *Am J Med Genet* 80:145, 1998.

Ozonoff S, et al: Behavioral phenotype of FG syndrome: Cognition, personality, and behavior in eleven affected boys, *Am J Med Genet* 97:112, 2000.

Risheg H, et al: A recurrent mutation in MED12 leading to R961W causes Opitz-Kaveggia syndrome, *Nat Genet* 39:451, 2007.

Graham JM, et al: Behavior of 10 patients with FG syndrome (Opitz-Kaveggia syndrome) and the p.R961W mutation in the *MED12* gene, *Am J Med Genet* 146:3011, 2008.

Clark RD, et al: FG syndrome, an X-linked multiple congenital anomaly syndrome: The clinical phenotype and an algorithm for diagnostic testing, *Genet Med* 11:769, 2009.

Graham JM, et al: Behavioral testing in young adults with FG syndrome (Opitz-Kaveggia syndrome), *Am J Med Genet C Semin Med Genet* 154C:477, 2010.

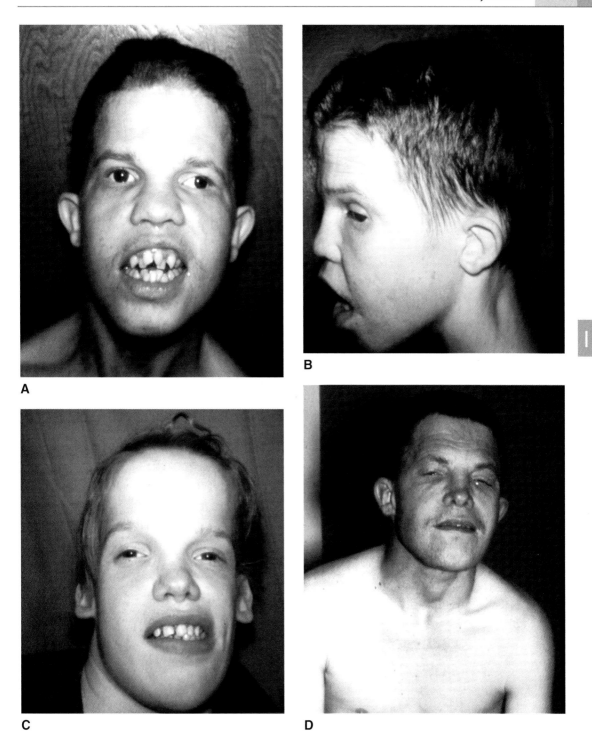

FIGURE 1. FG syndrome. Three affected male siblings, ages 27 (**A** and **B**), 17 (**C**), and 29 (**D**). Note the frontal upsweep, lateral displacement of the medial canthi, and small ears.

STICKLER SYNDROME (HEREDITARY ARTHRO-OPHTHALMOPATHY)
Flat Facies, Myopia, Spondyloepiphyseal Dysplasia

In 1965, Stickler and colleagues reported the initial observations on affected individuals in five generations of one family; the skeletal aspects have been further documented by Spranger, and the total spectrum of the disorder has been set forth by Herrmann and colleagues. Based on the ocular phenotype and molecular linkage, Stickler syndrome has been subclassified into four types.

ABNORMALITIES

Orofacial. Flat facies with depressed nasal bridge, prominent eyes, epicanthal folds, a short nose and anteverted nares, midfacial or mandibular hypoplasia; clefts of hard and/or soft palate and occasionally of uvula; Robin sequence; deafness (both sensorineural and conductive); hypermobile tympanic membranes; dental anomalies.

Ocular. Myopia, usually present before age 6, is nonprogressive and of high degree. Retinal detachment and cataracts also occur. Abnormalities of vitreous formation and gel architecture are manifest in the majority of patients. A vestigial vitreous gel, which occupies the immediate retrolental space, and is bordered by a distinct folded membrane constitutes the type I phenotype. In the type 2 phenotype, sparse and irregularly thickened bundles of fibers exist throughout the vitreous cavity. Type 3 lacks ocular findings. In type 4, a degenerative shrinkage of the vitreous occurs in which the gel breaks into liquid-filled particles, which coalesce and render it partially or completely fluid.

Musculoskeletal. Hypotonia, hyperextensible joints, talipes equinovarus. Prominence of large joints may be present at birth, severe arthropathy can occur in childhood, lesser joint pains simulate juvenile rheumatoid arthritis, and subluxation of the hip is present.

Imaging. In childhood, mild to moderate spondyloepiphyseal dysplasia (i.e., flat vertebrae with anterior wedging, underdevelopment of the distal tibial epiphyses, and flat irregular femoral epiphyses). Long bones show disproportionately narrow shafts relative to their metaphyseal width. Secondary degeneration of articular surfaces occurs in adulthood.

Other. Mitral valve prolapse.

OCCASIONAL ABNORMALITIES

Scoliosis, kyphosis, and increased lumbar lordosis; arachnodactyly with marfanoid habitus; pectus excavatum; thoracic disk herniation; thoracic myelopathy; pes planus; genu valgus; mental deficiency; short stature; lens dislocation; glaucoma.

NATURAL HISTORY

Arthritis, if present, most commonly becomes a problem after 30 years of age. Symptoms become more severe with advancing years, leading in some cases to total hip replacement. Spinal abnormalities, which occur almost universally, progress with age and are associated with back pain. Progressive myopia may give rise to retinal detachment and lead to blindness, the most severe complication of this disorder. Although myopia develops in 40% of patients before 10 years of age and 75% by age 20, it does not occur in some patients until after age 50. Retinal detachment can occur in childhood but usually not until after 20 years of age. The detachment often can be corrected surgically if recognized early. Affected individuals with mitral valve prolapse should be evaluated periodically.

ETIOLOGY

Types 1, 2, and 3 have an autosomal dominant inheritance pattern. Although highly variable expression of Stickler syndrome has been documented, the variability is mostly between families. The majority of cases are associated with the type 1 vitreous phenotype and show linkage to the gene encoding type II collagen (*COL2AI*) located on chromosome 12q13. Most patients with the type 2 vitreous phenotype have mutations in the gene encoding the a1 chain of type XI collagen (*COL11A1*) on chromosome 1p21. Mutations in the gene encoding the a2 chain of type XI collagen (*COL11A2*) on chromosome 6q21.3 result in a nonocular variant of Stickler syndrome (type 3). Mutations in *COL9A1* and *COL9A2* result in an autosomal recessive form of Stickler syndrome (types 4 and 5). As opposed to types 1 or 2, the vitreous in type 4 is described as degenerated due to progressive gel liquefaction.

COMMENT

The Stickler syndrome should be considered in any neonate with the Robin sequence, particularly in those with a family history of cleft palate and in patients with dominantly inherited myopia, nontraumatic retinal detachment, and/or mild spondyloepiphyseal dysplasia.

References

Stickler GB, et al: Hereditary progressive arthroophthalmopathy, *Mayo Clin Proc* 40:433, 1965.

Stickler GB, Pugh DG: Hereditary progressive arthroophthalmopathy. II. Additional observations on vertebral abnormalities, a hearing defect, and a report of a similar case, *Mayo Clin Proc* 42:495, 1967.

Spranger J: Arthro-ophthalmopathia hereditaria, *Ann Radiol (Paris)* 11:359, 1968.

Herrmann J, et al: The Stickler syndrome (hereditary arthroophthalmopathy), *Birth Defects* 11(2):76, 1975.

Temple IK: Stickler's syndrome, *J Med Genet* 26:119, 1989.

Zlotogora J, et al: Variability of Stickler syndrome, *Am J Med Genet* 42:337, 1992.

Snead MP, Yates JRW: Clinical and molecular genetics of Stickler syndrome, *J Med Genet* 36:353, 1999.

Rose PS, et al: The hip in Stickler syndrome, *J Pediatr Orthop* 21:657, 2001.

Rose PS, et al: Thoracolumbar spinal abnormalities in Stickler syndrome, *Spine* 26:403, 2001.

Rose PS, et al: Stickler syndrome: Clinical characteristics and diagnostic criteria, *Am J Med Genet* 138:199, 2005.

Hoornaert KP, et al: Stickler syndrome caused by *COL2A1* mutations: Genotype-phenotype correlation in a series of 100 patients, *Eur J Hum Genet* 18:872, 2010.

Baker S, et al: A loss of function mutation in the *COL9A2* gene causes autosomal recessive Stickler syndrome, *Am J Med Genet* 155:1668, 2011.

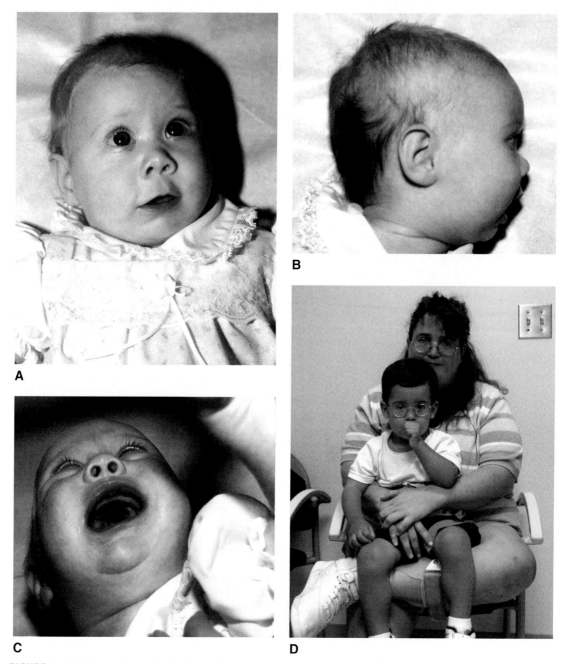

FIGURE 1.   Stickler syndrome. **A–C,** Infant girl showing flat face, depressed nasal bridge, epicanthal folds, a short nose with anteverted nares, maxillary hypoplasia, micrognathia, and U-shaped palatal cleft (Robin sequence). **D,** Mother and her affected son.

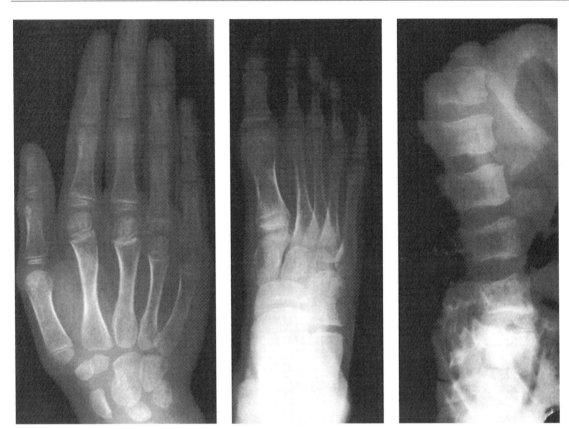

FIGURE 2. Radiographs showing arachnodactyly, fusion of some carpal centers, and mild spondyloepiphyseal dysplasia.

CATEL-MANZKE SYNDROME
(PALATODIGITAL SYNDROME–TYPE CATEL-MANZKE)
Micrognathia, Cleft Palate, Hyperphalangy of Index Finger

First reported by Catel in 1961 in a patient who was reevaluated by Manzke in 1966, more than 30 patients with this condition have been described.

ABNORMALITIES

Growth. Postnatal growth deficiency (75%).
Facies. Cleft palate (78%), micrognathia (72%), malformed ears (33%), high arched eyebrows.
Limbs. Hyperphalangy of index finger in 100% (an accessory bone between proximal phalanges of fingers 2 and 3), fifth-finger clinodactyly (39%), single palmar crease (40%).
Other. Cardiac defects (39%), primarily septal defects accompanied by overriding aorta, aortic coarctation, or dextrocardia.

OCCASIONAL ABNORMALITIES

Developmental delay, seizures, prenatal growth deficiency, short neck, cleft lip with or without cleft palate, naso-lacrimal duct obstruction, vertebral/rib anomalies, pectus excavatum/carinatum, talipes equinovarus, joint laxity/dislocation, camptodactyly, cryptorchidism, umbilical and inguinal hernias, facial paresis.

NATURAL HISTORY

Careful observation to recognize upper airway obstruction secondary to the Robin sequence should be part of routine care of newborns with this disorder. Failure to thrive is related to respiratory or cardiac problems. The vast majority of cases have normal intelligence. With advancing age, the accessory bone fuses to the proximal phalangeal epiphysis.

ETIOLOGY

The cause of this disorder is unknown. The majority of cases have been sporadic. Although most cases have been males, at least four affected females have been reported.

References

Catel W: *Differentialdiagnose von Krankheitssymptomen bei Kindern und Jugendlichen*, vol. 1, ed 3, Stuttgart, 1961, Thieme.

Manzke VH: Symmetrische Hyperphalangie des zweiten Fingers durch ein akzessorisches Metacarpale, *Fortschr Roentgenstr* 105:425, 1966.

Skinner SA, et al: Catel-Manzke syndrome, *Proc Greenwood Genet Center* 8:60, 1989.

Wilson GN, et al: Index finger hyperphalangy and multiple anomalies: Catel-Manzke syndrome? *Am J Med Genet* 46:176, 1993.

Kant SG, et al: The Catel-Manzke syndrome in a female infant, *Genet Couns* 9:187, 1998.

Manzke H, et al: Catel-Manzke syndrome: Two new patients and a critical review of the literature, *Eur J Med Genet* 51:452, 2008.

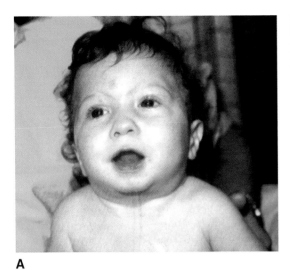

A

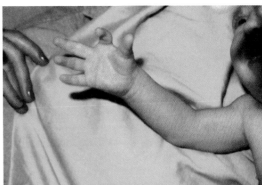

B

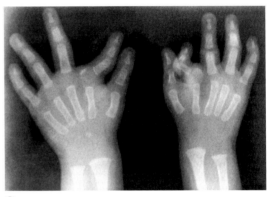

C

FIGURE 1. Catel-Manzke syndrome. **A–C,** A 15-month-old boy. Note the micrognathia and typical hand anomalies with accessory bones at the base of the index finger and hypoplasia of the second metacarpal. (From Stevenson RE et al: *J Med Genet* 17:238, 1980, with permission.)

LANGER-GIEDION SYNDROME
(TRICHO-RHINO-PHALANGEAL SYNDROME, TYPE II; TRP II)
Multiple Exostoses, Bulbous Nose with Peculiar Facies, Loose Redundant Skin in Infancy

Hall and colleagues in 1974 reported five new cases of this disorder and included two additional sporadic cases from the literature. An extensive review of the literature, including data from more than 30 patients, has been published by Langer and colleagues. Although the facies of these patients resemble the facies of tricho-rhino-phalangeal syndrome, type I, other features allow for separation of the two syndromes.

ABNORMALITIES

Growth. Postnatal onset of mild growth deficiency.
Performance. Mild to severe intellectual disability in 70%, with the remaining patients in the normal to dull-normal range; delayed onset of speech; sensorineural hearing loss.
Cranium. Microcephaly.
Facies. Large laterally protruding ears; heavy eyebrows; deep-set eyes; large bulbous nose with thickened alae nasi and septum, dorsally tented nares, and broad nasal bridge; simple philtrum, which is prominent and elongated; thin upper lip; recessed mandible.
Hair. Sparse scalp hair.
Skin. Redundancy or looseness in infancy, which regresses with age; maculopapular nevi around the scalp, face, neck, upper trunk, and upper limbs.
Hands. Cone-shaped epiphyses, which become radiologically evident at approximately 3 to 4 years of age; lack of normal modeling in metaphyseal regions; poor funnelization at proximal ends of phalanges; metaphyseal hooking over the lateral edges of the cone-shaped epiphyses; exostoses; brittle nails.
Imaging. Multiple exostoses of long tubular bones, with onset and distribution similar to the autosomal dominant variety of multiple cartilaginous exostoses; exostoses can involve other areas, such as the ribs, scapulae, and pelvic bones.
Other. Perthes-like changes in capital femoral epiphysis, segmentation defects of vertebrae with scoliosis, narrow posterior ribs; winged scapulae; syndactyly; lax joints; hypotonia; exotropia; recurrent upper respiratory tract infections; malocclusion; dental abnormalities.

OCCASIONAL ABNORMALITIES

Tendency toward fractures, thin hypomineralized bones, clinobrachydactyly, simian crease, bowed femurs, tibial hemimelia, ocular hypotelorism, ptosis, prominent eyes, epicanthal folds, iris coloboma, abducens palsy, tragal skin tag, cardiac defects, inguinal and umbilical hernia, ureteral reflux, widely spaced nipples, delayed sexual development, small phallus, cryptorchidism, premature thelarche and pubarche, hydrometrocolpos, abnormal electroencephalograph, seizures, conductive hearing loss, hypochromic anemia, severe short stature, and growth hormone deficiency.

NATURAL HISTORY

Some of these children have such redundancy or looseness to their skin at birth that they are misdiagnosed as having the Ehlers-Danlos syndrome. The children experience recurrent respiratory tract infections until they are 4 to 5 years old. General health is usually good after that except for a tendency toward fractures and the usual problems of multiple exostoses with their variable effects on bone growth. Severe upper cervical cord compression and tetraparesis have been described in an affected adult secondary to a large cervical exostotic osteochondroma.

ETIOLOGY

This disorder is caused by a deletion in the region 8q24.11-q24.13. In most cases, the deletion is visible with cytogenetic studies. A few cases of vertical transmission have been described. However, the vast majority have been sporadic. Langer-Giedion syndrome is a contiguous gene syndrome involving the tricho-rhino-phalangeal (*TRPS1*) gene and the gene involved in multiple exostosis (*EXT1*), both located within 8q24.11-q24.13. Additional features, such as intellectual disability and loose skin, are the result of deletion of genes outside the *TRPS1-EXT1* interval.

References

Hall BD, et al: Langer-Giedion syndrome, *Birth Defects* 10(12):147, 1974.
Langer LO, et al: The tricho-rhino-phalangeal syndrome with exostosis (or Langer-Giedion syndrome): Four additional patients without mental retardation and review of the literature, *Am J Med Genet* 19:81, 1984.

Bühler EM, et al: A final word on the tricho-rhino-phalangeal syndromes, *Clin Genet* 31:273, 1987.

Nardmann J, et al: The tricho-rhino-phalangeal syndromes: Frequency and parental origin of 8q deletions, *Hum Genet* 99:638, 1997.

Stevens CA, Moore CA: Tibial hemimelia in Lange-Giedion syndrome—possible gene location for the tibial hemimelia at 8q, *Am J Med Genet* 85:409, 1999.

Riedl S, et al: Pronounced short stature in a girl with tricho-rhino-phalangeal syndrome II (TRPS II, Langer-Giedion syndrome) and growth hormone deficiency, *Am J Med Genet* 131:200, 2004.

Miyamoto K, et al: Tetraparesis due to exostotic osteochondroma at upper cervical cord in a patient with multiple exostosis-mental retardation syndrome (Langer-Giedion syndrome), *Spinal Cord* 43:190, 2005.

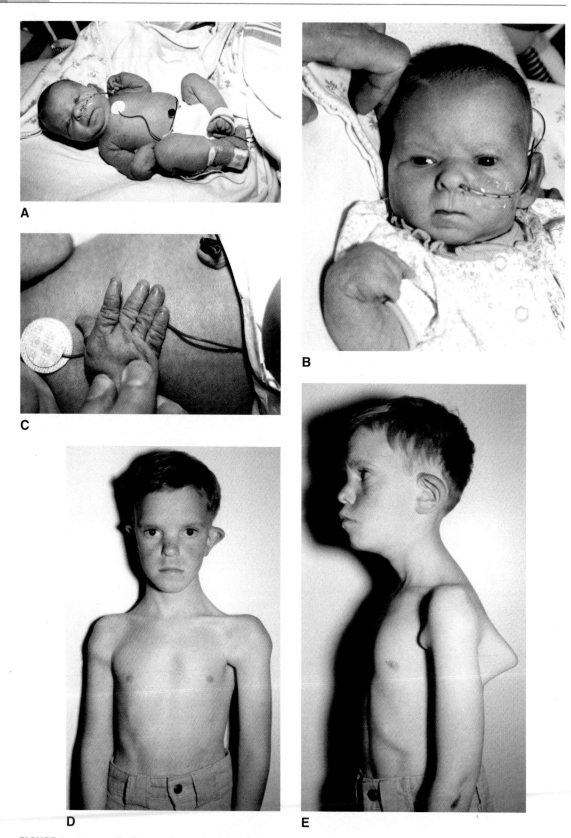

FIGURE 1.   Langer-Giedion syndrome. **A–C,** Newborn. Note the loose skin, bulbous nose with notching of the ala nasi, and simple but prominent philtrum. **D** and **E,** A 7-year-old child. Note the sparseness of hair, bulbous nose, simple but prominent philtrum, superiorly tented nares, thin upper lip, prominent ears, and exostoses on the scapula and proximal humerus. (**D** and **E,** Courtesy Dr. Bryan Hall, University of Kentucky, Lexington.)

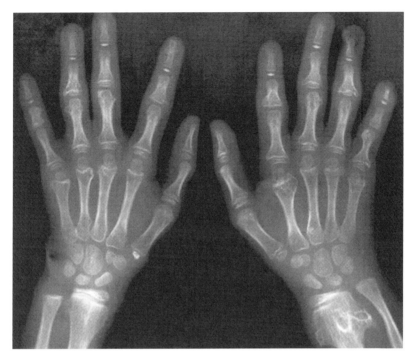

FIGURE 2. An 11½-year-old with exostoses, cone-shaped epiphyses, and metaphyseal hooking at the proximal ends of several of the middle phalanges.

TRICHO-RHINO-PHALANGEAL SYNDROME, TYPE I (TRP I)
Bulbous Nose, Sparse Hair, Epiphyseal Coning

Klingmüller reported two siblings with this pattern of malformation in 1956. Giedion further established the syndrome and set forth the tricho-rhino-phalangeal designation for it.

ABNORMALITIES

Growth. Mild growth deficiency (3rd to 10th percentiles).

Facial. Pear-shaped nose, prominent and long philtrum, narrow palate with or without micrognathia, large prominent ears; small, carious teeth with dental malocclusion; horizontal groove on chin.

Hair. Sparse, thin hair with relative hypopigmentation.

Nails. Thin.

Skeletal. Short metacarpals and metatarsals, especially the fourth and fifth; development of broadened middle phalangeal joint with cone-shaped epiphyses, especially the second through fourth fingers and toes; split distal radial epiphyses; winged scapulae.

OCCASIONAL ABNORMALITIES

Coxa plana and coxa magna, flattening of capital femoral epiphysis, partial syndactyly, pectus carinatum, pes planus, short stature, intellectual disability, craniosynostosis, mitral valve prolapse, deep voice, hypotonia during infancy, partial growth hormone deficiency.

NATURAL HISTORY

The hair is usually sparse at birth. Osseous changes, such as cone-shaped epiphyses, may develop in early childhood and become worse until adolescent growth is complete. Increased frequency of upper respiratory tract infections has been noted in some cases. Reduced bone mass and quality is common and may lead to osteoporosis in adults. Reports suggesting that growth hormone therapy leads to increased bone mass in affected individuals are conflicting. Osteoarthritis may involve multiple joints.

ETIOLOGY

This disorder has an autosomal dominant inheritance pattern. Mutations in *TRPS1*, a gene encoding a zinc finger transcription factor, have been found in the majority of patients with tricho-rhino-phalangeal syndrome, type I. The gene is located on chromosome band 8q24.1.

COMMENT

In addition to TRP types I and II, a disorder has been recognized that represents the severe end of the TRP spectrum, manifest by features of TRP type I plus severe shortness of all phalanges and metacarpals and short stature. Intelligence is normal, and there are no exostoses. This disorder, referred to as TRP type III, is caused by missense mutations in exon 6 of the *TRPS1* gene.

References

Klingmüller G: Über eigentümliche Konstitutions-anomalien bei 2 Schwestern und ihre Beziehungen zu neueren entwicklungspathologischen Befunden, *Hautarzt* 7:105, 1956.

Giedion A: Das tricho-rhino-phalangeale Syndrom, *Helv Paediatr Acta* 21:475, 1966.

Gorlin RJ, Cohen MM, Wolfson J: Tricho-rhino-phalangeal syndrome, *Am J Dis Child* 118:585, 1969.

Fontaine G, et al: Le syndrome trichorhinophalangien, *Arch Fr Pediatr* 27:635, 1970.

Felman AH, Frias JL: The trichorhinophalangeal syndrome: Study of 16 patients in one family, *AJR Am J Roentgenol* 129:631, 1977.

Goodman RM, et al: New clinical observations in the trichorhinophalangeal syndrome, *J Craniofac Genet Dev Biol* 1:15, 1981.

Buhler EM, et al: A final word on the tricho-rhino-phalangeal syndromes, *Clin Genet* 31:273, 1987.

Momeni P, et al: Mutations in a new gene, encoding a zinc-finger protein, cause tricho-rhino-phalangeal syndrome type I, *Nat Genet* 24:71, 2000.

Ludecke H-J, et al: Genotype and phenotype spectrum in the tricho-rhino-phalangeal syndromes types I and III, *Am J Hum Genet* 68:81, 2001.

Stagi S, et al: Partial growth hormone deficiency and changed bone quality and mass in type I trichorhino-phalangeal syndrome, *Am J Med Genet* 146:1598, 2008.

Izumi K, et al: Late manifestations of the tricho-rhino-phalangeal syndrome in a patient: Expanded skeletal phenotype in adulthood, *Am J Med Genet* 152:2115, 2010.

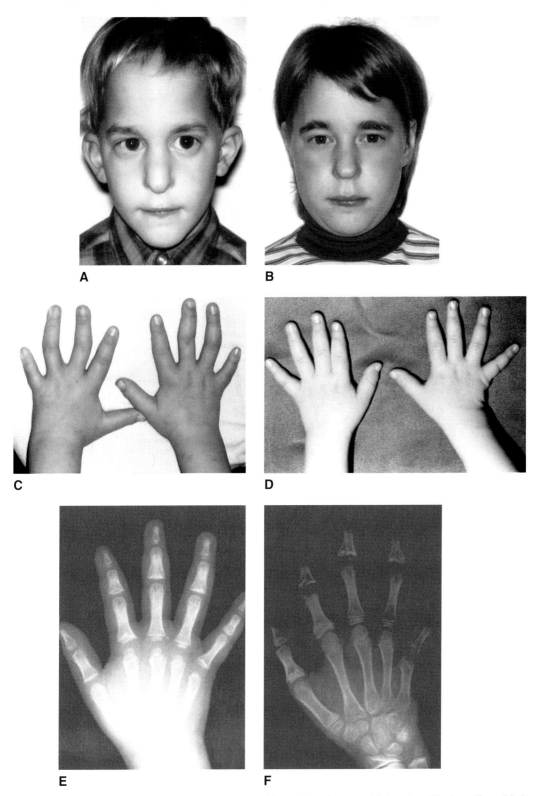

FIGURE 1. Tricho-rhino-phalangeal syndrome. A 6-year-old son (**A**) and 9-year-old daughter (**B**) of an affected father who became bald at 21 years of age. The children have fine, slow-growing hair. Note the tented hypoplastic nares and prominent philtrum. **C–F,** Note, too, the asymmetric length of fingers related to radiographic evidence of irregular metaphyseal cupping with cone-shaped epiphyses. (**A–F,** Courtesy of D. Weaver, Indiana University, Indianapolis.)

ECTRODACTYLY–ECTODERMAL DYSPLASIA–CLEFTING SYNDROME (EEC SYNDROME)
Ectrodactyly, Ectodermal Dysplasia, Cleft Lip-Palate

Although the association of ectrodactyly and cleft lip had been noted, it was not until 1970 that Rüdiger and colleagues appreciated that at least some of these patients also had features of ectodermal dysplasia and named the disorder the EEC syndrome. Bixler and colleagues added two cases and summarized the past observations. Well over 200 cases have been reported.

ABNORMALITIES

All features are variable.

Skin. Fair and thin, with mild hyperkeratosis; hypoplastic nipples.
Hair. Light-colored, sparse, thin, wiry hair on all hair-bearing areas; distortion of the hair bulb and longitudinal grooving of hair shaft is seen on scanning electron microscopic observation.
Teeth. Partial anodontia, microdontia, caries.
Eyes. Blue irides, photophobia, blepharophimosis, defects of lacrimal duct system (59%), blepharitis, dacryocystitis.
Face. Cleft lip, with or without cleft palate (68%); maxillary hypoplasia; mild malar hypoplasia, downslanting palpebral fissures, short philtrum.

Limbs. Defects in midportion of hands and feet, varying from syndactyly to ectrodactyly (84%); mild nail dysplasia.
Genitourinary. Anomalies in 52%, including megaureter, duplicated collecting system, vesicoureteral reflux, ureterocele, bladder diverticula, renal agenesis/dysplasia, hydronephrosis, micropenis, cryptorchidism, transverse vaginal septum.

OCCASIONAL ABNORMALITIES
Conductive hearing loss (14%), intellectual disability (7%), microcephaly, small or malformed auricles, broad nasal tip, perioral lesions associated with fissures at the oral commissures, choanal atresia, semilobar holoprosencephaly, polydactyly, clinodactyly, ear dysplasia, telecanthus/hypertelorism, inguinal hernia, anal atresia/rectovaginal fistula, growth hormone deficiency, hypogonadotropic hypogonadism, central diabetes insipidus.

NATURAL HISTORY
These individuals are usually of normal intelligence and adapt reasonably well with surgical closure of the facial clefts plus (as needed) limb surgery, dentures, and wigs. Chronic/recurrent respiratory infections occur in 6% of cases. Early and continued ophthalmologic evaluation and management are

critical. The major ocular problem involves defects of the meibomian gland resulting in an unstable tear film. The lacrimal drainage system defects lead to chronic dacryocystitis with subsequent corneal scarring.

ETIOLOGY

This disorder has an autosomal dominant inheritance with variable expression. No single feature, including ectrodactyly, is obligatory. Mutations of the p63 gene, *TP63*, at 3q27 have been identified in the vast majority of cases. Most are amino acid substitutions in the DNA-binding domain. *TP63* is a homologue of the tumor-suppressor gene p53.

COMMENT

Hartsfield holoprosencephaly-ectrodactyly syndrome includes ectrodactyly holoprosencephaly, cleft lip and palate and hypertelorism. It is likely that patients previously identified as having EEC syndrome—who, in addition, have holoprosencephaly, central diabetes insipidus and perhaps growth hormone deficiency, and hypogonadotrophic hypogonadism—actually have this disorder.

References

Cockayne EA: Cleft palate, harelip, dacryocystitis and cleft hand and feet, *Biometrika* 28:60, 1936.

Walker JC, Clodius L: The syndromes of cleft lip, cleft palate and lobster-claw deformities of hands and feet, *Plast Reconstr Surg* 32:627, 1963.

Rüdiger RA, Haase W, Passarge E: Association of ectrodactyly, ectodermal dysplasia, and cleft lip-palate, *Am J Dis Child* 120:160, 1970.

Bixler D, et al: The ectrodactyly-ectodermal dysplasia-clefting (EEC) syndrome, *Clin Genet* 3:43, 1972.

Rodini ESO, Richieri-Costa A: EEC syndrome: Report on 20 new patients, clinical and genetic considerations, *Am J Med Genet* 37:42, 1990.

Roelfsema NM, Cobben JM, et al: The EEC syndrome: A literature study, *Clin Dysmorphol* 5:115, 1996.

Celli J, et al: Heterozygous germline mutations in the p53 homolog p63 are the cause of EEC syndrome, *Cell* 99:143, 1999.

Barrow LL, et al: Analysis of *p63* gene in the classical EEC syndrome, related syndromes, and non-syndromic orofacial clefts, *J Med Genet* 39:559, 2002.

Akahoshi K, et al: EEC syndrome type 3 with a heterozygous germline mutation in the *P63* gene and B cell lymphoma, *Am J Med Genet* 120:370, 2003.

Vilain C, et al: Hartsfield holoprosencephaly-ectrodactyly syndrome in five male patients: Further delineation and review, *Am J Med Genet* 149:1476, 2009.

Pierre-Louis M, et al: Perioral lesions in ectrodactyly, ectodermal dysplasia, clefting syndrome, *Ped Derm* 27:658, 2010.

Di Iorio E, et al: Limbal stem cell deficiency and ocular phenotype in ectrodactyly-ectodermal dysplasia-clefting syndrome caused by p63 mutations, *Ophthalmology* 119:74, 2012.

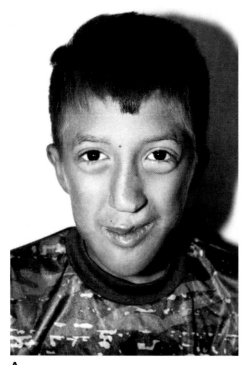

A

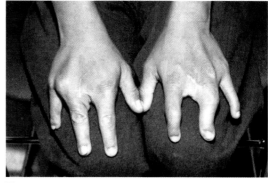

B

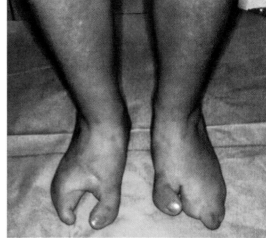

D

C

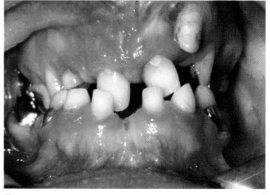

F

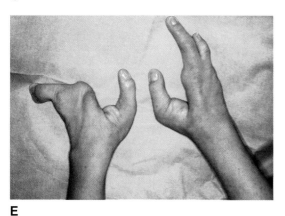

E

FIGURE 1. Ectrodactyly-ectodermal dysplasia–clefting syndrome. **A–C,** A 13-year-old boy and adult woman, both with thin, dry, lightly pigmented skin; sparse, fine hair; repaired cleft lip; and ectrodactyly. Note the inflammation of the conjunctiva in the adult who has photophobia. (**C,** Courtesy Dr. Michael Bamshad, University Utah, Salt Lake City.) **D–F,** Note the variability of the ectrodactyly, the partial anodontia, and microdontia.

HAY-WELLS SYNDROME OF ECTODERMAL DYSPLASIA
(ANKYLOBLEPHARON–ECTODERMAL DYSPLASIA–CLEFTING SYNDROME, AEC SYNDROME)
Ankyloblepharon, Ectodermal Dysplasia, Cleft Lip-Palate

In 1976, Hay and Wells described a specific type of ectodermal dysplasia associated with cleft lip or cleft palate and congenital filiform fusion of the eyelids. The association of facial clefting with ankyloblepharon filiforme adnatum had previously been documented in several case reports.

ABNORMALITIES

Growth. Short stature.

Craniofacial. Oval face; absence of lacrimal puncta; ocular hypotelorism; broadened nasal bridge; maxillary hypoplasia; micrognathia; thin vermillion border; cleft lip, cleft palate, or both; short philtrum; conical, widely spaced teeth; hypodontia to partial anodontia; ankyloblepharon filiforme adnatum; hypoplastic alae nasi; small ears.

Skin. Palmar and plantar keratoderma; peeling erythematous, eroded skin at birth from limited to high percentage of body surface area; hyperkeratosis; patchy, partial deficiency of sweat glands; partial anhidrosis; hyperpigmentation.

Nails. Absent or dystrophic.

Hair. Wiry and sparse to alopecia; head and/or eyelashes both affected; hypoplasia of lateral one third of eyebrows.

Hands and Feet. Syndactyly of the second and third toe and of the third and fourth toe; syndactyly of the third and fourth finger; internal toe deviation; broad first toe.

OCCASIONAL ABNORMALITIES

Deafness; trismus; atretic external auditory canal; cup-shaped auricles; supernumerary nipples; in rare cases, ventricular septal defect or patent ductus arteriosus; hypospadias; micropenis; split hand/split foot; camptodactyly; hypoplasia of toes; vaginal dryness or erosions; Wilms tumor.

NATURAL HISTORY

Surgical excision of the ankyloblepharon filiforme adnatum is required during the early neonatal period. Anomalies of the eye are not associated with these tissue bands. However, photophobia is common. Surgical closure of facial clefting and early ophthalmologic evaluation of the lacrimal duct system are required. Otitis media occurs frequently. Severe chronic granulomas of the scalp, which begin as infections, have been a serious problem and, in one case, have required multiple skin grafts. Careful monitoring of skin erosions because of difficult healing is critical. Although these patients have a partial capacity to produce sweat from fewer glands so that hyperthermia is not a serious threat, heat intolerance is common. Intelligence is normal.

ETIOLOGY

This disorder has an autosomal dominant inheritance pattern with marked variability of expression. Mutations in the p63 gene *(TP63)*, which give rise to amino acid substitutions in the sterile alpha motif (SAM) domain, are responsible for this disorder. The gene is a homologue of the tumor-suppressor p53 gene and is located at 3q27.

COMMENT

Ankyloblepharon filiforme adnatum is not a simple failure of eyelid separation. The eyelid fusion bands histologically are composed of a central core of vascular connective tissue entirely surrounded by epithelium. Muscle fibers may be observed as well. These bands may represent abnormal proliferation of mesenchymal tissue at certain points on the lid margin or an ectodermal deficit allowing mesodermal union.

References

Duke-Elder S: *Textbook of Ophthalmology*, vol 5, London, 1952, Kimpton.

Khanna VN: Ankyloblepharon filiforme adnatum, *Am J Ophthalmol* 43:774, 1957.

Rogers JW: Ankyloblepharon filiforme adnatum, *Arch Ophthalmol* 65:114, 1961.

Long JC, Blandford SE: Ankyloblepharon filiforme adnatum with cleft lip and palate, *Am J Ophthalmol* 53:126, 1962.

Hay RJ, Wells RS: The syndrome of ankyloblepharon, ectodermal defects, and cleft lip and palate: An autosomal dominant condition, *Br J Dermatol* 94:277, 1976.

Spiegel J, Colton A: AEC syndrome: Ankyloblepharon, ectodermal defects, and cleft lip and palate, *J Am Acad Dermatol* 12:810, 1985.

Vanderhooft SL, et al: Severe skin erosions and scalp infections in AEC syndrome, *Pediatr Dermatol* 10:334, 1993.

McGrath JA, et al: Hay-Wells syndrome is caused by heterozygous missense mutations in the SAM domain of p63, *Hum Mol Genet* 10:221, 2001.

Fomenkov K, et al: P63 Mutations lead to aberrant splicing of the keratinocyte growth factor receptor in the Hay-Wells syndrome, *J Biol Chem* 278:23906, 2003.

Julapalli MR, et al: Dermatologic findings of ankyloblepharon-ectodermal defects-cleft lip/palate (AEC) syndrome, *Am J Med Genet* 149:1900, 2009.

Sutton VR, et al: Craniofacial and anthropometric phenotype in ankyloblepharon-ectodermal defects-cleft lip/palate syndrome (Hay-Wells syndrome) in a cohort of 17 patients, *Am J Med Genet* 149:1916, 2009.

Lane MM, et al: Psychosocial functioning and quality of life in children affected by AEC syndrome, *Am J Med Genet* 149:1926, 2009.

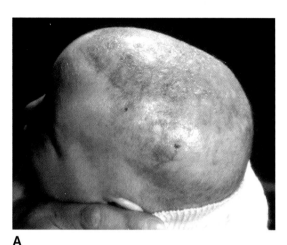

A

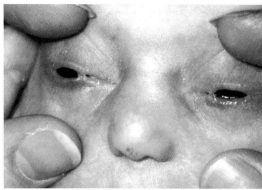

B

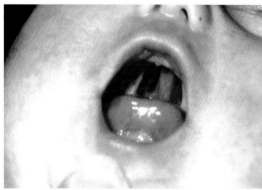

C

FIGURE 1. Hay-Wells syndrome. **A–C,** Ectodermal dysplasia with folliculitis of scalp, adhesions between eyelids, and cleft palate. (Courtesy of Dr. Mark Stephan, Madigan General Hospital, Tacoma, Wash.)

ROBERTS SYNDROME
(ROBERTS–SC PHOCOMELIA SYNDROME, SC PHOCOMELIA SYNDROME)
Hypomelia, Midfacial Defect, Severe Growth Deficiency

This disorder was initially described by Roberts in 1919 and more recently by Appelt and colleagues. Freeman and colleagues reported five cases and reviewed the features in the 17 previously recognized patients. The cases reported by Herrmann and colleagues as "pseudothalidomide or SC syndrome" and the case reported by Hall and Greenberg as "hypomelia-hypotrichosis–facial hemangioma syndrome" are caused by mutations in the same gene and thus represent variable expression of the same disorder.

ABNORMALITIES

Performance. Microcephaly (80%), severe to mild/borderline intellectual disability.

Growth. Profound growth deficiency of prenatal onset, birth weight in full-term infants 1.5 to 2.2 kg (88%) and birth length frequently less than 40 cm, mild or severe postnatal growth deficiency.

Facial. Cleft lip with or without cleft palate and prominent premaxilla, hypertelorism (87%), midfacial capillary hemangioma (78%), thin nares, shallow orbits and prominent eyes (69%), bluish sclerae, corneal clouding (68%), micrognathia, malformed ears with hypoplastic lobules.

Hair. Sparse, often silvery blond in some survivors.

Limbs. Hypomelia, more severe in upper limbs, varying from tetra-amelia to tetraphocomelia to lesser degrees of limb reduction, often including reduction in length or absence of the humerus (77%), radius (98%), or ulna (96%); reduction in number or length of fingers (75%), syndactyly (42%), or clinodactyly; reduction or absence of femur (65%), tibia (74%), or fibula (80%); reduction in number of toes (27%); incomplete development of dermal ridges; flexion contractures of knees, ankles, wrists, or elbows.

Genitalia. Cryptorchidism; phallus may appear relatively large in relation to body size.

OCCASIONAL ABNORMALITIES
Frontal encephalocele, hydrocephalus, brachycephaly, craniosynostosis, microphthalmia, cataract, lid coloboma, cranial nerve paralysis, short neck, nuchal cystic-hygroma, cardiac anomaly (atrial septal defect), renal anomaly (polycystic or horseshoe kidney), bicornuate uterus, rudimentary gallbladder, accessory spleen, splenogonadal fusion, polyhydramnios, thrombocytopenia, hypospadias.

NATURAL HISTORY
Most individuals born at term with birth length less than 37 cm and severe defects in midfacial and limb development were stillborn or died in early infancy. The majority of the survivors have had marked growth deficiency, and some have had severe intellectual disability. Birth length greater than 37 cm, less severe limb defects, absence of cleft palate, and presence of thin nares have been associated with a better prognosis. Ten adults, the majority of whom have had typical limb defects, craniofacial anomalies, growth retardation, and intellectual disabilities, have been reported. Additional features noted in adults include cardiac defects, particularly aortic stenosis; ocular findings in addition to corneal clouding, including cavernous hemangioma, paracentral scotoma and pits, tilting of the optic nerve, and bilateral optic nerve atrophy; one case of malignant melanoma and a possible increased risk for veno-occlusive disease. Only one of three adult females who have become pregnant has had a full-term baby.

ETIOLOGY
This disorder has an autosomal recessive inheritance pattern with great variability of expression within families. Mutations in establishment of cohesion 1 homologue 2 (*ESCO2*), on 8p21.1 are responsible. *ESCO2* is a human homologue of yeast ECO1, which is critically involved in sister chromatid cohesion. Roberts syndrome and SC phocomelia are both caused by mutations in *ESCO2*.

COMMENT
Premature centromere separation, which consists of "puffing" or "repulsion" of the constitutive heterochromatin of many chromosomes can be demonstrated in patients with this disorder. It is best demonstrated using the C-band staining technique.

References

Roberts JB: A child with double cleft of lip and palate, protrusion of the intermaxillary portion of the upper jaw and imperfect development of the bones of the four extremities, *Ann Surg* 70:252, 1919.

Appelt H, Gerken H, Lenz W: Tetraphokomelie mit Lippen-Kiefer-Gaumenspalte und Clitorishypertrophie—Ein Syndrome, *Paediatr Paedol* 2:119, 1966.

Fraser FC, et al: Pectoralis major defect and Poland sequence in second cousins: Extension of the Poland sequence spectrum, *Am J Med Genet* 33:468, 1989.

Martínez-Frias ML, et al: Smoking during pregnancy and Poland sequence: Results of a population-based registry and case-control registry, *Teratology* 59:35, 1999.

Torre M, et al: Dextrocardia in patients with Poland syndrome: Phenotypic characterization provides insight into the pathogenesis, *J Thorac Cardiovasc Surg* 139: 1177, 2010.

Baban A, et al: Familial Poland syndrome revisited, *Am J Med Genet* 158:140, 2012.

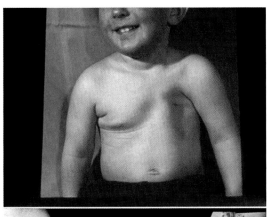
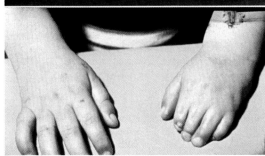

FIGURE 1. Poland sequence. The absence of the pectoralis minor and the sternal portion of the pectoralis major plus the ipsilateral syndactyly of the hand are the more usual features of this complex sequence. The bony thoracic anomaly and the hypoplasia of the hand, as noted in this otherwise normal boy, are more severe expressions of this defect.

J

ULNAR-MAMMARY SYNDROME
Ulnar Ray Defects, Absence/Hypoplasia of Breast Development, Diminished/Absent Axillary Hair and Perspiration

Originally described in 1882 by Gilly in a woman with mammary hypoplasia, inability to lactate, and absence of the third, fourth, and fifth fingers and ulna, this disorder has been reported in more than 80 patients, both male and female. The clinical phenotype and the molecular characterization have been most extensively delineated by Bamshad and colleagues.

ABNORMALITIES

Facies. Broad nasal tip; underdeveloped alae nasi; full cheeks with wide midface; downturned corners of mouth; pointed, prominent chin.

Limb. Hypoplasia of phalanges of fifth digits, partial or complete fifth-digit phalangeal fusion with absent interphalangeal creases, postaxial polydactyly, absence of digits 3 to 5, partial ventral duplication of fifth fingernail, aplasia/hypoplasia of ulna, short radius, absent/hypoplasia of metacarpals 3 to 5.

Apocrine. Diminished/absent axillary hair and perspiration, lack of body odor.

Mammary. Hypopigmentation and hypoplasia of areola, nipple, and breast; normal to absent lactation.

Other. Delayed puberty and skeletal maturation, particularly in males; genital anomalies, including shawl scrotum, micropenis, and cryptorchidism.

OCCASIONAL ABNORMALITIES

Intellectual disability, anophthalmia, absent or ectopic canine teeth, cleft palate, bifid uvula, lingual frenulum extending to tip of tongue, subglottic stenosis, upslanting palpebral fissures, wide nasal base, imperforate hymen, bicornuate uterus, complete absence of forearm and hand, patent ductus arteriosus, mitral valve prolapse, ventricular septal defect with pulmonic stenosis, cardiac conduction defect, accessory nipples, inverted nipple, carpal bone absence or fusion on ulnar side, hypoplastic flexion creases of first and second digits, short terminal phalanges of toes 4 and 5, hypoplastic

humerus, hypoplastic scapula, hypoplastic clavicle, absent/short xiphisternum, obesity, inguinal hernia, renal agenesis, pyloric stenosis, anal atresia/stenosis, anatomic abnormality of pituitary, gonadotropin deficiency, growth hormone deficiency.

NATURAL HISTORY

Significant delay in growth and skeletal maturation. Puberty and catch-up growth occur but frequently affected individuals are 5 to 7 years delayed. Testing for growth hormone deficiency as well as screening for cardiac arrhythmias should be offered.

ETIOLOGY

This disorder has an autosomal dominant inheritance pattern. Mutations in *TBX3*, a member of the T-box gene family that has been mapped to 12q23-24.1 are responsible. A submicroscopic deletion encompassing the *TBX3* gene has been documented in at least one affected individual.

References

Gilly E: Absence complète des mamelles chez une femme mère: Atrophie du membre supérieur droit, *Courrier Med* 32:27, 1882.

Pallister PD, et al: Studies of malformation syndrome in man XXXXII: A pleiotropic dominant mutation affecting skeletal, sexual and apocrine-mammary development, *Birth Defects Orig Artic Ser* 12(5):247, 1976.

Schinzel A: Ulnar-mammary syndrome, *J Med Genet* 24:778, 1987.

Bamshad M, et al: Clinical analysis of a large kindred with the Pallister ulnar mammary syndrome, *Am J Med Genet* 65:325, 1996.

Bamshad M, et al: Mutations in human *BX3* alter limb, apocrine and genital development in ulnar-mammary syndrome, *Nat Genet* 16:311, 1997.

Klopocki E, et al: Ulnar-mammary syndrome with dysmorphic facies and mental retardation caused by a novel 1.28Mb deletion encompassing the *TBX3* gene, *Eur J Hum Genet* 14:1274, 2006.

Linden H, et al: Ulnar mammary syndrome and *TBX3*: Expanding the phenotype, *Mer J Med Genet* 149:2809, 2009.

Joss S, et al: The face of ulnar mammary syndrome? *Eur J Med Genet* 54:301, 2011.

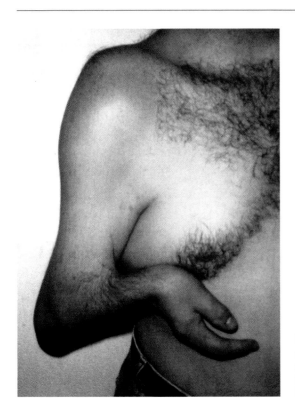

FIGURE 1. Ulnar-mammary syndrome. There is an absent ulna, short radius, absence of metacarpals 3 to 5, diminished axillary hair, and hypoplasia of the breast. (Courtesy Dr. Michael Bamshad, University of Utah, Salt Lake City.)

J

POPLITEAL PTERYGIUM SYNDROME
(FACIO-GENITO-POPLITEAL SYNDROME)
Popliteal Web, Cleft Palate, Lower Lip Pits

This disorder was first reported by Trelat in 1869. More than 80 cases have been recorded.

ABNORMALITIES

Oral. Cleft palate with or without cleft lip (90%), salivary lower lip pits (46%), intraoral fibrous band connecting maxillary and mandibular alveolar ridges (43%), thin upper lip.

Limbs. Popliteal web, in extreme form from heel to ischium (90%). Toenail dysplasia, pyramidal skinfold extending from base to tip of great toe (33%), syndactyly of toes.

Genitalia. Anomalies in 51%, including hypoplastic labia majora, scrotal dysplasia, cryptorchidism.

OCCASIONAL ABNORMALITIES

Unusual oral frenula, hypodontia, cutaneous webs between eyelids (20%), atresia of external ear canal, intercrural pterygium (9%), syndactyly of fingers most commonly digits 3 to 4, bifid toenail, hypoplasia or aplasia of digits, reduction defect of thumb, fusion of distal interphalangeal joints, valgus deformity of feet, talipes equinovarus, hypoplasia of tibia, bifid or absent patella, posterior dislocation of fibulae, low acetabular angle, spina bifida occulta, other vertebral anomalies, bifid ribs, short sternum, scoliosis, renal agenesis, ambiguous external genitalia, penile ectopia or torsion, ectopic testes, underdevelopment of vagina or uterus, inguinal hernia, abnormal scalp hair.

NATURAL HISTORY

There is usually a dense fibrous cord in the posterior portion of the popliteal pterygium. Magnetic resonance imaging has been successfully used to locate the peroneal nerve and popliteal artery, which often run through the fibrous band, prior to surgical repair. There may be associated defects of muscle in the lower extremities, with limitation of function despite repair of the pterygium. The genital anomalies are most likely due to distortion by intercrural webs that often run from medial thigh to the base of the phallus. Other webbing across the eyelids or in the mouth may require excision. Although a number of cosmetic and orthopedic corrective procedures are frequently required, normal intelligence and good ambulation should be anticipated in the majority of affected individuals.

ETIOLOGY

An autosomal dominant inheritance pattern is implied, with wide variability in severity. Mutations in the gene encoding interferon regulatory factor 6 *(IRF6),* located at chromosome 1q32-q41, are responsible for 97% of cases of this disorder as well as 68% of cases of Van der Woude syndrome, indicating that these two disorders are allelic. The function of *IRF6* is at present uncertain.

References

Trelat U: Sur un vice conformation très rare de la lèvre-inférieure, *J Med Chir Prat* 40:442, 1869.

Hecht F, Jarvinen JM: Heritable dysmorphic syndrome with normal intelligence, *J Pediatr* 70:927, 1967.

Escobar V, Weaver D: The facio-genito-popliteal syndrome, *Birth Defects* 14:185, 1978.

Raithel H, Schweckendiek W, Hillig U: The popliteal pterygium syndrome in three generations, *Z Kinderchir* 26:56, 1979.

Hall JG, et al: Limb pterygium syndromes: A review and report of eleven patients, *Am J Med Genet* 12:377, 1982.

Froster-Iskenius UG: Popliteal pterygium syndrome, *J Med Genet* 27:320, 1990.

Hunter A: The popliteal pterygium syndrome: Report of a new family and review of the literature, *Am J Med Genet* 36:196, 1990.

Lees MM, et al: Popliteal pterygium syndrome: A clinical study of three families and report of linkage to the Van der Woude syndrome locus at 1q32, *J Med Genet* 36:888, 1999.

Donnelly LF, et al: MR imaging of popliteal pterygium syndrome in pediatric patients, *AJR Am J Roentgenol* 178:1281, 2002.

Kondo S, et al: Mutations in IRF6 cause Van der Woude and popliteal pterygium syndromes, *Nat Genet* 32:285, 2002.

Ferreira RLL, et al: Prevalence and nonrandom distribution of exonic mutations in interferon regulatory factor 6 in 307 families with Van der Woude syndrome and 37 families with popliteal pterygium syndrome, *Genet Med* 11:241, 2009.

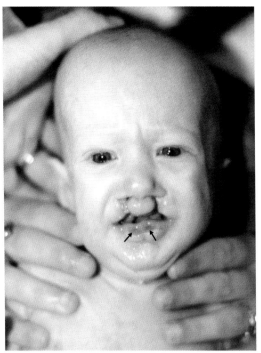

A

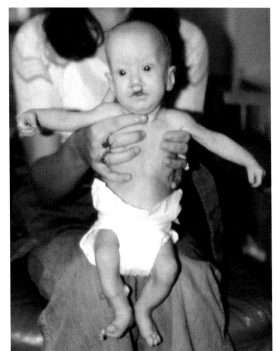

B

J

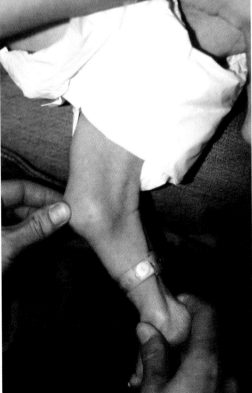

C

FIGURE 1. Popliteal pterygium syndrome. **A–C,** Infant with bilateral cleft lip, lip pits, and popliteal web. Note the rod-like taut core. (Courtesy Dr. David Weaver, Indiana University, Indianapolis.)

ESCOBAR SYNDROME (MULTIPLE PTERYGIUM SYNDROME)
Multiple Pterygia, Camptodactyly, Syndactyly

Originally described by Bussière in 1902, this disorder was fully delineated by Escobar and colleagues in 1978.

ABNORMALITIES

Growth. Small stature.

Facies. Ptosis of eyelids with downslant of palpebral fissures; inner canthal folds; hypertelorism; micrognathia with downturning corners of mouth; difficulty opening mouth widely; long philtrum; cleft palate; sad, flat, emotionless face; low-set ears.

Pterygia. Pterygia of neck, axillae, antecubital, popliteal, and intercrural areas.

Limbs. Pterygia plus camptodactyly, syndactyly, equinovarus, or rocker-bottom feet.

Genitalia. Cryptorchidism, absence of labia majora.

Other. Scoliosis, kyphosis, fusion of vertebrae or fused laminae, rib anomalies, absent or dysplastic patella.

OCCASIONAL ABNORMALITIES

Intrauterine growth restriction; anterior clefts of vertebral bodies, tall vertebral bodies with decreased anteroposterior diameter, failed fusion of posterior neural arches; rib fusion; long clavicles with lateral hooks; modeled scapulae; dislocated radial head; distal radioulnar separation; vertical talus; muscle atrophy; dislocation of hip; hypoplastic and/or widely spaced nipples; conductive hearing loss; abnormal ossicles; diaphragmatic eventration; hypospadias; cardiac defects.

NATURAL HISTORY

The majority of affected individuals become ambulatory. Intelligence is normal. Respiratory problems, including pneumonia, plus episodes of dyspnea and apnea presumably secondary to the kyphoscoliosis and small chest size lead to significant morbidity as well as death in the first year of life in approximately 6% of patients.

The pterygia may become more obvious with time, leading to fixed contractures. Early, vigorous physical therapy is indicated to retain the greatest joint mobility. Scoliosis occurs before 5 years of age in the majority of patients and frequently requires surgical fusion. Formal hearing evaluation is indicated in all individuals.

ETIOLOGY

This disorder has an autosomal recessive inheritance pattern. Mutations in the γ-subunit gene (*CHRNG*) of the acetylcholine receptor (AChR) are responsible for 27% of cases. These mutations lead to fetal akinesia with arthrogryposis and multiple pterygia. However, the γ-subunit is not a constituent part of the adult acetylcholine receptor, which takes over from the embryonal acetylcholine receptor in the third trimester. Therefore, postnatal muscle weakness and fatigue are not seen in *CHRNG*-positive patients with Escobar syndrome.

COMMENT

Mutations in *CHRNG* have also been seen in the lethal multiple pterygium syndrome (page 232). Although the lethal multiple pterygium syndrome and the Escobar syndrome phenotypes are seen in different families with the same *CHRNG* mutation, it is estimated that that there is a 95% chance that subsequent siblings in the same family will have the same phenotype as the proband.

References

Escobar V, et al: Multiple pterygium syndrome, *Am J Dis Child* 132:609, 1978.

Hall JG, et al: Limb pterygium syndromes: A review and report of eleven patients, *Am J Med Genet* 12:377, 1982.

Thompson EM, et al: Multiple pterygium syndrome: Evolution of the phenotype, *J Med Genet* 24:733, 1987.

Ramer JC, et al: Multiple pterygium syndrome: An overview, *Am J Dis Child* 142:794, 1988.

Hoffman K, et al: Escobar syndrome is a prenatal myasthenia caused by disruption of the acetylcholine receptor fetal γ subunit, *Am J Hum Genet* 79:303, 2006.

Vogt J, et al: CHRNG genotype-phenotype correlations in the multiple pterygium syndromes, *J Med Genet* 49:21, 2012.

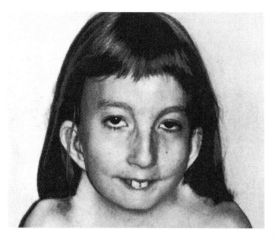
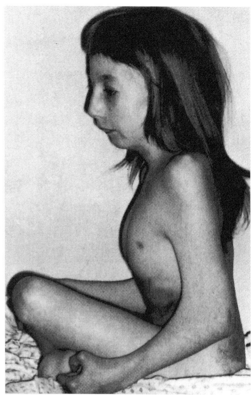
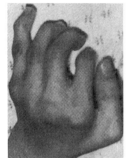
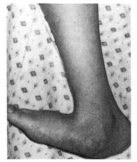

FIGURE 1. A 12-year-old girl showing features of Escobar syndrome. (From Escobar V, et al: *Am J Dis Child* 132:609, 1978, with permission.)

J

CHILD SYNDROME
Unilateral Hypomelia and Skin Hypoplasia, Cardiac Defect

Falek and colleagues reported two female siblings with this unique pattern of malformation in 1968, and Shear noted a comparable case. The term CHILD is an acronym for *c*ongenital *h*emidysplasia with *i*chthyosiform erythroderma and *l*imb *d*efects.

ABNORMALITIES

Growth. Mild prenatal growth deficiency.

Limbs. Unilateral hypomelia varying from absence of a limb to hypoplasia of some metacarpals and phalanges, webbing at elbows and knees, joint contractures.

Skin. Unilateral ichthyosiform skin lesion, sometimes referred to as an ichthyosiform nevus or inflammatory epidermal nevus, with sharp midline demarcation; small patches of involved skin may occur on opposite side; unilateral alopecia, hyperkeratosis, and nail destruction; histologically, there is a thick parakeratotic stratum corneum overlying a psoriasiform, acanthotic epidermis, often with inflammatory infiltration and lipid-laden histiocytes.

Other Skeletal. Ipsilateral hypoplasia of bones involving any part of the skeleton, including mandible, clavicle, scapula, ribs, and vertebrae; ipsilateral punctate epiphyseal calcifications during infancy.

Other. Cardiac septal defects, single coronary ostium, single ventricle, unilateral renal agenesis.

OCCASIONAL ABNORMALITIES

Ipsilateral hypoplasia of brain, cranial nerves, spinal cord, lung, thyroid, adrenal gland, ovary, and fallopian tube; mild intellectual disability; mild contralateral anomalies of skin, bone, or viscera; scoliosis; cleft lip; umbilical hernia; hearing loss; meningomyelocele.

NATURAL HISTORY

The skin lesions, usually present at birth, may develop during the first few weeks of life. New areas of involvement may occur as late as 9 years. The face is spared. Early death is due primarily to cardiac defects. When the left side of the body is involved, which occurs far less frequently than the right, severity is far greater. Treatment with etretinate, an aromatic retinoid, has been successful in management of the skin problems in some cases.

ETIOLOGY

This disorder has an X-linked dominant inheritance pattern with lethality in males. Although the majority of cases are sporadic, rare familial cases with mother-daughter transmission have been reported. The majority of cases are caused by mutations in the *NSDHL* (NADH steroid dehydrogenase-like) gene located at Xq28. A deletion of the coding region of *NSDHL* was responsible in one patient.

References

Falek A, et al: Unilateral limb and skin deformities with congenital heart disease in twin siblings: A lethal syndrome, *J Pediatr* 73:910, 1968.

Shear CS, et al: Syndrome of unilateral ectromelia, psoriasis, and central nervous system anomalies, *Birth Defects* 7:197, 1971.

Happle R, Koch H, Lenz W: The CHILD syndrome, *Eur J Pediatr* 134:27, 1980.

Christiansen JR, Petersen HO, Søgaard H: The CHILD syndrome—congenital hemidysplasia with ichthyosiform erythroderma and limb defects: A case report, *Acta Dermatol Venereol (Stockh)* 64:165, 1984.

Hebert A, et al: The CHILD syndrome: Histologic and ultrastructural studies, *Arch Dermatol* 123:503, 1987.

Emami S, et al: Peroxisomal abnormality in fibroblasts from involved skin of CHILD syndrome: Case study and review of peroxisomal disorders in relation to skin disease, *Arch Dermatol* 128:1213, 1992.

Konig A, et al: Mutations in the *NSDHL* gene, encoding a 3b-hydroxysteroid dehydrogenase, cause CHILD syndrome, *Am J Med Genet* 90:339, 2000.

Kelley RI, et al: Inborn errors of sterol biosynthesis, *Annu Rev Genomics Hum Genet* 2:299, 2001.

Bornholdt D, et al: Mutational spectrum of NSDHL in CHILD syndrome, *J Med Genet* 42:e17, 2005.

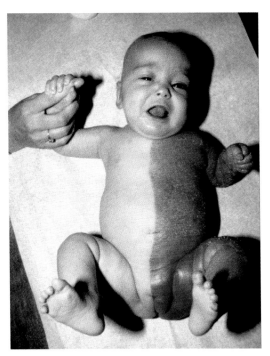

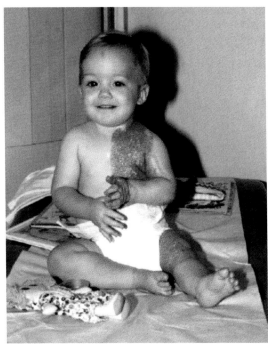

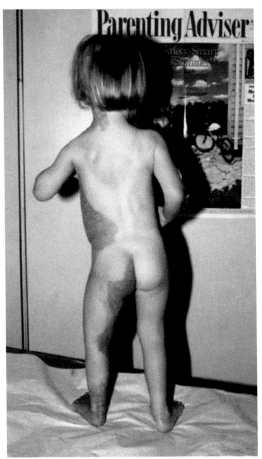

J

FIGURE 1. CHILD syndrome. Affected child at 3 months, 13 months, and 23 months of age. Note the unilateral erythema and scaling with ipsilateral hypoplasia.

FEMORAL HYPOPLASIA–UNUSUAL FACIES SYNDROME
Femoral Hypoplasia, Short Nose, Cleft Palate

Following single case reports in 1961 by Franz and O'Rahilly and in 1965 by Kucera and colleagues, Daentl and colleagues recognized four additional patients and set forth this unique syndrome in 1975.

ABNORMALITIES

Growth. Small stature, predominantly the result of short lower limbs.

Facial. Short nose with hypoplastic alae nasi, long philtrum, and thin upper lip; micrognathia, cleft palate; upslanting palpebral fissures; low-set, poorly formed pinnae.

Limbs. Bilateral, usually asymmetric involvement; hypoplastic to absent femora and variable asymmetric involvement of fibula and tibia; variable hypoplasia of humeri with restricted elbow movement, including radioulnar and radiohumeral synostosis and limited shoulder movement; Sprengel deformity; talipes equinovarus.

Pelvis. Hypoplastic acetabulae, constricted iliac base with vertical ischial axis, and large obturator foramina.

Spine. Dysplastic sacrum, missing vertebrae or hemivertebrae, sacralization of lumbar vertebrae, scoliosis.

Genitourinary. Cryptorchidism; inguinal hernia; small penis, testes, or labia majora; polycystic kidneys, absent kidneys, abnormal collecting system.

OCCASIONAL ABNORMALITIES
Astigmatism; esotropia; short third, fourth, and fifth metatarsals; preaxial polydactyly of feet; tapered, fused, or missing ribs; inguinal hernia; cardiac defects, including ventricular septal defect, pulmonary stenosis, and truncus arteriosus; craniosynostosis; central nervous system anomalies, including hydrocephalus; agenesis of the corpus callosum, hypoplasia of falx cerebri, absent septum pellucidum, and colpocephaly.

NATURAL HISTORY
Although there may be problems in speech development, the patients have been of normal intelligence; most of them have been ambulatory.

ETIOLOGY
The cause of this disorder is unknown. Although the vast majority of cases are sporadic, an affected male whose daughter is similarly affected raises the possibility of autosomal dominant inheritance. Maternal diabetes has been documented in 38% of cases.

References

Franz CH, O'Rahilly R: Congenital skeletal limb deficiencies, *J Bone Joint Surg Am* 43:1202, 1961.

Kucera VJ, Lenz W, Maier W: Missbildungen der Beine und der kaudalen Wirbelsaeule bei Kindern diabetischer Muetter, *Dtsch Med Wochenschr* 90:901, 1965.

Daentl DL, et al: Femoral hypoplasia–unusual facies syndrome, *J Pediatr* 86:107, 1975.

Lampert RP: Dominant inheritance of femoral hypoplasia–unusual facies syndrome, *Clin Genet* 17:255, 1980.

Johnson JP, et al: Femoral hypoplasia–unusual facies syndrome in infants of diabetic mothers, *J Pediatr* 102:866, 1983.

Baraitser M, et al: Femoral hypoplasia–unusual facies syndrome with preaxial polydactyly, *Clin Dysmorphol* 3:40, 1994.

Leal E, et al: Femoral-facial syndrome with malformations in the central nervous system, *J Clin Imaging* 27:23, 2003.

Ho AI, et al: Femoral facial syndrome: A case report with coexistent hydrocephaly, *Clin Dysmorphol* 17:259, 2008.

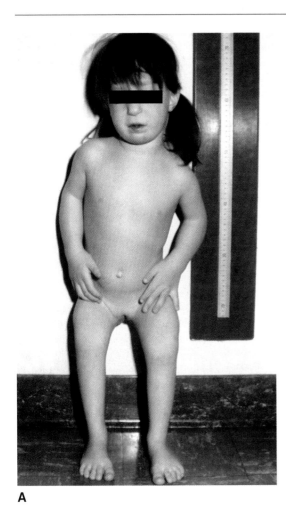

A

FIGURE 1.   **A** and **B,** Girl showing short humeri with synostosis at the elbow, in addition to femoral shortness.

Continued

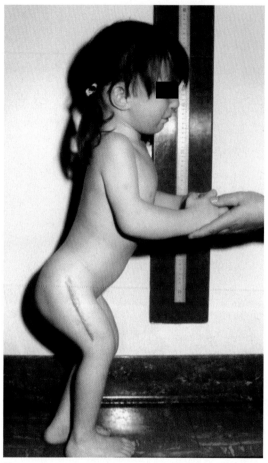

B

FIGURE 1, cont'd

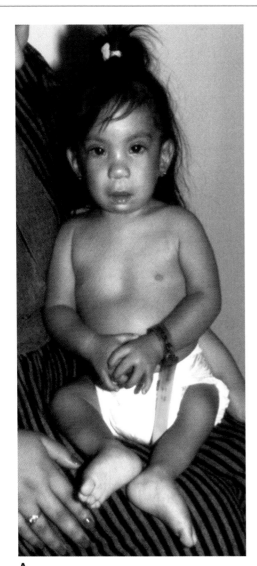

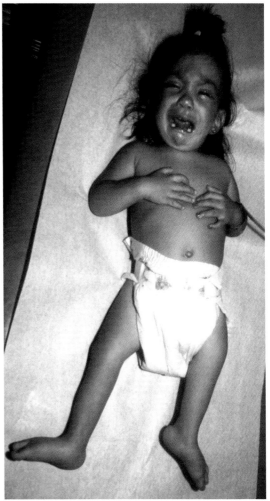

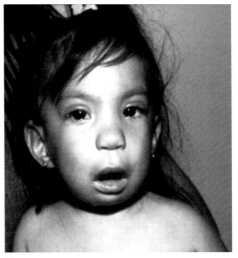

FIGURE 2. Femoral hypoplasia–unusual facies syndrome. **A–C,** Photograph of a 21-month-old girl. Note the short nose, small mandible, variable and asymmetric hypoplasia of the femurs and humeri, and inability to extend the elbow fully.

TIBIAL APLASIA–ECTRODACTYLY SYNDROME
(SPLIT-HAND/FOOT MALFORMATION AND LONG-BONE DEFICIENCY [SHFLD])
Split-Hand/Split-Foot, Absence of Long Bones of Arms and Legs

A single patient with this pattern of malformation was described in 1575 by Ambroise Paré. Subsequently, more than 100 affected individuals have been reported. The complete spectrum of this condition has been set forth by Majewski and colleagues and by Hoyme and colleagues.

ABNORMALITIES

Hands. Abnormalities in 68%, most commonly ectrodactyly (split hand); absence of multiple fingers.

Feet. Abnormalities in 64%, most commonly variable absence of tarsals, metatarsals, and toes.

Limbs. Absence of long bone of legs in 55%, most commonly tibial aplasia; tibial hypoplasia; fibular hypoplasia or aplasia.

OCCASIONAL ABNORMALITIES

Cup-shaped ears; aplasia of ulna, radius, or humerus; monodactyly; absence of multiple fingers; syndactyly; proximally placed thumbs; ectrodactyly of feet; metatarsus adductus; talipes equinovarus; supernumerary preaxial digit; postaxial polydactyly; absence of entire leg; bifid or hypoplastic femur; contracted knee joint with patellar hypoplasia; hypoplasia of great toe; craniosynostosis; bifid xiphoid.

ETIOLOGY

Duplications of *BHLHA9* located at chromosome 17p13.3 are responsible. *BHLHA9* is a putative basic loop helix transcription factor. There is widely variable expression and frequent examples of nonpenetrance in structurally normal obligate carriers that is sex biased that more males who carry the duplication are clinically affected. Because of the frequency of clinically normal individuals who carry the gene for this disorder, prenatal ultrasonographic studies should be performed in all pregnancies in affected families even if neither parent is clinically affected.

References

Majewski F, et al: Aplasia of tibia with split-hand/split-foot deformity: Report of six families with 35 cases and considerations about variability and penetrance, *Hum Genet* 70:136, 1985.

Hoyme HE, et al: Autosomal dominant ectrodactyly and absence of long bones of upper or lower limbs: Further clinical delineation, *J Pediatr* 111:538, 1987.

Richieri-Costa A, et al: Tibial hemimelia: Report on 37 new cases. Clinical and genetic considerations, *Am J Med Genet* 27:867, 1987.

Majewski F, et al: Ectrodactyly and absence (hypoplasia) of the tibia: Are there dominant and recessive types? *Am J Med Genet* 63:185, 1996.

Armour AM, et al: 17p13.3 microduplications are associated with split-hand/foot malformation and long-bone deficiency (SHFLD), *Eur J Hum Genet* 19:1144, 2011.

Klopocki E, et al: Duplications of BHLHA9 are associated with ectrodactyly and tibia hemimelia inherited in non-Mendelian fashion, *J Med Genet* 49:119, 2012.

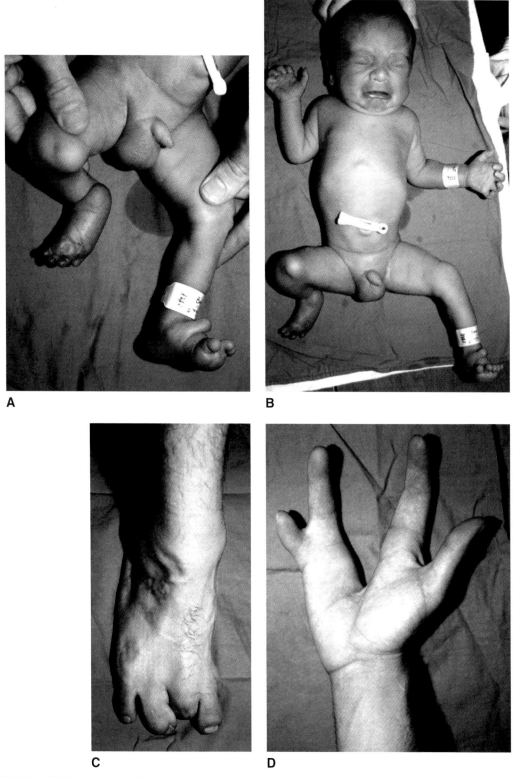

FIGURE 1. Tibial aplasia–ectrodactyly syndrome. **A** and **B,** Newborn infant with absent right tibia and great toe and supernumerary preaxial digit arising from dorsum of right foot. **C** and **D,** Father of newborn infant pictured in **A** and **B.** Note the typical split hand. Ectrodactyly of the foot has been surgically repaired. (**A–D,** From Hoyme HE, et al: *Pediatrics* 111:538, 1987, with permission.)

ADAMS-OLIVER SYNDROME
Aplasia Cutis Congenita, Terminal Transverse Defects of Limbs

Adams and Oliver described eight members of a family with this disorder in 1945. More than 100 affected individuals have been reported.

ABNORMALITIES

Growth. Mild growth deficiency (3rd to 10th percentile).

Scalp. Aplasia cutis congenita over posterior parietal region, with or without an underlying defect of bone; in older individuals, solitary or multiple, round-oval hairless scars are found in the parietal region; tortuous veins over posterior scalp.

Limbs. Variable degrees of terminal transverse defects, including those of lower legs, feet, hands, fingers, toes, or distal phalanges; short fingers; small toenails.

Cardiac. Defects in 20%, including atrial septal defect, ventricular septal defect, aortic coarctation, obstructive lesions of the left heart, hypoplastic left and right ventricles, double-outlet right ventricle, and double-outlet left ventricle.

Skin. Cutis marmorata telangiectasia congenital (20%).

OCCASIONAL ABNORMALITIES

Intrauterine growth restriction; esotropia; microphthalmia; epilepsy; cleft lip; cleft palate; micrognathia; syndactyly; talipes equinovarus; accessory nipples; duplicated collecting system; imperforate vaginal hymen; cryptorchidism; aplasia cutis congenita on trunk and limbs; thin, hyperpigmented skin; Poland sequence; chylothorax; pulmonary and portal hypertension; low IGF-1 levels; partial growth hormone deficiency; neurologic abnormalities, including encephalocele, acrania, microcephaly, and arrhinencephaly; defects of neuronal migration with combined focal pachygyria and polymicrogyria; dysplastic cerebral cortex; hypoplastic optic nerve; small pituitary; intellectual disability; spastic hemiplegia.

NATURAL HISTORY

Although prognosis is excellent in the vast majority of cases, larger scalp defects are more likely to be associated with underlying defects of bone and, where the superior sagittal sinus or dura are exposed, an increased risk of hemorrhage or meningitis. For those cases, early surgical intervention with grafting is indicated. For the usual case in which the sagittal sinus or dura is not exposed, healing without need for grafting almost always occurs.

ETIOLOGY

The majority of cases of this disorder have an autosomal dominant inheritance pattern with marked variability in expression and lack of penetrance in some cases. Gain-of-function mutations of *ARHGAP31*, a Cdc42/Rac1 GTPase regulator, are responsible for a small proportion of the cases. A careful physical examination and radiographs of hands and feet are indicated in first-degree relatives of affected individuals.

COMMENT

Autosomal recessive inheritance has been suggested in a few families with more than one affected child born to unaffected parents. These cases are far more likely to have a severe phenotype with neurologic abnormalities and intellectual disability. Recessive mutations in the dedicator of cytokinesis 6 (*DOCK6*) gene have been identified. *DOCK6* encodes a guanidine nucleotide exchange factor, which is known to activate Cdc42 and Rac1, two members of the Rho GTPase family.

References

Adams FH, Oliver CP: Hereditary deformities in man due to arrested development, *J Hered* 36:3, 1945.

Scribanu N, Tamtamy SA: The syndrome of aplasia cutis congenita with terminal transverse defects of limbs, *J Pediatr* 87:79, 1975.

Bonafede RP, Beighton P: Autosomal dominant inheritance of scalp defects with ectrodactyly, *Am J Med Genet* 3:35, 1979.

Kuster W, et al: Congenital scalp defects with distal limb anomalies (Adams-Oliver syndrome): Report of ten cases and review of the literature, *Am J Med Genet* 31:99, 1988.

Toriello HW, et al: Scalp and limb defects with cutis marmorata telangiectatica congenita: Adams-Oliver syndrome? *Am J Med Genet* 29:269, 1988.

Der Kaloustian VM, et al: Possible common pathogenetic mechanisms for Poland sequence and Adams-Oliver syndrome, *Am J Med Genet* 38:69, 1991.

Whitely CB, Gorlin RJ: Adams-Oliver syndrome revisited, *Am J Med Genet* 40:319, 1991.

Bamforth JS, et al: Adams-Oliver syndrome: A family with extreme variability in clinical expression, *Am J Med Genet* 49:393, 1994.

J

Lin AE, et al: Adams-Oliver syndrome associated with cardiovascular malformations, *Am J Med Genet* 7:235, 1999.

Snape KMG, et al: The spectra of clinical phenotypes in aplasia cutis congenita and terminal transverse limb defects, *Am J Med Genet* 149:1860, 2009.

Kalian MA, et al: Do children with Adams-Oliver syndrome require endocrine follow-up? New information on the phenotype and management, *Clin Genet* 78:227, 2010.

Shaheen B, et al: Recessive mutations in *DOCK6*, encoding the guanidine nucleotide exchange factor DOCK6 lead to abnormal actin cytoskeleton organization and Adams-Oliver syndrome, *Am J Hum Genet* 89:328, 2011.

Southgate L, et al: Gain-of function mutations of ARHGAP31, a Cdc42/Rac1 GTPase regulator, cause syndromic cutis aplasia and limb anomalies, *Am J Hum Genet* 88:574, 2011.

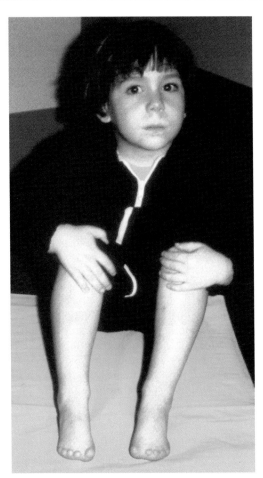

A

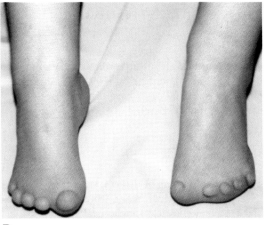

B

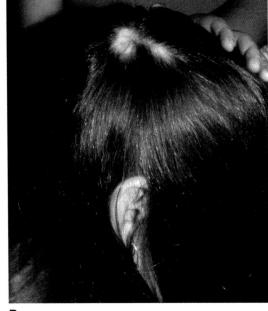

D

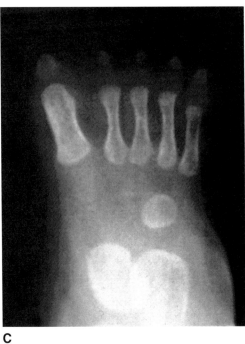

C

FIGURE 1. Adams-Oliver syndrome. **A–D,** Boy, 3½ years old, and his mother's sister. Note the terminal transverse defects involving the toes (**A–C**) and the area of aplasia cutis congenita over his maternal aunt's posterior scalp (**D**). The maternal aunt was otherwise normal.

J

HOLT-ORAM SYNDROME (CARDIAC-LIMB SYNDROME)
Upper Limb Defect, Cardiac Anomaly, Narrow Shoulders

This syndrome of skeletal and cardiovascular abnormalities was first described by Holt and Oram in 1960. More than 200 cases have been reported. Its prevalence is approximately 1 in 100,000 live births.

ABNORMALITIES

Skeletal. All gradations of defect in the upper limb and shoulder girdle. The thumbs may be absent, hypoplastic, triphalangeal, or bifid; syndactyly often occurs between thumb and index finger; phocomelia (10%); asymmetric involvement with left side more severely affected is frequently seen; clinodactyly; brachydactyly; hypoplasia to absence of first metacarpal and radius; defects of ulna, humerus, clavicle, scapula, sternum; decreased range of motion at elbows and shoulders, which are often narrow and sloping; carpal anomalies, particularly involving the scaphoid, which is often hypoplastic or has a bipartite ossification; proximal as well as distal epiphyses of metacarpals, particularly the first.

Cardiovascular. Ventricular septal defect and ostium secundum atrial septal defect have been the most common defects, and about one third of patients have had other types of congenital heart defects; conduction defects; hypoplasia of distal blood vessels.

OCCASIONAL ABNORMALITIES
Hypertelorism, absent pectoralis major muscle, pectus excavatum, thoracic scoliosis, vertebral anomalies, absence of one or more ossification centers in the wrist, Sprengel deformity, postaxial and central polydactyly, foot abnormalities including bifid distal phalanges of third toes and absence of distal phalanges of fourth toes (one patient), lung hypoplasia, refractive errors.

NATURAL HISTORY
Conduction defects can get worse with time. Pacemakers are sometimes required. Sudden death from heart block has been reported.

ETIOLOGY
This disorder has an autosomal dominant inheritance pattern with marked intra- and interfamilial variation. A correlation has been observed between the severity of the limb and heart defects in a given patient. Mutations of the *TBX5* gene, a member of the T-box transcription factor family, which is linked to chromosome 12q24.1 and is expressed in embryonic heart and limb tissues, are detected in approximately 25% of familial cases and in up to 50% of sporadic cases. Consistent with the concept of anticipation, increasing severity has occurred in succeeding generations.

COMMENT
Because of the marked variability in expression, at-risk individuals with a normal physical exam should have radiographs of wrists, arms, and hands to check for subtle changes of the thumb and carpal bones and an echocardiogram. Skeletal defects involve the upper limbs exclusively. Although bilateral, the limb defects are more prominent on the left.

References

Holt M, Oram S: Familial heart disease with skeletal malformations, *Br Heart J* 22:236, 1960.

Poznauski A, et al: Objective evaluation of the hand in the Holt-Oram syndrome, *Birth Defects* 8:125, 1972.

Kaufman RL, et al: Variable expression of the Holt-Oram syndrome, *Am J Dis Child* 127:21, 1974.

Hurst JA, et al: The Holt-Oram syndrome, *J Med Genet* 28:406, 1991.

Moens P, et al: Holt-Oram syndrome: Postaxial and central polydactyly as variable manifestations in a four generation family, *Genet Couns* 4:277, 1993.

Basson CT, et al: The clinical and genetic spectrum of the Holt-Oram syndrome (heart-hand syndrome), *N Engl J Med* 330:885, 1994.

Newbury-Ecob RA, et al: Holt-Oram syndrome: A clinical genetic study, *J Med Genet* 33:300, 1996.

Yi Li Q, et al: Holt-Oram syndrome is caused by mutations in *TBX5*, a member of the Brachyury (T) gene family, *Nat Genet* 15:21, 1997.

Garavelli L, et al: Holt-Oram syndrome associated with anomalies of the feet, *Am J Med Genet* 146:1185, 2008.

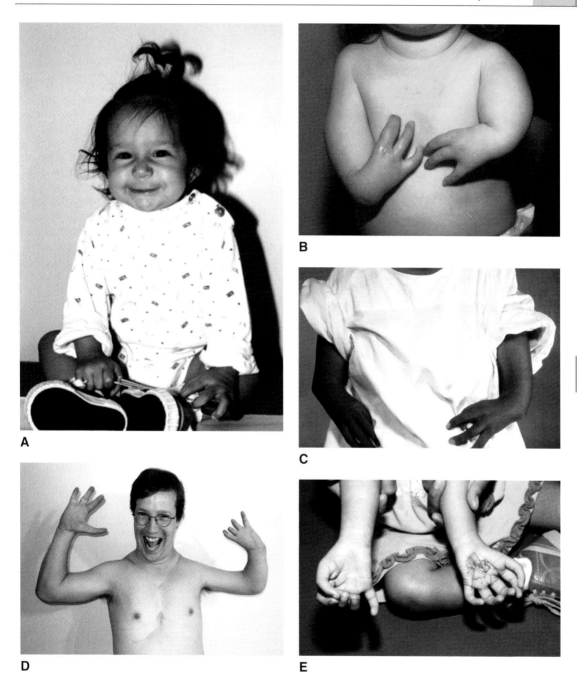

FIGURE 1.   Holt-Oram syndrome. **A–E,** Note radial defects that vary from severe forearm hypoplasia to thumb anomalies, including absent, hypoplastic, and triphalangeal thumbs, and the altered shoulder girdle. (**C,** Courtesy Dr. Mark Stephan, Madigan General Hospital, Tacoma, Wash.; **D,** courtesy Dr. Michael Bamshad, University of Utah, Salt Lake City.)

LEVY-HOLLISTER SYNDROME
(Lacrimo-Auriculo-Dento-Digital Syndrome, LADD Syndrome)

Although Levy described the first affected patient in 1967, this disorder was first delineated by Hollister and colleagues in 1973. More than 50 cases have been reported.

ABNORMALITIES

Lacrimal Anomalies. Nasolacrimal duct obstruction; aplasia or hypoplasia of lacrimal puncta (45%); alacrima due to hypoplasia or aplasia of lacrimal glands (40%).

Ears. Simple, cup-shaped ears with short helix and underdeveloped antihelix (70%).

Hearing. Mild to severe mixed conductive and sensorineural hearing loss (55%).

Dental. Abnormalities in 90%, including hypodontia, peg-shaped incisors, enamel hypoplasia of both deciduous and permanent teeth; delayed eruption of primary teeth.

Limb. Digital abnormalities in 95%, including digitalization of thumb, deficiency of bone and soft tissue of thumb and index finger, preaxial polydactyly, triphalangeal thumb, duplication of distal phalanx of thumb, thenar muscle hypoplasia, syndactyly between index and middle fingers, clinodactyly of third and fifth fingers, absent radius and thumb, and broad first toe. Shortening of radius and ulna.

OCCASIONAL ABNORMALITIES

Absence of parotid glands and Stensen ducts, nasolacrimal fistulae, cleft lip with or without cleft palate, hypoplastic epiglottis, hypertelorism or telecanthus, downslanting palpebral fissures, coronal hypospadias, renal agenesis or nephrosclerosis, hydronephrosis, vesicoureteral reflux, congenital hip dislocation, hiatal hernia, diaphragmatic hernia, syndactyly of toes 2 and 3 and 3 and 4, camptodactyly, distal thumb symphalangism, bicornuate uterus, cystic ovarian disease.

NATURAL HISTORY

A persistent dry mouth with eating difficulties and a propensity to develop inflammation of the oral mucosa and candidiasis frequently occur early in life. Because of decreased salivation and enamel hypoplasia, severe dental caries occur. A lack of tears and chronic dacryocystitis result from hypoplasia of the nasolacrimal duct system. Decreased tear production also can occur. Although the hearing loss is usually mild to moderate, it has been severe in a few cases. Multiple middle and inner ear malformations have been noted on computed tomography of the temporal bone. In rare cases, neonatal death secondary to bilateral renal agenesis has occurred.

ETIOLOGY

This disorder has an autosomal dominant inheritance pattern with marked variability of expression. It is caused by heterozygous mutations in the tyrosine kinase domains of the genes encoding fibroblast growth factor receptors 2 and 3 (*FGFR2* and *FGFR3*) and in mutations in the gene encoding fibroblast growth factor 10 (*FGF10*).

References

Levy WJ: Mesoectodermal dysplasia, *Am J Ophthalmol* 63:978, 1967.

Hollister DW, et al: The lacrimo-auriculo-dento-digital syndrome, *J Pediatr* 83:438, 1973.

Shiang EL, Holmes LB: The lacrimo-auriculo-dentodigital syndrome, *Pediatrics* 59:927, 1977.

Thompson E, Pembrey M, Graham JM: Phenotypic variation in LADD syndrome, *J Med Genet* 22:382, 1985.

Wiedemann HR, Drescher J: LADD syndrome: Report of new cases and review of the clinical spectrum, *Eur J Pediatr* 144:579, 1986.

Heinz GW, et al: Ocular manifestations of the lacrimoauriculo-dento-digital syndrome, *Am J Ophthalmol* 115:243, 1993.

Ramirez D, Lammer EJ: Lacrimoauriculodentodigital syndrome with cleft lip/palate and renal manifestations, *Cleft Palate Craniofac J* 41:501, 2004.

Milunsky JM, et al: LADD syndrome is caused by *FGF10* mutations, *Clin Genet* 69:349, 2006.

Rohmann E, et al: Mutations in different components of FGF signaling in LADD syndrome, *Nat Genet* 3:414, 2006.

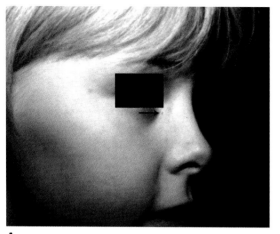

A

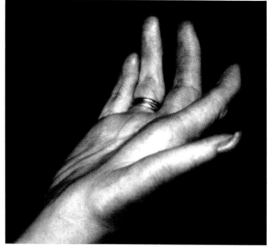

B

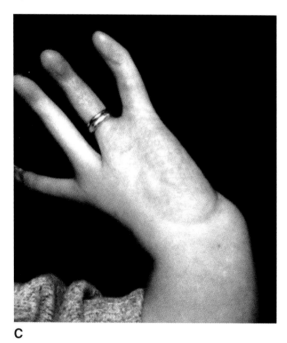

C

FIGURE 1. Levy-Hollister syndrome. A 9-year-old girl showing a nasolacrimal fistula caused by nasolacrimal duct obstruction (**A;** see *arrow*), digitalized thumb plus fifth finger clinodactyly (**B),** and a long tapering thumb with absent creases and surgically removed index finger (**C**). (Courtesy Dr. H. E. Hoyme, Stanford University, Palo Alto, Calif.)

J

OKIHIRO SYNDROME
(DUANE SYNDROME WITH UPPER LIMB ANOMALIES, ACRO-RENAL-OCULAR SYNDROME)
Duane Anomaly, Radial Ray Defects, Renal Anomaly

Okihiro and colleagues described a three-generation family in which multiple members were affected with the Duane anomaly, a congenital disorder of ocular motility, with or without radial ray defects. Several prior cases were reported in series of patients with radial ray defects or Duane anomaly.

ABNORMALITIES

Growth. Normal pre- and postnatal growth.

Performance. Normal cognitive performance. Sensorineural, mixed, or conductive hearing loss.

Craniofacial. Unilateral or bilateral Duane anomaly (limited abduction associated with widening of the palpebral fissure; retraction of the globe and narrowing of the palpebral fissure with adduction); nystagmus.

Limbs. Hypoplastic/absent thumb, altered thenar crease, decreased movement in interphalangeal thumb joint, hypoplastic radius and ulna, metatarsus adductus.

Renal. Crossed renal ectopia, double collecting system, malrotation, vesicoureteral reflux, bladder diverticula.

Imaging. Small navicular and multangular bones; hypoplasia of radius, ulna, first metacarpal, and thumb; phalangealization of the thumb; hypoplastic scaphoid; fused cervical vertebrae; spina bifida occulta.

OCCASIONAL ABNORMALITIES

Ptosis. Coloboma of iris and/or optic nerve, choroidal atrophy, microcornea, microphthalmia, cataract, conjunctival lipodermoid, choanal atresia, preauricular tag, microtia, atresia or slit-like openings of external auditory canal, facial asymmetry, preaxial polydactyly, severe upper limb reduction defects, shoulder dislocation, short neck, pectus excavatum, tibial hemimelia, talipes equinovarus, Hirschsprung disease, anal stenosis, hiatal hernia, atrial septal defect, pulmonic stenosis, ventricular septal defect, onychodystrophy, renal agenesis, pilonidal sinus, lumbosacral meningocele, pigmentary abnormalities of skin.

NATURAL HISTORY

Growth and cognitive functioning are normal. Some individuals face challenges based on the nature of the ocular anomalies and hearing impairment. Hypertension and recurrent urinary tract infections are common. Upper limb function is typically good since most affected individuals do not have severe reduction defects.

ETIOLOGY

Mutations in *SALL4* that result in haploinsufficiency (either through truncating mutations or deletion of the whole gene or specific coding exons) account for the majority of cases.

COMMENT

Many patients, particularly those with more severe limb malformations, have been initially considered to have Holt-Oram syndrome until reexamination revealed a Duane anomaly in one family member. At least two affected individuals have been initially diagnosed with thalidomide embryopathy, including a family reported by McBride, as evidence of the mutagenicity of thalidomide.

References

Al-Baradie R, et al: Duane radial ray syndrome (Okihiro syndrome) maps to 20q13 and results from mutations in *SALL4,* a new member of the SAL family, *Am J Hum Genet* 71:1195, 2002.

Borozdin W, et al: *SALL4* deletions are a common cause of Okihiro and acro-renal-ocular syndrome and confirm haploinsufficiency as the pathogenetic mechanism, *J Med Genet* 41:e113. doi:10.1136/jmg.2004.019901.

Borozdin W, et al: Multigene deletions on chromosome 20q13.3-q13, including *SALL4,* result in an expanded phenotype of Okihiro syndrome plus developmental delay, *Hum Mutat* 28:830, 2007.

Hayes A, Costa T, Polomeno RC: The Okihiro syndrome of Duane anomaly, radial ray abnormalities, and deafness, *Am J Med Genet* 22:273, 1985.

Kohlhase J, et al: Mutations at the *SALL4* locus on chromosome 20 result in a range of clinically overlapping phenotypes, including Okihiro syndrome, Holt-Oram syndrome, acro-renal-ocular syndrome, and patients previously reported to represent thalidomide embryopathy, *J Med Genet* 40:473, 2003.

Okihiro MM, et al: Duane syndrome and congenital upper-limb anomalies, *Arch Neurol* 34:174, 1977. (Original report)

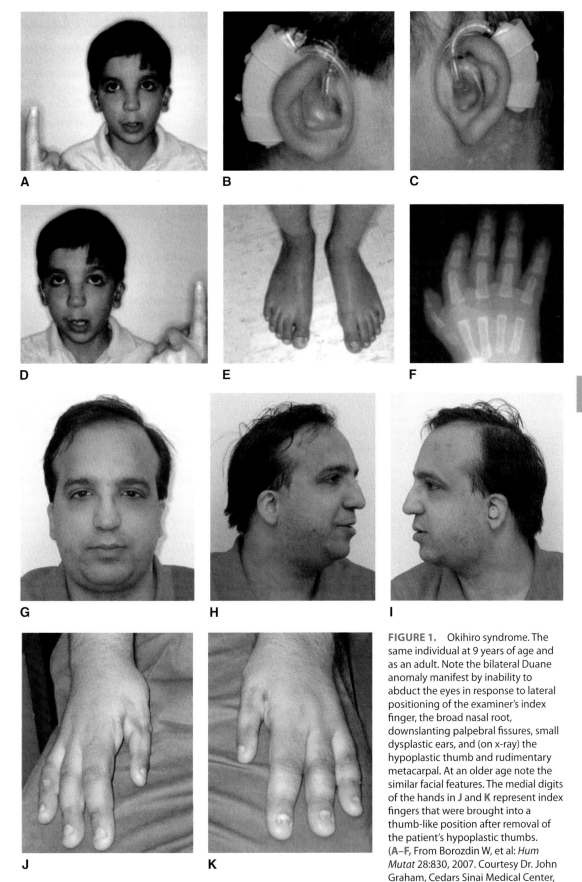

FIGURE 1. Okihiro syndrome. The same individual at 9 years of age and as an adult. Note the bilateral Duane anomaly manifest by inability to abduct the eyes in response to lateral positioning of the examiner's index finger, the broad nasal root, downslanting palpebral fissures, small dysplastic ears, and (on x-ray) the hypoplastic thumb and rudimentary metacarpal. At an older age note the similar facial features. The medial digits of the hands in **J** and **K** represent index fingers that were brought into a thumb-like position after removal of the patient's hypoplastic thumbs. (**A–F,** From Borozdin W, et al: *Hum Mutat* 28:830, 2007. Courtesy Dr. John Graham, Cedars Sinai Medical Center, Los Angeles, Calif. **G–K,** Courtesy Dr. Leah Burke, University of Vermont, Burlington.)

FANCONI PANCYTOPENIA SYNDROME
Radial Hypoplasia, Hyperpigmentation, Pancytopenia

Since Fanconi's original description of three affected siblings in 1927, numerous cases have been reported. Glanz and Fraser as well as Giampietro and colleagues have documented the marked variability of the clinical phenotype. Because 25% of affected individuals are structurally normal, the importance of considering this diagnosis in any anemic child with chromosome breaks, even in the absence of dysmorphic features on the physical examination, has been emphasized. Conversely, since the median age of onset of the hematologic abnormalities is 7 years (range, birth–31 years), this diagnosis should be considered in all children with the characteristic dysmorphic features, even in the absence of hematologic abnormalities. At least five cases have presented in the neonatal period. The carrier frequency for this disorder in the United States is 1 in 181.

ABNORMALITIES

Growth. Short stature, frequently of prenatal onset.
Performance. Microcephaly (25%–37%), intellectual disability in 25%.
Eye. Anomalies in 41%, including ptosis of eyelid, strabismus, nystagmus, and microphthalmos.
Skeletal. Radial ray defect in 49%, including hypoplasia to aplasia of thumb, with supernumerary thumbs in some cases or hypoplastic or aplastic radii.
Urogenital. Renal and urinary tract anomalies in 34%, including hypoplastic or malformed kidneys and double ureters; abnormalities in males, including hypospadias, small penis, small testes, or cryptorchidism in 20%.
Hematologic. Pancytopenia manifested by poikilocytosis, anisocytosis, reticulocytopenia, thrombocytopenia, and leukopenia; decreased bone marrow cellularity; leukemia; myelodysplastic syndrome.
Skin. Brownish pigmentation (64%).

OCCASIONAL ABNORMALITIES
Central Nervous System. Abnormalities in 8%, including hydrocephalus, absent septum pellucidum, absent corpus callosum, neural tube closure defect, migration defect, Arnold-Chiari malformation, or single ventricle.
Gastrointestinal. Abnormalities in 14%, including anorectal, duodenal atresia, tracheoesophageal fistula with or without esophageal atresia, annular pancreas, intestinal malrotation, intestinal obstruction, and duodenal web.

Other Skeletal. Defects occurring in 22%, including congenital hip dislocation, scoliosis, rib anomalies, talipes equinovarus, broad base of proximal phalanges, sacral agenesis or hypoplasia, Perthes disease, Sprengel deformity, genu valgum, leg length discrepancy, and kyphosis.
Other. Cardiac defect (13%), auricular anomaly (15%), deafness (11%), syndactyly.

NATURAL HISTORY
The majority of patients are relatively small at birth. Respiratory tract infections may be a frequent problem. The uneven brownish pigmentation of the skin tends to increase with age, being most evident in the anogenital area, groin, axillae, and trunk.

Life expectancy averages 20 years (range, birth–50 years). The usual presentation is progressive bone marrow failure and the development of malignancy, especially acute myeloid leukemia and, to a lesser extent, solid tumors, particularly squamous cell carcinomas. Progressive bone marrow failure, which usually leads to transfusion-dependent anemia, often occurs in the first two decades. Survivors frequently develop solid cancers later in life. Successful pregnancies after bone marrow transplantation have been reported.

ETIOLOGY
This disorder has an autosomal recessive inheritance pattern. At least 15 complementation groups have been identified, and corresponding genes have been identified for all of them. There is very little correlation between the complementation group and differences in phenotype.

COMMENT
Successful prenatal and postnatal diagnoses of this disorder can be accomplished by demonstrating a high frequency of spontaneous diepoxybutane-induced chromosomal breakage in peripheral blood lymphocytes as well as in cultured amniotic fluid cells.

References

Fanconi G: Familiäre infantile pernizosaaritige anämie, *Z Kinderheilkd* 117:257, 1927.
Garriga S, Crosby WH: The incidence of leukemia in families of patients with hypoplasia of the marrow, *Blood* 14:1008, 1959.
Nilsson LR: Chronic pancytopenia with multiple congenital abnormalities (Fanconi's anaemia), *Acta Paediatr* 49:518, 1960.
Schmid WK, et al: Chromosomenbrüchigkeit bei der familiären Panmyelopathie (Typus Fanconi), *Schweiz Med Wochenschr* 95:1461, 1965.

Glanz A, Fraser FC: Spectrum of anomalies in Fanconi anemia, *J Med Genet* 19:412, 1982.

Giampietro PF, et al: The need for more accurate and timely diagnosis in Fanconi anemia: A report from the International Fanconi Anemia Registry, *Pediatrics* 91:1116, 1993.

Landmann E, et al: Fanconi anemia in a neonate with pancytopenia, *J Pediatr* 145:125, 2004.

Dalle JH, et al: Successful pregnancies after bone marrow transplantation for Fanconi anemia, *Bone Marrow Transplant* 34:1099, 2004.

Rosenberg PS, et al: How high are carrier frequencies of rare recessive syndromes? Contemporary estimates for Fanconi anemia in the United States and Israel, *Mer J Med Genet* 155:1877, 2011.

Joenje H, Patel KJ: The emerging genetic and molecular basis of Fanconi anaemia, *Nat Rev Genet* 2:446, 2001.

Kutler DI, et al: A 20-year perspective on the International Fanconi anemia registry (IFAR), *Blood* 101:1249, 2003.

Rosenberg PS, et al: Cancer incidence in persons with Fanconi anemia, *Blood* 101:822, 2003.

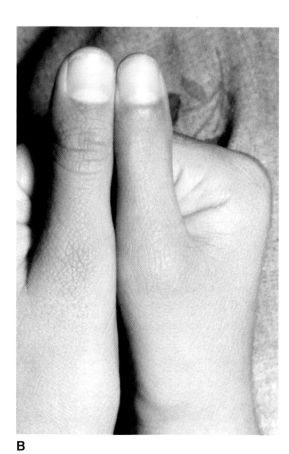

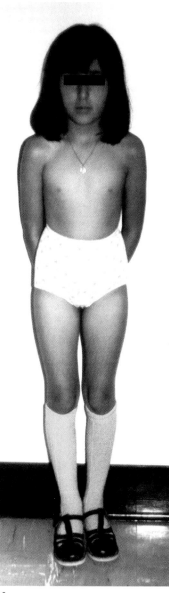

FIGURE 1. Fanconi pancytopenia syndrome.
A and **B,** A 7-year-old child with brownish pigmentation of the skin and hypoplasia of the right thumb with absent creases.

RADIAL APLASIA–THROMBOCYTOPENIA SYNDROME
(TAR SYNDROME)

Gross, Groh, and Weippl described this entity in siblings in 1956; subsequently, more than 100 cases have been reported.

ABNORMALITIES

Hematologic. Most severe in early infancy; thrombocytopenia with absence or hypoplasia of megakaryocytes (absent in 66%, decreased in 12%, inactive in 12%); "leukemoid" granulocytosis in 62% of patients, especially during bleeding episodes; eosinophilia in 53%; anemia, often out of proportion to apparent blood loss.

Limbs.

Arms: Bilateral absence of radius (100%); ulna abnormalities, including hypoplasia (100%), bilateral absence (20%) or unilateral absence (10%); abnormal humerus (50%) with bilateral absence in 5% to 10%; possible abnormal shoulder joint; thumbs are always present.

Legs: Abnormalities in 50%, including hip dislocation, subluxation of knees, coxa valga, dislocation of small patella, femoral and tibial torsion, abnormal tibiofibular joint, ankylosis of knee, small feet, abnormal toe placement; absence of fibula.

OCCASIONAL ABNORMALITIES

Cleft palate; congenital heart defect (15%), primarily tetralogy of Fallot and atrial septal defect; small stature; central facial capillary hemangioma; strabismus; ptosis; dysseborrheic dermatitis; excessive perspiration; pedal and dorsal edema; pes valgus; talipes equinovarus; fourth and fifth metatarsal synostosis; fourth and fifth toe syndactyly; phocomelia; agenesis of cruciate ligament and hypoplasia of menisci with knee dysplasia; renal anomaly (23%); absent uterus, cervix, and upper two thirds of the vagina (Mayer-Rokitansky-Küster-Hauser anomaly); ovarian agenesis; spina bifida; scoliosis; brachycephaly; micrognathia; lateral clavicular hook; pancreatic cyst; Meckel diverticulum; hypogammaglobulinemia; sensorineural hearing loss; intellectual disability (7%) that is usually related to intracranial bleeding; delayed myelination; hypoplasia of cerebellum, particularly the vermis; a cavum septum pellucidum; cerebellar dysgenesis with or without agenesis of corpus callosum on magnetic resonance imaging of brain.

NATURAL HISTORY

Approximately 40% of the patients have died, usually as a result of hemorrhage during early infancy. Thrombocytopenia during that time, most likely associated with a dysmegakaryocytopoiesis characterized by cells blocked at an early stage of differentiation, is precipitated by viral illness, particularly gastrointestinal. With advancing age, the severity of the hematologic disorder usually becomes less profound; therefore, vigorous early management is indicated. With the exception of menorrhagia, affected adults usually have no problem. Intracranial bleeding, when present, almost always occurs before 1 year of age. Delayed motor development is due to skeletal abnormalities. Bracing, splinting, or stabilization of the wrist centrally should be considered. Arthritis of wrist and knees is a late complication. The presence of an abnormal brachiocarpalis muscle, which originates on the anterolateral aspect of the humerus and inserts into the radial side of the carpus, may influence the surgical treatment. Cow's milk allergy or intolerance (47%) can be a significant problem with introduction of cow's milk precipitating thrombocytopenia, eosinophilia, or leukemoid reactions.

ETIOLOGY

This disorder has an autosomal recessive inheritance pattern. The disorder is the result of the concurrent presence of one of two noncoding single nucleotide polymorphisms on one allele of the *RBM8A* gene and a deletion of 1q21.1 at the other. *RBM8A*, which is located at 1q21.1, encodes Y14, which is a critical part of the exon junction complex. The reduced expression of *RBM8A* results in deficiency of Y14, which subsequently leads to the TAR syndrome.

References

Gross H, Groh C, Weippl G: Congenitale hypoplastische Thrombopenie mit Radialaplasie, *Neue Osterr Z Kinderheilkd* 1:574, 1956.

Shaw S, Oliver RAM: Congenital hypoplastic thrombocytopenia with skeletal deformities in siblings, *Blood* 14:374, 1956.

Hall JG, et al: Thrombocytopenia with absent radius (TAR), *Medicine* 48:441, 1969.

Anyane-Yeboa K, et al: Brief clinical report: Tetraphocomelia in the syndrome of thrombocytopenia with absent radii (TAR syndrome), *Am J Med Genet* 20:571, 1985.

Hall JG: Thrombocytopenia and absent radius (TAR) syndrome, *J Med Genet* 24:79, 1987.

MacDonald MR, et al: Hypoplasia of the cerebellar vermis and corpus callosum in thrombocytopenia with absent radius syndrome on MRI studies, *Am J Med Genet* 50:46, 1994.

Letestu R, et al: Existence of a differentiation blockage at the stage of a megakaryocyte precursor in the thrombocytopenia and absent radii (TAR) syndrome, *Blood* 95:1633, 2000.

Greenhalgh KL, et al: Thrombocytopenia-absent radius: A clinical genetic study, *J Med Genet* 39:876, 2002.

Oishi SN, et al: Thrombocytopenia absent radius syndrome: Presence of brachiocarpalis muscle and its importance, *J Hand Surg* 34:1696, 2009.

Toriello HV: Thrombocytopenia-absent radius syndrome, *Semin Thromb Hemost* 37:707, 2011.

Albers CA, et al: Compound inheritance of a low-frequency regulatory SNP and a rare null mutation in exon-junction complex subunit RBM8A causes TAR syndrome, *Nat Genet* 44:435, 2012.

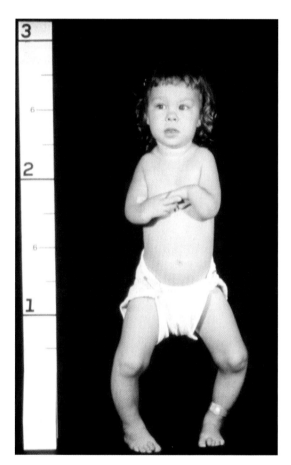

FIGURE 1. Radial aplasia–thrombocytopenia syndrome. Child with serious bleeding and thrombocytopenia as an infant. Note the presence of thumbs despite the bilateral absence of radii, abnormal shoulders, and subluxation of the knees.

AASE SYNDROME (DIAMOND-BLACKFAN ANEMIA)
Triphalangeal Thumb, Congenital Anemia

Aase and Smith described two male siblings with triphalangeal thumbs and a congenital anemia in 1969. Diamond-Blackfan anemia, initially described in 1938, is a pure red cell aplasia that is sometimes associated with features seen in Aase syndrome. It is now clear that Aase syndrome should not be separated from Diamond-Blackfan anemia.

ABNORMALITIES

Growth. Mild growth deficiency, about 3rd percentile.

Hematologic. Hypoplastic anemia that tends to improve with age.

Skeletal. Triphalangeal thumbs, mild radial hypoplasia, narrow shoulders, late closure of fontanels.

OCCASIONAL ABNORMALITIES

Intellectual disability; downslanting palpebral fissures; cleft lip; cleft palate; retinopathy; cataracts; glaucoma; webbed neck; 11 pairs of ribs; bifid thoracic vertebra; agenesis of clavicle; underdeveloped ilia, distal sacrum, and coccygeal vertebrae; dysplastic middle phalanx of fifth finger; cardiac defects; urogenital anomalies.

NATURAL HISTORY

The anemia, which has been responsive to prednisone therapy, tends to improve with age.

ETIOLOGY

This disorder has an autosomal dominant inheritance pattern. Of all cases of Aase syndrome, 55% are sporadic. Mutations in one of nine ribosomal protein (RP) genes are responsible, accounting for approximately 53% of patients with this syndrome. The *RPS19* gene accounts for about 25% of the cases.

COMMENT

Of all cases of Diamond-Blackfan syndrome, 30% to 50% have craniofacial, upper limb, heart, and urinary tract defects that are consistent with Aase syndrome.

References

Aase JM, Smith DW: Congenital anemia and triphalangeal thumbs: A new syndrome, *J Pediatr* 74:417, 1969.

Murphy S, Lubin B: Triphalangeal thumbs and congenital erythroid hypoplasia: Report of a case with unusual features, *J Pediatr* 81:987, 1972.

Higginbottom MC, et al: Case report: The Aase syndrome in a female patient, *J Med Genet* 15:484, 1978.

Muis N, et al: The Aase syndrome: Case report and review of the literature, *Eur J Pediatr* 145:153, 1986.

Hurst JA, et al: Autosomal dominant transmission of congenital erythroid hypoplastic anemia with radial abnormalities, *Am J Med Genet* 40:482, 1991.

Hing AV, Dowton SB: Aase syndrome: Novel radiographic features, *Am J Med Genet* 45:413, 1993.

Draptchinskaia N, et al: The gene encoding ribosomal protein S19 is mutated in Diamond-Blackfan anaemia, *Nat Genet* 21:169, 1999.

Doherty L, et al: Ribosomal protein genes *RPS10* and *RPS26* are commonly mutated in Diamond-Blackfan anemia, *Am J Hum Genet* 86:222, 2010.

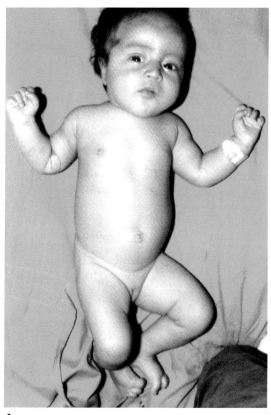

A

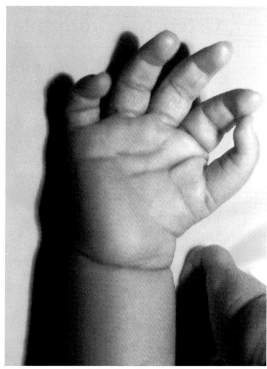

B

FIGURE 1. Aase syndrome. **A** and **B,** Newborn female infant with triphalangeal thumbs and thenar hypoplasia.

J

K Osteochondrodysplasias

ACHONDROGENESIS TYPES IA AND IB
Low Nasal Bridge, Very Short Limbs, Incomplete Ossification of Lower Spine

This early lethal disorder was described in 1925 by Donath and Vogl and termed *achondrogenesis* by Fraccaro in 1952. More than 20 cases have been reported. Studies by Borochowitz and colleagues indicate that achondrogenesis type I (previously referred to as Parenti-Fraccaro type) represents two radiographically and histopathologically distinct disorders, referred to as types IA and IB. In the classification set forth by Whitley and Gorlin, type I is synonymous with type IA and type II with type IB.

ABNORMALITIES

Growth. Extremely small stature (22 to 30 cm).
Craniofacial. Cranium large for gestational age, low nasal bridge, micrognathia.
Limbs. Severe micromelia.
Radiographs. In both types, the skull, vertebral bodies, fibula, talus, and calcaneus are poorly ossified; the ilia are crenated; the long bones are stellate; and the ribs are extremely short. In type IA, multiple rib fractures are present, and the proximal femora have metaphyseal spikes. Conversely, in type IB, rib fractures do not occur, and the distal femora have metaphyseal irregularities.

NATURAL HISTORY AND COMMENT
The defect in the development of cartilage and bone is severe. In type IA, normal-appearing but hypervascular cartilage matrix is present with increased cellular density. Large lacunae surround the chondrocytes, which contain round cytoplasmic inclusion bodies. In type IB, sparse interterritorial cartilaginous matrix is present, with a marked deficiency of collagen fibers. The chondrocytes are large, have a central round nucleus, and are surrounded by a dense collagenous ring. Developmental pathology beyond the skeletal system is implied by the frequent findings of polyhydramnios, hydrops, and early lethality. Most infants are stillborn or die shortly after birth. Occipital encephalocele has been reported in one child with type IA disease.

ETIOLOGY
This disorder has an autosomal recessive inheritance pattern. Achondrogenesis type IA is caused by mutations in the thyroid hormone receptor interactor gene (*TRIP11*), which leads to deficiency of Golgi microtubule-associated protein 210 (GMAP-210). Achondrogenesis type IB is caused by mutations in the diastrophic dysplasia sulfatase transporter (DTDST) gene (*SLC26A2*). Inactivation of the gene product, a sulfate-chloride exchanger of the cell membrane, leads to intracellular sulfate depletion and to synthesis of undersulfated proteoglycans in susceptible cells. Mutations in this gene are responsible for four recessively inherited chondrodysplasias, including achondrogenesis type IB, diastrophic dysplasia, multiple epiphyseal dysplasia, and atelosteogenesis type II.

References

Donath J, Vogl A: Untersuchungen über den chondrodystrophischen Zwergwuchs, *Wien Arch Intern Med* 10:1, 1925.

Fraccaro M: Contributo allo studio delle malattie del mesenchima osteopoietico: I achondrogenesi, *Folia Hered Pathol (Milano)* 1:190, 1952.

Maroteaux P, Lamy M: Le diagnostic des nanismes chondrodystrophiques chez les nouveau-nés, *Arch Fr Pediatr* 25:241, 1968.

Whitley CB, Gorlin RJ: Achondrogenesis: New nosology with evidence of genetic heterogeneity, *Radiology* 148:693, 1983.

Borochowitz Z, et al: Achondrogenesis type I—further heterogeneity, *J Pediatr* 112:23, 1988.

Freisinger P, et al: Achondrogenesis type IB (Fraccaro): Study of collagen in the tissue and in chondrocytes cultured in agarose, *Am J Med Genet* 49:439, 1994.

Superti-Furga A: Achondrogenesis type 1B, *J Med Genet* 33:957, 1996.

Superti-Furga A et al: Achondrogenesis type IB is caused by mutations in the diastrophic dysplasia sulfate transporter gene, *Nat Genet* 2:100, 1996.

Karniski LP: Mutations in the diastrophic dysplasia sulfate transporter (DTDST) gene: Correlation between sulfate transport activity and chondrodysplasia phenotype, *Hum Mol Genet* 10:1485, 2001.

Smits P, et al: Lethal skeletal dysplasia in mice and humans lacking the Golgin GMAP-210, *N Eng J Med* 362:206, 2010.

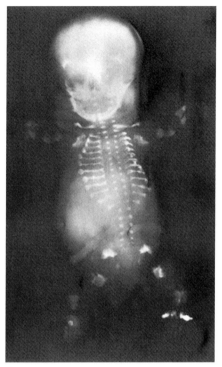

A

K

Type	Achondrogenesis IA	Achondrogenesis IB
Skull	Poorly ossified	Poorly ossified
Ribs	Short and fractured	Short, no fractures, cupped ends
Spine	Completely unossified	Posterior pedicles only
Illium	Arched	Crenated
Ischium	*Ossified-hypoplastic	Unossified
Femur	Wedged with metaph. spike	Trapezoid
Tibia	Short with	Crenated
Fibula	metaph. flare	Unossified
	*Unossified 30 weeks' gestation	

B

FIGURE 1.   **A,** Stillborn infant at 30 weeks' gestation with achondrogenesis type IA. **B,** Radiographic features that differentiate type IA from type IB are delineated on the drawings. (**A** and **B,** Courtesy Dr. R. Lachman, Harbor-UCLA Medical Center, and Dr. D. L. Rimoin, Cedars-Sinai Medical Center, Los Angeles.)

TYPE II ACHONDROGENESIS-HYPOCHONDROGENESIS
(LANGER-SALDINO ACHONDROGENESIS, HYPOCHONDROGENESIS)

Initially described by Langer and colleagues and Saldino, this early lethal disorder has been more completely delineated by Chen and colleagues and Borochowitz and colleagues.

ABNORMALITIES

Growth. Extremely short stature (27 to 36 cm).
Craniofacial. Large calvarium with large anterior and posterior fontanels, flat nasal bridge, small anteverted nostrils, micrognathia.
Limbs. Short.
Radiographs. Normal cranial ossification; short ribs without fractures; short, broad long bones with disproportionately long fibula and metaphyseal irregularity of distal ulna; variable degrees of failure of ossification of lumbar spine, cervical spine, sacrum, ischial and pubic bones, and calcaneus and talus.
Other. Polyhydramnios.

OCCASIONAL ABNORMALITIES

Cleft soft palate, microtia, postaxial polydactyly of feet, cystic hygroma, hydrops, diverticulosis of proximal small bowel, atrial septal defect, atrioventricular canal defect.

NATURAL HISTORY

Although one child survived to 3 months, the majority are stillborn or die in the first few hours of life from pulmonary hypoplasia.

ETIOLOGY

The vast majority of cases are sporadic. Molecular studies have documented mutations of *COL2A1*, the gene encoding type II collagen. In all cases where mutations have been identified, they have been heterozygous, indicating an autosomal dominant mode of inheritance. A number of examples of more than one affected child in a family born to unaffected parents have been reported and are felt to be the result of germline mosaicism. Mutations in the gene for type II collagen result in distinct clinical disorders known as type II collagenopathies, with a clinical spectrum ranging from mild to perinatal lethal, including Stickler syndrome, spondyloepimetaphyseal dysplasia, Strudwick type, Kniest dysplasia, spondyloepiphyseal dysplasia congenita, and type II achondrogenesis-hypochondrogenesis.

COMMENT

Hypochondrogenesis, previously thought to be a distinct disorder, and achondrogenesis type II represent a spectrum of the same disorder referred to as type II achondrogenesis-hypochondrogenesis. Patients with the most severe radiographic and pathologic features have been labeled achondrogenesis type II, while those with less severe, although similar features, hypochondrogenesis.

References

Langer LO, et al: Thanatophoric dwarfism: A condition confused with achondroplasia in the neonate, with brief comments on achondrogenesis and homozygous achondroplasia, *Radiology* 92:285, 1969.

Saldino RM: Lethal short-limbed dwarfism: Achondrogenesis and thanatophoric dwarfism, *Am J Roentgenol Radium Ther Nucl Med* 112:185, 1971.

Chen H, Lin CT, Yang SS: Achondrogenesis: A review with special consideration of achondrogenesis type II (Langer-Saldino), *Am J Med Genet* 10:379, 1981.

Borochowitz Z, et al: Achondrogenesis II-hypochondrogenesis: Variability versus heterogeneity, *Am J Med Genet* 24:273, 1986.

Godfrey M, Hollister DW: Type II achondrogenesis-hypochondrogenesis: Identification of abnormal type II collagen, *Am J Hum Genet* 43:904, 1988.

Horton WA: Characterization of a type II collagen gene (COL2A1) mutation identified in cultured chondrocytes from human hypochondrogenesis, *Proc Natl Acad Sci U S A* 89:4583, 1992.

Wainwright H, Beighton P: Visceral manifestations of hypochondrogenesis, *Virchows Arch* 453:203, 2008.

Nagendran S, et al: Somatic mosaicism and the phenotypic expression of COL2A1 mutations, *Am J Med Genet* 158:1204, 2012.

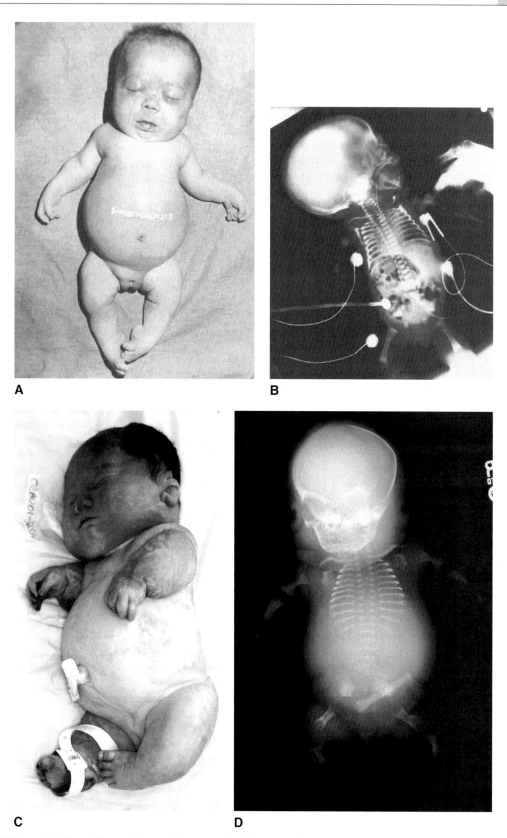

FIGURE 1.   A–D, Two stillborn infants with type II achondrogenesis-hypochondrogenesis, showing the variation in severity of the disorder. Note the relatively normal cranial ossification, short ribs, and variable degrees of failure of ossification of lumbar and cervical spines, sacrum, and ischial and pubic bones. (**A** and **B,** Courtesy Dr. R. Lachman, Harbor-UCLA Medical Center, and Dr. D. L. Rimoin, Cedars-Sinai Medical Center, Los Angeles; **C** and **D,** courtesy Dr. Lynne M. Bird, Children's Hospital, San Diego.)

FIBROCHONDROGENESIS

Lazzaroni-Fossati described a patient with this early lethal disorder in 1978. Subsequently, approximately 13 additional patients have been reported. A distinctive fibrosis of the growth-plate cartilage led to the designation fibrochondrogenesis.

ABNORMALITIES

Growth. Short stature.

Craniofacial. Widely patent anterior fontanel, coronal and sagittal sutures; protuberant eyes with large corneae; hypoplastic nose with flat nasal bridge and anteverted nares; long philtrum; small mouth; cleft palate; short neck; low-set, malformed ears.

Trunk. Flattened vertebrae with posterior vertebral hypoplasia and a sagittal midline cleft; short, thin ribs with anterior and posterior cupping; long, thin clavicles; small chest; small/elevated scapula.

Limbs. Rhizomelic shortening; small hands and feet; camptodactyly; fifth-finger clinodactyly; hypoplastic finger and toenails; short, dumbbell-shaped long bones with broad, irregular metaphyses; prominent metaphyseal spurs adjacent to growth plates; short fibulae.

Pelvis. Hypoplastic with ovoid ilia, irregular flattened acetabula with medial spikes and narrow sacrosciatic notches; broad, hypoplastic ischii.

Other. Omphalocele, hydrops.

NATURAL HISTORY

The vast majority of affected individuals have been stillborn or have died in the neonatal period.

ETIOLOGY

There are both autosomal dominant and autosomal recessive forms of this disorder. Mutations in the gene encoding the proa1(XI) chain of type XI collagen, *COL11A1,* are responsible for the recessively inherited mutations, and mutations in the gene encoding the proa2 (XI) chain of type XI collagen, *COL11A2,* are responsible for the dominantly inherited mutations.

COMMENT

Microscopic examination of long bones demonstrates gross disorganization of growth plate cartilage, fibrous appearance of the matrix, and normal metaphyseal and diaphyseal bone formation.

References

Lazzaroni-Fossati F, et al: La fibrochondrogenese, *Arch Fr Pediatr* 35:1096, 1978.

Eteson DJ, et al: Fibrochondrogenesis: Radiologic and histologic studies, *Am J Med Genet* 19:277, 1984.

Whitely CB, et al: Fibrochondrogenesis: Lethal, autosomal recessive chondrodysplasia with distinctive cartilage histopathology, *Am J Med Genet* 19:265, 1984.

Bankier A, et al: Fibrochondrogenesis in male twins at 24 weeks gestation, *Am J Med Genet* 38:95, 1991.

Al-Gazali LI, et al: Fibrochondrogenesis: Clinical and radiological features, *Clin Dysmorphol* 6:157, 1997.

Al-Gazali LI, et al: Recurrence of fibrochondrogenesis in a consanguineous family, *Clin Dysmorphol* 8:59, 1999.

Thompson SW, et al: Fibrochondrogenesis results from mutations in the COL11A1 type XI collagen gene, *Am J Hum Genet* 87:708, 2010.

Thompson SW, et al: Dominant and recessive forms of fibrochondrogenesis resulting from mutations at a second locus, COL11A2, *Am J Med Genet* 158:309, 2012

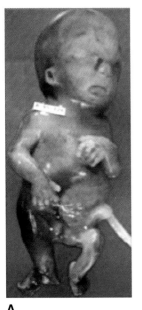

A

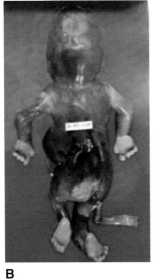

B

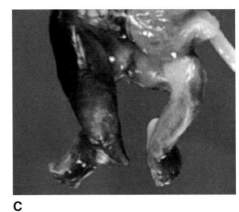

C

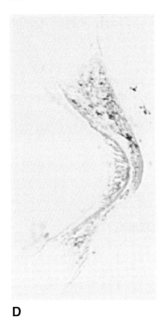

D

K

FIGURE 1. A fetus with boomerang dysplasia. Note full forehead, hypertelorism, markedly depressed nasal bridge and hypoplastic nasal septum, micrognathia, short neck, and omphalocele (A and B), extremely incurved tibia (C). Histologically, the tibia is the single bone in the middle segment of the lower limb and shows delayed ossification, with a central fibrocartilaginous area with a boomerang shape seen with trichromic stain (D). (Courtesy Prof. Nuria Torán, Hospital Vall d'Hebron, Barcelona.)

SHORT RIB–POLYDACTYLY SYNDROMES

The short rib–polydactyly syndromes (SRPs) represent a group of conditions belonging to the ciliopathies. Primary cilia play an important role in transduction of signals in the hedgehog pathway that is of critical importance in skeletal development. The eight disorders belonging to this group are SRP I (Saldino-Noonan type), SRP II (Majewski type), SRP III (Verma-Naumoff type), SRP IV (Beemer-Langer type), Jeune thoracic dystrophy, Ellis–van Creveld (EvC) syndrome, Sensenbrenner syndrome, and Weyer acrofacial dyostosis. Weyer acrofacial dysostosis is not covered in this book. All of the SRPs are autosomal recessive lethal conditions. Death from respiratory insufficiency secondary to pulmonary hypoplasia has occurred in all infants in the first few days of life.

SRP TYPE I

ABNORMALITIES

Growth. Short stature.

Limbs. Short; postaxial polydactyly of hands or feet; syndactyly; metaphyseal irregularities of long bones, with spurs extending longitudinally from medial and lateral segments; underossified phalanges.

Trunk. Short, horizontal ribs; notch-like ossification defects around periphery of vertebral bodies.

Pelvis. Small iliac bones with horizontal acetabular roof, triangular ossification defect above lateral aspect of acetabulum.

Other. Cardiac defects, including transposition of great vessels, double-outlet left ventricle, double-outlet right ventricle, endocardial cushion defect, and hypoplastic right heart; polycystic kidneys; hypoplasia of penis; defects of cloacal development; imperforate anus.

OCCASIONAL ABNORMALITIES

Natal teeth, preaxial polydactyly, sex-reversal (phenotypic females with a 46XY karyotype).

ETIOLOGY

This disorder has an autosomal recessive inheritance pattern. The causative gene has not been identified.

SRP TYPE II

ABNORMALITIES

Growth. Short stature with disproportionately short limbs.

Craniofacial. Midline cleft lip; cleft palate; short, flat nose; low-set, small, malformed ears.

Limbs. Both preaxial and postaxial polysyndactyly of hands or feet; brachydactyly; disproportionately short, oval-shaped tibiae; short, rounded metacarpals and metatarsals; premature ossification of proximal epiphyses of humeri, femora, and lateral cuboids; underossified phalanges.

Trunk. Narrow thorax; short, horizontal ribs; high clavicles.

Other. Ambiguous genitalia; hypoplasia of epiglottis and larynx; multiple glomerular cysts and focal dilatation of distal tubules of kidney.

OCCASIONAL ABNORMALITIES

Microglossia; lobulated tongue; absent gallbladder; brain anomalies, including pachygyria, a small vermis, and absence of olfactory bulbs; persisting left superior vena cava; hydrops; polyhydramnios.

ETIOLOGY

This disorder has an autosomal recessive inheritance pattern. Mutations in *NEK1* and *DYNC2H1* are both responsible for SRP type II. *NEK1* encodes a protein that functions in DNA-double strand repair, neuronal development, and coordination of cell-cycle-associated ciliogenesis. *DYNC2H1* encodes a cytoplasmic dynein protein involved in retrograde transport in the cilia and functions in intraflagellar transport. Mutations in *DYNC2H1* are also responsible for Jeune thoracic dystrophy.

SRP TYPE III

ABNORMALITIES

Growth. Short stature.

Limbs. Short, bowed femora and humeri with cortical thickening of inner midshaft; metaphyses are broad and cupped with osseous spurs projecting laterally in femora, humeri, and phalanges.

Trunk. Narrow and cylindrical with short, horizontal ribs; normally structured vertebral bodies although pedicles of the vertebral arches appear plump; scapulae are square.

Pelvis. Small, square-shaped iliac bones.

Other. Anomalies of heart, intestine, genitalia, liver, and pancreas.

OCCASIONAL ABNORMALITIES
Postaxial polydactyly.

ETIOLOGY
This disorder has an autosomal recessive inheritance pattern. Mutations in *IFT80* and *DYNC2H1* are responsible. *IFT80* encodes a protein that is important in intraflagellar transport and is essential for the development and maintenance of motile and sensory cilia. *DYNC2H1* encodes a cytoplasmic dynein protein involved in retrograde transport in the cilia and functions in intraflagellar transport. Mutations in both of these genes have been identified in Jeune thoracic dystrophy, suggesting that they are variants of the same condition.

SRP TYPE IV

ABNORMALITIES

Growth. Short stature.

Limbs. Short, with smooth metaphyseal margins; nonovoid tibia; tibial bones longer than fibular bones; bowed radius and ulna.

Trunk. Narrow and cylindrical with short, horizontal ribs; high clavicles; small scapulae.

Pelvis. Small ilia.

Other. Anomalies of cardiovascular system, intestinal malrotation, multicystic pancreas, accessory spleen, omphalocele.

OCCASIONAL ABNORMALITIES
Ocular hypertelorism, retinal coloboma, lobulated tongue, midline cleft lip and palate, micropenis, multicystic kidneys, polymicrogyria, corpus callosum agenesis, hydrocephaly, cerebellar hypoplasia, hamartoma of hypothalamus.

ETIOLOGY
This disorder has an autosomal recessive pattern of inheritance. The causative gene has not been identified.

K

References

Majewski F, et al: Polysyndaktylie, verkürzte Gliedmassen und Genitalfehlbildungen: Kennzeichen eines selbständigen Syndroms? *Z Kinderheilkd* 111:118, 1971.

Saldino RM, Noonan CD: Severe thoracic dystrophy with striking micromelia, abnormal osseous development, including the spine, and multiple visceral anomalies, *Am J Roentgenol Radium Ther Nucl Med* 114:257, 1972.

Spranger J, et al: Short rib-polydactyly (SRP) syndromes, types Majewski and Saldino-Noonan, *Z Kinderheilkd* 116:73, 1974.

Naumoff P, et al: Short rib-polydactyly syndrome type 3, *Radiology* 122:443, 1977.

Beemer FA, et al: A new short rib syndrome: Report of two cases, *Am J Med Genet* 14:115, 1983.

Dagoneau N, et al: *DYNC2H1* mutations cause asphyxiating thoracic dystrophy and short rib-polydactyly syndrome type III, *Am J Hum Genet* 84:706, 2009.

Cavalcanti DP, et al: Mutation in *IFT80* in a fetus with the phenotype of Verma-Naumoff provides molecular evidence for the Jeune-Verma-Naumoff dysplasia spectrum, *J Med Genet* 48:653, 2011.

Thiel C, et al: *NEK1* mutations cause short-rib polydactyly syndrome type Majewski, *Am J Hum Genet* 88:106, 2011.

Huber C, Cormier-Daire V: Ciliary disorder of the skeleton, *Am J Med Genet C Semin Med Genet* 160C:165, 2012.

Hokayem JE, et al: *NEK1* and *DYNC2H1* are both involved in short rib polydactyly Majewski type but not in Beemer-Langer cases, *J Med Genet* 49:227, 2012.

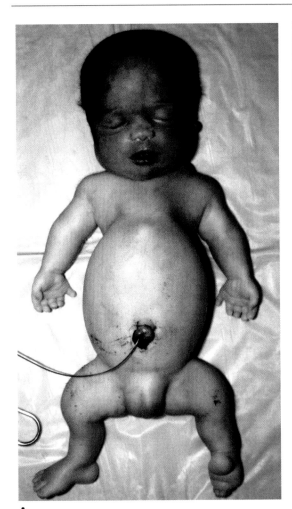

A

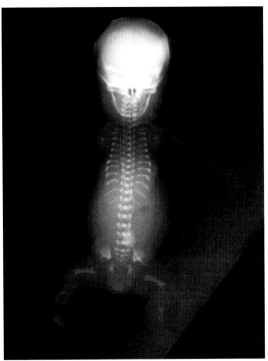

B

K

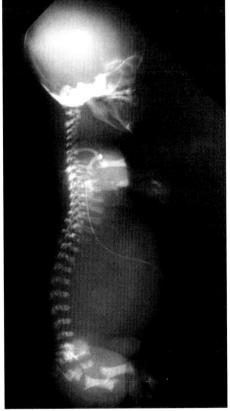

C

FIGURE 1.   Short rib–polydactyly syndrome, Saldino-Noonan type. **A,** Stillborn male infant. Note the narrow thorax, short limbs, postaxial polydactyly, and hypoplastic penis. **B** and **C,** Radiographs show short, horizontal ribs; metaphyseal irregularities of long bones, with spurs extending from medial and lateral segments; and triangular ossification defects above lateral aspect of acetabulum.

THANATOPHORIC DYSPLASIA
Short Limbs, Flat Vertebrae, Large Cranium with Low Nasal Bridge

Maroteaux and colleagues set forth this disorder in 1967 and used the Greek term *thanatophoric* ("death-bringing") to emphasize that such patients usually die shortly after birth. Langer and colleagues separated this condition into two types. Type I (TDI) is most common and is characterized by curved long bones (most obviously the femora), and very flat vertebral bodies (35% or less of the adjacent disk space in the lumbar region). Type II (TDII) is characterized by straight femora and taller vertebral bodies. Almost all cases of thanatophoric dysplasia with a severe cloverleaf skull (the kleeblattschädel anomaly) are TDII.

ABNORMALITIES

Central Nervous System. Severe abnormalities, the most common of which is temporal lobe dysplasia; other defects include megalencephaly, hydrocephalus, encephalocele; brainstem hypoplasia, maldevelopment of inferior olivary and cerebellar dentate nuclei; hypotonia; severe intellectual disability in the few survivors.

Growth. Severe growth deficiency; 36 to 46 cm tall, with an average of 40 cm.

Craniofacial. Large cranium and fontanel; 36 to 47 cm, average of 37 cm; small foramen magnum and short base of skull, with full forehead, low nasal bridge, bulging eyes, and small facies; cloverleaf skull.

Limbs. Short, with small sausage-like fingers, bowed long bones with cupped spur-like irregular flaring of metaphyses, and lack of ossification in secondary centers at knee; fibulae are shorter than tibiae; disorganized chondrocytes and bony trabeculae, especially in central epiphyseal-metaphyseal region.

Thorax. Narrow with short ribs.

Spine. Short, flattened vertebrae with relatively wide intervertebral disk space; lack of caudal widening of spinal canal.

Scapulae. Small and square.

Pelvis. Square and short, with small sciatic notch and medial spurs; accessory ossification centers in the ischia and ilia at gestational age younger than 24 weeks.

OCCASIONAL ABNORMALITIES

Patent ductus arteriosus, atrial septal defect, horseshoe kidney, hydronephrosis, imperforate anus, radioulnar synostosis, soft tissue syndactyly of fingers and toes, acanthosis nigricans in long-term survivors.

NATURAL HISTORY

Feeble fetal activity and polyhydramnios are frequent in this disorder. These patients usually die shortly after birth, partially owing to the small thoracic cage and respiratory insufficiency. Although survival beyond the neonatal period is rare, three affected children (two 9-year-olds and one 10-year-old) have been reported. All had profound developmental delay, severe growth deficiency, and were ventilatory-dependent.

ETIOLOGY

This disorder has an autosomal dominant inheritance pattern. All cases represent fresh gene mutations, and most, if not all, are due to mutations in the fibroblast growth factor receptor 3 (*FGFR3*) gene. All cases with a Lys650Glu substitution had straight femora with craniosynostosis and frequently a cloverleaf skull (TDII). All other mutations were associated with curved femora, and cloverleaf skull was only infrequently present (TDI).

References

Maroteaux P, Lamy M, Robert JM: Le nanisme thanatophore, *Presse Med* 75:2519, 1967.

Giedion A: Thanatophoric dwarfism, *Helv Paediatr Acta* 23:175, 1968.

Goutières F, Aicardi J, Farkas-Bargeton E: Une malformation cérébrale particulière associée au nanisme thanatophore, *Presse Med* 79:960, 1971.

Thompson BH, Parmley TH: Obstetric features of thanatophoric dwarfism, *Am J Obstet Gynecol* 109:396, 1971.

Horton WA, Harris DJ, Collins DL: Discordance for the kleeblattschädel anomaly in monozygotic twins with thanatophoric dysplasia, *Am J Med Genet* 15:97, 1983.

Langer LO, et al: Thanatophoric dysplasia and cloverleaf skull, *Am J Med Genet Suppl* 3:167, 1987.

Knisely AS, Amber MW: Temporal lobe abnormalities in thanatophoric dysplasia, *Pediatr Neurosci* 14:169, 1988.

Martínez-Frías ML, et al: Thanatophoric dysplasia: An autosomal dominant condition? *Am J Med Genet* 31:815, 1988.

MacDonald IM, et al: Growth and development in thanatophoric dysplasia, *Am J Med Genet* 33:508, 1989.

Tavorima PL, et al: Thanatophoric dysplasia (types I and II) caused by distinct mutations in fibroblast growth factor receptor 3, *Nat Genet* 9:321, 1995.

Baker KM, et al: Long-term survival in typical thanatophoric dysplasia type I, *Am J Med Genet* 70:427, 1997.

Wilcox WR, et al: Molecular, radiologic, and histologic correlations in thanatophoric dysplasia, *Am J Med Genet* 78:274, 1998.

Li D, et al: Thanatophoric dysplasia type 2 with encephalocele during the second trimester. *Am J Med Genet* 140:1476, 2006.

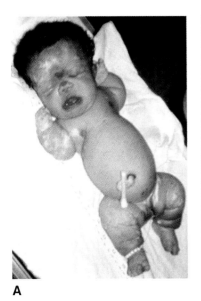
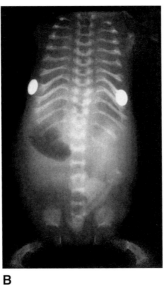

A   **B**

FIGURE 1. Thanatophoric dysplasia type I. **A,** Note the large cranium with full forehead, low nasal bridge, short limbs, narrow thorax. **B,** Note the curved femora and very flat vertebrae.

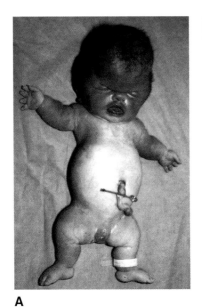

A

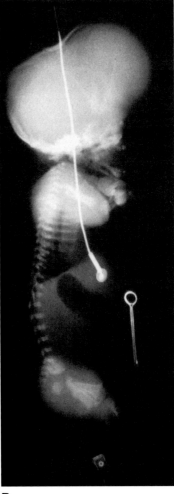

FIGURE 2. Thanatophoric dysplasia type II. **A,** Note the cloverleaf skull in addition to the other features of type I. **B,** Note the straight femora and taller vertebral bodies.

B

K

JEUNE THORACIC DYSTROPHY (ASPHYXIATING THORACIC DYSTROPHY)
Small Thorax, Short Limbs, Hypoplastic Iliac Wings

First described by Jeune and colleagues in 1955, more than 100 cases have now been reported.

ABNORMALITIES

Growth. Short stature (72%).

Skeletal. Infancy: Short horizontal ribs with irregular costochondral junctions and small thoracic cage (95%), hypoplastic iliac wings, horizontal acetabular roofs with spur-like projections at lower margins of sciatic notches, early ossification of capital femoral epiphysis. Childhood: Irregular epiphyses and metaphyses with rhizomelic shortening of limbs (88%), brachydactyly/micromelia (76%); relatively short ulnae and fibulae; cone-shaped epiphyses and early fusion between epiphyses and metaphyses of distal and middle phalanges.

Respiratory. Lung hypoplasia, presumably secondary to the small thoracic cage, is the major cause of death in early infancy.

Renal. Cystic tubular dysplasia or glomerular sclerosis (34%).

Hepatic. Biliary dysgenesis with portal fibrosis and bile duct proliferation (28%).

OCCASIONAL ABNORMALITIES

Polydactyly, usually of hands and feet, notching of distal end of metacarpal and metatarsal bones; lacunar skull; direct hyperbilirubinemia with prolonged jaundice; pancreatic defects, including fibrosis and cysts; Hirschsprung disease; retinal dysplasia/foveal hypoplasia (15%); lobation of the tongue and gingiva; cardiac defects (1.6%) ; abdominal muscle dysplasia; foregut dysmotility and malrotation; situs inversus; intellectual disability; Dandy-Walker complex.

NATURAL HISTORY

Early death, usually the consequence of asphyxia with or without pneumonia, occurs frequently, almost always prior to 2 years of age. Procedures to expand the chest have been successful and should be considered in select cases. For those who survive, progressive improvement in the relative growth of the thoracic cage occurs and there may be only slight to moderate shortness of stature. However, respiratory difficulties occur in all survivors. Chronic nephritis leading to renal failure is a serious potential feature of this disorder occurring in approximately one third of the 30% who have renal abnormalities. Renal insufficiency may be evident by 2 years of age and accounts for most deaths between 3 and 10 years of age. Although infrequent, progressive hepatic dysfunction also occurs and may contribute to the relatively poor long-term prognosis for individuals with this disorder. Survival to the fourth decade has occurred. However, little information is available for affected individuals older than 20 years.

ETIOLOGY

This disorder has an autosomal recessive inheritance pattern. Mutations in *IFT80, DYNC2H,* and *TTC21B* are responsible. *IFT80* encodes a protein that is important in intraflagellar transport and is essential for the development and maintenance of motile and sensory cilia. *DYNC2H1* encodes a cytoplasmic dynein protein involved in retrograde transport in the cilia and functions in intraflagellar transport. *TTC21B* encodes the retrograde intraflagellar transport protein IFT139. Mutations of both *IFT80* and *DYNC2H* have also been identified in short rib–polydactyly type III, suggesting that these two disorders are variants of the same condition.

COMMENT

A follow-up protocol has been proposed. In the first 2 years of life, focus should be on treatment of severe respiratory problems. Laboratory evaluation of urine and blood should be done twice a year and abdominal ultrasound should be performed at 2, 5, 10, and 15 years. Spirometry should be done yearly, and an ophthalmology exam should be performed at 5 and 10 years of age.

References

Jeune M, Beraud C, Carron R: Dystrophie thoracique asphyxiante de caractère familial, *Arch Fr Pediatr* 12:886, 1955.

Pirnar T, Neuhauser EBD: Asphyxiating thoracic dystrophy of the newborn, *Am J Roentgenol Radium Ther Nucl Med* 98:358, 1966.

Herdman RC, Langer LO: The thoracic asphyxiant dystrophy and renal disease, *Am J Dis Child* 116:192, 1968.

Langer LO: Thoracic-pelvic-phalangeal dystrophy, *Radiology* 91:447, 1968.

Friedman JM, Kaplan HG, Hall JG: The Jeune syndrome in an adult, *Am J Med* 59:857, 1975.

Allen AW, et al: Ocular findings in thoracic-pelvic-phalangeal dystrophy, *Arch Ophthalmol* 97:489, 1979.

Shah KJ: Renal lesions in Jeune's syndrome, *Br J Radiol* 53:432, 1980.

Hudgins L, et al: Early cirrhosis in survivors with Jeune thoracic dystrophy, *J Pediatr* 120:754, 1992.

Beals PL, et al: IFT80, which encodes a conserved intraflagellar transport protein, is mutated in Jeune asphyxiating thoracic dystrophy, *Nat Genet* 39:727, 2007.

Dagoneau N, et al: *DYNC2H1* mutations cause asphyxiating thoracic dystrophy and short rib-polydactyly syndrome, type III, *Am J Hum Genet* 84:706, 2009.

de Vries J, et al: Jeune syndrome: Description of 13 cases and a proposal for follow-up protocol, *Eur J Pediatr* 169:77, 2010.

Keppler-Noreuil KM, et al: Clinical insights gained from eight new cases and review of reported cases with Jeune syndrome (asphyxiating thoracic dystrophy), *Am J Med Genet* 155:1021, 2011.

Davis EE, et al: *TTC21B* contributes both causal and modifying alleles across the ciliopathy spectrum, *Nat Genet* 43:189, 2011.

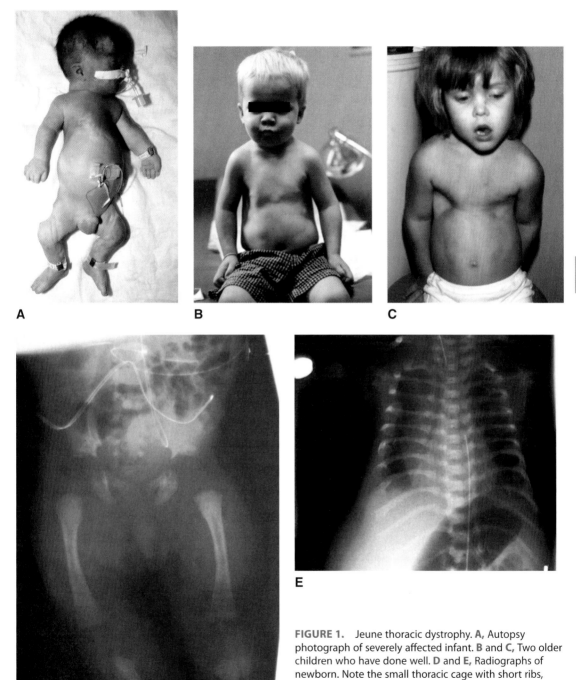

K

FIGURE 1. Jeune thoracic dystrophy. **A,** Autopsy photograph of severely affected infant. **B** and **C,** Two older children who have done well. **D** and **E,** Radiographs of newborn. Note the small thoracic cage with short ribs, hypoplastic iliac wings, and horizontal acetabular roofs with spur-like projections at lower margins of sciatic notches. (**B** and **C,** Courtesy Dr. Bryan Hall, University of Kentucky, Lexington.)

CAMPOMELIC DYSPLASIA
Bowed Tibiae, Hypoplastic Scapulae, Flat Facies

Although reports of this condition appeared in the 1950s by Bound and colleagues and Bain and Barrett, it was not until the 1970s that the syndrome became more broadly recognized by Spranger and colleagues and Maroteaux and colleagues, who used the term *campomélique,* meaning "bent limb," to epitomize the disorder.

ABNORMALITIES

Growth. Prenatal onset of growth deficiency with retarded osseous maturation and large head; birth length, 35 to 49 cm; average occipitofrontal circumference is 37 cm.

Central Nervous System. Tendency toward having large brain with gross cellular disorganization, most evident in cerebral cortex, thalamus, and caudate nucleus; absence or hypoplasia of olfactory tract or bulbs; hydrocephalus.

Facies. Flat-appearing small face with high forehead, anterior frontal hair upsweep, large anterior fontanel, low nasal bridge, micrognathia, cleft palate, short palpebral fissures, and malformed or low-set ears.

Limbs. Anterior bowing of tibiae with skin dimpling over convex area, short fibulae, mild bowing of femora and tibiae, congenital hip dislocation, and talipes equinovarus.

Radiographic. Short and somewhat flat vertebrae, particularly cervical; hypoplastic scapulae, small thoracic cage with slender or decreased number of ribs, kyphoscoliosis, small iliac wings with relatively wide pelvic outlet; absent mineralization of sternum; lack of ossification of proximal tibial and distal femoral epiphysis and talus; short first metacarpal.

Tracheobronchial. Incomplete cartilaginous development with tracheobronchiomalacia.

Genitalia. Sex reversal or ambiguous genitalia in about two thirds of genetic males.

OCCASIONAL ABNORMALITIES

Cardiac defects, renal anomalies, polyhydramnios, hypoplastic cochlea and semicircular canals, anomalies of incus and stapes, hearing loss.

NATURAL HISTORY

The great majority of patients die in the neonatal period from respiratory insufficiency. Although there have been some survivors with normal intelligence, the majority have mild to moderate intellectual disability. At birth the limbs are short with a trunk of normal length, but with development of the kyphoscoliosis, which is progressive, the trunk becomes short relative to the arms. Conductive hearing loss, myopia, dental caries, and recurrent apnea and respiratory problems are complications with advancing age.

ETIOLOGY

Campomelic dysplasia (CD) has an autosomal dominant inheritance pattern, with most cases representing fresh gene mutations. The small number of recurrences are due to gonadal mosaicism. Mutations in *SOX9,* a member of the SRY-related gene family, are responsible for the majority of cases. Acampomelic campomelic dysplasia (ACD) is associated with similar but milder skeletal abnormalities and lacks long bone curvature. Although both CD and ACD can be caused by heterozygous mutations in *SOX9* or chromosomal aberration affecting *SOX9* or the putative enhancer region, the type of mutations and chromosomal aberrations are different. CD is primarily caused by nonsense or frameshift mutations or by chromosomal aberrations disrupting *SOX9.* ACD, on the other hand, is more often caused by missense mutations or by chromosomal aberrations affecting the enhancer region. *SOX9* is involved in both bone formation and control of testes development. It regulates the expression of COL2A1 and is a transcription factor essential for chondrocyte differentiation and formation of cartilage.

References

Bound JP, Finlay HVL, Rose FC: Congenital anterior angulation of the tibia, *Arch Dis Child* 27:179, 1952.

Bain AD, Barrett HS: Congenital bowing of the long bones: Report of a case, *Arch Dis Child* 34:516, 1959.

Spranger J, Langer LO, Maroteaux P: Increasing frequency of a syndrome of multiple osseous defects? *Lancet* 2:716, 1970.

Maroteaux P, et al: Le syndrome campomélique, *Presse Med* 79:1157, 1971.

Hoefnagel D, et al: Campomelic dwarfism, *Lancet* 1:1068, 1972.

Schmickel RD, Heidelberger KP, Poznanski AK: The campomelique syndrome, *J Pediatr* 82:299, 1973.

Hall BD, Spranger JW: Campomelic dysplasia, *Am J Dis Child* 134:285, 1980.

Houston CS, et al: The campomelic syndrome: Review, report of 17 cases, and follow-up on the currently 17-year-old boy first reported by Maroteaux et al in 1971, *Am J Med Genet* 15:3, 1983.

Normann EK, et al: Campomelic dysplasia—an underdiagnosed condition? *Eur J Pediatr* 152:331, 1993.

Foster JW, et al: Campomelic dysplasia and autosomal sex reversal caused by mutations in an SRY-related gene, *Nature* 372:525, 1994.

Mansour S, et al: A clinical and genetic study of campomelic dysplasia, *J Med Genet* 32:415, 1995.

Mansour S, et al: The phenotype of survivors of campomelic dysplasia, *J Med Genet* 39:597, 2002.

Wada Y, et al: Mutation analysis of *SOX9* and single copy number variant analysis of the upstream region in eight patients with campomelic dysplasia and acampomelic campomelic dysplasia, *Am J Med Genet* 149: 2882, 2009.

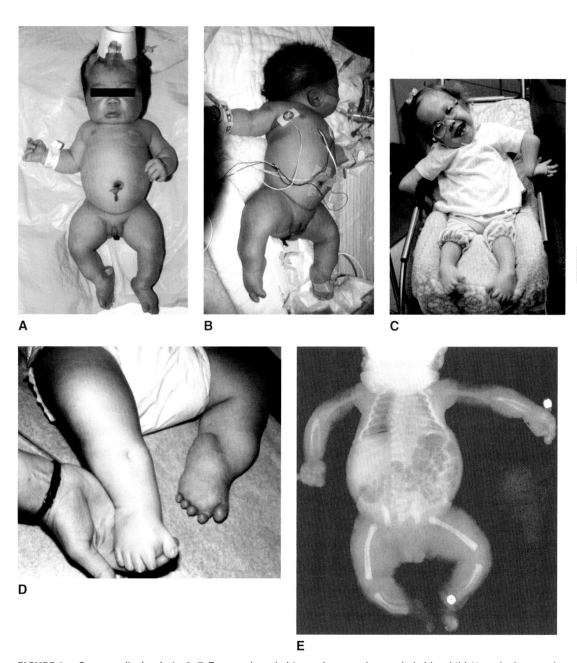

FIGURE 1. Campomelic dysplasia. **A–E,** Two newborn babies and a severely retarded older child. Note the low nasal bridge, micrognathia, small thorax, aberrant hand positioning, and bowed tibiae with dimples at the maximal point of bowing. Roentgenogram shows the slim, poorly developed bones and osseous immaturity (knee and foot). (**C** and **D,** Courtesy Dr. Bryan Hall, University of Kentucky, Lexington; **E,** from Hoefnagel D et al: *Lancet* 1:1068, 1972, with permission. Copyrighted by The Lancet Ltd., 1972.)

ACHONDROPLASIA
Short Limbs, Low Nasal Bridge, Caudal Narrowing of Spinal Canal

The most common chondrodysplasia, true achondroplasia, occurs with a frequency of approximately 1 in 15,000.

ABNORMALITIES

Growth. Small stature, mean adult height in males is 131 ± 5.6 cm and in females is 124 ± 5.9 cm.

Craniofacial. Megalocephaly, small foramen magnum, short cranial base with early spheno-occipital closure, low nasal bridge with prominent forehead, mild midfacial hypoplasia with narrow nasal passages.

Skeletal. Small cuboid-shaped vertebral bodies with short pedicles and progressive narrowing of lumbar interpedicular distance; lumbar lordosis, mild thoracolumbar kyphosis with anterior beaking of first or second lumbar vertebra; small iliac wings with narrow greater sciatic notch; short tubular bones, especially humeri; metaphyseal flare with ball-and-socket arrangement of epiphysis to metaphysis; short trident hand, fingers being similar in length, with short proximal and midphalanges; short femoral neck; incomplete extension of elbow.

Other. Mild hypotonia; early motor progress is often slow, although eventual intelligence is usually normal; relative glucose intolerance evident with an oral glucose tolerance test.

OCCASIONAL ABNORMALITIES

Hydrocephalus, spinal cord or root compression; pulmonary hypertension, synostosis of multiple sutures.

NATURAL HISTORY

Macrocephaly may represent mild hydrocephaly relating to a small foramen magnum. Therefore, ultrasound studies of the brain should be performed if the fontanel size is particularly large, the occipitofrontal circumference increases too rapidly, head circumference above the 95th percentile, or any symptoms of hydrocephalus develop. Respiratory problems secondary to a small chest, upper airway obstruction, and sleep-disordered breathing are common. Cervical cord compression occurs frequently. Indications for decompression include lower limb hyper-reflexia, central apnea, and foramen magnum measurements below the mean for achondroplasia. Computed tomography dimensions for the foramen magnum of children with achondroplasia have been established by Hecht and colleagues. It is important to recognize that evaluation of affected children with symptoms relating to cervical cord compression should be performed by individuals experienced with, and aware of, the natural history of achondroplasia. Osteotomies for severe bowlegs are usually deferred until full growth has occurred. By discouraging the sitting position or other positions that cause the trunk to curve anteriorly until an age when good trunk strength has developed, a permanent gibbus or kyphosis, which is due to anterior wedging of the first two lumbar vertebrae, can be prevented as well as obviating many of the problems with spinal stenosis and spinal cord compression that are so debilitating to adults with this condition. Exercises may also be used in an attempt to flatten the lumbosacral curve. Relative overgrowth of the fibula may accentuate bowing and require early stapling. Short eustachian tubes may lead to middle ear infection and conductive hearing loss. Tympanic membrane tubes may be indicated. Verbal comprehension is frequently impaired. Sleep-related respiratory disturbances, primarily hypoxemia, is common. The mandibular teeth may become crowded, possibly requiring removal of one or more. Todorov and colleagues developed a screening test that establishes normal milestones for children with achondroplasia up to 2 years of age. Some degree of developmental delay, primarily motor, is common, as is a decrease in IQ score compared with siblings. There is a tendency toward late childhood obesity, and females are more prone to have menorrhagia, fibroids, and large breasts. Complications from spinal stenosis increase in adults. By 10 years of age, a significant number of affected children have developed neurologic symptoms with claudication and increased reflexes in their legs. There is no clear evidence of long-term benefit from growth hormone therapy. Surgical leg lengthening is controversial because of the need for repeated surgeries, the long period of time that orthopedic appliances must be used, superficial infections, and the stretching of nonskeletal tissues. The average life expectancy is decreased by 15 years.

ETIOLOGY

This disorder has an autosomal dominant inheritance pattern; approximately 90% of the cases represent a fresh gene mutation. Older paternal age has been a contributing factor in these cases. Because of gonadal mosaicism, there is a 0.2% recurrence risk for siblings of achondroplastic children with unaffected parents. Mutations in the gene encoding fibroblast growth factor receptor 3 (*FGFR3*), located at 4p16.3, have been documented in all cases reported to date. Interestingly, virtually all cases demonstrate the same single base pair substitution, possibly accounting for the consistency of the phenotype seen in this disorder.

COMMENT

Health Supervision Guidelines for Children with Achondroplasia have been established by the American Academy of Pediatrics.

References

Maroteaux P, Lamy M: Achondroplasia in man and animals, *Clin Orthop* 33:91, 1964.

Caffey J: *Pediatric X-Ray Diagnosis*, ed 5, Chicago, 1967, Year Book Medical Publishers.

Cohen ME, Rosenthal AD, Matson DD: Neurological abnormalities in achondroplastic children, *J Pediatr* 71:367, 1967.

Nelson MA: Spinal stenosis in achondroplasia, *Proc R Soc Med* 65:1028, 1972.

Horton WA, et al: Standard growth curves for achondroplasia, *J Pediatr* 93:435, 1978.

Oberklaid F, et al: Achondroplasia and hypochondroplasia, *J Med Genet* 16:140, 1979.

Todorov AB, et al: Developmental screening tests in achondroplastic children, *Am J Med Genet* 9:19, 1981.

Hall JG, et al: Letter to the editor. Head growth in achondroplasia: Use of ultrasound studies, *Am J Med Genet* 13:105, 1982.

Stokes DC, et al: Respiratory complications of achondroplasia, *J Pediatr* 102:534, 1983.

Hecht JT, et al: Computerized tomography of the foramen magnum: Achondroplastic values compared to normal standards, *Am J Med Genet* 20:355, 1985.

Reid CS, et al: Cervicomedullary compression in young patients with achondroplasia: Value of comprehensive neurologic and respiratory evaluation, *J Pediatr* 110:522, 1987.

Hall JG: Kyphosis in achondroplasia: Probably preventable, *J Pediatr* 112:166, 1988.

Brinkman G, et al: Cognitive skills in achondroplasia, *Am J Med Genet* 47:800, 1993.

Shiang R, et al: Mutations in the transmembrane domain of *FGFR3* cause the most common genetic form of dwarfism, achondroplasia, *Cell* 78:335, 1994.

Pauli RM, et al: Prospective assessment of risk for cervicomedullary junction compression in infants with achondroplasia, *Am J Hum Genet* 56:732, 1995.

Rimoin DL: Invited editorial. Cervicomedullary junction compression in infants with achondroplasia: When to perform neurosurgical decompression, *Am J Hum Genet* 56:824, 1995.

Hunter AGW, et al: Medical complications of achondroplasia: A multicentre patient review, *J Med Genet* 35:705, 1998.

Mettler G, Fraser FC: Recurrence risk for sibs of children with "sporadic" achondroplasia, *Am J Med Genet* 90:250, 2000.

Trotter TL, et al: Health supervision for children with achondroplasia, *Pediatrics* 116:771, 2005.

Horton EA, et al: Achondroplasia, *Lancet* 370:162, 2007.

Georgoulis G, et al: Achondroplasia with synostosis of multiple sutures, *Am J Med Genet* 155:1969, 2011.

Ireland PJ, et al: Development of children with achondroplasia: A prospective clinical cohort study, *Dev Med Child Neurol* 54:532, 2012.

K

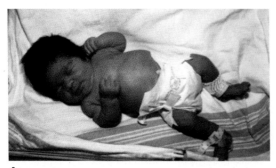

A

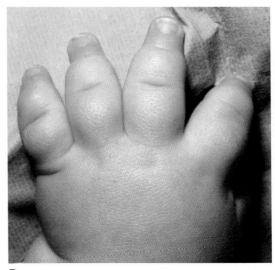

B

FIGURE 1.   Achondroplasia. **A,** Newborn infant with achondroplasia, showing macrocephaly, low nasal bridge, relatively small thoracic cage, shortness of humeri and femora (rhizomelia). (Courtesy Dr. Lynne M. Bird, Children's Hospital, San Diego.) **B,** "Trident" position of the open, small hand.

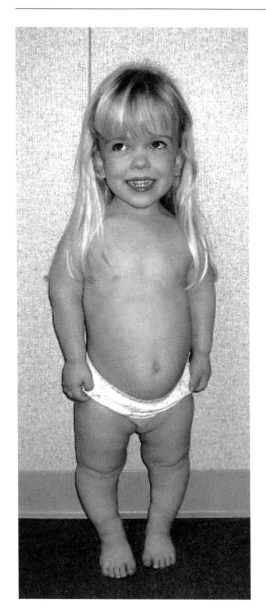

FIGURE 2. Photograph of a 1-year-old girl showing relative macrocephaly, small thoracic cage, and rhizomelic shortening. (Courtesy Dr. Stephen Braddock, St. Louis University.)

K

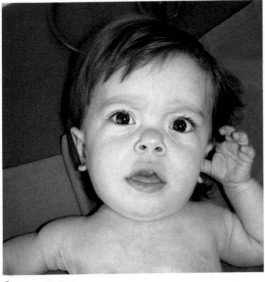

A

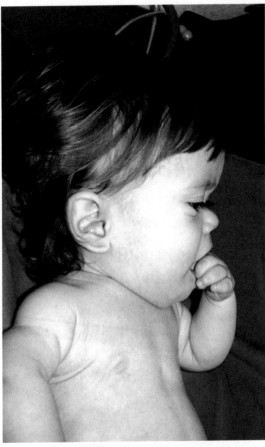

B

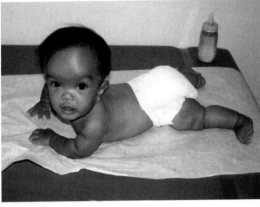

C

FIGURE 3.   A–C, Two affected 6-month-old children.
Note low nasal bridge, relative macrocephaly with
prominent forehead, and midface hypoplasia. (Courtesy
Dr. Lynne M. Bird, Children's Hospital, San Diego.)

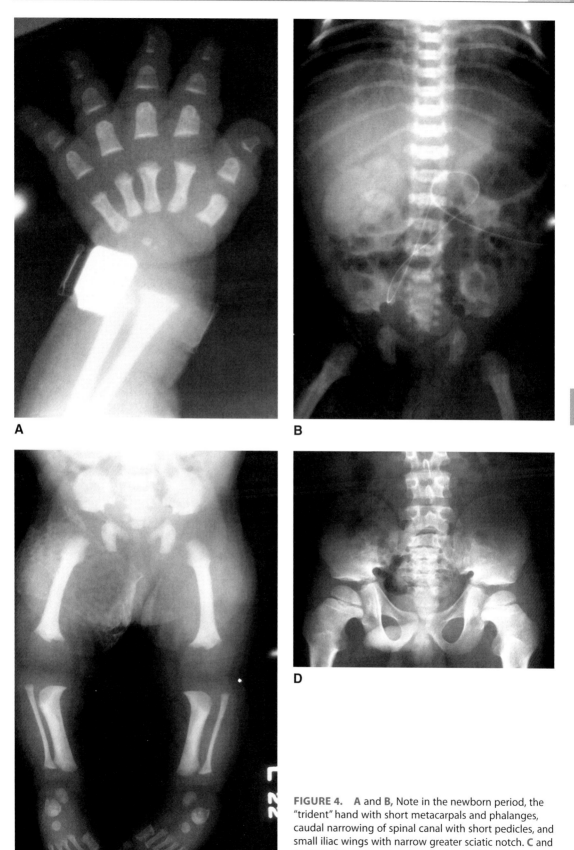

A

B

C

D

K

FIGURE 4. **A** and **B,** Note in the newborn period, the "trident" hand with short metacarpals and phalanges, caudal narrowing of spinal canal with short pedicles, and small iliac wings with narrow greater sciatic notch. **C** and **D,** Note the progressive changes in an older child and an adult.

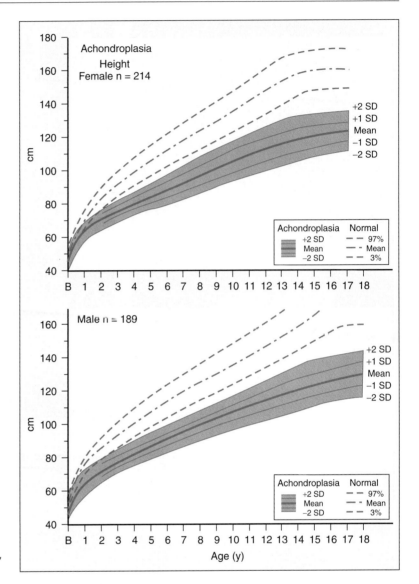

FIGURE 5.   Note that approximately one half of the newborn babies with achondroplasia are within normal limits for length at birth, but there is a progressive deceleration of growth rate beginning in infancy. (From Horton WA et al: *J Pediatr* 93:435, 1978, with permission.)

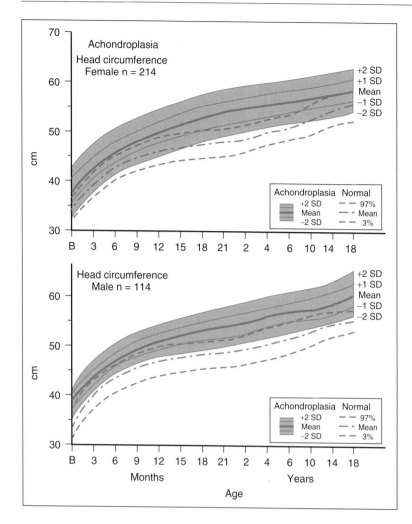

FIGURE 6. Macrocephaly, predominantly caused by a large brain, is a usual feature of individuals with achondroplasia. (From Horton WA et al: *J Pediatr* 93:435, 1978, with permission.)

K

HYPOCHONDROPLASIA
Short Limbs, Caudal Narrowing of Spine, Near-Normal Craniofacial

Although the features of this disorder were described by Ravenna in 1913, and its designation as hypochondroplasia and mode of inheritance were set forth in 1924, the majority of cases have been misdiagnosed as achondroplasia until recently.

Hypochondroplasia has an incidence of approximately one twelfth that of achondroplasia and can be distinguished from it by the relative lack of craniofacial involvement and milder features in the hands and spine.

ABNORMALITIES

Growth. Small stature, usually of postnatal onset; mean birth length, 47.7 cm; mean birth weight, 2.9 kg; macrocephaly.

Limbs. Relatively short without rhizomelic, mesomelic, or acromelic predominance; short tubular bones with mild metaphyseal flare; short, broad femoral necks; long distal fibulae, short distal ulnae, and long ulnar styloids; brachydactyly; bowing of legs; stubby hands and feet; mild limitation in elbow extension and supination.

Spine. Anteroposterior shortening of lumbar pedicles on lateral view; spinal canal narrowing or unchanged caudally, with or without lumbar lordosis.

Pelvis. Squared and short ilia.

OCCASIONAL ABNORMALITIES

Intellectual disability, bilateral dysgenesis of the medial temporal lobe structures, brachycephaly with short base of skull, mild frontal bossing, esotropia, cataract, ptosis, postaxial polydactyly of feet, high vertebrae, flat vertebrae, acanthosis nigricans.

NATURAL HISTORY

Slow growth, if not evident by birth, is usually obvious by 3 years of age. Final height attainment in adults ranges from 118 to 152 cm. Outward bowing of the lower limbs and genu varum may become pronounced with weight-bearing. Although this may improve in childhood, the condition may merit surgical straightening. The relatively long fibulae can result in inversion of the feet. Exercise may provoke mild aching in the knees, ankles, or elbows during childhood, and such discomfort is usually worse and may include the low back in the adult. Cesarean section is often required for delivery in pregnant women with this disorder. Improved growth and reduced body disproportion have been reported following growth hormone treatment in children with the N540K mutation in *FGFR3*. Intellectual disability, a rare feature in achondroplasia, was noted in 4 of the 13 cases reported in one study, with IQs ranging from 50 to 80, and in 9% of the patients reported by Hall and Spranger.

ETIOLOGY

This disorder has an autosomal dominant inheritance pattern. Older paternal age has been documented in presumed fresh mutation cases. Approximately 50% of affected patients carry an N540K mutation in the fibroblast growth factor receptor 3 (FGFR3) gene located at 4p16.3.

COMMENT

In contrast to achondroplasia, hypochondroplasia is clinically and genetically heterogeneous. Patients with the N540K mutation have a more severe phenotype associated with disproportionate short stature, macrocephaly, and with radiologic evidence of unchanged/narrow interpedicular distance and fibula longer than tibia. In contrast, patients with hypochondroplasia unlinked to chromosome 4p16.3 have milder radiologic anomalies with normal hand and long bones and no metaphyseal flaring.

References

Ravenna F: Achondroplasie et chondrohypoplasie: Contribution clinique, *N Iconog Salpêtrière* 26:157, 1913.

Léri A, Linossier (Mlle): Hypochondroplasia héréditaire, *Bull Mem Soc Med Hop (Paris)* 48:1780, 1924.

Beals RK: Hypochondroplasia: A report of five kindred, *J Bone Joint Surg Am* 51:728, 1969.

Walker BA, et al: Hypochondroplasia, *Am J Dis Child* 122:95, 1971.

Hall BD, Spranger J: Hypochondroplasia: Clinical and radiological aspects in 39 cases, *Radiology* 133:95, 1979.

Bellus GA, et al: A recurrent mutation in the tyrosine kinase domain of fibroblast growth factor receptor 3 causes hypochondroplasia, *Nat Genet* 10:357, 1995.

Prinster C, et al: Diagnosis of hypochondroplasia: The role of radiological interpretation, *Pediatr Radiol* 31:203, 2001.

Alatzoglou KS, et al: Acanthosis nigricans and insulin insensitivity in patients with achondroplasia and hypochondroplasia due to *FGFR3* mutations, *J Clin Endocrinol Metab* 94:3959, 2009.

Rothenbuhler A, et al: A pilot study of discontinuous, insulin-like growth factor 1-dosing growth hormone treatment in young children with FGFR3 N540K-mutated hypochondroplasia, *J Pediatr* 160:849, 2012.

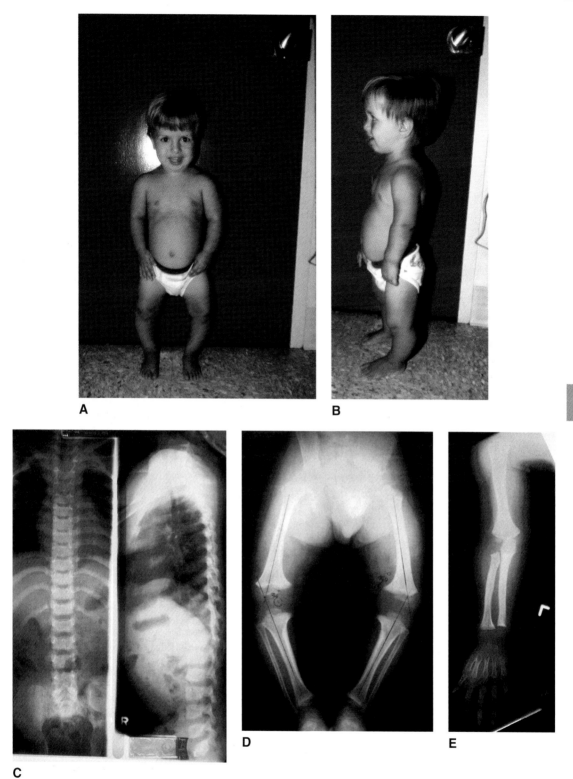

FIGURE 1.   Hypochondroplasia. **A** and **B,** A 2½-year-old boy showing short stature, short arms with mild limitation in elbow extension, bowed legs, and relative macrocephaly. **C–E,** Radiographs of the same child at 2½ years of age. Note the anterior-posterior shortening of lumbar pedicles on lateral view and mild degree of caudal narrowing of the spinal canal (**C**) and the relatively short tubular bones with mild metaphyseal flare, short, broad femoral necks, long distal fibula, and short distal ulna (**D** and **E**).

PSEUDOACHONDROPLASIA
(PSEUDOACHONDROPLASTIC SPONDYLOEPIPHYSEAL DYSPLASIA)
Small Irregular Epiphyses, Irregular Mushroomed Metaphyses, Flattening or Anterior Beaking of Vertebrae, Normal Craniofacial Appearance

Maroteaux and Lamy described three individuals with this pattern of altered bone morphogenesis in 1959. Numerous cases have been published.

ABNORMALITIES

Growth. Postnatal onset of short-limbed growth deficiency that becomes obvious between 18 months and 2 years; adult stature, 82 to 130 cm.

Craniofacial. Normal head size and face.

Limbs. Disproportionately short; hypermobility of major joints except elbows leading to genu varum, valgum, and recurvatum; ulnar deviation of hands; short fingers that are hypermobile.

Radiographs. Short long bones with wide metaphyses; epiphyses are small, irregular, or "fragmented," especially the capital femoral epiphyses; vertebral abnormalities consist of variable degrees of flattening with biconvex end plates and a central anterior bony protrusion from the anterior surface of the body; there is normal widening of the interpedicular distance from upper to lower lumbar spine; odontoid aplasia or hypoplasia; short sacral notches; ribs tend to be spatulate; terminal phalanges small.

Other. Lumbar lordosis, kyphosis, scoliosis.

NATURAL HISTORY

The patients have been described as "normal" at birth, with small size, short arms, and waddling gait becoming evident between 6 months and 4 years of age. Bowed lower extremities with waddling gait and scoliosis are the principal orthopedic problems, and there may be some limitation in joint motility. Intelligence is normal. Odontoid hypoplasia in association with hypermobility can result in increased motion of C1 on C2, leading to cord damage. Although the vertebral changes resolve with age, the epiphyseal changes of the long bones become more severe, leading to progressive degeneration and severe osteoarthritis. About one third to one half require total hip replacement in their mid-30s. Neurologic complications, most commonly numbness or tingling of the limbs, occur in 28%. Mild and severe forms have been described.

ETIOLOGY

This disorder has an autosomal dominant inheritance pattern. Mutations in the cartilage oligomeric matrix protein gene (COMP), which has been localized to chromosome 19p13.1, lead to both mild and severe forms of this disorder which are part of a continuum. Most of the cases have been sporadic and presumably represent fresh mutations. Based on what may well be an increased risk of gonadal mosaicism in this disorder, it has been estimated that unaffected parents who have had one affected child have a recurrence risk in the range of 4%.

COMMENT

Mutations in COMP are also responsible for the majority of cases of multiple epiphyseal dysplasia. It has been suggested that these two disorders comprise a clinical spectrum with mild multiple epiphyseal dysplasia at one end and pseudoachondroplasia at the other.

References

Maroteaux P, Lamy M: Les formes pseudoachondroplastiques des dysplasies spondyloépiphysaires, *Presse Med* 67:383, 1959.

Ford N, Silverman FN, Kozlowski K: Spondyloepiphyseal dysplasia (pseudoachondroplastic type), *Am J Roentgenol Radium Ther Nucl Med* 86:462, 1961.

Hall JG, et al: Gonadal mosaicism in pseudoachondroplasia, *Am J Med Genet* 28:143, 1987.

Briggs MD, et al: Genetic linkage of mild pseudoachondroplasia (PSACH) to markers in the pericentromeric region of chromosome 19, *Genomics* 18:656, 1993.

Hecht JT, et al: Linkage of typical pseudoachondroplasia to chromosome 19, *Genomics* 18:661, 1993.

Langer LO, et al: Patients with double heterozygosity for achondroplasia and pseudoachondroplasia, with comments on these conditions and the relationship between pseudoachondroplasia and multiple epiphyseal dysplasia, Fairbank type, *Am J Med Genet* 47:772, 1993.

Hecht JL, et al: Mutations in exon 17B of cartilage oligomeric matrix protein (COMP) cause pseudoachondroplasia, *Nat Genet* 10:325, 1995.

McKeand J, et al: Natural history study of pseudoachondroplasia, *Am J Med Genet* 63:406, 1996.

Mabuchi A, et al: Novel types of *COMP* mutations and genotype-phenotype association in pseudoachondroplasia and multiple epiphyseal dysplasia, *Hum Genet* 112:84, 2003.

Jackson GC, et al: Pseudoachondroplasia and multiple epiphyseal dysplasia: A 7-year comprehensive analysis of the known disease genes identify novel and recurrent mutations and provides an accurate assessment of their relative contribution, *Hum Mutat* 33:44, 2012.

K

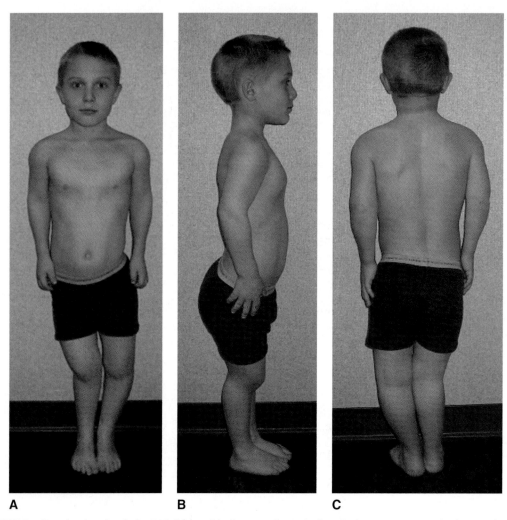

A   **B**   **C**

FIGURE 1. Pseudoachondroplasia. **A–C,** A boy with disproportionately short limbs, genu varus and valgus, and scoliosis. (Courtesy Dr. Stephen Braddock, St. Louis University.)

Continued

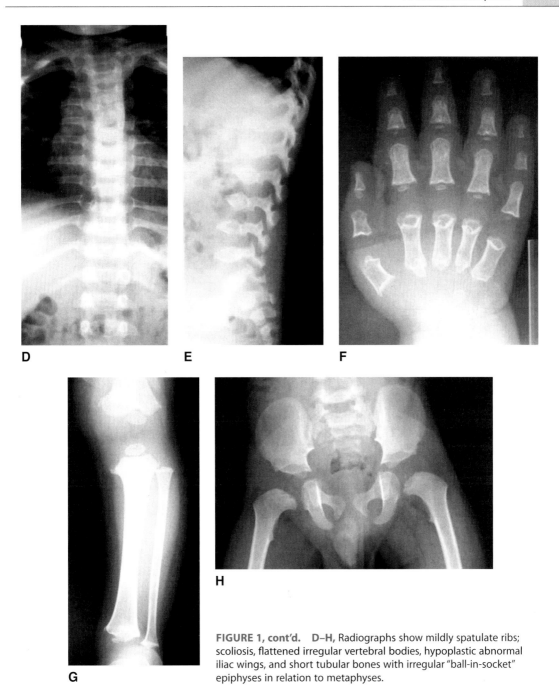

D

E

F

H

G

K

FIGURE 1, cont'd.   D–H, Radiographs show mildly spatulate ribs; scoliosis, flattened irregular vertebral bodies, hypoplastic abnormal iliac wings, and short tubular bones with irregular "ball-in-socket" epiphyses in relation to metaphyses.

ACROMESOMELIC DYSPLASIA
(ACROMESOMELIC DYSPLASIA, TYPE MAROTEAUX)
Short Distal Limbs, Frontal Prominence, Low Thoracic Kyphosis

Maroteaux and colleagues recognized this disorder in 1971, and Langer and colleagues summarized the manifestations in 19 patients in 1977. More than 40 cases have been reported.

ABNORMALITIES

Craniofacial. Disproportionately large head with relative frontal prominence, with or without relatively short nose.

Limbs. Short limbs with short hands and feet, bowed forearms that are relatively shorter than upper arms, limited elbow extension, short fingers and toes with short but not dysplastic nails, redundant skin developing over fingers in childhood.

Spine. Development of lower thoracic kyphosis.

Radiographs. Metacarpals and phalanges become increasingly shorter during the first year; middle and proximal phalanges are broad; cone-shaped epiphyses develop; shortening of humerus, radius, and ulna progresses during first year; bowed radius; vertebral bodies are oval-shaped in infancy, but with advancing age the lumbar vertebrae become wedge-shaped with the posterior aspect of the bodies shorter than the anterior; by 24 months, a central protrusion of bone develops anteriorly; superiorly curved clavicles that appear located high; flared metaphyses of long tubular bones; hypoplasia of basilar portion of ilia and irregular ossification of lateral superior acetabular region in childhood.

OCCASIONAL ABNORMALITIES
Relatively large great toe, corneal clouding, hydrocephalus, mild intellectual disability.

NATURAL HISTORY
Birth weight may be normal, and the linear growth deficiency becomes more evident during the first year. Radiographs frequently do not show abnormal bones or growth plates in the newborn period. However, radiologic skeletal changes are diagnostic by 2 years of age. Lower thoracic kyphosis, increased lumbar lordosis, and prominent buttocks are common. Most joints tend to be relatively lax. There may be some lag in gross motor performance because of the relatively large head and short limbs, but intelligence is normal. Final height in nine adults ranged from 96.5 to 124.5 cm.

ETIOLOGY
This disorder has an autosomal recessive inheritance pattern. Mutations in *NPR2* which encodes the transmembrane natriuretic peptide receptor NPR-B is responsible. The average height of obligate carrier adults is significantly shorter (5.7 cm) than matched controls.

References

Maroteaux P, Martinelli B, Campailla E: Le nanisme acro-mésomélique, *Presse Med* 79:1838, 1971.

Langer LO, et al: Acromesomelic dwarfism: Manifestations in childhood, *Am J Med Genet* 1:87, 1977.

Langer LO, Garrett RT: Acromesomelic dysplasia, *Radiology* 137:349, 1980.

Fernández del Moral R, et al: Report of a case: Acromesomelic dysplasia. Radiologic, clinical and pathological study, *Am J Med Genet* 33:415, 1989.

Kant SG, et al: Acromesomelic dysplasia, Maroteaux type, maps to human chromosome 9, *J Med Genet* 63:155, 1998.

Bartels CF, et al: Mutations in the transmembrane natriuretic peptide receptor NPR-B impair skeletal growth and cause acromesomelic dysplasia, type Maroteaux, *Am J Hum Genet* 75:27, 2004.

K

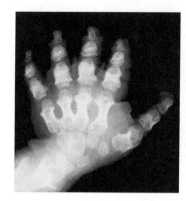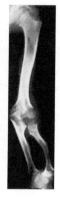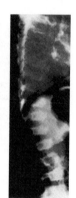

FIGURE 1.   Characteristic radiologic findings. (From Langer LO et al: *Am J Med Genet* 1:87, 1977. Copyright 1977. Reprinted with permission of Wiley-Liss, Inc., a subsidiary of John Wiley & Sons, Inc.)

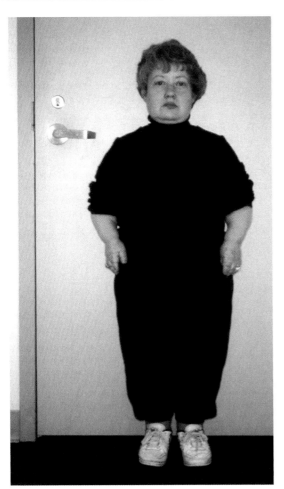

A

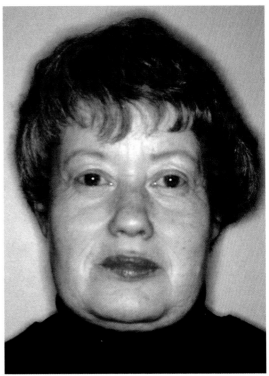

B

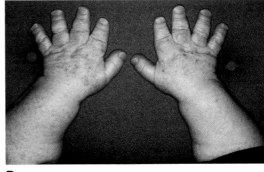

D

K

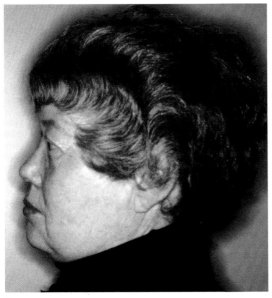

C

FIGURE 2.   A–D, A 57-year-old woman with acromesomelic dysplasia. Note the relative macrocephaly with frontal prominence without short nose and the short limbs with short hands, particularly the fingers.

SPONDYLOEPIPHYSEAL DYSPLASIA CONGENITA
Short Trunk, Lag in Epiphyseal Mineralization, Myopia

Spranger and Wiedemann established this disorder in 1966 when they reported 6 new cases and summarized 14 from the literature. Numerous additional cases have been reported subsequently.

ABNORMALITIES

Onset at birth.

Growth. Prenatal onset of growth deficiency; final height, 34 to 132 cm.

Facies. Variable flat facies, malar hypoplasia, cleft palate.

Eyes. Myopia, retinal detachment (50%).

Spine. Short, including neck with ovoid flattened vertebrae with narrow intervertebral disk spaces, odontoid hypoplasia, kyphoscoliosis, lumbar lordosis.

Chest. Barrel chest with pectus carinatum.

Limbs. Lag in mineralization of epiphyses, which tend to be flat, with no os pubis, talus, calcaneus, or knee centers mineralized at birth; coxa vara; diminished joint mobility at elbows, knees, and hips; conductive hearing loss.

Muscles. Weakness, easy fatigability, hypoplasia of abdominal muscles.

OCCASIONAL ABNORMALITIES

Talipes equinovarus, dislocation of hip.

NATURAL HISTORY

The hypotonic weakness and orthopedic situation contribute to a late onset of walking, usually with a waddling gait. Myopia should be suspected, and frequent ophthalmologic evaluation is merited to guard against retinal detachment. Conductive hearing loss is common. Morning stiffness may be a feature; however, there is usually no undue joint pain.

ETIOLOGY

This disorder has an autosomal dominant inheritance pattern. A variety of alterations in the *COL2A1* gene, which codes for type II collagen, lead to spondyloepiphyseal dysplasia congenita. Instances of affected siblings born to unaffected parents are most likely due to gonadal mosaicism.

COMMENT

A number of disorders are caused by mutations in *COL2A1,* including achondrogenesis II/hypochondrogenesis, spondyloepiphyseal dysplasias congenita, Kniest dysplasia, and Stickler syndrome.

References

Spranger J, Wiedemann HR: Dysplasia spondyloepiphysaria congenita, *Helv Paediatr Acta* 21:598, 1966.

Spranger J, Langer LO: Spondyloepiphyseal dysplasia congenita, *Radiology* 94:313, 1970.

Harrod MJE, et al: Genetic heterogeneity in spondyloepiphyseal dysplasia congenita, *Am J Med Genet* 18:311, 1984.

Spranger J, et al: The type II collagenopathies: A spectrum of chondrodysplasias, *Eur J Pediatr* 153:56, 1994.

Dahiya R, et al: Spondyloepiphyseal dysplasia congenita associated with conductive hearing loss, *Ear Nose Throat J* 79:178, 2000.

K

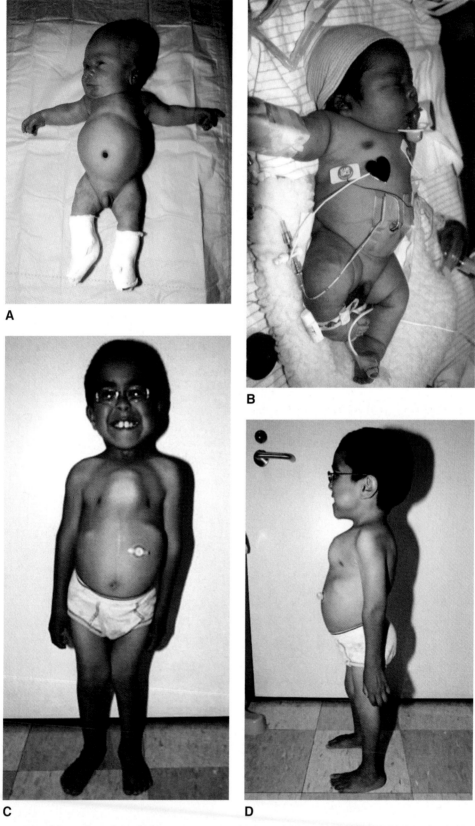

FIGURE 1.   Spondyloepiphyseal dysplasia congenita. **A** and **B,** Two children as newborns. **C** and **D,** The child in **B** at 10 years of age. Note the lumbar lordosis and flat midface.

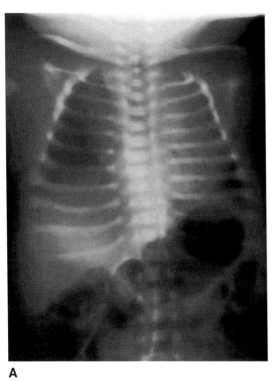

A

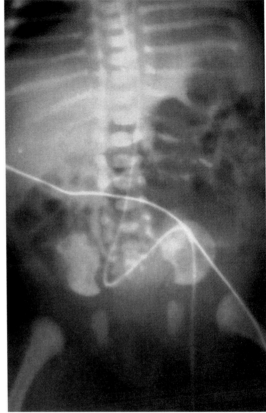

B

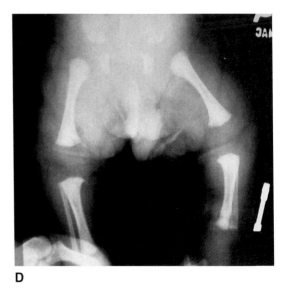

D

C

K

FIGURE 2.   A–D, Radiographs of child in Figure 1 at 1 day of life showing ovoid vertebrae, no os pubis, severe ossification delays, and lag in mineralization of the epiphyses.

KNIEST DYSPLASIA
Flat Facies, Thick Joints, Platyspondyly

Although Kniest described this disorder in 1952, it has been more generally recognized only in recent years.

ABNORMALITIES

Growth. Disproportionate short stature with short, barrel-shaped chest.

Craniofacial. Flat facies with prominent eyes, low nasal bridge, myopia that may progress to retinal detachment, vitreoretinal degeneration, cataract, cleft palate with frequent ear infections; the head, which is of normal size, is relatively large with respect to height.

Limbs. Enlarged joints with limited joint mobility and variable pain and stiffness; short limbs, often with bowing; some irregularity of epiphyses with late ossification of femoral heads; flexion contractures in hips; inability to form fist secondary to bony enlargements and soft tissue swelling at interphalangeal joints.

Radiographs. Dumbbell-shaped femora, hypoplastic pelvic bones, platyspondyly, and vertical clefts of vertebrae in newborn period; by age 3, pelvis becomes "dessert-cup shaped," ends of bones reveal irregular epiphyses, diffuse osteoporosis, and cloud-like radiodensities on both sides of epiphyseal plates; thereafter, platyspondyly remains, intervertebral disk space is narrow, odontoid is large and wide; flared metaphyses; large epiphyses.

Other. Lumbar kyphoscoliosis, inguinal and umbilical hernias, small pelvis, short clavicles, hearing loss, tracheomalacia, cataracts, lens dislocation, glaucoma.

NATURAL HISTORY

Marked clinical variability is the rule, with some individuals dying in the newborn period with respiratory failure and others living a relatively normal life with mild disproportionate short stature and kyphoscoliosis. Short extremities and stiff joints occur in the newborn period; marked lumbar lordosis and kyphoscoliosis lead to disproportionate shortening of the trunk in childhood; late walking because of orthopedic disability with contracted hips; limitation of joint motion with pain, stiffness, and flexion contractures of major joints develops; chronic otitis media related to cleft palate; normal intelligence despite delayed motor milestones and delayed speech; final height, 106 to 145 cm; frequent ophthalmologic evaluations are indicated in order to prevent retinal detachment.

ETIOLOGY

This disorder has an autosomal dominant inheritance pattern. Most cases represent a fresh gene mutation. This disorder represents one of a spectrum of chondrodysplasias caused by defects in the gene for type II collagen, COL2A1. Others include type II achondrogenesis-hypochondrogenesis, spondyloepiphyseal dysplasia congenita, and Stickler syndrome.

COMMENT

The original patient described by Wilhelm Kniest was 42 years of age at last report. She had short stature, restricted joint mobility, and blindness, but she was mentally alert and leading an active life.

References

Kniest W: Zur Abgrenzung der Dysostosis enchondralis von der Chondrodystrophie, *Z Kinderheilkd* 70:633, 1952.

Kim HJ, et al: Kniest syndrome with dominant inheritance and mucopolysacchariduria, *Am J Hum Genet* 77:755, 1975.

Rimoin DL, et al: Metatropic dwarfism, the Kniest syndrome and the pseudoachondroplastic dysplasias, *Clin Orthop* 114:70, 1976.

Maumenee IH, Traboulsi EI: The ocular findings in Kniest dysplasia, *Am J Ophthalmol* 100:155, 1985.

Spranger J, et al: The type II collagenopathies: A spectrum of chondrodysplasias, *Eur J Pediatr* 153:56, 1994.

Cole WG: Abnormal skeletal growth in Kniest dysplasia caused by type II collagen mutations, *Clin Orthop* 341:162, 1997.

Spranger J, et al: Kniest dysplasia: Dr. W. Kniest, his patient, the molecular defect, *Am J Med Genet* 69:79, 1997.

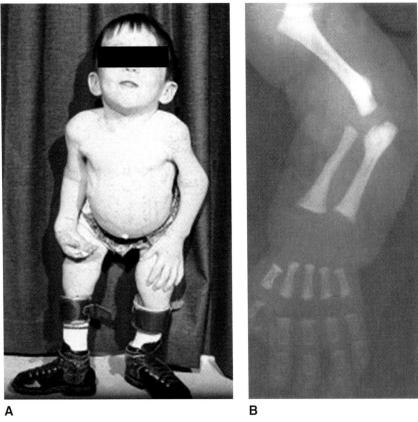

A   **B**

FIGURE 1.   **A** and **B,** A 3-year-old boy with Kniest dysplasia. (Courtesy Dr. D. L. Rimoin, Cedars-Sinai Medical Center, Los Angeles.)

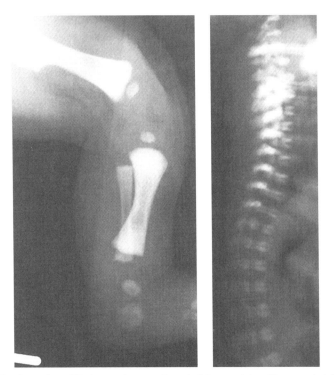

FIGURE 2.   Radiographs show altered limb morphogenesis and platyspondyly with coronal clefting. (Courtesy Dr. J. H. Graham, Cedars-Sinai Medical Center, Los Angeles.)

K

DYGGVE-MELCHIOR-CLAUSEN SYNDROME

Initially described in 1962 by Dyggve and colleagues, the clinical and radiographic features were set forth more completely in 1975 by Spranger and colleagues. The disorder is characterized as a progressive spondyloepimetaphyseal dysplasia associated with intellectual disability.

ABNORMALITIES

Growth. Deficiency of postnatal onset, with short trunk dwarfism becoming evident before 18 months.

Performance. Intellectual disability.

Craniofacial. Microcephaly, coarse facies, prognathism, facial bones large for cranium.

Spine. Platyspondyly, vertebral bodies show double-humped appearance with central constriction, short neck, odontoid hypoplasia, scoliosis, kyphosis, lordosis.

Thorax. Sternal protrusion, barrel chest.

Pelvis. Small ilia with irregularly calcified (lacelike) iliac crests in childhood developing into a marginal irregularity in adulthood; lateral displacement of capital femoral epiphyses; sloping, dysplastic acetabulae; wide pubic ramus.

Limbs. Restricted joint mobility; waddling gait; dislocated hips; genu valga and vera; rhizomelic limb shortening with irregular metaphyses and epiphyses; malformed olecranons and radial heads; broad hands and feet; short metacarpals, particularly the first, and short notched phalanges; cone-shaped epiphyses; small carpals.

NATURAL HISTORY

Manifestations become evident between 1 and 18 months and are progressive. Feeding problems frequently occur during infancy. Restriction of joint mobility primarily affects the elbows, hips, and knees. Spinal cord compression due to atlantoaxial instability is a preventable complication. The degree of intellectual disability has varied from moderate to severe. Three known adults measured 128 cm, 127 cm, and 119 cm in height, respectively.

ETIOLOGY

This disorder has an autosomal recessive inheritance pattern. Mutations in *DYM* located at 18q21.1 are responsible. *DYM* encodes dymeclin, a novel peripheral membrane protein dynamically associated with the Golgi apparatus. *DYM* is expressed in brain, cartilage, and bone, the three tissues most affected by Dyggve-Melchior-Clausen syndrome (DMC).

COMMENT

Smith-McCort dysplasia (SMC) has identical radiographic findings but is associated with normal intelligence. Mutations in DYM are also responsible for SMC, indicating that DMC and SMC are allelic. Of particular interest, lower levels of the dymeclin protein product are found in DMC. This suggests that decreased levels initially lead to abnormalities of cartilage and bone, but once the levels of functional protein drop below a certain threshold, the brain becomes affected.

References

Dyggve HV, Melchior JC, Clausen J: Morquio-Ullrich's disease: An inborn error of metabolism? *Arch Dis Child* 37:525, 1962.

Spranger J, Maroteaux P, Der Kaloustian VM: The Dyggve-Melchior-Clausen syndrome, *Radiology* 114:415, 1975.

Naffah J: The Dyggve-Melchior-Clausen syndrome, *Am J Hum Genet* 28:607, 1976.

Spranger J, Bierbaum B, Herrmann J: Heterogeneity of Dyggve-Melchior-Clausen dwarfism, *Hum Genet* 33:279, 1976.

Bonafede RP, Beighton P: The Dyggve-Melchior-Clausen syndrome in adult siblings, *Clin Genet* 14:24, 1978.

Beighton P: Dyggve-Melchior-Clausen syndrome, *J Med Genet* 27:512, 1990.

Cohn DH, et al: Mental retardation and abnormal skeletal development (Dyggve-Melchior-Clausen) due to mutations in a novel evolutionary conserved gene, *Am J Hum Genet* 72:419, 2003.

Ghouzzi VE, et al: Mutations in a novel gene dymeclin (*FLJ20071*) are responsible for Dyggve-Melchior-Clausen syndrome, *Mol Genet* 12:357, 2003.

Dimitrov A, et al: The gene responsible for Dyggve-Melchior-Clausen syndrome encodes a novel peripheral membrane protein dynamically associated with the Golgi apparatus, *Hum Mol Genet* 18:440, 2009.

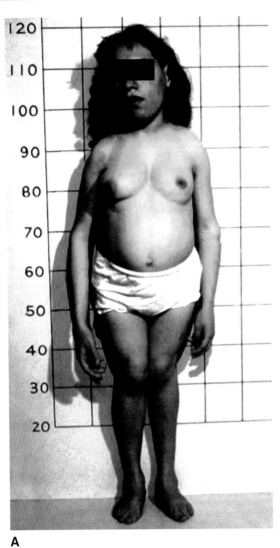

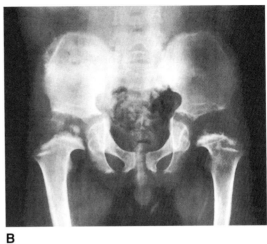

B

A

FIGURE 1.   A and **B,** Adolescent with Dyggve-Melchior-Clausen syndrome. Note the irregularly calcified iliac crests. (Courtesy Dr. R. Lachman, Harbor-UCLA Medical Center, and Dr. D. L. Rimoin, Cedars-Sinai Medical Center, Los Angeles.)

K

SPONDYLOMETAPHYSEAL DYSPLASIA, KOZLOWSKI TYPE
(KOZLOWSKI SPONDYLOMETAPHYSEAL CHONDRODYSPLASIA)
Early-Childhood-Onset Short Spine, Irregular Metaphyses, Pectus Carinatum

Kozlowski and colleagues established this disorder in 1967. Spondylometaphyseal dysplasia comprises a group of disorders in which the spine and metaphyses of the tubular bones are affected. At least seven types have been classified based on minor radiographic differences and mode of transmission. The Kozlowski type is the most known and the most common.

ABNORMALITIES

Growth. Growth deficiency, especially of trunk, with onset from 1 to 4 years of age; adult height, 129.5 to 152 cm.

Spine. Short neck and trunk with dorsal kyphosis; generalized platyspondyly with anterior narrowing in thoracolumbar region on lateral roentgenograms; on anteroposterior view, vertebral bodies extend more laterally to pedicles producing an "open-staircase" appearance; odontoid hypoplasia.

Thorax. Pectus carinatum.

Pelvis. Square, short iliac wings; flat, irregular acetabulae.

Limbs. Irregular rachitic-like metaphyses, especially the proximal femur with very short femoral necks; short, stocky hands; hypoplastic carpal bones with late ossification (delayed bone age).

NATURAL HISTORY

Affected patients are usually normal at birth. A noticeably waddling gait with limitation of joint mobility becomes apparent at 15 to 20 months and is often the first sign of the disorder. Degenerative joint changes leading to discomfort occur at a relatively early age. The elbows are often more affected than the knees. Final adult height is 130 to 150 cm.

ETIOLOGY

This disorder has an autosomal dominant inheritance pattern, with most cases representing fresh mutations. Mutations in the gene encoding the calcium-permeable ion channel (*TRPV4*) are responsible. In addition to being responsible for a number of skeletal dysplasias including metatrophic dysplasia, *TRPV4* mutations can also cause neurodegenerative disorders. A small group of patients with *TRPV4*-related skeletal dysplasias have had signs of motor neuron disease or peripheral neuropathy.

References

Kozlowski K, Maroteaux P, Spranger J: La dysostose spondylo-métaphysaire, *Presse Med* 75:2769, 1967.

Riggs W Jr, Summitt RL: Spondylometaphyseal dysplasia (Kozlowski): Report of affected mother and son, *Radiology* 101:375, 1971.

Le Quesne GW, Kozlowski K: Spondylometaphyseal dysplasia, *Br J Radiol* 46:685, 1973.

Kozlowski K, et al: Spondylo-metaphyseal dysplasia. (Report of 7 cases and essay of classification.) In Papadatos CJ, Bartsocas CS (eds): Skeletal Dysplasias, New York, 1982, Alan R. Liss, pp 89–101.

Keakow D, et al: Mutations in the gene encoding the calcium-permeable ion channel TRPV4 produce spondylometaphyseal dysplasia, Kozlowski type and metatrophic dysplasia, *Am J Hum Genet* 84:307, 2009.

Nishimura G, et al: *TRPV4*-associated skeletal dysplasias, *Am J Med Genet C Semin Med Genet* 160C:190, 2012.

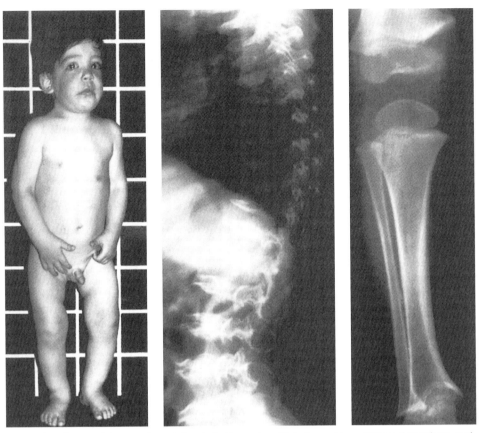

FIGURE 1.   Kozlowski spondylometaphyseal dysplasia. Young boy. Note bowed legs, flattened vertebrae, and metaphyseal flare. (From Riggs W Jr, Summitt RL: *Radiology* 101:375, 1971, with permission.)

K

METATROPIC DYSPLASIA (METATROPIC DWARFISM SYNDROME)
Small Thorax, Thoracic Kyphoscoliosis, Metaphyseal Flaring

Maroteaux and colleagues set forth this entity with 5 cases of their own and 12 unrecognized cases from the literature. *Metatropic* derives from the Greek word *metatropos*, which means "changing patterns" and refers to the change in body proportions from short limb/long trunk to short trunk/long limb as kyphoscoliosis becomes more progressive. More than 90 cases have been reported.

ABNORMALITIES

Growth. Birth weight normal; birth length greater than 97th percentile; trunk, initially long relative to the limbs, becomes progressively short with the development of kyphoscoliosis, leading to short-trunk dwarfism.

Facies. Prominent forehead, midface hypoplasia, square jaw.

Skeletal. Early platyspondyly with progressive kyphosis and scoliosis in infancy to early childhood; odontoid hypoplasia; delayed ossification/hypoplasia of the anterior portion of the first cervical vertebra, C1-C2 subluxation; narrow thorax with short ribs; short limbs with metaphyseal flaring and epiphyseal irregularity with hyperplastic trochanters; prominent joints with restricted mobility at knee and hip but increased extensibility of finger joints; irregular and squared-off calcaneal bones and precocious calcification of the hyoid and cricoid cartilage; erratic areas of microcalcifications in vertebral bodies and epiphyses; hypoplasia of basilar pelvis with horizontal acetabula, short deep sacroiliac notch, and squared iliac wings.

OCCASIONAL ABNORMALITIES

Macrocephaly, enlarged ventricles, small foramen magnum, clinical evidence of cord compression, ocular hypertelorism, thyroid agenesis, excess vertebrae.

NATURAL HISTORY

Often evident at birth, the vertebral changes become severe during infancy. The trunk, originally long, becomes extremely short secondary to rapidly progressing kyphoscoliosis. Odontoid hypoplasia with C1-C2 subluxation can lead to cord compression, quadriplegia, and sometimes death. Cervical (C1-C2) fusion should be considered in all such cases. Measurements of the foramen magnum are indicated. There are multiple causes of the respiratory difficulties, including abnormalities of the thorax, abnormal vocal cords with arytenoid fusion, and laryngotracheomalacia. Sensorineural hearing loss is common. Adult height ranges from 110 cm to 145.5 cm. Pelvic outlet constriction has led to colonic obstruction in at least one case. The major cause of death is cardiorespiratory failure caused by kyphoscoliosis and the narrow thorax.

ETIOLOGY

This disorder has an autosomal dominant mode of inheritance. The small number of recurrences are due to gonadal mosaicism. Mutations in the gene encoding TRPV4, a calcium permeable ion channel, are responsible. All cases ranging from perinatal lethality to mild forms are due to mutations of the same gene.

References

Fleury J, et al: Un cas singulier de dystrophie ostéochondrale congénitale (nanisme métatropique de Maroteaux), *Ann Pediatr (Paris)* 13:453, 1966.

Maroteaux P, Spranger I, Wiedemann HR: Der metatropische Zwergwucks, *Arch Kinderheilkd* 173:211, 1966.

Larose JH, Gay BG: Metatropic dwarfism, *Am J Roentgenol Radium Ther Nucl Med* 106:156, 1969.

Beck M, et al: Heterogeneity of metatropic dysplasia, *Eur J Pediatr* 140:231, 1983.

Shohat M, et al: Odontoid hypoplasia with vertebral cervical subluxation and ventriculomegaly in metatropic dysplasia, *J Pediatr* 114:239, 1989.

O'Sullivan MJ, et al: Morphologic observations in a case of lethal variant (type I) metatropic dysplasia with atypical features: Morphology of lethal metatropic dysplasia, *Pediatr Dev Pathol* 1:405, 1998.

Kannu P, et al: Metatrophic dysplasia: Clinical and radiographic findings in 11 patients demonstrating long-term natural history, *Am Med Genet* 143:2512, 2007.

Genevieve D, et al: Revisiting metatropic dysplasia: Presentation of a series of 19 novel patients and review of the literature, *Am J Med Genet* 146:992, 2008.

Krakow D, et al: Mutations in the gene encoding the calcium-permeable ion channel TRPV4 produce spondylometaphyseal dysplasia, Kozlowski type and metatrophic dysplasia, *Am J Hum Genet* 84:307, 2009.

Camacho N, et al: Dominant TRPV4 mutations in nonlethal and lethal metatropic dysplasia, *Am J Med Genet* 152:1169, 2010.

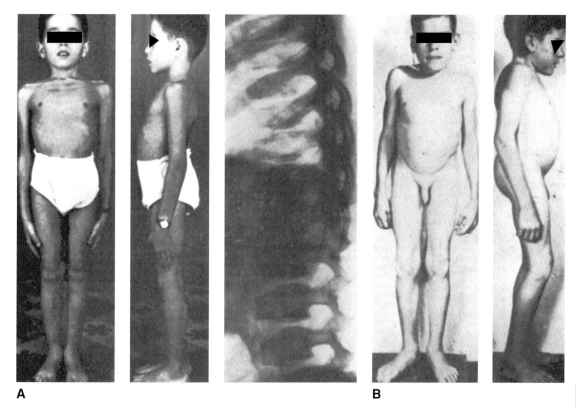

A   B

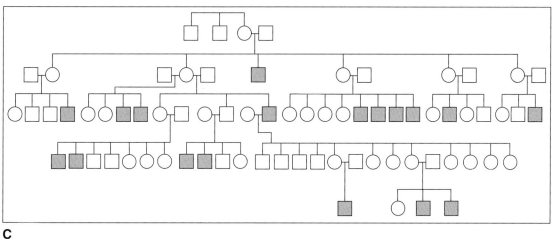

C

FIGURE 1. Spondyloepiphyseal dysplasia tarda. **A,** A 12-year-old child. Note shortening of trunk caused by flattened vertebrae, each of which has a central "hump" in the area of its epiphyses. (Courtesy P. Maroteaux, Hospital for Sick Infants, Paris.) **B,** A 15-year-old child. (From Jacobsen AW: *JAMA* 113:121, 1939, with permission.) **C,** Pedigree, of which patient shown in **B** is a member, showing evidence of X-linked recessive inheritance. (Courtesy R. Bannaman, Buffalo General Hospital, Buffalo, New York.)

MULTIPLE EPIPHYSEAL DYSPLASIA
Small Irregular Epiphyses, Pain and Stiffness in Hips, Short Stature

This condition was described by Ribbing in 1937 and by Fairbank in 1947. It is frequently misdiagnosed as bilateral Legg-Perthes disease.

ABNORMALITIES

Growth. Normal to slight shortness of stature; adult stature, 145 to 170 cm.

Limbs. Late ossifying, small, irregular, mottled epiphyses with eventual osteoarthritis caused by loss of articular cartilage in many large joints, especially in hips and knees; short femoral neck; mild metaphyseal flare; shortness of metacarpals and phalanges leading to short stubby fingers; approximately one third have symmetrical shoulder problems; double-layered patellae that often dislocate laterally; genu varum or genu valgus.

Spine. Although vertebral bodies are usually spared, they can be blunted, slightly ovoid, sometimes flattened.

NATURAL HISTORY

Not usually apparent at birth or through the first 2 years of life. Evident from 2 to 10 years because of waddling gait, easy fatigue, joint pain after exercise and slow growth. Mild to moderate growth deficiency is the rule; however, stature within the normal range occurs in some adults. Muscular hypotonia, even to the extent of myopathy, is frequent in young children. Back pain is common; slow, progressive pain and stiffness in joints, particularly in the hips, may be a complaint as early as 5 years, but usually not until 30 to 35 years; joint replacement is often required.

ETIOLOGY

This disorder has an autosomal dominant inheritance pattern with wide variability in expression. Mutations in the cartilage oligomeric matrix protein (COMP) gene, which has been localized to chromosome 19p13.1, have been identified in some cases. Point mutations in the three type IX collagen genes (COL9A1, COL9A2, and COL9A3) located on 6q13, 1p33-p32.2, and the von Willebrand factor A domain of matrilin-3 located on chromosome 2p24-23, can cause a distinctive mild type. Finally, homozygous mutations in the diastrophic dysplasia sulfate transporter (DTDST) gene located on chromosome 5q32-q33.1 are responsible for an autosomal recessive form of multiple epiphyseal dysplasia. It has been suggested that mutations in the known genes are responsible for less than one half of the cases of this disorder.

COMMENT

Radiographic abnormalities are correlated with genotype. Type IX collagen defects are associated with more severe joint involvement at the knees and relative hip sparing. Significant involvement at the capital femoral epiphysis and irregular acetabuli are associated with COMP mutations. Radiographic evidence of a "double-layered" patella is characteristic of mutations in the DTDST gene.

References

Ribbing S: Studien über hereditäre multiple ëpiphysenstörungen, Acta Radiol (Suppl):34, 1937.

Fairbank T: Dysplasia epiphysialis multiplex, Br J Surg 34:225, 1947.

Maudsley RH: Dysplasia epiphysialis multiplex: A report of fourteen cases in three families, J Bone Joint Surg 37B:228, 1955.

Hoefnagel D, et al: Hereditary multiple epiphysial dysplasia, Ann Hum Genet 30:201, 1967.

Spranger J: The epiphyseal dysplasias, Clin Orthop Rel Res 114:46, 1976.

Ingram RR: The shoulder in multiple epiphyseal dysplasia, J Bone Joint Surg 73B:277, 1991.

Unger SL, et al: Multiple epiphyseal dysplasia: Radiographic abnormalities correlated with genotype, Pediatr Radiol 31:10, 2001.

Briggs MD, Chapman KL: Pseudoachondroplasia and multiple epiphyseal dysplasia: Mutation review, molecular interactions, and genotype to phenotype correlations, Hum Mutat 19:465, 2002.

Chapman KL, et al: Review: Clinical variability and genetic heterogeneity in multiple epiphyseal dysplasia, Pediatr Pathol Mol Med 22:53, 2003.

Makitie O, et al: Autosomal recessive multiple epiphyseal dysplasia with homozygosity for C653S in the DTDST gene: Double-layer patella as a reliable sign, Am J Med Genet 122A:187, 2003.

Jakkula E, et al: Mutations in the known genes are not the major cause of MED: Distinctive phenotypic entities among patients with no identified mutations, Eur J Hum Genet 13:292, 2005.

Unger S, et al: Multiple epiphyseal dysplasia: Clinical and radiographic features, differential diagnosis and molecular basis, Best Pract Res Clin Rheumatol 22:19, 2008.

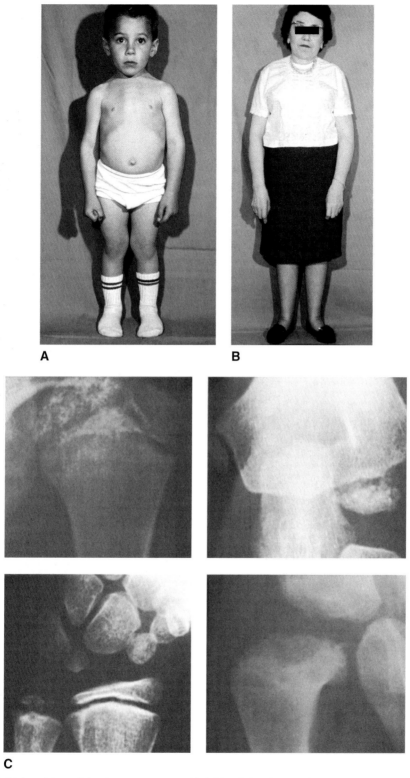

FIGURE 1. Multiple epiphyseal dysplasia. **A,** A 5-year-old child with height age of 2½ years. Patient had occasional aching in legs. **B,** Affected mother of patient shown in **A**. She is short of stature and has hip discomfort. **C,** Late and irregular mineralization of epiphyses, which may be small or aberrant in shape or both.

K

METAPHYSEAL DYSPLASIA, SCHMID TYPE

Since the initial description by Schmid in 1949, several large pedigrees of affected individuals have been reported.

ABNORMALITIES

Growth. Mild to moderate shortness of stature; adult height, 130 to 160 cm.

Skeletal. Relatively short tubular bones; tibial bowing, especially at ankle; waddling gait with coxa vara and genu varum; flare to lower rib cage.

Radiographic. Enlarged capital femoral epiphyses before 10 years of age; coxa vara beginning at 3 years; femoral bowing; metaphyseal abnormalities of distal and proximal femora, proximal tibiae, proximal fibulae, distal radius and ulna; anterior cupping, splaying, and sclerosis of ribs; abnormalities of the hands, including shortening of tubular bones and metaphyseal cupping of the proximal metacarpals and phalanges, are common; the spine is normal in the majority of cases; there is mild irregularity of acetabular roof.

OCCASIONAL ABNORMALITIES

Mild platyspondyly, vertebral body abnormalities, and end plate irregularities.

NATURAL HISTORY

Bowed legs with waddling gait, the usual presenting sign, is usually evident in second year; height, usually less than the 5th percentile, is rarely less than 7 SD below the mean; pain in legs during childhood; symptomatic and radiographic improvement beginning as early as 3 years of age, with orthopedic measures indicated only for unusual degrees of deformity and usually not until growth is complete; because the epiphyses are not affected, there are usually no osteoarthritic symptoms; intelligence and life expectancy are not affected.

ETIOLOGY

This disorder has an autosomal dominant inheritance pattern with variable expression. Mutations of the type X collagen (*COL10A1*) gene, which has been mapped to 6q22.3, are responsible for this pattern of malformation. Type X collagen expression is restricted to hypertrophic chondrocytes in areas undergoing endochondral ossification, such as growth plates. It has been suggested that reduction in the amount of normal type X collagen results in the phenotype.

References

Schmid F: Beitrag zur Dysostosis enchondralis metaphysaria, *Monatsschr Kinderheilkd* 97:393, 1949.

Stickler GB, et al: Familial bone disease resembling rickets (hereditary metaphysial dysostosis), *Pediatrics* 29:996, 1962.

Rosenbloom AL, Smith DW: The natural history of metaphyseal dysostosis, *J Pediatr* 66:857, 1965.

Lachman RS, et al: Metaphyseal chondrodysplasia: Schmid type. Clinical and radiographic delineation with review of the literature, *Pediatr Radiol* 18:93, 1988.

Warman ML, et al: A type X collagen mutation causes Schmid metaphyseal chondrodysplasia, *Nat Genet* 5:79, 1993.

Savarirayan R, et al: Schmid type metaphyseal chondrodysplasia: A spondylometaphyseal dysplasia identical to the "Japanese" type, *Pediatr Radiol* 30:460, 2000.

Elliot AM, et al: Hand involvement in Schmid metaphyseal chondrodysplasia, *Am J Med Genet* 132:191, 2005.

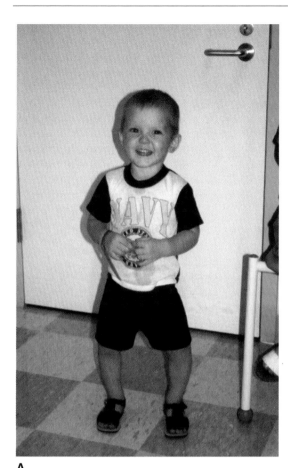

A

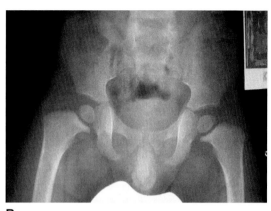

B

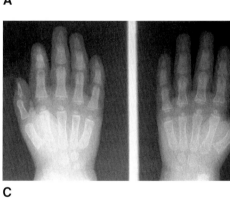

C

D

K

FIGURE 1. Metaphyseal dysplasia, Schmid type.
A–D, Image of a 27-month-old boy. Note the bowing of
legs, enlarged capital femoral epiphyses, and
metaphyseal abnormalities.

METAPHYSEAL DYSPLASIA, MCKUSICK TYPE
(CARTILAGE-HAIR HYPOPLASIA SYNDROME)
Mild Bowing of Legs, Wide Irregular Metaphyses, Fine Sparse Hair

Discovered by McKusick and colleagues among an inbred Amish population, this condition has subsequently been detected in non-Amish individuals, particularly in the Finnish population.

ABNORMALITIES

Growth. Prenatal onset of short limb, long trunk, short stature evident neonatally in 76% of cases and in 98% by 1 year; adult height, 104 to 149 cm; decreased or absent pubertal growth spurt; obesity in adults.

Hair. Fine, sparse, light, relatively fragile; eyebrows, eyelashes, and body hair are also affected.

Skeletal. Relatively short limbs, mild bowing of legs; prominent heel; flat feet; short hands, fingernails, toenails; loose-jointed "limp" hands and feet; incomplete extension of elbow; mild flaring of lower rib cage with prominent sternum; lumbar lordosis, scoliosis, small pelvic inlet.

Radiographic. Flared, scalloped, irregularly sclerotic metaphyses noted before closing of epiphyses primarily in knees and ankles, less frequently in hips; epiphyses only minimally affected; short tibia in relation to fibula.

Other. Diminished cellular immune response manifest by lymphopenia, decreased delayed hypersensitivity, and impaired in vitro responsiveness of lymphocytes to Phytohemagglutinin (PHA); mild macrocytic anemia; neutropenia.

OCCASIONAL ABNORMALITIES

Brachycephaly; malignancies (6%–10%), particularly non–Hodgkin lymphoma; esophageal atresia; Hirschsprung disease, particularly in severe cases; intestinal malabsorption in infancy; impaired humoral immunity; autoimmune hypoparathyroidism, congenital hypoplastic anemia; impaired spermatogenesis.

NATURAL HISTORY

The early history is often indicative of an intestinal malabsorption problem, which tends to improve with time. Postoperative mortality following surgery for Hirschsprung disease is as high as 38%, primarily related to severe enterocolitis-related septicemia. The diminished cellular immunity often leads to severe or fatal response to varicella as well as other infections. Even those patients for whom in vitro immunologic competence has been documented should be followed carefully. The rare congenital hypoplastic anemia can occasionally be fatal. However, in most cases, spontaneous recovery occurs before adulthood. The presence of anemia correlates with severity of the immunodeficiency and growth failure and to the neutropenia.

ETIOLOGY

This disorder has an autosomal recessive inheritance pattern. Mutations in the *RMRP* gene, which encodes the untranslated RNA that is a component of mitochondrial RNA-processing endoribonuclease and is mapped to the proximal part of 9p, are responsible.

COMMENT

The diagnosis is difficult in infancy. Widened metaphyses, short long bones, elongated fibulae, and anterior angulation of the sternum should raise concern regarding this disorder in the neonatal period.

References

McKusick VA, et al: Dwarfism in the Amish. II. Cartilage-hair hypoplasia, *Bull Johns Hopkins Hosp* 116:285, 1965.

Lux SE, et al: Chronic neutropenia and abnormal cellular immunity in cartilage-hair hypoplasia, *N Engl J Med* 282:231, 1970.

Van der Burgt I, et al: Cartilage hair hypoplasia, metaphyseal chondrodysplasia type McKusick: Description of seven patients and review of the literature, *Am J Med Genet* 41:371, 1991.

Makitie O, Kaitila I: Cartilage-hair hypoplasia—clinical manifestations in 108 Finnish patients, *Eur J Pediatr* 152:211, 1993.

Sulisalo T, et al: Cartilage-hair hypoplasia gene assigned to chromosome 9 by linkage analysis, *Nat Genet* 3:338, 1993.

Makitie O, et al: Cartilage-hair hypoplasia, *J Med Genet* 32:39, 1995.

Glass RBJ, et al: Radiologic changes in infancy in McKusick cartilage hair hypoplasia, *Am J Med Genet* 86:312, 1999.

Ridanpaa M, et al: Mutations in the RNA component of RNase MRP cause a pleiotropic human disease, cartilage-hair hypoplasia, *Cell* 104:195, 2001.

Makitie O, et al: Hirschsprung's disease in cartilage-hair hypoplasia has poor prognosis, *J Pediatr Surg* 37:1585, 2002.

Bacchetta J, et al: Autoimmune hypoparathyroidism in a 12-year-old girl with McKusick cartilage hair hypoplasia, *Pediatr Nephrol* 24:2449, 2009.

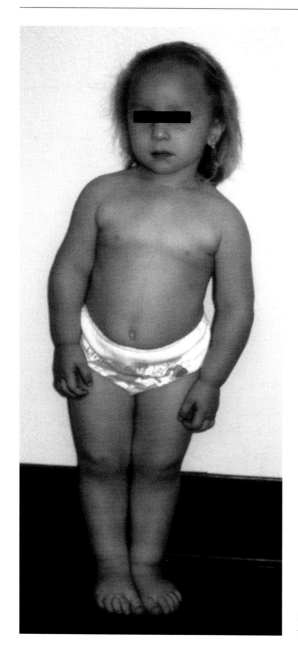

K

FIGURE 1.   Metaphyseal dysplasia, McKusick type. Note the fine, sparse hair and short limbs.

CHONDRODYSPLASIA PUNCTATA, X-LINKED DOMINANT TYPE
(CONRADI-HÜNERMANN SYNDROME)
Asymmetric Limb Shortness, Early Punctate Mineralization, Large Skin Pores

Initially described by Conradi and later by Hünermann, this disorder was clearly distinguished from the autosomal recessive type of chondrodysplasia punctata by Spranger and colleagues. The disorder occurs almost exclusively in girls.

ABNORMALITIES

Growth. Mild to moderate growth deficiency.

Facies. Variable low nasal bridge with flat facies; hypoplasia of malar eminences with downslanting palpebral fissures; cataracts.

Limbs. Asymmetric shortening related to areas of punctate mineralization in epiphyses, variable joint contractures.

Spine. Frequent scoliosis, even in infancy, related to areas of punctate mineralization.

Skin. In newborns, severe erythroderma and scaling arranged on the back in whorls and swirls following the lines of Blaschko. In older children, variable follicular atrophoderma with large pores resembling "orange peel" and ichthyosis predominate; sparse hair that tends to be coarse, and patchy areas of alopecia.

OCCASIONAL ABNORMALITIES

Dysplastic auricles; minor nail anomalies; nystagmus; cataracts; microphthalmos; glaucoma; atrophy of retina and optic nerve; short neck; hydramnios; hydrops; mild to moderate mental deficiency; tracheal calcifications with associated tracheal stenosis; cardiac defects; dislocated patella; hexadactyly; vertebral anomalies, including clefting, wedging, or absence.

NATURAL HISTORY

Failure to thrive and infection may occur in early infancy. If the patient survives the first few months, the prognosis for survival is good. Stippling of the epiphyses of the long bones frequently resolves by 9 months. Orthopedic problems including scoliosis are frequent, and there is an enhanced risk of cataract formation.

ETIOLOGY

This disorder has an X-linked dominant inheritance pattern. Mutations of an X-linked gene encoding Δ^8,Δ^7 sterol isomerase emopamil-binding protein (EBP), leading to a deficiency of sterol-Δ^1-isomerase, are responsible. Recognition that abnormal cholesterol biosynthesis is a feature of this disorder permits a definitive biochemical diagnosis. Strong intrafamilial variation exists in this syndrome making genetic counseling difficult. Increases in disease expression occur in succeeding generation (anticipation).

COMMENT

In addition to this disorder and the autosomal recessive chondrodysplasia punctata, an X-linked recessive type exists. That condition is characterized by skeletal manifestation of chondrodysplasia punctata, ichthyosis caused by steroid sulfatase deficiency, short stature, microcephaly, developmental delay, cataracts, and hearing loss. In addition, some affected males have anosmia and hypogonadism (Kallmann syndrome). The majority of patients have documented deletions and translocations of Xp22.3. Point mutations in the gene encoding arylsulfatase E (*ARSE*), which maps to Xp22.3, have been identified in a number of patients with this disorder, suggesting that the skeletal abnormalities are the result of altered *ARSE* activity.

References

Conradi E: Vorzeitiges Auftreten von Knochen und eigenartigen Verkalkungskernen bei Chondrodystrophia foetalis hypoplastica, *Jahrb Kinderheilkd* 80:86, 1914.

Hünermann C: Chondrodystrophia calcificans congenita als abortive Form der Chondrodystrophie, *Z Kinderheilkd* 51:1, 1931.

Spranger J, Opitz JM, Bidder U: Heterogeneity of chondrodysplasia punctate, *Humangenetik* 11:190, 1971.

Happle R: X-linked dominant chondrodysplasia punctata: Review of literature and report of a case, *Hum Genet* 53:65, 1979.

Curry CJR, et al: Inherited chondrodysplasia punctata due to a deletion of the terminal short arm of an X chromosome, *N Engl J Med* 311:1010, 1984.

Ballabio A, Andria G: Deletions and translocations involving the distal short arm of the human X chromosome: Review and hypothesis, *Hum Mol Genet* 1:221, 1992.

Wulfsberg EA, et al: Chondrodysplasia punctata: A boy with X-linked recessive chondrodysplasia punctata due to an inherited X-Y translocation with a current classification of these disorders, *Am J Med Genet* 43:823, 1992.

Franco B, et al: A cluster of sulfatase genes on Xp22.3: Mutations in chondrodysplasia punctata (CDPX) and implications for warfarin embryopathy, *Cell* 81:15, 1995.

Derry JM, et al: Mutations in a delta 8-delta 7 sterol isomerase in the tattered mouse and X-linked dominant chondrodysplasia punctata, *Nat Genet* 22:286, 1999.

Kelley RI, et al: Abnormal sterol metabolism in patients with Conradi-Hünermann-Happle syndrome and sporadic lethal chondrodysplasia punctata, *Am J Med Genet* 83:213, 1999.

Has C, et al: The Conradi-Hünermann-Happle syndrome (CDPX2) and emopamil binding protein: Novel mutations, and somatic and gonadal mosaicism, *Hum Mol Genet* 9:1951, 2000.

K

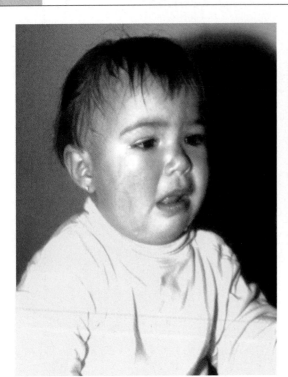

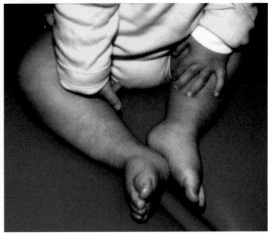

B

A

FIGURE 1.   Chondrodysplasia punctata, X-linked dominant type. **A** and **B,** Image of a 19-month-old girl. Note the flat face, low nasal bridge, sparse hair with patchy alopecia, and leg asymmetry.

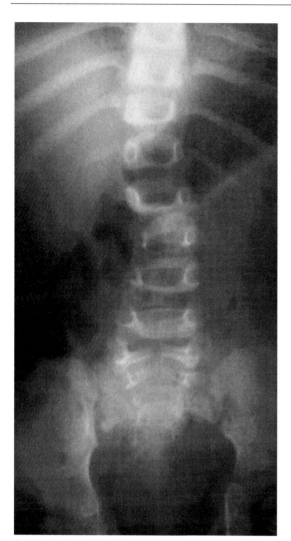

A

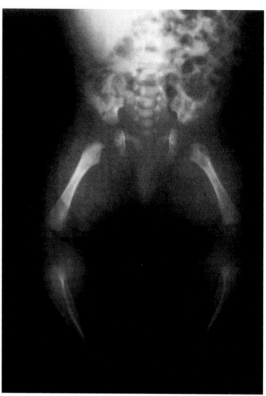

B

K

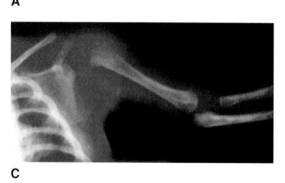

C

FIGURE 2.   A–C, Radiographs of child in Figure 1. Note the scoliosis and ectopic calcifications, most evident in the shoulder.

AUTOSOMAL RECESSIVE CHONDRODYSPLASIA PUNCTATA
(CHONDRODYSPLASIA PUNCTATA, RHIZOMELIC TYPE)
Short Humeri and Femora, Coronal Cleft in Vertebrae, Punctate Epiphyseal Mineralization

Spranger and colleagues clearly distinguished the rhizomelic (short proximal limb) type of chondrodysplasia punctata as a separate entity from the Conradi-Hünermann or X-linked dominant type of chondrodysplasia punctata.

ABNORMALITIES

Growth. Mean birth weight 2.9 kg; birth length 46.6 cm and occipitofrontal circumference (OFC) 32.4 cm; postnatal growth slow, averaging 1 kg in the first 6 months, 0.5 kg in the second 6 months, and 0.5 kg per year thereafter to at least 3 years of age.

Central Nervous System. Intellectual disabilities, with or without spasticity, microcephaly; although delayed, skills such as smiling, laughing, and recognition of familiar voices do develop; more advanced milestones, such as walking, sitting without support, speaking in phrases, and toilet training, never occur; seizures.

Craniofacial. Low nasal bridge and flat facies with or without upward slanting palpebral fissures; cataracts.

Limbs. Symmetric proximal shortening of humeri and femora; metaphyseal splaying and cupping, especially at the knee, with sparse and irregular trabeculae; epiphyseal and extraepiphyseal foci of calcification in early infancy with later epiphyseal irregularity; multiple joint contractures.

Spine. Coronal cleft noted on lateral roentgenogram with dysplasia and irregularity of vertebrae.

Pelvis. Trapeziform dysplasia of upper ilium.

OCCASIONAL ABNORMALITIES

Ichthyosiform skin dysplasia (28%), lipomas, craniocervical junction anomalies, cardiac defects, hip dislocation, delayed myelination, cerebellar atrophy, hemifacial paralysis, diaphragmatic hernia, cleft palate, hypospadias, cryptorchidism.

NATURAL HISTORY

Survival beyond infancy occurs in 90% and to age 6 to 6½ years in 50% of children. Respiratory problems are the major cause of death. Severe feeding problems are common. In children who live beyond 2 months of age, seizures occur in over 80%. Temperature instability is common. Cataract extraction is recommended for visual stimulation and to improve environmental interaction. Otitis media with hearing loss is common. Delayed eruption of teeth as well as dental caries occur frequently. Joint contractures improve with time and benefit from physical therapy. Curvature of the spine occurs in the majority of children who live beyond 2 months of age. Skin problems, most commonly eczema, miscellaneous rashes, and mild ichthyosis occur in half of these children.

ETIOLOGY

This disorder has an autosomal recessive inheritance pattern. Three types, all of which are associated with alterations of peroxisomal metabolism and are clinically indistinguishable, have been identified: type I: those with mutations in the PEX7 gene that encodes peroxin 7, the cytosolic PTS2-receptor protein required for targeting a subset of enzymes to peroxisomes; type II: those with mutations in the gene that encodes peroxisomal dihydroxyacetonephosphate acyltransferase; and type III: those with mutations in the gene that encodes peroxisomal alkyl-dihydroxyacetonephosphatate synthase. The vast majority of cases are due to mutations in the PRX7 gene. One case of type II has been reported due to paternal isodisomy of chromosome 1.

COMMENT

It is now clear that chondrodysplasia punctata is etiologically heterogeneous. In addition to genetic causes, punctate calcifications occur in chromosomal abnormalities such as trisomies 13, 18, and 21, as well as peroxisomal disorders, abnormalities of cholesterol metabolism, lysosomal storage disorders, abnormalities of vitamin K metabolism, and exposure to certain teratogens such as warfarin. It has also been seen in the offspring of women with autoimmune disease.

References

Spranger JW, Opitz JM, Bidder U: Heterogeneity of chondrodysplasia punctata, *Humangenetik* 11:190, 1970.

Spranger JW, Bidder U, Voelz C: Chondrodysplasia punctata (Chondrodystrophia calcifans). II. Der rhizomele Type, *Fortschr Geb Roentgenstr Nuklearmed* 114:327, 1971.

Gilbert EF, et al: Chondrodysplasia punctata: Rhizomelic form, *Eur J Pediatr* 123:89, 1976.

Heselson NG, Cremin BJ, Beighton P: Lethal chondrodysplasia punctata, *Clin Radiol* 29:679, 1978.

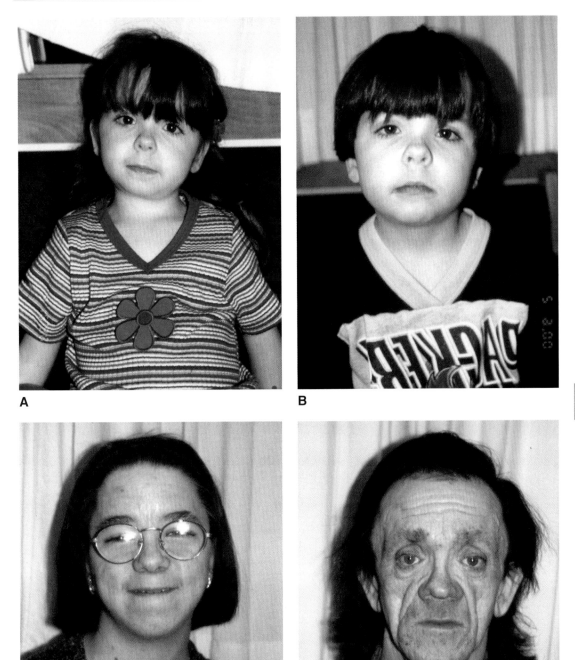

A

B

K

C

D

FIGURE 1. Hajdu-Cheney syndrome. **A** and **B,** Same child at 4 and 5 years of age. **C,** The boy's half-sister at 18 years of age. **D,** The children's father at 56 years of age. Note the progressive coarsening of facial features. (**A–D,** From Brennan AM, Pauli RM: *Am J Med Genet* 100:292, 2001, with permission.)

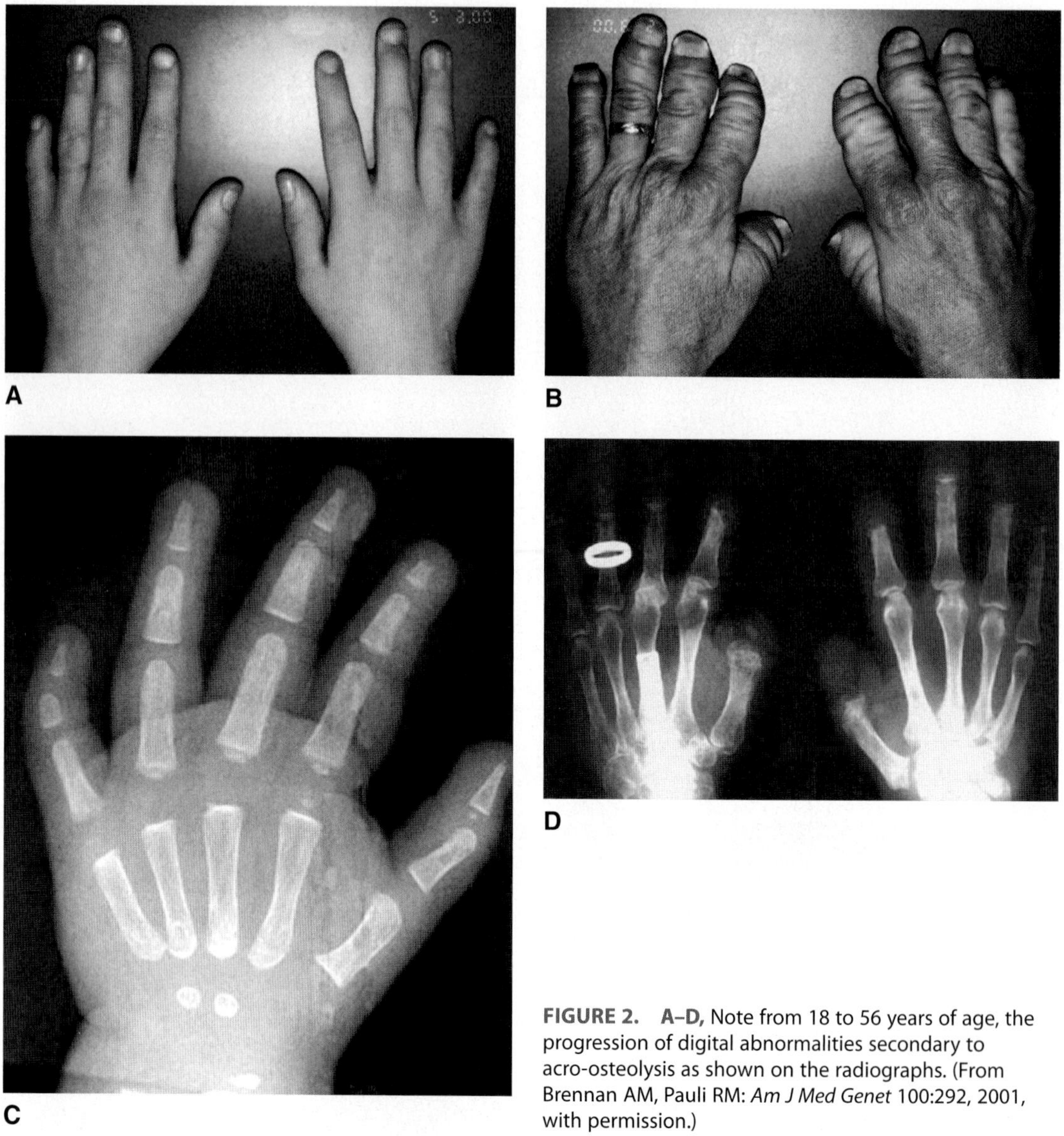

A

B

C

D

FIGURE 2.   **A–D,** Note from 18 to 56 years of age, the progression of digital abnormalities secondary to acro-osteolysis as shown on the radiographs. (From Brennan AM, Pauli RM: *Am J Med Genet* 100:292, 2001, with permission.)

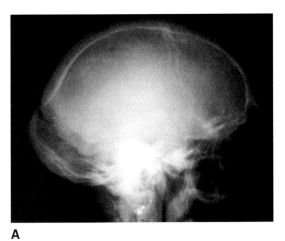

A

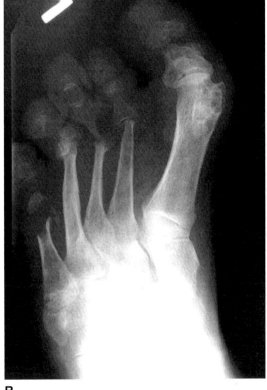

B

FIGURE 3. **A** and **B,** Lateral skull and foot in 56-year-old man showing thickening of the calvarium, prominent occiput and platybasia, and severe acro-osteolysis of virtually all phalanges and metatarsals. (From Brennan AM, Pauli RM: *Am J Med Genet* 100:292, 2001, with permission.)

K

CRANIOMETAPHYSEAL DYSPLASIA
Bony Wedge over Bridge of Nose, Mild Splaying of Metaphyses

Often confused with the Pyle metaphyseal dysplasia syndrome, this disorder has more profound craniofacial hyperostosis and less metaphyseal broadening than in Pyle disease. An autosomal dominant and a much rarer and more severe autosomal recessive form have been reported.

ABNORMALITIES

Craniofacial. Thick calvarium with dense base of cranial vault, facial bones, and mandible; macrocephaly; variable absence of pneumatization; unusual thick bony wedge over bridge of nose and supraorbital area with hypertelorism and relatively small nose; variable proptosis of eyes; compression of foramina with cranial nerve deficits, headache, and narrow nasal passages with rhinitis.

Limbs. Mild to moderate metaphyseal broadening with diaphyseal sclerosis, most evident in the distal femora; genu valgum.

OCCASIONAL ABNORMALITIES

Chiari I malformation, syringomyelia, intellectual disability.

NATURAL HISTORY

The above features are evident from infancy in both the autosomal dominant and the autosomal recessive forms. In adults with autosomal dominant craniometaphyseal dysplasia, the typical craniofacial appearance becomes less obvious. Clinical features, if present, are mild and consist of compression of cranial nerves, particularly the seventh and eighth. Sclerosis along the suture lines may be the only finding. In the autosomal recessive form, the craniofacial features progress. The skull base becomes more sclerotic with overgrowth and the calvarium becomes progressively hyperostotic with bony encroachment around the orbits and nasal bones. In those cases, severe visual handicaps, bilateral hearing loss, malocclusion, and facial paralysis occur. Prognathism becomes more pronounced with age. Truncal ataxia, responsive to posterior cranial fossa decompression, occurs. In some cases, intellectual disability occurs.

ETIOLOGY

Both autosomal dominant and autosomal recessive types of disease have been delineated, the latter being more severe in degree. The autosomal dominant type is caused by mutations in the human ortholog (ANKH) of the mouse progressive ankylosis gene located on human chromosome 5p15.2-p14.1. The ANK protein spans the outer cell membrane and shuttles inorganic pyrophosphate, a major inhibitor of physiologic and pathologic calcification, bone mineralization, and bone resorption. A candidate locus at 6q21-22.1 has been mapped for the recessive type, but the causative gene has not been identified.

References

Spranger J, Paulsen K, Lehmann W: Die kraniometaphysare Dysplasia, *Z Kinderheilkd* 93:64, 1965.

Millard DR Jr, et al: Craniofacial surgery in craniometaphyseal dysplasia, *Am J Surg* 113:615, 1967.

Gorlin RJ, Spranger J, Koszalka M: Genetic craniotubular bone dysplasias and hyperostoses: A critical analysis, *Birth Defects* 5:79, 1969.

Gorlin RJ, et al: Pyle's disease (familial metaphyseal dysplasia), *J Bone Joint Surg Am* 52:347, 1970.

Penchaszadeh VB, Gutierrez ER, Figuero P: Autosomal recessive craniometaphyseal dysplasia, *Am J Med Genet* 5:43, 1980.

Beighton P: Pyle disease (metaphyseal dysplasia), *J Med Genet* 24:321, 1987.

Hudgins RJ, Edwards MSB: Craniometaphyseal dysplasia associated with hydrocephalus: Case report, *Neurosurgery* 20:617, 1987.

Cole DEC, Cohen MM: A new look at craniometaphyseal dysplasia, *J Pediatr* 112:577, 1988.

Elcioglu N, Hall CM: Temporal aspects in craniometaphyseal dysplasia: Autosomal recessive type, *Am J Med Genet* 76:245, 1998.

Nurnberg P, et al: Heterozygous mutations in ANKH, the human ortholog of the mouse progressive ankylosis gene, result in craniometaphyseal dysplasia, *Nat Genet* 28:37, 2001.

Prontero P, et al: Craniometaphyseal dysplasia with severe craniofacial involvement shows homozygosity at the 6q21-22.1 locus, *Am J Med Genet* 155:1106, 2011.

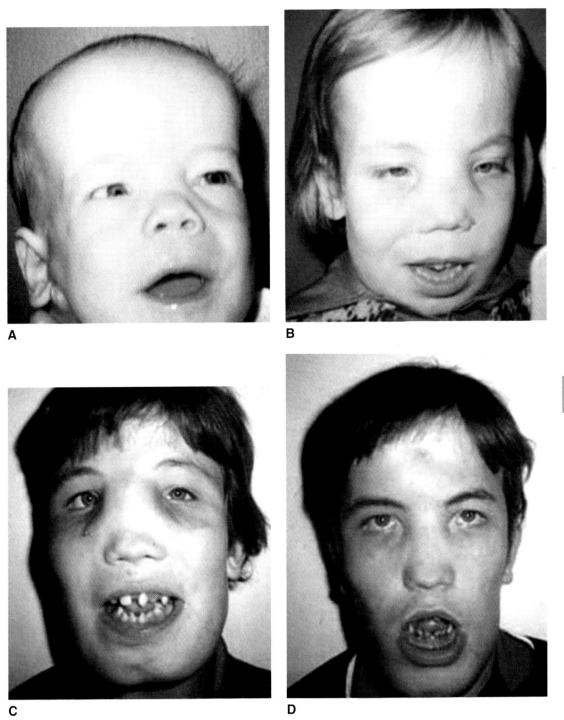

FIGURE 1.   Craniometaphyseal dysplasia. **A–D,** An affected child showing the facial changes that took place over time. Note the craniofacial findings at 7 months, 3 years, 12 years, and 16 years of age, respectively. (From Feingold M: *Am J Med Genet* 86:501, 1999, with permission.)

FRONTOMETAPHYSEAL DYSPLASIA
Prominent Supraorbital Ridges, Joint Limitations, Splayed Metaphyses

More than 30 cases of this disorder have been reported since Gorlin and Cohen's initial description in 1969.

ABNORMALITIES

Craniofacial. Thickened calvarium, coarse facies with wide nasal bridge, ocular hypertelorism, and prominent supraorbital ridges; incomplete sinus development; downslanting palpebral fissures, partial anodontia, delayed eruption, and retained deciduous teeth; high palate; small mandible with decreased angle and prominent antegonial notch.

Limbs. Flexion contracture of fingers, wrists, elbows, knees, and ankles; arachnodactyly with disproportionately wide and elongated phalanges; increased density in diaphyseal region with lack of modeling in metaphyseal region, giving Erlenmeyer-flask appearance to femur and tibia; partial fusion of carpal and of tarsal bones.

Other Skeletal. Wide foramen magnum with various cervical vertebral anomalies and wide interpedicular distance of vertebrae, flared pelvis with constriction of supra acetabular area, chest cage deformities, winged scapulae, scoliosis.

Cardiac. Arial septal defects, ventricular septal defects, pulmonary stenosis, mitral valve prolapse, aneurysm of aortic sinus of Valsalva, unruptured cerebral aneurysm.

Other. Mixed conductive and sensorineural hearing loss, which progresses; wasting of muscles of arms and legs, especially hypothenar and interosseous muscles of hands.

OCCASIONAL ABNORMALITIES

Intellectual disability, subglottic tracheal narrowing, ureteric and urethral stenosis.

NATURAL HISTORY

Affected individuals are usually asymptomatic at birth. The restriction of joint mobility and development of contractures are progressive. Respiratory difficulties, including subglottic stenosis, can lead to significant morbidity and even death. Severe progressive scoliosis has occurred. Anesthesia can be a significant problem. All patients should be evaluated to rule out urologic abnormalities.

ETIOLOGY

This disorder has an X-linked inheritance pattern with severe manifestations in males and variable but more mildly affected females. Mutations in the gene *FLNA,* located at Xq28, are responsible. *FLNA* codes for filamin A, a widely expressed protein that regulates reorganization of the actin cytoskeleton.

COMMENT

Mutations in *FLNA* are responsible for three additional X-linked disorders, oto-palato-digital syndrome (types I and II) and Melnick-Needles syndrome. All four of these disorders have a number of clinically overlapping features.

References

Gorlin RJ, Cohen MM: Frontometaphyseal dysplasia: A new syndrome, *Am J Dis Child* 118:487, 1969.

Danks DM, et al: Fronto-metaphyseal dysplasia: A progressive disease of bone and connective tissue, *Am J Dis Child* 123:254, 1972.

Gorlin RJ, Winder RB: Frontometaphyseal dysplasia-evidence for X-linked inheritance, *Am J Med Genet* 5:81, 1980.

Fitzsimmons JS, et al: Frontometaphyseal dysplasia: Further delineation of the clinical syndrome, *Clin Genet* 22:195, 1982.

Verloes A, et al: Fronto-otopalatodigital dysplasia: Clinical evidence for a single entity encompassing Melnick-Needles syndrome, otopalatodigital syndrome types 1 and 2, and frontometaphyseal dysplasia, *Am J Med Genet* 90:407, 2000.

Takahashi K, et al: Frontometaphyseal dysplasia: Patient with ruptured aneurysm of the aortic sinus of Valsalva and cerebral aneurysm, *Am J Med Genet* 108:249, 2002.

Morava E, et al: Clinical and genetic heterogeneity in frontometaphyseal dysplasia: Severe progressive scoliosis in two families, *Am J Med Genet* 116:272, 2003.

Robertson SP, et al: Localized mutations in the gene encoding the cytoskeletal protein filamin A cause diverse malformations in humans, *Nat Genet* 33:487, 2003.

Robertson SP, et al: Frontometaphyseal dysplasia: Mutations in *FLNA* and phenotypic diversity, *Am J Med Genet* 140:1726, 2006.

K

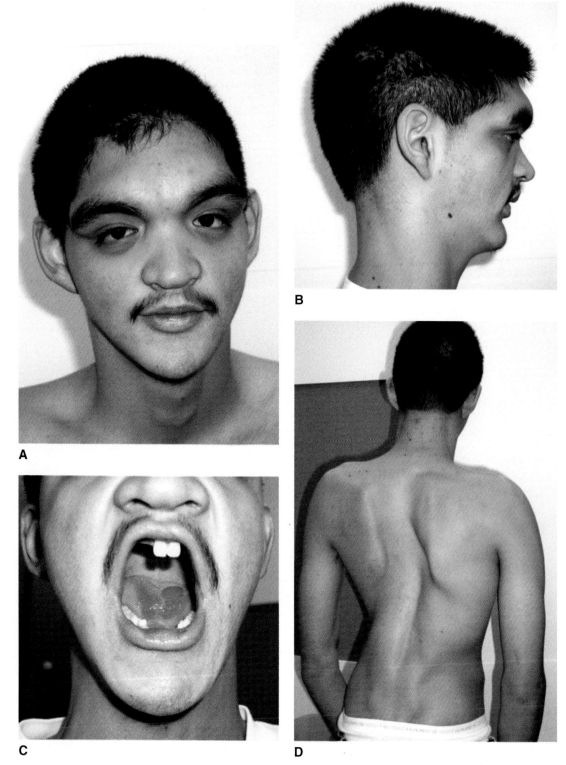

FIGURE 1. Frontometaphyseal dysplasia. **A–D,** Note wide nasal bridge, prominent supraorbital ridges, micrognathia, partial anodontia, and scoliosis. (Courtesy Dr. H. Eugene Hoyme, Sanford School of Medicine of the University of South Dakota, Sioux Falls, SD.)

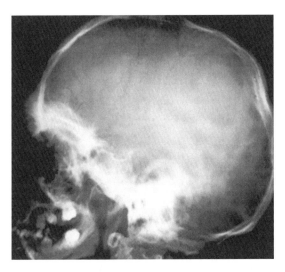

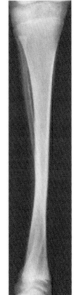
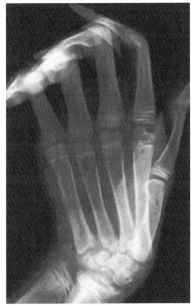

K

FIGURE 2. The skull shows supraorbital bossing with small paranasal sinuses. Note metaphyseal flaring of tibia; long, poorly modeled tubular bones of hands; and partial lysis of carpal bones. (From Danks DM et al: *Am J Dis Child* 123:254, 1972, with permission.)

L Osteochondrodysplasia with Osteopetrosis

OSTEOPETROSIS: AUTOSOMAL RECESSIVE—LETHAL
(INFANTILE MALIGNANT OSTEOPETROSIS)
Dense, Thick, Fragile Bone; Secondary Pancytopenia; Cranial Nerve Compression

More than 100 cases of this genetically heterogeneous and commonly lethal group of disorders have been reported since the first cases were described. Two different subsets of patients are recognized based on bone morphology: (1) osteoclast-rich, associated with a high number of mature but nonfunctional osteoclasts, and (2) osteoclast–poor, in which these cells are absent because of defect in differentiation. In both cases there is absence of proper bone resorption and an increased bone mass. It is estimated to occur in 1 out of 250,000 births. Several genotypes of autosomal recessive osteopetrosis (ARO) have specific natural histories.

ABNORMALITIES

Growth. Normal birth parameters with subsequent failure to thrive and progressive macrocephaly. Short stature in untreated survivors.

Performance. Seizures secondary to hypocalcemia; blindness; hearing loss; intellectual disability (depends on genotype).

Craniofacial. Frontal bossing; open fontanel; progressive proptosis; strabismus; choanal stenosis; facial palsy; a tendency for primary molars and permanent dentition to be distorted and for teeth to fail to erupt; poor periodontal attachment, allowing for exfoliation; early decay.

Imaging. Thick, dense, fragile bone with modeling alterations such as obtuse mandibular angle, partial aplasia of distal phalanges, straight femora, block-like "bone within a bone" metacarpals, obliteration of bone marrow space.

Metabolic. Serum calcium level may be low and serum phosphorus level elevated, increased alkaline phosphatase.

Other. Hepatosplenomegaly secondary to extramedullary hematopoiesis; immunodeficiency.

NATURAL HISTORY

Marrow impingement leads to pancytopenia. Compression of cranial foramina may lead to deafness, blindness, vestibular nerve dysfunction, extraocular muscle paralysis, other cranial nerve palsies, and hydrocephalus. Fractures are common. Ocular involvement, occurring at a median age of 2 months, is the most common presenting sign followed by seizures from hypocalcemia. Failure to thrive secondary to airway compromise occurs. Without treatment, life expectancy rarely exceeds adolescence for most forms. Problems with dentition and dental infection may include recurrent mandibular osteomyelitis.

ETIOLOGY

This disorder has primarily an autosomal recessive inheritance pattern.

Osteoclast-Rich Forms

TCIRG1 mutations account for 50% and present with classic phenotype and a predominantly hematologic presentation. Neurologic issues are the result of compression of neural foramina rather than primary brain involvement. Hematopoietic stem cell transplant (HSCT) is effective. Founder mutations in Costa Rica make this form of ARO more common in this population.

CLCN7 mutations account for 15% of cases. Homozygous or compound heterozygous patients have a classic hematologic presentation; however, this mutation may cause severe primary involvement of the nervous system, specifically the brain and retina, that may not be mitigated by HSCT. Long-term survival without HSCT has been reported. Heterozygous mutations in this gene cause a spectrum of anomalies from bone sclerosis, fractures, and dental abscesses to asymptomatic increased bone mass. This gene is responsible for Albers-Schönberg disease.

OSTM1 mutations account for 5% of cases and include ARO associated with a lysosomal storage disorder and a particularly poor prognosis due to severe brain anomalies and seizures. This condition is analogous to the gray-lethal phenotype in mice. HSCT has not been recommended in these patients.

PLEKHM1 mutations are rare (<1%) but produce an ARO phenotype associated with much milder bone disease such that affected individuals have not needed HSCT.

Carbonic anhydrase II–dependent ARO is distinguished by its association with renal tubular acidosis and cerebral calcifications. HSCT is a therapeutic option.

NEMO-dependent osteopetrosis is rare, X-linked, and distinguished by the occurrence of lymphedema, immunodeficiency, and anhidrotic ectodermal dysplasia in affected males. HSCT is a therapeutic option.

SNX10 mutations, thus far reported only in the Palestinian population, cause a classical ARO that is ameliorated by HSCT. Mutations in this gene result in small osteoclasts with reduced reabsorptive capacity.

Osteoclast-Poor Forms

TNFSF11 (RANKL) encodes the main osteoclast-differentiating factor produced by osteoblasts and stromal cells. Homozygous mutations in this gene cause a classical phenotype that is not rescued by HSCT because *RANKL* is not produced by hematopoietic lineages. Mutations in this gene account for 5% of cases.

TNFRSF11A (RANK) encodes the receptor for *RANKL*. Mutations in this gene account for 5% of ARO cases. Affected individuals have a severe skeletal phenotype with a milder hematologic presentation. It is recommended that this group be considered for HSCT early on the basis of severe skeletal rather than hematologic involvement. Affected individuals may have severe, prolonged hypercalcemia following transplantation.

References

Albers-Schönberg H: Eine bisher nicht beschriebene Allgemeinekrankung des Skelettes im Röntgenbilde, *Fortschr Geb Roentgenstrahlen Nuklearmed* 11:261, 1907.

Gerritsen EJA, et al: Autosomal recessive osteopetrosis: Variability of findings at diagnosis and during the natural course, *Pediatrics* 93:247, 1994.

Cleiren E, et al: Albers-Schönberg disease (autosomal dominant osteopetrosis, type II) results from mutations in the (*CLCN7*) chloride channel gene, *Hum Mol Genet* 10:2861, 2001.

Villa A, et al: Infantile malignant, autosomal recessive osteopetrosis: The rich and the poor, *Calcif Tissue Int* 84:1, 2009.

Pangrazio A, et al: RANK-dependent autosomal recessive osteopetrosis: Characterization of five new cases with novel mutations, *J Bone Min Res* 27:342, 2012.

Aker M, et al: An *SNX10* mutation causes malignant osteopetrosis of infancy, *J Med Genet* 49:221, 2012.

L

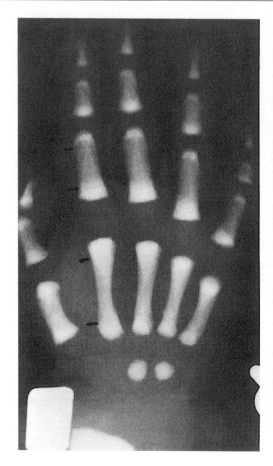

FIGURE 1. Osteopetrosis: autosomal recessive—lethal. An 8-month-old child. The sclerotic skeleton shows the "bone within a bone" (endobone) appearance, vertical striations at the metaphyseal-diaphyseal juncture, and broad metaphyses.

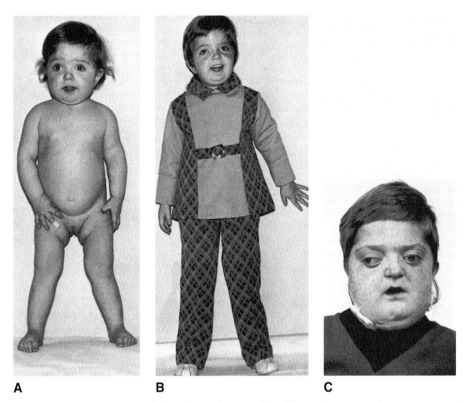

A   **B**   **C**

FIGURE 2.   Same child at 2 years (**A**), with length at 3rd percentile and beginning genu valgum; at 3½ years (**B**), with vision lost, despite attempted decompression of optic nerve; and at 10½ years (**C**), with proptosis and mandibular osteitis. Her death at 11 years resulted from carotid artery compression. (Courtesy Dr. Dag Aarskog, Bergen, Norway.)

L

LENZ-MAJEWSKI HYPEROSTOSIS SYNDROME
Dense, Thick Bone; Symphalangism; Hypotrophic Skin

Since 1974, when Lenz and Majewski first proposed this condition as a distinct syndrome, only nine patient reports have appeared in the literature. However, at least three other isolated cases have been published as "unknown" multiple malformation syndromes. The features in infancy differ greatly from those in older childhood, producing difficulties in early diagnosis.

ABNORMALITIES

Growth. Intrauterine growth retardation, postnatal short stature, eventual severe emaciation.

Performance. Moderate to severe intellectual disability.

Craniofacial. Disproportionately large cranium with broad and prominent forehead; late closure of large fontanels; hypertelorism with protuberant eyes; frequent choanal stenosis or atresia; nasolacrimal duct stenosis; dysplastic enamel; late eruption of deciduous and permanent teeth.

Skin. Cutis laxa in infancy; later, skin becomes hypotrophic and thin with prominent, subcutaneous veins, especially over the scalp, creating appearance of premature aging; cutaneous syndactyly of the digits; absence of elastic fibers on skin biopsy; sparse hair in infancy.

Limbs. Syndactyly, brachydactyly, dorsiflexion of fingers, hyperextensible joints.

Imaging. Proximal symphalangism, delayed ossification of ulnar rays, short or absent middle phalanges; broad, thick ribs and clavicles; widespread cortical sclerosis and thickening of bone in diaphyses, calvarium, vertebrae, and skull base; shallow and distorted orbits; long, flared, and radiolucent metaphyses, osteopenic epiphyses, long-bone hyperostosis; delayed bone age.

Other. Cryptorchidism and inguinal hernia in boys.

OCCASIONAL ABNORMALITIES

Facial palsy, cleft palate, large, floppy ears, small tongue, micrognathia, cerebral atrophy, dysgenesis of corpus callosum, hydrocephalus, flexion contractures at elbows and knees, hypospadias/chordee, dislocated hips (one case), early death.

NATURAL HISTORY

At birth, cutis laxa, large fontanels, and syndactyly are the most prominent features. Progressive hyperostosis becomes evident only after the first 6 months of life, often leading to erroneous diagnosis in infancy. Choanal stenosis may cause respiratory insufficiency and repeated episodes of pneumonia. Later, this problem may be aggravated by relative thoracic immobility caused by rib widening. Poor weight gain and slow statural growth persist even after resolution of infantile feeding difficulties. The original patient described by Lenz and Majewski was 30 years of age when last reported. She was 120 cm tall, spoke only a few words, and was ambulatory.

ETIOLOGY

The cause of this disorder is unknown. All cases have been sporadic. New mutation for a dominant gene has been suggested because of a tendency toward increased parental age.

References

Kaye CI, Fischer DE, Esterly BE: Cutis laxa, skeletal anomalies and ambiguous genitalia, *Am J Dis Child* 127:115, 1974.

Lenz WD, Majewski FA: A generalized disorder of the connective tissues with progeria, choanal atresia, symphalangism, hypoplasia of dentine and craniodiaphyseal hyperostosis, *Birth Defects* 10(12):133, 1974.

Majewski F: Lenz-Majewski hyperostotic dwarfism: Reexamination of the original patient, *Am J Med Genet* 93:335, 2000.

Dateki S, et al: A Japanese patient with a mild Lenz-Majewski syndrome, *J Hum Genet* 52:686, 2007.

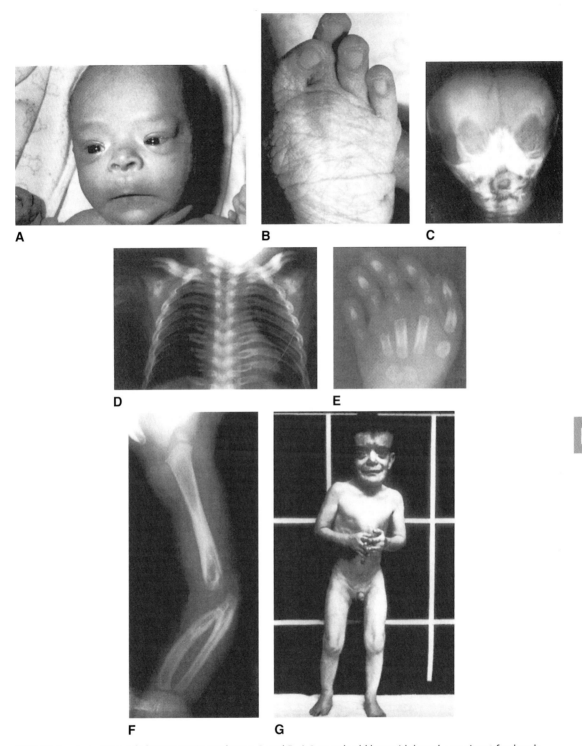

FIGURE 1. Lenz-Majewski hyperostosis syndrome. **A** and **B,** A 2-month-old boy with broad, prominent forehead; ocular hypertelorism; cutaneous syndactyly with dorsiflexed fingers; and cutis laxa. Radiographs of the same patient at 1 year reveal sclerosis of skull base (**C**), broad ribs and clavicles (**D**), symphalangism and hypoplasia of middle phalanges (**E**), and diaphyseal undermodeling and cortical thickening with radiolucent metaphyses and epiphyses (**F**). **G,** The changing phenotype is demonstrated by a boy, 4½ years old, who has a square forehead with bifrontal bossing, ocular hypertelorism, and flexion contractures at elbows and knees. (**A–F,** Courtesy Dr. Jon Aase, University of New Mexico, Albuquerque. **G,** Courtesy Dr. Meinhard Robinow, Children's Medical Center, Dayton, Ohio.)

PYKNODYSOSTOSIS
Osteosclerosis, Short Distal Phalanges, Delayed Closure of Fontanels

Although cleidocranial dysostosis associated with osteosclerosis and bone fragility had been recognized before 1962, this condition was not well clarified until Maroteaux and Lamy described it as a distinct condition and called it pyknodysostosis (*pyknos* meaning "dense"). Fewer than 200 cases have been reported.

ABNORMALITIES

Growth. Small stature with adult height of less than 150 cm.

Performance. Normal cognitive function.

Craniofacial. Frontal and occipital prominence, delayed closure of sutures, persistence of anterior fontanel; proptosis; blue sclerae; facial hypoplasia with prominent nose and narrow grooved palate; obtuse angle to mandible, which may be small; irregular permanent teeth with or without partial anodontia, delayed dental eruption, crowding, caries.

Skeletal. Stubby hands with broad distal phalanges, wrinkled skin over dorsa of distal fingers, flattened and grooved nails.

Imaging. Osteosclerosis with tendency toward transverse fracture; clavicular dysplasia to loss of acromion end; acro-osteolytic dysplasia of distal phalanges, especially of index finger; Wormian bones; lack of frontal sinus.

OCCASIONAL ABNORMALITIES

Intellectual disability, craniosynostosis, hearing loss, obstructive sleep apnea, giant-cell granuloma of maxilla, pseudarthrosis of clavicle, scoliosis, spondylolysis, vertebral arch defects in the interarticular parts or pedicles (most frequently at L5), bone marrow hypoplasia with compensatory splenomegaly.

NATURAL HISTORY

Life span is normal. Approximately two thirds of the patients have had fractures (which heal poorly), most commonly of the mandible, clavicle, and lower extremities, including the metatarsals. There may be progressive degeneration of the distal phalanges and outer clavicle and persistent open fontanels, especially posteriorly. Special dental care is often indicated. Osteomyelitis of the jaw occurs frequently. Obstructive sleep apnea from airway obstruction at multiple levels may need to be addressed. Three patients have had favorable responses to growth hormone treatment.

ETIOLOGY

This disorder has an autosomal recessive inheritance pattern. Homozygous or compound heterozygous mutations in the cathepsin K gene (*CTSK*) located at chromosome 1q21 are responsible. There are several reports of uniparental disomy (UPD) causing this condition. Cathepsin K is involved in the process of bone resorption and extracellular matrix remodeling.

COMMENT

The artist Toulouse-Lautrec may have had pyknodysostosis.

References

Thomsen G, Guttadauro M: Cleidocranial dysostosis associated with osteosclerosis and bone fragility, *Acta Radiol* 37:559, 1952.

Maroteaux P, Lamy M: La pycnodysostose, *Presse Med* 70:999, 1962.

Gelb BD, et al: Pycnodysostosis, a lysosomal disease caused by cathepsin K deficiency, *Science* 273:1236, 1996.

Bertola D, et al: Craniosynostosis in pycnodysostosis: Broadening the spectrum of the cranial flat bone abnormalities, *Am J Med Genet Part A* 152A:2599, 2010.

Rothenbühler A, et al: Near normalization of adult height and body proportions by growth hormone in pyknodysostosis, *J Clin Endocrinol Metab* 95:2827, 2010.

Xue Y, et al: Clinical and animal research findings in pycnodysostosis and gene mutations of cathepsin K from 1996 to 2011, *Orphanet J Rare Dis* 6:20, 2011.

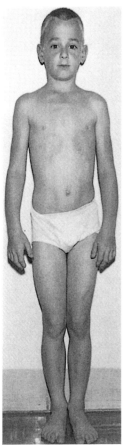

A

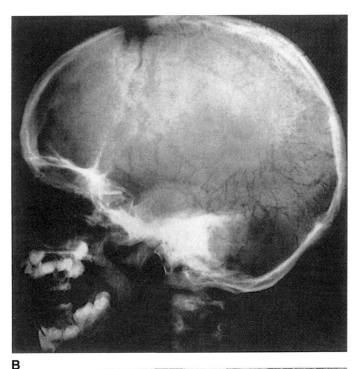

B

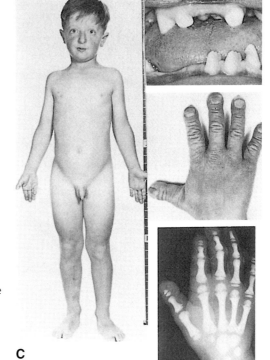

C

FIGURE 1. Pyknodysostosis. **A,** A 10-year-old child with height age of 8½ years. **B,** Same patient shown in **A.** Note the open fontanel and lamboid suture, absence of frontal sinus or mastoid air cells, obtuse angle of mandible, and delay in eruption of permanent dentition. **C,** A 7½-year-old with height age of 4½ years. Note the generally dense bone and partial loss of several distal phalanges. (**C,** From Shuler SE: *Arch Dis Child* 38:620, 1963, with permission.)

L

CLEIDOCRANIAL DYSOSTOSIS
Defect of Clavicle, Late Ossification of Cranial Sutures, Delayed Eruption of Teeth

A possible example of this rather generalized dysplasia of osseous and dental tissues was detected in the skull of a Neanderthal man. The more obvious features of the defect in the clavicle and cranium prompted Marie and Sainton to use the term "cleidocranial dysostosis" for this condition. However, the more generalized dysplasia of bone and teeth has been emphasized, and the term "cleidocranial dysostosis" depicts only a portion of the abnormal development. Well over 500 cases have been reported. A prevalence of 0.12 per 10,000 births has been documented.

ABNORMALITIES

Growth. Slight to moderate shortness of stature.

Craniofacial. Brachycephaly with bossing of frontal, parietal, and occipital bones; delayed calvarial ossification; midfacial hypoplasia with low nasal bridge, narrow high-arched palate; hypertelorism; late dental eruption, especially the permanent teeth, which are often abnormal with aplasia, malformed roots, retention cysts, enamel hypoplasia, enhanced caries, and supernumerary teeth.

Skeletal. Palpably absent clavicle with associated muscle defects, small thorax; hand anomalies, including asymmetric length of fingers with long second metacarpal, short middle phalanges of second and fifth fingers, short and tapering distal phalanges with or without down-curving nails.

Imaging. Late closure of fontanels and mineralization of sutures; late or incomplete development of accessory sinuses and mastoid air cells; Wormian bones; small sphenoid bones; calvarial thickening; partial to complete clavicular aplasia; short oblique ribs; cone-shaped phalangeal epiphyses in childhood, accessory proximal metacarpal epiphyses that fuse in childhood, and slow rate of carpal ossification; delayed mineralization of pubic bone with wide symphysis pubis, narrow pelvis, broad femoral head with short femoral neck (with or without coxa vara), lateral notching of proximal femoral ossification centers, spondylolysis, spondylolisthesis.

OCCASIONAL ABNORMALITIES

Absent ossification of parietal bones, atlantoaxial subluxation, cervical rib, small scapulae, syringomyelia, kyphosis, flat acetabula, genu valga, scoliosis, pes planus, osteosclerosis, increased bone fragility, deafness, cleft palate, micrognathia.

NATURAL HISTORY

Although stature is often reduced, cognitive function is usually normal. Hearing should be assessed, and dental problems should be anticipated. Removal of deciduous teeth does not seem to hasten the eruption of permanent teeth, and the permanent teeth may be difficult to extract because of malformed roots. A narrow pelvis may necessitate cesarean section in the pregnant woman with this condition. A narrow thorax may lead to respiratory distress in early infancy. Upper respiratory complications and sinus infections are common.

ETIOLOGY

Autosomal dominant inheritance with wide variability in expression. Heterozygous point mutations in *RUNX2*, formerly known as the core-binding factor a-1 (*CBFA1*) gene, located at 6p21, are responsible for most cases, although 10% will have an intragenic deletion or duplication. *RUNX2* plays an important role in osteogenesis and differentiation of precursor cells of the clavicular anlage, as well as having an important role in regulating many genes involved in osteogenesis and chondrocyte differentiation.

References

Marie P, Sainton P: Observation d'hydrocephalie héréditaire (père et fils) par vice de développement du crane et du cerveau, *Bull Mem Soc Med Hop (Paris)* 14:706, 1897.

Grieg DM: Neanderthal skull presenting features of cleidocranial dysostosis and other peculiarities, *Edinburgh Med J* 40:407, 1933.

Mundlos S, et al: Genetic mapping of cleidocranial dysplasia and evidence of a microdeletion in one family, *Hum Mol Genet* 4:71, 1995.

Mundlos S: Cleidocranial dysplasia: Clinical and molecular genetics, *J Med Genet* 36:177, 1999.

Ott CE, et al: Deletions of the *RUNX2* gene are present in about 10% of individuals with cleidocranial dysplasia, *Hum Mut* 31:E1587, 2010.

Cohen MM: RUNX genes, neoplasia, and cleidocranial dysplasia, *Am J Med Genet* 104:185, 2001.

Cooper SC, et al: A natural history of cleidocranial dysplasia, *Am J Med Genet* 104:1, 2001.

L

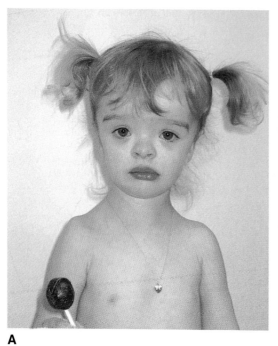
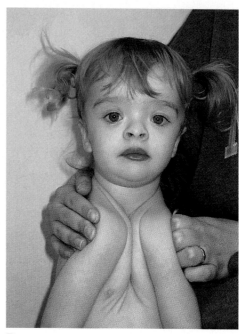

A   **B**

FIGURE 1.   A–E, Cleidocranial dysostosis in a 4-year-old girl and 11-year-old boy. Note the absent clavicles and hypoplasia of the ilia with widespread pubic rami. (**A** and **B,** Courtesy Dr. Stephen Braddock, Saint Louis University, St. Louis, Missouri.

Continued

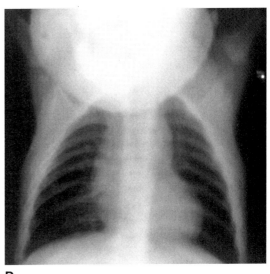

D

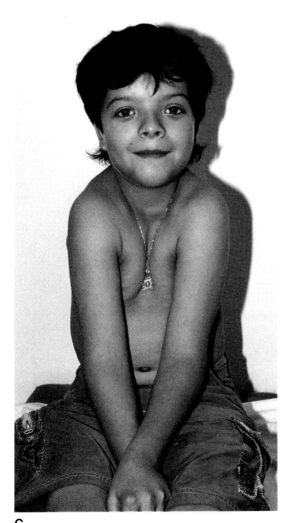

C

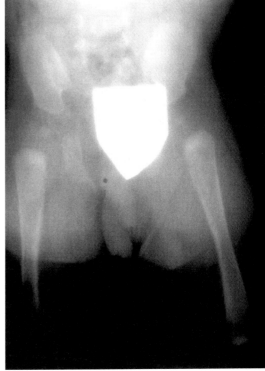

E

L

FIGURE 1, cont'd. **C,** Courtesy Dr. Marilyn C. Jones, Children's Hospital, San Diego.)

SAETHRE-CHOTZEN SYNDROME (ACROCEPHALOSYNDACTYLY TYPE III)
Brachycephaly with Maxillary Hypoplasia, Prominent Ear Crus, Syndactyly

Originally described by Saethre and by Chotzen in the early 1930s, this disorder was more recently appreciated as a distinct entity.

ABNORMALITIES

Craniofacial. Craniosynostosis of most commonly coronal but also sagittal, lambdoidal, metopic, or multiple sutures; late closing fontanels; brachycephaly with high flat forehead; low frontal hairline; shallow orbits; hypertelorism; downslanting palpebral fissures; ptosis of eyelids; lacrimal duct abnormalities; maxillary hypoplasia with narrow palate; facial asymmetry with deviation of nasal septum; prominent ear crus extending from the root of the helix across the concha; small, posteriorly rotated ears.

Limbs. Cutaneous syndactyly, usually partial, most commonly of second and third fingers or third and fourth toes; mild to moderate brachydactyly with small distal phalanges and clinodactyly of fifth finger; single upper palmar crease; short angulated or flattened thumbs; broad great toes with valgus deformity; finger-like thumbs; limited elbow extension.

Imaging. Both ossification defects and hyperostosis of the calvarium; parietal foramina; short clavicles with distal hypoplasia; delayed bone age; triangular epiphysis and duplicated terminal phalanx of the hallux.

OCCASIONAL ABNORMALITIES

Short stature; intellectual disability; lacrimal duct stenosis; bifid uvula; cleft palate; teeth with broad, bulbous crowns, thin, narrow tapering roots, and diffuse pulp stones in the pulp chambers of all posterior teeth; deafness; microtia; strabismus; radioulnar synostosis; vertebral anomalies, particularly of the cervical spine; short fourth metacarpals; hallucal reduplication; presumed cardiac anomaly (murmur); cryptorchidism; renal anomaly.

NATURAL HISTORY

Craniosynostosis is not an obligate feature. Although most patients are apparently of normal intelligence, intellectual disability of mild to moderate degree has been described. Facial appearance tends to improve during childhood. Increased intracranial pressure (as manifest by papilledema) has been seen in up to 28% of patients, even following surgical release of craniosynostosis. Obstructive sleep apnea is documented in 5%. Fluctuating hearing loss, usually conductive in nature, is common as is strabismus. Midface advancement is typically not necessary.

ETIOLOGY

This disorder has an autosomal dominant inheritance pattern. Truncating mutations of the *TWIST* gene located at 7p21-p22 are detectable in over half of affected individuals. An extremely wide variance in expression exists. Exonic or whole-gene deletions account for 11% to 28% of cases. Visible cytogenetic rearrangements may be seen in 4%. Those with large deletions in this region have, in addition to the characteristic features of Saethre-Chotzen syndrome, significant intellectual disability.

References

Saethre H: Ein Beitrag zum Turmschaedelproblem (Pathogenese, Erblichkeit und Symptomatologie), *Z Nervenheilkd* 117:533, 1931.

Chotzen F: Eine eigenartige familiare Entwicklungsstörung (Akrocephalosyndaktylie, Dysostosis craniofacialis und Hypertelorismus), *Monatsschr Kinderheilkd* 55:97, 1932.

El Ghouzzi V, et al: Mutations of the *TWIST* gene in the Saethre-Chotzen syndrome, *Nat Genet* 15:42, 1997.

Howard TD, et al: Mutations in *TWIST*, a basic helix-loop-helix transcription factor, in Saethre-Chotzen syndrome, *Nat Genet* 15:36, 1997.

Johnson D, et al: A comprehensive screen for *TWIST* mutations in patients with craniosynostosis identified a new microdeletion syndrome of chromosome band 7p21.1, *Am J Hum Genet* 63:1282, 1998.

Trusen A, et al: The pattern of skeletal anomalies in the cervical spine, hands, and feet in patients with Saethre-Chotzen syndrome, *Pediatr Radiol* 33:168, 2003.

Foo R, et al: The natural history of patients treated for *TWIST1*-confirmed Saethre-Chotzen syndrome, *Plast Reconstr Surg* 124:2085, 2009.

de Jong T, et al: Long-term functional outcome in 167 patients with syndromic craniosynostosis: Defining a syndrome-specific risk profile, *J Plast Reconstr Aesthet Surg* 63:1635, 2012.

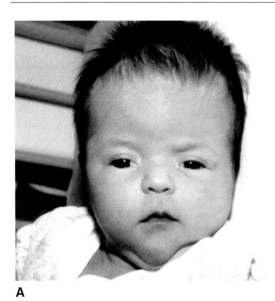

A

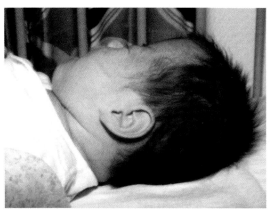

B

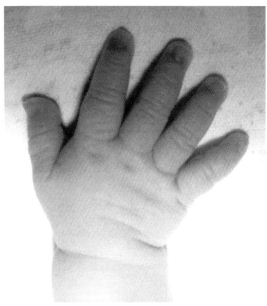

C

FIGURE 1. Saethre-Chotzen syndrome. **A–C**, A 1-month-old child showing brachycephaly with high flat forehead, shallow orbits, prominent ear crus, and brachydactyly.

M

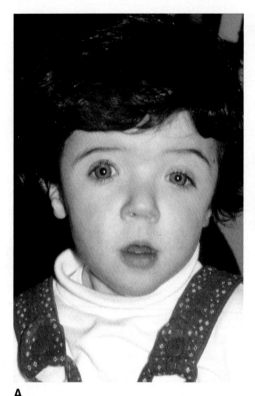

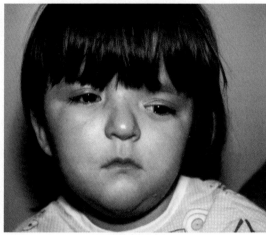

B

A

FIGURE 2.   **A–E,** Two children and an adult. Note ocular hypertelorism, high flat forehead, maxillary hypoplasia, ptosis, prominent ear crus extending from the root of the helix across the concha, cutaneous syndactyly, and fifth-finger clinodactyly. (Courtesy Dr. Michael Cohen, Dalhousie University, Halifax, Nova Scotia.)

Continued

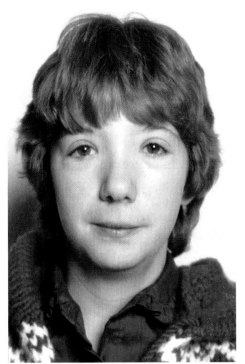

C

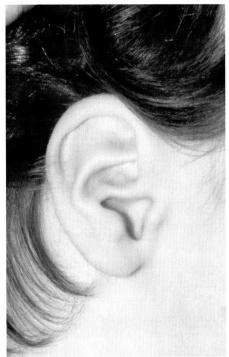

D

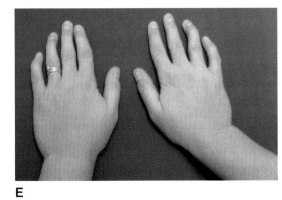

E

FIGURE 2, cont'd

M

PFEIFFER SYNDROME (PFEIFFER-TYPE ACROCEPHALOSYNDACTYLY)
Brachycephaly, Mild Syndactyly, Broad Thumbs and Toes

Since this disorder was reported by Pfeiffer in 1964, many cases have been published.

ABNORMALITIES

Craniofacial. Brachycephaly with craniosynostosis of coronal, with or without sagittal sutures with full high forehead; multisutural synostosis; ocular hypertelorism; shallow orbits; proptosis; strabismus; small nose with low nasal bridge; choanal stenosis; narrow maxilla; high arched palate.

Limbs. Broad, medially deviated distal phalanges of thumb and big toe; proximal phalanx of thumb and great toe frequently a delta phalanx; small middle phalanges of fingers; partial syndactyly of second and third fingers and second, third, and fourth toes.

OCCASIONAL ABNORMALITIES

Choanal atresia; ocular anterior chamber dysgenesis; exophthalmos; sensorineural hearing loss; cartilaginous trachea; laryngo-, tracheo-, and bronchomalacia; cleft palate; kleeblattschädel anomaly (cloverleaf skull); radiohumeral synostosis of elbow; symphalangism of index finger; brachydactyly; fused vertebrae; hydrocephalus; Chiari type I malformation; seizures; fifth-finger clinodactyly; arthrogryposis; intestinal malrotation; imperforate anus; cryptorchidism; sacrococcygeal eversion resembling a human tail; tethered cord.

NATURAL HISTORY AND COMMENT

Cohen delineated three clinical subtypes of Pfeiffer syndrome (PS) that are significant with respect to prognosis. Patients with type 1 have the "classic" phenotype, with craniosynostosis, broad thumbs and great toes, variable degrees of syndactyly, and normal to near normal intelligence. Long-term outcome is excellent. Type 2 is associated with cloverleaf skull, severe ocular proptosis, severe central nervous system involvement, elbow ankylosis/ synostosis, broad thumbs and great toes, and a variety of low-frequency visceral anomalies. Affected children generally do poorly, often with early death. Type 3 PS is similar to type 2 but lacks the cloverleaf skull. Although the vast majority of children with types 2 and 3 do very poorly, survival is possible, especially with aggressive medical and surgical treatment, particularly as it relates to the upper airway. Fluctuating hearing loss secondary to middle ear disease is common in all types. Patients with types 2 and 3 PS have significant risk for exposure keratopathy, obstructive sleep apnea, and persistent increased intracranial pressure after release of craniosynostosis. Midface advancement, often at a young age, may be necessary to address airway concerns. Intellectual disability is common in PS types 2 and 3.

ETIOLOGY

Autosomal dominant inheritance as well as sporadic cases, presumably caused by fresh gene mutation, have been seen in type 1. All cases of PS types 2 and 3 reported to date have been sporadic. Pfeiffer syndrome is genetically heterogeneous. Mutations of the fibroblast growth factor receptor 1 (*FGFR1*) gene, which maps to chromosome 8p11.22-p12, and of the fibroblast growth factor receptor 2 (*FGFR2*) gene, which maps to chromosome 10q25-q26, have been documented. Changes in the hands and feet tend to be less severe in children with *FGFR1* mutations than in those with *FGFR2* mutations. Five percent of individuals with PS type 1 have mutations in *FGFR1*. The remaining cases, as well as all cases of PS types 2 and 3, have mutations in *FGFR2*. Three mutations in *FGFR2* (p.Ser351Cys, p.Trp290Cys, and p.Cys342Arg) have been associated with severe phenotypes.

References

Pfeiffer RA: Dominant erbliche Akrocephalosyndactylie, *Z Kinderheilkd* 90:301, 1964.

Martsolf JT, et al: Pfeiffer syndrome: An unusual type of acrocephalosyndactyly with broad thumbs and great toes, *Am J Dis Child* 121:257, 1971.

Cohen MC: Pfeiffer syndrome update, clinical subtypes, and guidelines for differential diagnosis, *Am J Med Genet* 45:300, 1993.

Muenke M, et al: A common mutation in the fibroblast growth factor receptor 1 gene in Pfeiffer syndrome, *Nat Genet* 8:268, 1994.

Rutland P, et al: Identical mutations in the *FGFR2* gene cause both Pfeiffer and Crouzon syndrome phenotypes, *Nat Genet* 9:173, 1995.

de Jong T, et al: Long-term functional outcome in 167 patients with syndromic craniosynostosis: Defining a syndrome-specific risk profile, *J Plast Reconstr Aesthet Surg* 63:1635, 2010.

Wilkinson CC, et al: Syndromic craniosynostosis, fibroblastic growth factor receptor 2 (*FGFR2*) mutations, and sacrococcygeal eversion presenting as human tails, *Childs Nerv Syst* 28:1221, 2012.

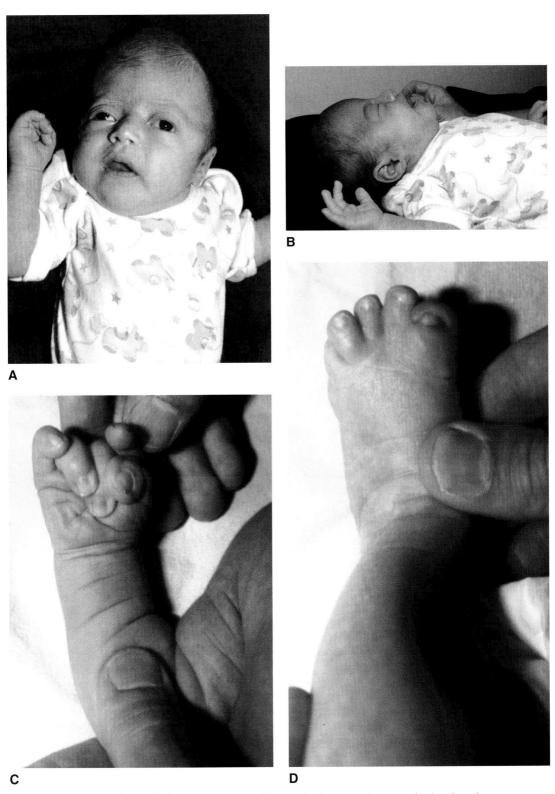

FIGURE 1.   Pfeiffer syndrome. **A–D,** A 1-month-old child. Note the brachycephaly, high forehead, ocular hypertelorism, broad thumbs and great toes with syndactyly of feet.

M

APERT SYNDROME (ACROCEPHALOSYNDACTYLY TYPE 1)

Irregular Craniosynostosis, Midfacial Hypoplasia, Syndactyly, Broad Distal Phalanx of Thumb and Big Toe

The condition was reported by Wheaton in 1894. In 1906, Apert summarized nine cases, and in 1920, Park and Powers published an exceptional essay on this entity. Numerous cases have been reported. The birth prevalence is 1 in 80,000 live births.

ABNORMALITIES

Growth. Mean birth length and weight above the 50th percentile; in childhood, deceleration of linear growth occurs such that most values are between the 5th and 50th percentiles; deceleration becomes more pronounced after adolescence.

Performance. Intellectual disability is present in a significant number of patients although normal intelligence has been seen. In two separate studies, mean IQ was 74 with a range from 52 to 89, and 61 with a range from 44 to 90, respectively; in a third study, 52% had an IQ less than 70.

Craniofacial. Brachyturricephaly with high, full forehead and flat occiput; craniosynostosis, especially of coronal suture; fontanels may be large and late in closure; flat facies, supraorbital horizontal groove, shallow orbits, interrupted eyebrows; hypertelorism, strabismus, downslanting of palpebral fissures, small nose, maxillary hypoplasia; narrow palate with median groove, with or without cleft palate or bifid uvula; dental anomalies, including delayed or ectopic eruption and shovel-shaped incisors; malocclusion.

Limbs. Osseous or cutaneous syndactyly, varying from total fusion to partial fusion, most commonly with complete fusion of second, third, and fourth fingers; distal phalanges of the thumbs are often broad and in valgus position; fingers may be short; cutaneous syndactyly of all toes with or without osseous syndactyly; distal hallux may be broad and malformed.

Skin. Hyperhidrosis; moderate to severe acne, including the forearms, at adolescence.

Imaging. A variety of brain malformations, including agenesis of corpus callosum, nonprogressive ventriculomegaly, progressive hydrocephalus, absent or defective septum pellucidum, gyral abnormalities, hippocampal abnormalities, and megalencephaly; fusion of cervical vertebrae usually at C5 to C6; radiohumeral synostosis; abnormal semicircular canals.

OCCASIONAL ABNORMALITIES

Kleeblattschädel anomaly (cloverleaf skull); Chiari I malformation; optic atrophy; short humerus, limitation of joint mobility especially elbow, pre- and postaxial polydactyly; genu valga; gastrointestinal anomalies in 1.5%, including pyloric stenosis, esophageal atresia, and ectopic anus; respiratory anomalies in 1.5%, including pulmonary aplasia and anomalous tracheal cartilage; cardiac defects in 10%, including pulmonic stenosis, overriding aorta, ventricular septal defect, and endocardial fibroelastosis; genitourinary anomalies in 10%, including polycystic kidney, hydronephrosis, bicornuate uterus, vaginal atresia, and cryptorchidism; diaphragmatic hernia; ovarian dysgerminoma.

NATURAL HISTORY

Early surgery for craniosynostosis does not appear to prevent intellectual disability, which is most likely related to malformations of the central nervous system. Moderate to severe language problems, as well as expressive language difficulties, occur frequently. Upper airway compromise, caused by a combination of reduction in size of the nasopharynx and reduction in patency of the choanae, and lower airway compromise, caused by anomalies of the tracheal cartilage, may be responsible for early death. Exposure keratopathy may occur secondary to proptosis. When the thumb is immobilized, early surgery to allow for a pincer grasp is indicated, with later attempts at further improvement of hand function. Hearing loss secondary to chronic otitis media or congenital fixation of the stapedial footplate is common. Multiple surgeries are typically necessary to improve structure and function. Increased intracranial pressure, obstructive sleep apnea, refractive visual errors, and strabismus dictate ongoing surveillance. Preliminary assessment of quality of life suggests resilience in this group of individuals.

ETIOLOGY

This disorder has an autosomal dominant inheritance pattern. The vast majority of cases are sporadic and have been associated with older paternal age. Mutations in the fibroblast growth factor receptor 2 gene (*FGFR2*), which maps to chromosome 10q25-10q26, cause Apert syndrome. Individuals with the p.Pro253Arg mutation respond better to craniofacial surgery but have more pronounced severity of syndactyly than those with the p.Ser252Trp mutation, the mutations that account for more than 98% of cases. Different mutations in *FGFR2* cause Crouzon syndrome as well as Pfeiffer syndrome.

References

Wheaton SW: Two specimens of congenital cranial deformity in infants associated with fusion of the fingers and toes, *Trans Pathol Soc Lond* 45:238, 1894.

Apert E: De l'acrocephalosyndactylie, *Bull Soc Med* 23:1310, 1906.

Park EA, Powers GF: Acrocephaly and scaphocephaly with symmetrically distributed malformations of the extremities: A study of the so-called acrocephalosyndactylism, *Am J Dis Child* 20:235, 1920.

Cohen MM, Kreiborg S: The central nervous system in the Apert syndrome, *Am J Med Genet* 35:36, 1990.

Wilkie AOM, et al: Apert syndrome results from localized mutations of *FGFR2* and is allelic with Crouzon syndrome, *Nat Genet* 9:165, 1995.

Allam KA, et al: Treatment of Apert syndrome: A long-term follow-up study, *Plast Reconstr Surg* 127:1601, 2011.

Raposo-Amaral CE, et al: Apert syndrome: Quality of life and challenges in a management protocol in Brazil, *J Craniofac Surg* 23:1104, 2012.

M

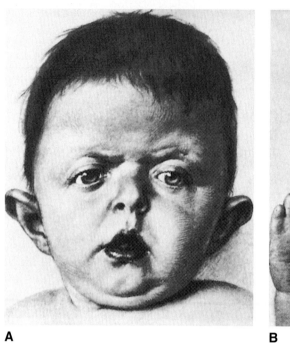
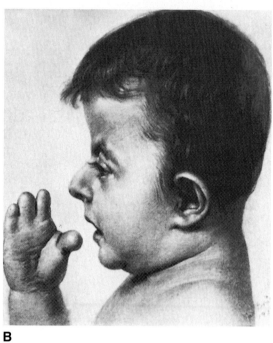

A   B

FIGURE 1.   Apert syndrome. **A** and **B,** A girl, drawn by the late M. Brödel. (**A** and **B,** From Park EA, Powers GF: *Am J Dis Child* 20:235, 1920.)

Continued

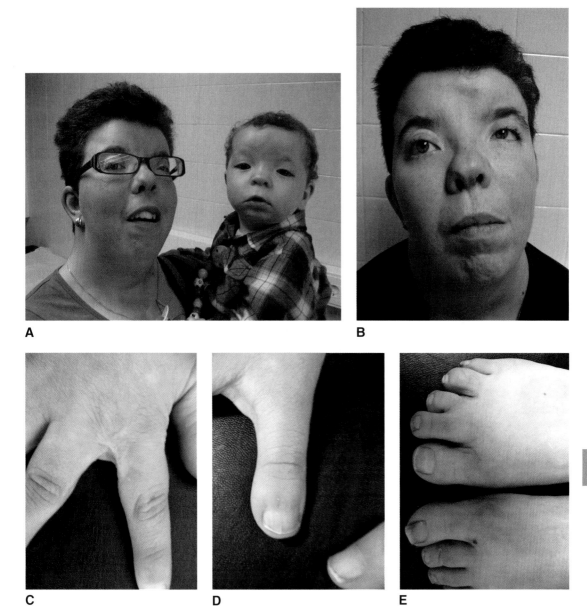

M

FIGURE 2.   A, Affected mother and her son. **B,** The mother, who had surgery for metopic synostosis in infancy, has hypertelorism, a broad nasal root, a bifid nasal tip, repaired partial cutaneous syndactyly of the hands (**C**), longitudinal splitting of the nails (**D**), broad halluces and 2-3 syndactyly of the feet (**E**). Her son has a broad forehead, hypertelorism, and telecanthus but no craniosynostosis. Both have dry curly hair.

CARPENTER SYNDROME
Acrocephaly, Polydactyly and Syndactyly of Feet, Lateral Displacement of Inner Canthi

Although Carpenter described this condition in 1901, it was not firmly established as an entity until Temtamy's report in 1966. More than 60 cases have been reported.

ABNORMALITIES

Growth. Increased birth weight, postnatal growth less than 25th percentile, obesity.

Performance. Intellectual disability in half of patients; IQs have ranged from 52 to 104.

Craniofacial. Brachycephaly with variable synostosis of sagittal, metopic, coronal, and lambdoid sutures; shallow supraorbital ridges; temporal bulging; flat nasal bridge; lateral displacement of the inner canthi with or without epicanthal folds; arched eyebrows; corneal opacity, maldeveloped cornea or microcornea, optic atrophy and/or blurring of disk margins; anteverted nares; low-set and malformed ears; hypoplastic mandible or maxilla; narrow, highly arched palate.

Limbs. Brachydactyly of hands with clinodactyly, partial syndactyly, camptodactyly; postaxial polydactyly; broad bifid thumbs; single flexion crease; subluxation at distal interphalangeal joints; angulation deformities at knees; preaxial or central polydactyly of the feet with partial syndactyly; short or missing middle phalanges of fingers and toes; clubfeet.

Cardiovascular. Defects in 50%, including ventricular septal defect, atrial septal defect, patent ductus arteriosus, pulmonic stenosis, tetralogy of Fallot, and transposition of great vessels.

Other. Hypogenitalism, cryptorchidism, umbilical hernia, omphalocele.

Imaging. Hydrocephalus, ventriculomegaly, agenesis of corpus callosum, midline cyst, split epiphyses at base of several proximal phalanges, biphalangeal digits, flat acetabulum, flare to pelvis, coxa valga.

OCCASIONAL ABNORMALITIES

Brain abnormalities, including atrophy, abnormal gyral patterns, enlarged foramen magnum; kleeblattschädel anomaly (cloverleaf skull); meningomyelocele; preauricular pits; cleft palate; short muscular neck; delayed loss of deciduous teeth; partial anodontia; duplication of second phalanx of thumb; kyphoscoliosis; metatarsus varus; genu valgum; lateral displacement of patellae; pilonidal dimple; accessory spleen; laterality defect; Meckel diverticulum; hydronephrosis with or without hydroureter; precocious puberty; conductive and sensorineural hearing loss.

NATURAL HISTORY

Intellectual disability is not an invariable feature despite the frequent imaging findings in the brain and significant cranial deformity. The sagittal and metopic sutures are most commonly involved. Fine motor dysfunction secondary to the digital anomalies is a continuing problem. Articulation errors attributed to inability to perform rapidly alternating movements of the lips and tongue can lead to speech problems. Eustachian tube dysfunction is secondary to the short cranial base. Mild short stature and obesity are common.

ETIOLOGY

This disorder has an autosomal recessive inheritance pattern. Homozygous or compound heterozygous mutations in *RAB23* cause this condition. Truncating mutations produce a protein that is subject to nonsense-mediated decay, a mechanism that is felt to play a role in the pathogenesis of this condition.

References

Carpenter G: Two sisters showing malformations of the skull and other congenital abnormalities, *Rep Soc Study Dis Child Lond* 1:110, 1901.

Temtamy SA: Carpenter's syndrome: Acrocephalopolysyndactyly, an autosomal recessive syndrome, *J Pediatr* 69:111, 1966.

Jenkins D, et al: *RAB23* mutations in Carpenter syndrome imply an unexpected role for hedgehog signaling in cranial-suture development and obesity, *Am J Hum Genet* 80:1162, 2007.

Perlyn CA, Marsh JL: Craniofacial dysmorphology of Carpenter syndrome: Lessons from three affected siblings, *Plast Reconstr Surg* 121:971, 2008.

Jenkins D, et al: Carpenter syndrome: Extended *RAB23* mutation spectrum and analysis of nonsense-mediated mRNA decay, *Hum Mut* 32:E2069, 2011.

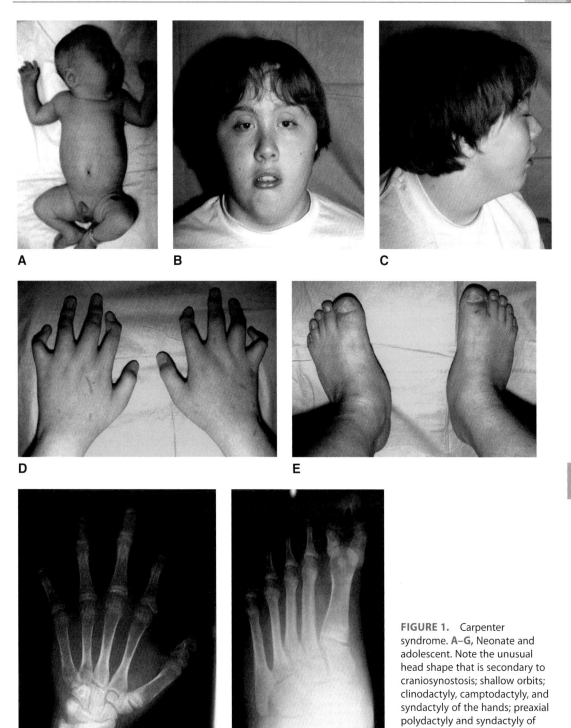

FIGURE 1. Carpenter syndrome. **A–G,** Neonate and adolescent. Note the unusual head shape that is secondary to craniosynostosis; shallow orbits; clinodactyly, camptodactyly, and syndactyly of the hands; preaxial polydactyly and syndactyly of the feet; and short middle phalanges of the fingers and toes. (From Robinson LK et al: *Am J Med Genet* 20:461, 1985.)

M

GREIG CEPHALOPOLYSYNDACTYLY SYNDROME
Preaxial and Postaxial Polydactyly, Syndactyly, Frontal Bossing

Initially described by Greig in 1926, additional cases were reported by Temtamy and McKusick, Marshall and Smith, and Hootnick and Holmes. Although highly penetrant, the disorder has a great degree of interfamilial and intrafamilial variability. The incidence is estimated to be 1 to 9 per 1,000,000.

ABNORMALITIES

Craniofacial. High forehead (70%); frontal bossing (58%); macrocephaly (52%); apparent hypertelorism; telecanthus; broad nasal root (79%).

Limbs. Hands: postaxial polydactyly (78%); broad thumbs (90%); syndactyly, primarily fingers 3 and 4 (82%). Feet: Preaxial polydactyly (81%); broad halluces (89%); syndactyly, primarily toes 1 to 3 (90%).

Imaging. Absence or dysgenesis of the corpus callosum, ventriculomegaly, preaxial polydactyly of hands and postaxial polydactyly of feet, osseous syndactyly, advanced bone age.

OCCASIONAL ABNORMALITIES

Intellectual disability, seizures, broad late-closing cranial sutures, trigonocephaly, craniosynostosis (metopic and sagittal), short or downslanting palpebral fissures, mild muscle fiber anomalies, camptodactyly, cardiac defect, hyperglycemia, hirsutism, inguinal and umbilical hernia, cryptorchidism, hypospadias.

ETIOLOGY

This disorder has an autosomal dominant inheritance pattern. Mutations in the *GLI3* gene located on chromosome 7p13 are responsible. In addition to mutations, translocations that interrupt the gene, microdeletions, and large cytogenetically detectable deletions have been described. The latter are associated with a more complex phenotype, involving some of the occasional abnormalities (cardiac defects, intellectual disability, seizures, and maturity onset diabetes of the young) noted previously, as a result of deletion of additional genes. *GLI3* is a downstream mediator of sonic hedgehog signaling. Functional haploinsufficiency produces the phenotype.

COMMENT

Mutations of *GLI3* cause Pallister-Hall syndrome and at least one case of acrocallosal syndrome. Some individuals presenting with metopic or sagittal craniosynostosis have been misdiagnosed with Carpenter syndrome.

References

Greig DM: Oxycephaly, *Edinburgh Med J* 33:189, 1926.

Temtamy S, McKusick VA: Synopsis of hand malformation with particular emphasis on genetic factors, *Birth Defects* 5(3):125, 1969.

Marshall RE, Smith DW: Frontodigital syndrome: A dominant inherited disorder with normal intelligence, *J Pediatr* 77:129, 1970.

Hootnick D, Holmes LB: Family polysyndactyly and craniofacial anomalies, *Clin Genet* 3:128, 1972.

Tommerup N, Nielsen F: A familial translocation t(3;7)(p21.1;p13) associated with the Greig polysyndactyly-craniofacial anomalies syndrome, *Am J Med Genet* 16:313, 1983.

Vortkamp A, et al: *GLI3* zinc-finger gene interrupted by translocations in Greig syndrome families, *Nature* 352:539, 1991.

Biesecker LG: The Greig cephalopolysyndactyly syndrome, *Orphanet J Rare Dis* 3:10, 2008.

Balk K, Biesecker LG: The clinical atlas of Greig cephalopolysyndactyly syndrome, *Am J Med Genet A* 146A:548, 2008.

Hurst JA, et al: Metopic and sagittal synostosis in Greig cephalopolysyndactyly syndrome: Five cases with intragenic mutations or complete deletions of *GLI3*, *Eur J Hum Genet* 19:757, 2011.

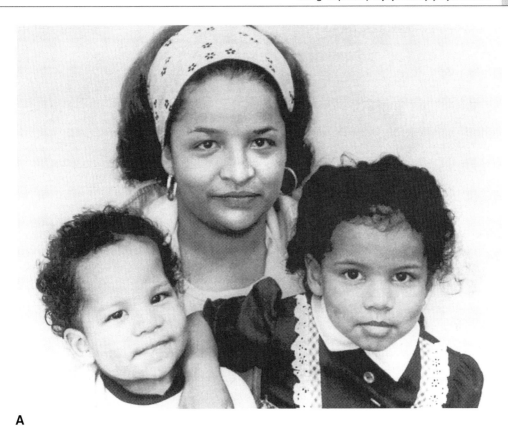

A

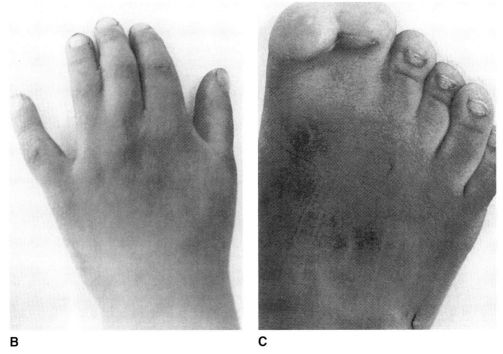

B   C

M

FIGURE 1.   A–C, Mother and her children with Greig cephalopolysyndactyly syndrome. Note the high forehead, syndactyly of fingers 3 and 4, and preaxial polydactyly of foot. (From Duncan PA et al: *Am J Dis Child* 133:818, 1979, with permission.)

ANTLEY-BIXLER SYNDROME
(MULTISYNOSTOTIC OSTEODYSGENESIS, TRAPEZOIDOCEPHALY/ MULTIPLE SYNOSTOSIS)
Craniosynostosis, Choanal Atresia, Radiohumeral Synostosis

This condition was first described by Antley and Bixler in 1975. Approximately 80 cases have been reported.

ABNORMALITIES

Craniofacial. Brachycephaly, frontal bossing, large anterior fontanel, craniosynostosis, midfacial hypoplasia, depressed nasal bridge, proptosis, choanal stenosis or atresia, dysplastic ears, stenotic external auditory canals.

Limbs. Radiohumeral synostosis; joint contractures, including inability to extend fingers and decreased range of motion at wrists, hips, knees, and ankles; arachnodactyly associated with enlarged interphalangeal joints, increased numbers of flexion creases, and distal tapering with narrow nails; femoral bowing; femoral fractures; rocker-bottom feet, clubfeet.

Imaging. Radiohumeral synostosis; carpal and tarsal synostoses; vertebral anomalies; tall vertebral bodies; vertebral clefts; spinal dysraphism.

OCCASIONAL ABNORMALITIES

Hydrocephalus, Arnold-Chiari malformation, kleeblattschädel anomaly (cloverleaf skull), preauricular tags, absent ossicular chain, ambiguous genitalia, vaginal atresia, hypoplastic labia majora, fused labia minora, clitoromegaly, anterior anus, atrial septal defects, renal defect, multiple hemangiomata, partial cutaneous syndactyly, narrow chest and pelvis.

NATURAL HISTORY

Respiratory compromise secondary to upper airway obstruction at multiple levels has varied from severe nasal congestion to multiple apneic episodes leading to death in the first few months of life. Survivors frequently require tracheostomy and placement of a gastrostomy tube until more definitive surgical management can be performed. Although gross and fine motor function have been difficult to assess because of joint contractures, prognosis may be reasonably good once the difficult perinatal period has passed. Joint contractures have improved with age and passive range-of-motion exercises. There has been no propensity to fracture postnatally. Individuals with mutations in P450 oxidoreductase (see Etiology) need long-term follow-up for congenital adrenal hyperplasia and surgery to correct genital anomalies.

ETIOLOGY

Three different causes of Antley-Bixler syndrome (ABS) have been identified: (1) Autosomal dominant mutations in the fibroblast growth factor receptor 2 (*FGFR2*) gene associated with a phenotype that includes the skeletal abnormalities and lacks manifestations of altered steroidogenesis or genital ambiguity. Rarely are mutations in *FGFR3* detected in this group. (2) Mutations in the cytochrome P450 oxidoreductase gene (POR) located on chromosome 7q11.23 resulting in autosomal recessive inheritance and an ABS phenotype that includes genital ambiguity and a characteristic urinary steroid profile (elevated excretion of metabolites of pregnenolone and progesterone; elevated metabolite levels associated with 17-α-hydroxylase deficiency; and elevated metabolites characteristic of 21-hydroxylase deficiency). POR mutations may also lead to the skeletal defects as a result of decreased lanosterol 14-α-demethylase activity. (3) In utero exposure to fluconazole, an antifungal medication that inhibits lanosterol 14-α-demethylase, an enzyme critical in sterol biosynthesis.

COMMENT

Undetectable unconjugated estriol implying abnormal fetal steroid or sterol metabolism has been demonstrated at mid-gestation maternal serum screening and may provide a prenatal marker for this disorder in some cases.

References

Antley RM, Bixler D: Trapezoidocephaly, midface hypoplasia, and cartilage abnormalities with multiple synostoses and skeletal fractures, *Birth Defects* 11(2):397, 1975.

DeLozier CD: Antley-Bixler syndrome from a prognostic perspective, *Am J Med Genet* 32:262, 1989.

Kelley RJ, et al: Abnormal sterol metabolism in a patient with Antley-Bixler syndrome and ambiguous genitalia, *Am J Med Genet* 110:95, 2002.

Adachi M, et al: Compound heterozygous mutations of cytochrome P450 oxidoreductase (POR) in two patients with Antley-Bixler syndrome, *Am J Med Genet* 128:333, 2004.

Cragun DL, et al: Undetectable maternal serum uE3 and postnatal abnormal sterol and steroid metabolism in Antley-Bixler syndrome, *Am J Med Genet* 129:1, 2004.

Huang N, et al: Diversity and function of mutations in P450 oxidoreductase in patients with Antley-Bixler syndrome and disordered steroidogenesis, *Am J Hum Genet* 76:729, 2005.

McGlaughlin KL, et al: Spectrum of Antley-Bixler syndrome, *J Craniofac Surg* 21:1560, 2010.

M

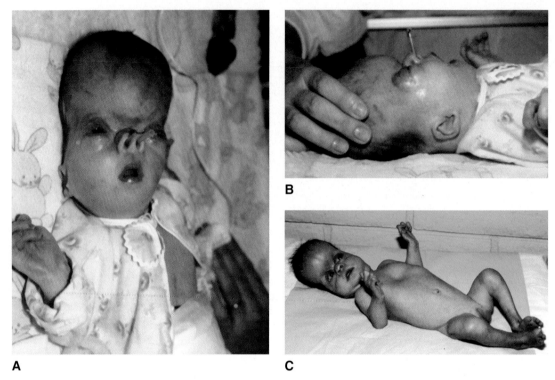

A
B
C

FIGURE 1.   Antley-Bixler syndrome. **A–E,** Newborn female infant with severe maxillary hypoplasia, depressed nasal bridge, proptosis, and dysplastic ears. Note the multiple joint contractures, radiohumeral synostosis, and femoral bowing. (From Robinson LK et al: *J Pediatr* 101:201, 1982, with permission.)

Continued

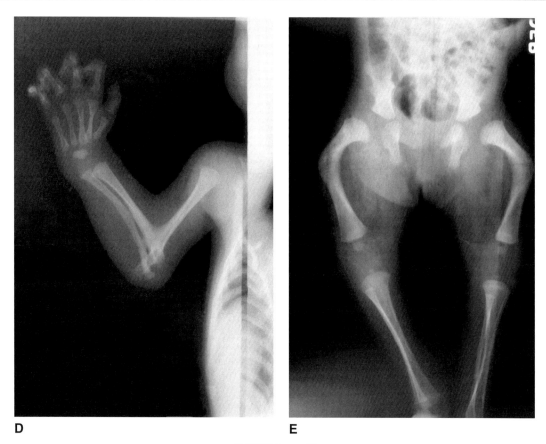

D   E

FIGURE 1, cont'd

M

BALLER-GEROLD SYNDROME
(CRANIOSYNOSTOSIS–RADIAL APLASIA SYNDROME)
Craniosynostosis, Radial Limb Reduction Defect, Anal Anomaly

Baller described a 26-year-old woman in 1950, and Gerold subsequently reported affected siblings. More than 30 cases have been reported.

ABNORMALITIES

Performance. Fifty percent of those followed beyond infancy have had intellectual disability.

Growth. Prenatal and postnatal growth deficiency.

Craniofacial. Craniosynostosis involving any or all sutures (100%), low-set and posteriorly rotated ears (64%), micrognathia (50%), prominent nasal bridge (32%), downslanting palpebral fissures (32%), microstomia (32%), epicanthal folds (27%), flattened forehead (27%).

Limbs. Radial aplasia/hypoplasia (77%); short, curved ulna (68%); missing carpals, metacarpals, and phalanges; fused carpals; absent or hypoplastic thumbs (100%).

Anal. Anomalies in 40%, including imperforate anus or anteriorly placed anus.

Urogenital. Anomalies in 35%, including ectopic, hypoplastic, dysplastic, or absent kidney, and persistence of the cloaca.

OCCASIONAL ABNORMALITIES

Epicanthal folds; bifid uvula; cleft palate; choanal stenosis; strabismus; optic atrophy; myopia; nystagmus; blue sclerae; seizures; polymicrogyria; hydrocephalus; absent corpus callosum; conductive hearing loss; capillary hemangiomata over nose and philtrum; hypoplastic ala nasi; vertebral defects; rib fusions; scoliosis; hypoplastic humerus; decreased range of motion at shoulders, elbows, and knees; postaxial polydactyly; hypoplastic patellae; coxa valga; spina bifida occulta; cardiac defects (25%), including subaortic valvular hypertrophy, ventricular septal defect, and tetralogy of Fallot; congenital portal venous malformation; poikiloderma; lymphoma (one case).

NATURAL HISTORY

Twenty percent of the live-born infants died unexpectedly during the first year of life. For the remainder, postnatal growth deficiency is common. Poikiloderma may develop in the first year of life. Although normal intelligence has been reported, variable degrees of cognitive impairment are more common. Although only one case of lymphoma has been reported, the allelic conditions (see Etiology) have an increased risk for osteosarcoma. Published information on natural history in Baller-Gerold syndrome is too limited to know if an increased risk exists for these patients as well.

ETIOLOGY

This disorder has an autosomal recessive inheritance pattern. Mutations in *RECQL4* account for most cases.

COMMENT

Before diagnosis of this disorder, other conditions with overlapping clinical features, including Fanconi pancytopenia syndrome and Roberts syndrome, should be excluded. Mutations in *RECQL4* also cause Rothmund-Thomson syndrome and RAPADILINO syndrome, a very rare condition seen almost exclusively in the Finnish population. Prenatal exposure to valproic acid produces a phenotype similar to Baller-Gerold syndrome.

References

Baller F: Radiusaplasie und Inzucht, *Z Menschl Vererb-Konstit-Lehre* 29:782, 1950.

Gerold M: Frakturheilung bei einem seltenen Fall kongenitaler Anomalie der oberen Gliedmassen, *Zentralbl Chir* 84:831, 1959.

Quarrell OWJ et al: Baller-Gerold syndrome and Fanconi anaemia, *Am J Med Genet* 75:228, 1998.

Maldergem LV, et al: Revisiting the craniosynostosis-radial ray hypoplasia association: Baller-Gerold syndrome caused by mutations in the *RECQL4* gene, *J Med Genet* 43:148, 2006.

Santos de Oliveira R et al: Fetal exposure to sodium valproate associated with Baller-Gerold syndrome: Case report and review of the literature, *Childs Nerv Syst* 22:90, 2006.

Debeljak M, et al: A patient with Baller-Gerold syndrome and midline NK/T lymphoma, *Am J Med Genet A* 149A:755, 2009.

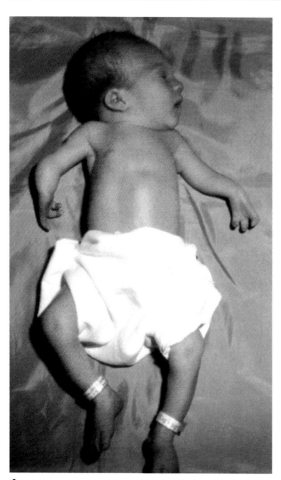

A

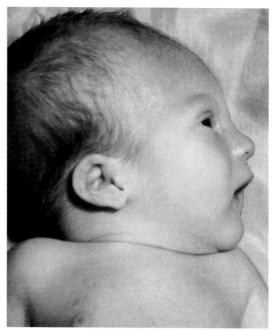

B

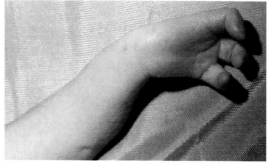

C

FIGURE 1. Baller-Gerold syndrome. **A–C,** Newborn infant with metopic craniosynostosis, mildly dysplastic ears, and radial dysplasia with absent thumbs. (From Greitzer LJ: *J Pediatr* 84:723, 1974, with permission.)

M

MULTIPLE SYNOSTOSIS SYNDROME (SYMPHALANGISM SYNDROME)
Symphalangism, Hypoplasia of Alae Nasi

In the past, this disorder was generally termed *symphalangism* (synostosis of finger joints), a nonspecific anomaly. The multiple synostosis character of the disorder herein set forth was emphasized by Maroteaux and colleagues, based on the presence of characteristic facial features and more severe and widespread joint involvement, especially in the vertebrae and hips.

ABNORMALITIES

Craniofacial. Sloping forehead, prominent supraorbital ridges, broad nasal bridge, hypoplastic nasal septum, bulbous tip of the nose with hypoplasia of alae nasi, malar flattening, short philtrum, asymmetric mouth, thin vermilion of upper lip, hyperopia, strabismus, conductive deafness.

Skeletal. Limited flexion, extension, and lateral bending of the neck; pectus excavatum or carinatum; prominent costochondral junction; limited rotation of hips and abduction of shoulders.

Limbs. Limited flexion of interphalangeal joints with faint or absent interphalangeal creases; variable clinodactyly, brachydactyly, and distal bone hypoplasia or aplasia of distal phalanges; absent, hypoplastic, or short fingernails/toenails; cutaneous syndactyly; broad, short thumbs; limited forearm flexion/extension and pronation/supination; short feet and broad hallux; inability to flex toes; deformity of heel; decreased range of motion of heel and foot; waddling gait.

Imaging. Multiple fusion of proximal and middle phalangeal joints (second to fifth digits); fusions of carpal and tarsal bones (especially navicular to talus); vertebral anomalies; fusion of the nasal bone and the frontal process of the maxilla; variable fusion of middle ear ossicles, most commonly fusion of stapes to the round window.

OCCASIONAL ABNORMALITIES

Moderate intellectual disability, Klippel-Feil anomaly, short sternum, humeroradial synostosis, good muscle development, short arms and legs.

NATURAL HISTORY

Hearing deficit typically presents in childhood and may progress later. Many cases are amenable to surgical correction. Hyperopia can be severe and should be looked for early in life. Symphalangism is not always present in childhood. Bony fusions are progressive and lead to increasing stiffness, and limitation of movement of the spine and/or limbs, which is sometimes painful. Neurologic complications secondary to spinal canal stenosis occurred in one patient.

ETIOLOGY

This disorder has an autosomal dominant inheritance pattern with appreciable variance in expression. Mutations in the *NOG* gene that encodes noggin, are responsible. Noggin is an antagonist of bone morphogenetic protein (BMP). Mice lacking noggin fail to initiate joint development suggesting that excess BMP leads to enhanced recruitment of cells into cartilage, resulting in oversized growth plates and failure of normal joint development. Genetic heterogeneity is present as mutations in two other genes, *GDF5* and *FGF9*, have been reported in a small number of families.

COMMENT

The term *NOG-related symphalangism spectrum disorder* has been proposed to include the many different phenotypes related to *NOG* mutations, which include proximal symphalangism, multiple synostoses syndrome, stapes ankylosis with broad thumbs and toes, tarsal-carpal coalition syndrome, and brachydactyly type B2.

References

Vesell ES: Symphalangism, strabismus and hearing loss in mother and daughter, *N Engl J Med* 263:839, 1960.

Maroteaux P, et al: La maladie des synostoses multiples, *Nouv Presse Med* 1:3041, 1972.

Gong Y, et al: Heterozygous mutations in the gene encoding noggin affect human joint morphogenesis, *Nat Genet* 21:302, 1999.

Dawson K, et al: GDF5 is a second locus for multiple-synostosis syndrome, *Am J Hum Genet* 78:708, 2006.

Wu XL, et al: Multiple synostoses syndrome is due to a missense mutation in exon 2 of *FGF9* gene, *Am J Hum Genet* 85:53, 2009.

Potti TA, et al: A comprehensive review of reported heritable noggin-associated syndromes and proposed clinical utility of one broadly inclusive diagnostic term: NOG-related-symphalangism spectrum disorder (NOG-SSD), *Hum Mutat* 32:877, 2011.

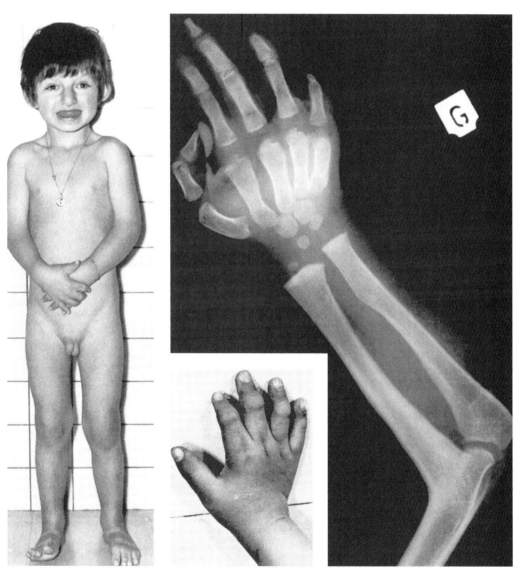

FIGURE 1.   Multiple synostosis syndrome. Note the narrow nose; prominent external ear; and variable brachydactyly, aplasia of distal phalanges, and synostoses. (From Maroteaux P et al: *Nouv Presse Med* 1:3041, 1972, with permission.)

SPONDYLOCARPOTARSAL SYNOSTOSIS SYNDROME
Disproportionate Short Stature, Block Vertebrae, Carpal Synostosis

This disorder was delineated in 1994 by Langer and colleagues, who described six affected individuals and reviewed an additional six from the literature. At least 25 cases have been reported to date. Diagnostic criteria were set forth by Coelho et al in 1998 and include fusion of multiple cervical, thoracic, or lumbar vertebral bodies; carpal and/or tarsal synostosis; short stature and scoliosis and/or lordosis; and absence of rib anomalies.

ABNORMALITIES

Growth. Disproportionate short stature with short trunk; increased upper-lower segment ratio.

Craniofacial. Mild dysmorphic features: round face with frontal bossing, anteverted nostrils; low-set, posteriorly rotated ears; conductive hearing loss due to recurrent otitis media, sensorineural hearing loss.

Skeletal. Variable degrees of scoliosis and lordosis, most commonly involving the thoracic spine; short trunk; short neck with low hairline.

Limbs. Single transverse palmar crease, absent interphalangeal flexion creases, fifth-finger clinodactyly, pes planus.

Imaging. Carpal synostosis, most commonly capitate-hamate and lunate-triquetrum; tarsal synostosis; block vertebrae; unsegmented bar.

OCCASIONAL ABNORMALITIES

Cleft palate; preauricular skin tag; ocular hypertelorism; short nose, with broad, square nasal tip; enamel hypoplasia; missing permanent teeth; decreased range of motion at elbows; odontoid hypoplasia; delayed ossification of many epiphyses as well as in carpal ossification; broad humerus; femoral epiphyseal dysplasia; postaxial polydactyly; clinodactyly; sacral anomaly; clubfoot; renal cyst and other kidney anomalies; mild developmental delay.

NATURAL HISTORY

Failure of normal spinal segmentation—which, when symmetric, leads to block vertebrae and when asymmetric, leads to unsegmented bars—causes most of the morbidity. Progressive scoliosis and lordosis are the major complications and are sometimes associated with restrictive lung disease. Cervical vertebral instability has been described. The unsegmented bar is difficult to identify on radiographs in early life because it is cartilaginous. Tomography is often helpful.

ETIOLOGY

This disorder has an autosomal recessive inheritance pattern. Mutations in the gene encoding filamin B (*FLNB*) are responsible. *FLNB* seems to have an important role in vertebral segmentation, joint formation, and endochondral ossification. An *FLNB* mutation–negative affected mother and son were recently reported. Genetic heterogeneity is suggested.

References

Langer LO, Moe JM: A recessive form of congenital scoliosis different from spondylothoracic dysplasia, *Birth Defects* 11(6):83, 1975.

Langer LO, et al: Spondylocarpotarsal synostosis syndrome (with or without unilateral unsegmented bar), *Am J Med Genet* 51:1, 1994.

Coelho KE, et al: Three new cases of spondylocarpotarsal synostosis syndrome: Clinical and radiographic studies, *Am J Med Genet* 77:12, 1998.

Krakow D, et al: Mutations in the gene encoding filamin B disrupt vertebral segmentation, joint formation, and skeletogenesis, *Nat Genet* 36:405, 2004.

Mitter D, et al: Expanded clinical spectrum of spondylocarpotarsal synostosis syndrome and possible manifestation in a heterozygous father, *Am J Med Genet A* 146A:779, 2008.

Isidor B, et al: Autosomal dominant spondylocarpotarsal synostosis syndrome: Phenotypic homogeneity and genetic heterogeneity, *Am J Med Genet A* 146A:1593, 2008.

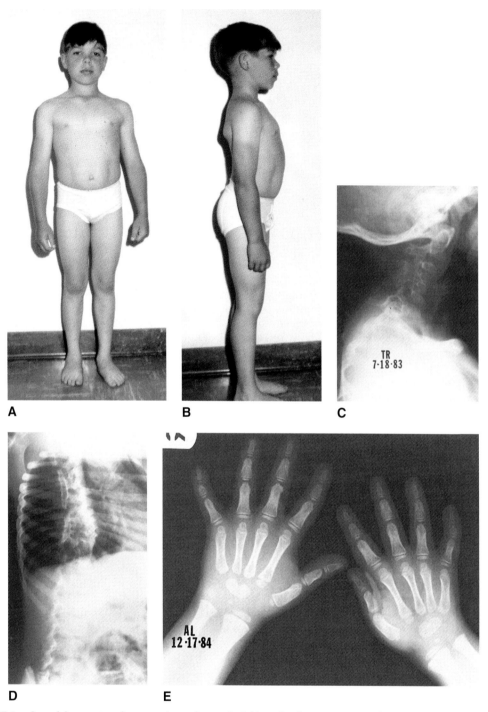

A   B   C

D   E

FIGURE 1.   Spondylocarpotarsal synostosis syndrome. **A–E,** Note the disproportionate short stature and short neck, synostosis of the cervical vertebrae, the unilateral unsegmented bar, and the carpal synostosis. (**A** and **B,** From Jones KL, Smith DW: *Syndrome Identification* 1:10, 1973; **C–E,** radiographs from Langer LO et al: *Am J Med Genet* 51:1, 1994. Copyright © 1994. Reprinted with permission of Wiley-Liss, Inc., a subsidiary of John Wiley & Sons, Inc.)

LARSEN SYNDROME
Multiple Joint Dislocation, Flat Facies, Short Fingernails

Larsen and colleagues described six sporadic cases of this condition in 1950. Two forms of Larsen syndrome (LS) share multiple joint dislocations at birth, but have significantly different clinical and radiographic findings, as well as different inheritance patterns and genetic etiologies.

ABNORMALITIES

Craniofacial. Autosomal dominant LS: flat face with depressed nasal bridge and prominent forehead, hypertelorism; cleft palate.

Skeletal. Dislocations of elbows, hips, knees, and wrists; long, nontapering fingers; talipes equinovalgus or varus; cervical kyphosis; scoliosis, lordosis, scoliosis of lumbar spine. Autosomal dominant LS: short, broad, spatulate distal phalanges, particularly the thumb; short nails.

Imaging. Dysplastic epiphyseal centers developing in childhood, short metacarpals and multiple carpal ossification centers, delayed coalescence of the two calcaneal ossification centers, spina bifida and hypoplastic bodies of cervical vertebrae, wedged vertebrae, spina bifida occulta of sacral spine, anomalies of posterior elements of thoracic spine, dysraphism, spondylolysis. *Autosomal dominant LS:* supernumerary carpal and tarsal bones, advanced bone age. *Autosomal recessive LS:* delayed or normal bone age, wide interpedicular distance at L1, shortening and clefting of the lumbar vertebrae in infancy, bifid distal humerus with dislocation or subluxation of the radial heads, short metacarpals and phalanges.

OCCASIONAL ABNORMALITIES
Intellectual disability; cleft lip; hypodontia; supernumerary teeth; gingival hyperplasia; periodontitis; conductive and sensorineural hearing loss; hypoplastic humerus; entropion of lower eyelids; anterior cortical lens opacities; simian crease; cardiovascular defect; mobile, infolding arytenoid cartilage; tracheomalacia; bronchomalacia; tracheal stenosis; cryptorchidism; malignant hyperthermia.

NATURAL HISTORY
Autosomal dominant LS: Prognosis is relatively good with aggressive orthopedic management. Many patients begin walking late. Osteoarthritis involving large joints and progressive kyphoscoliosis are potential complications. Airway obstruction caused

References

Solomon L: Hereditary multiple exostosis, *Am J Hum Genet* 16:351, 1964.

Ahn J, et al: Cloning of the putative tumour suppressor gene for hereditary multiple exostosis (EXT 1), *Nat Genet* 11:137, 1995.

Porter DE, et al: Severity of disease and risk of malignant change in hereditary multiple exostoses. A genotype-phenotype study, *J Bone Joint Surg Br* 86:1041, 2004.

Clement ND, et al: Skeletal growth patterns in hereditary multiple exostoses: A natural history, *J Pediatr Orthop B* 21:150, 2012.

Winston MJ, et al: Bisphosphonates for pain management in children with benign cartilage tumors, *Clin J Pain* 28:268, 2012.

Pedrini E, et al: Genotype-phenotype correlation study in 529 patients with multiple hereditary exostoses: Identification of "protective" and "risk" factors, *J Bone Joint Surg Am* 93:2294, 2012

N

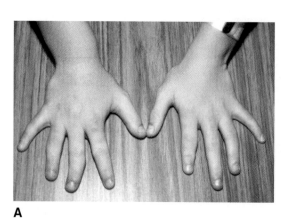

A

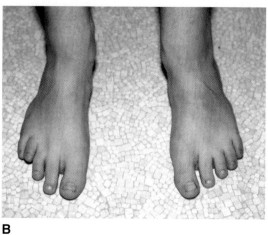

B

FIGURE 1.   Multiple exostoses syndrome. **A–F,** Note the grossly evident exostosis in the hand; altered angulation of the finger; short fourth and fifth toes, which are due to short fourth and fifth metatarsals; and, in the radiographs, the presence of exostoses at the ends of long bones as well as in the pelvis.

Continued

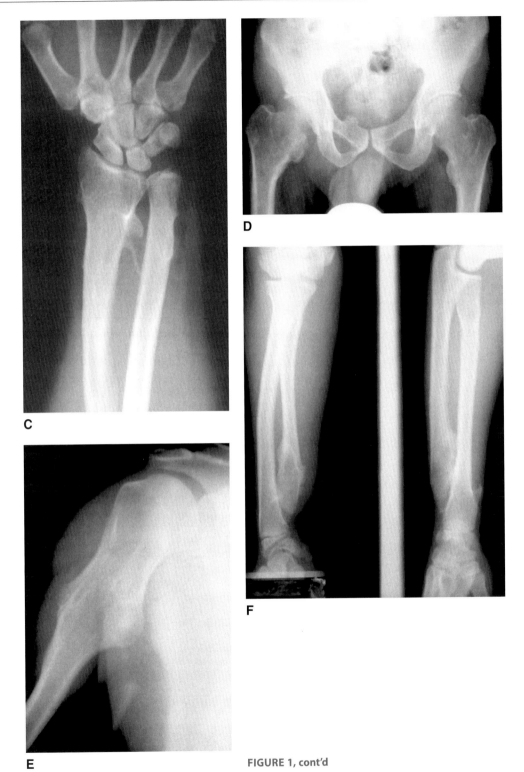

FIGURE 1, cont'd

NAIL-PATELLA SYNDROME (HEREDITARY OSTEO-ONYCHODYSPLASIA)
Nail Dysplasia, Patella Hypoplasia, Iliac Spurs

Little's report in 1897, limited to a presentation of the patellar defect, is usually credited as the initial description of this syndrome. This pattern is now known to include multiple other dysplasias of osseous and nonosseous mesenchymal tissues resulting in renal disease, glaucoma, and hearing impairment. The incidence of the disorder is estimated at 1 in 50,000.

ABNORMALITIES

Craniofacial. Glaucoma, ocular hypertension; dark pigmentation or iris centrally in cloverleaf or flower shape, particularly noticeable in blue eyes; sensorineural hearing impairment, unilateral or bilateral.

Skeletal. Incomplete elbow extension, pronation, and supination; cubitus valgus; palpable posterior iliac spur (81%); hypoplastic to absent patella; absence of distal phalangeal joints with missing creases; Madelung deformity; calcaneovalgus; talipes equinovalgus; tight Achilles tendons; scoliosis; lumbar lordosis.

Nails. Hypoplasia; splitting, most commonly of thumbnail; discoloration; longitudinal ridging; poorly formed lunulae and triangular lunulae.

Renal. Proteinuria with or without hematuria, casts, renal insufficiency.

Imaging. Hypoplastic capitellum, small head of radius (90%); hypoplastic to absent patella, hypoplasia of lateral femoral condyle, small head of fibula, and prominent tibial tuberosity; spur in midposterior ilium (71%); hypoplastic scapula with convex thick outer border (44%); delayed ossification of secondary centers of ossification; valgus deformity of femoral neck.

OCCASIONAL ABNORMALITIES

Intellectual disability, psychosis, attention deficit hyperactivity disorder, depressive disorder, peripheral neurologic symptoms; keratoconus, microcornea, microphakia, cataract, ptosis; cleft lip/palate, weak crumbling teeth; aplasia of pectoralis minor, biceps, triceps, quadriceps; antecubital or axillary pterygia, congenital hip dislocation, clinodactyly of fifth finger; polyarteritis-like vasculitis, irritable bowel or constipation; and, on imaging, prominent outer clavicle, hypoplasia of first ribs, malformed sternum, spina bifida, enlarged ulnar styloid process, dislocation of head of radius.

NATURAL HISTORY

Patients may have problems resulting from limitation of joint mobility, dislocation, or both, especially at the elbows and knee, where osteoarthritis may eventually limit function. Children should be closely followed for scoliosis. Proteinuria with or without hematuria is the most common early indication of a renal problem. Once proteinuria is present, it can remit spontaneously, remain asymptomatic, progress to nephrotic syndrome or nephritis. Renal involvement occurs in approximately 25% of cases and is clinically evident in one third of those older than 40 years. Most affected individuals have an accelerated age-related loss of filtration function, which may be exacerbated during pregnancy. Roughly 5% to 10% of individuals develop nephrotic-range proteinuria in childhood or young adulthood, progressing to end-stage kidney failure over variable periods of time.

ETIOLOGY

This disorder has an autosomal dominant inheritance pattern. Mutations and deletions in the LIM-homeodomain gene, *LMX1B*, located at 9q34, are responsible. Parental mosaicism in apparently unaffected fathers has been seen to cause recurrence. Nephropathy is more common with mutations affecting the home domain than in those affecting the LIM domains.

References

Little EM: Congenital absence or delayed development of the patella, *Lancet* 2:781, 1897.

Dreyer SD, et al: Mutations in *LMX1B* cause abnormal skeletal patterning and renal dysplasia in nail patella syndrome, *Nat Genet* 19:47, 1998.

Lemley KV: Kidney disease in nail-patella syndrome, *Pediatr Nephrol* 24:2345, 2009.

Marini M, et al: A spectrum of *LMX1B* mutations in nail-patella syndrome: New point mutations, deletion, and evidence of mosaicism in unaffected parents, *Genet Med* 12:431, 2010.

López-Arvizu C: Increased symptoms of attention deficit hyperactivity disorder and major depressive disorder symptoms in nail-patella syndrome: Potential association with *LMX1B* loss-of-function, *Am J Med Genet B Neuropsychiatr Genet* 156B:59, 2011.

N

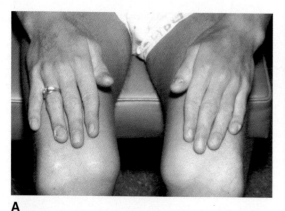

A

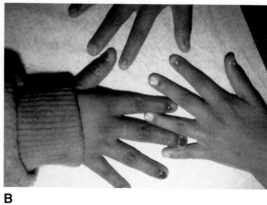

B

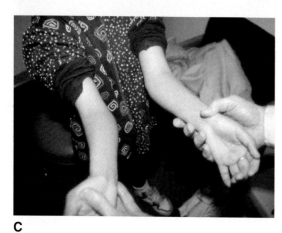

C

FIGURE 1.   Nail-patella syndrome. **A,** Adolescent showing nail hypoplasia, especially of thumbs, and displacement of small patellae. **B,** Two affected children showing nail dysplasia. **C,** Incomplete extension of the elbows.

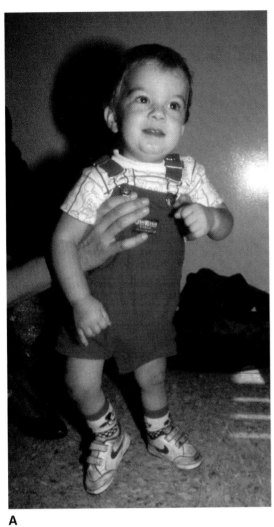

A

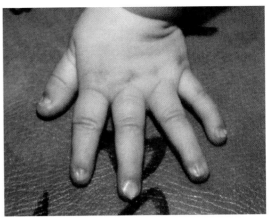

B

FIGURE 2.   **A** and **B,** A 15-month-old child. Note the striking nail dysplasia and evidence of joint dislocation at the knees.

MEIER-GORLIN SYNDROME
Absent/Hypoplastic Patella, Microtia, Short Stature

Initially described in two separate case reports in 1959 and by Gorlin and colleagues in 1975, this disorder has now been reported in more than 50 patients. De Munnik and colleagues reviewed 45 cases in 2012.

ABNORMALITIES

Growth. Prenatal and postnatal growth deficiency.

Performance. IQ is normal in close to 95%; a cheerful, friendly personality has been described.

Craniofacial. Microcephaly (less than 50% at birth) becomes more apparent with age; microtia; low-set abnormally formed ears; atretic/small external auditory canals; convex and narrow profile to the nose; high nasal bridge; small mouth with full lips; micrognathia; high-arched palate.

Skeletal. Absent/hypoplastic patella, dimples over the knees, hyperextensible joints, joint subluxations, genu recurvatum, clubfeet or other joint contractures, pectus carinatum, chest asymmetry.

Pulmonary. Emphysema, congenital or postnatal; laryngomalacia, tracheomalacia; bronchomalacia.

Genitalia. Cryptorchidism, small testes, micropenis, hypospadias, hypoplastic labia majora/ minora, clitoromegaly.

Other. Mammary hypoplasia reported in all postpubertal females, nipple hypoplasia, sparse axillary and pubic hair.

Imaging. Delayed bone age; absent/hypoplastic, slender, or short ribs; slender long bones; abnormal flattened epiphysis; lack of sternal ossification; hooked clavicles.

OCCASIONAL ABNORMALITIES

Moderate intellectual disability, expressive language delay (usually associated with normal hearing); decreased arm span for height, early closure of cranial sutures, cortical dysplasia, pachygyria and ventricular enlargement, maxillary hypoplasia, strabismus, bifid uvula, cleft palate, deafness with narrow external auditory canal, congenital labyrinthine anomalies, prominent veins over nose and forehead, thin skin, ventricular septal defect, patent ductus arteriosus, fifth-finger clinodactyly, hyperconvex nails, growth hormone deficiency.

NATURAL HISTORY

Failure to thrive secondary to feeding problems is common throughout the first 2 years. Respiratory difficulties can improve after the neonatal period. The typical facial features seen in infancy—including micrognathia, a small mouth, and full lips—change over time such that by adolescence, a high vertical forehead, narrow nose, and high nasal bridge are most characteristic. Growth hormone and estrogen treatment may be of some benefit relative to growth retardation and breast and genital hypoplasia.

ETIOLOGY

This disorder has an autosomal recessive inheritance pattern with marked genetic heterogeneity. Mutations in five genes encoding pre-replication complex proteins, *ORC1, ORC4, ORC6, CDT1,* and *CDC6,* produce this phenotype. A recent study of 45 individuals detected mutation in these genes in 35 (78%), suggesting further heterogeneity. Individuals with *ORC1* mutations had more severe short stature and smaller heads than the rest. A lethal phenotype with multiple congenital anomalies was seen in four individuals with compound heterozygous *ORC1* and *CDT1* mutations. Congenital pulmonary emphysema was reported in seven out of nine individuals with mutation in *CDT1.*

COMMENT

Mutations in *ORC1* encoding a subunit of the origin recognition complex (ORC) have also been seen in five patients with microcephalic primordial dwarfism.

References

Meier Z, et al: Ein Fall von Arthrogryposis multiplex congenita kombiniert mit Dysostosis mandibulofacialis (Franceschetti-Syndrom), *Helv Pediatr Acta* 14:213, 1959.

Gorlin RJ, et al: A selected miscellany, *Birth Defects* 11(2):39, 1975.

Guernsey DL, et al: Mutations in origin recognition complex gene *ORC4* cause Meier-Gorlin syndrome, *Nat Genet* 43:360, 2011

Bicknell LS, et al: Mutations in the pre-replication complex cause Meier-Gorlin syndrome, *Nat Genet* 43:356, 2011.

Bicknell LS, et al: Mutations in *ORC1,* encoding the largest subunit of the origin recognition complex, cause microcephalic primordial dwarfism, *Nat Genet* 43:350, 2011.

de Munnik SA, et al: Meier-Gorlin syndrome genotype-phenotype studies: 35 individuals with pre-replication complex gene mutations and 10 without molecular diagnosis, *Eur J Hum Genet* 20:598, 2012.

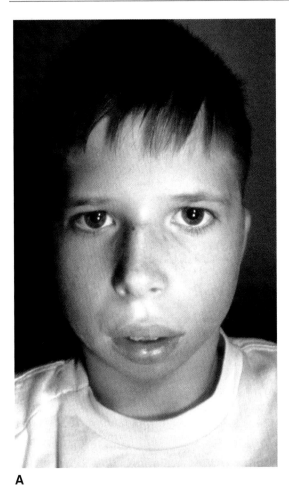

A

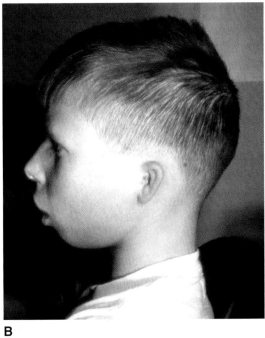

B

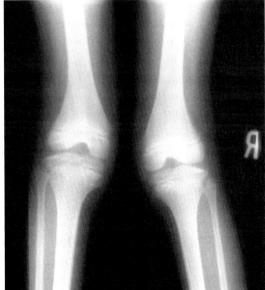

C

FIGURE 1. Meier-Gorlin syndrome. **A–C,** A 16-year-old boy. Note the small mouth with full lips, micrognathia, microtia, and absent patella. (From Gorlin RJ et al: *Birth Defects* 11:39, 1975.)

N

CANTÚ SYNDROME
Congenital Hypertrichosis, Cardiomegaly and Osteochondrodysplasia

In 1982 Cantú and colleagues described siblings and two unrelated individuals with a distinct disorder of hirsutism associated with a skeletal dysplasia. Fewer than 50 (33) cases have been reported worldwide; half of the cases are from Mexico.

ABNORMALITIES

Growth. Fetal macrosomia, which does not persist; muscular body build.
Performance. Mild motor delay, normal intelligence.
Behavior. Mood swings, anxiety.
Craniofacial. Macrocephaly, low frontal hairline, coarse facies, thick eyebrows and eyelashes, epicanthal folds, broad low nasal bridge, long philtrum, thick lips, dental malocclusion, thick alveolar ridge, high arched palate, macroglossia.
Heart. Cardiomegaly secondary to increased cardiac muscle mass, pericardial effusion, pulmonary hypertension, patent ductus arteriosus, bicuspid aortic valve.
Abdomen. Hepatomegaly.
Skeletal. Narrow thorax.
Limbs. Broad hands.
Skin. Striking hypertrichosis at birth, abundant scalp hair.
Imaging. Osteopenia, thick calvarium, vertical skull base, enlarged sella, narrow thorax with broad ribs, ovoid vertebral bodies, platyspondyly, hypoplastic ischium and pubis, coxa valga, expansion of the diaphyses of the long bones, metaphyseal widening with Erlenmeyer flask deformity, genu valga, proximal and distal megaepiphyses of long bones, broad first metatarsal, advanced bone age.

OCCASIONAL ABNORMALITIES

Mild intellectual disability, obsessive traits, tortuous retinal vessels, pulmonary venous obstruction, hypertrophic cardiomyopathy, coarctation of aorta pectus carinatum, umbilical hernia, peripheral edema, deep-set nails, fetal fingertip pads.

NATURAL HISTORY

The pericardial effusion may develop at any age and be recurrent, necessitating draining and/or pericardectomy. Cardiomegaly is due to increase in the mass of cardiac muscle although function and histology are typically normal. Nonspecific chronic inflammatory changes have been documented in pericardial biopsies. Childhood is characterized by recurrent infections with low immunoglobulin levels. Gastric bleeding has been seen in some individuals secondary to duodenitis and esophagitis. Some patients require treatment for gastroesophageal reflux.

ETIOLOGY

Heterozygous missense mutations in *ABCC9*, also called *SUR2*, have been documented in the majority of tested individuals. Prior reports of affected siblings born to unaffected parents likely represent unrecognized mosaicism in a parent. *ABCC9* encodes the sulfonylurea receptor that forms ATP-sensitive potassium channels. Mutations that product Cantú syndrome appear to be activating.

COMMENT

Loss of function mutations in *ABCC9* cause dilated cardiomyopathy. Side effects of the antihypertensive vasodilator, minoxidil, produce a phenotype similar to Cantú syndrome. Minoxidil is an agonist of the *ABCC9* related potassium channel.

References

Cantú JM, et al: A distinct osteochondrodysplasia with hypertrichosis—Individualization of a probable autosomal recessive entity, *Hum Genet* 60:36, 1982.

Lizalde B, et al: Autosomal dominant inheritance in Cantú syndrome (congenital hypertrichosis, osteochondrodysplasia, and cardiomegaly), *Am J Med Genet* 94:421, 2000.

Herman TE, McAlister WH: Cantú syndrome, *Pediatr Radiol* 35:550, 2005.

Scurr I, et al: Cantú syndrome: Report of nine new cases and expansion of the clinical phenotype, *Am J Med Genet A* 155:508, 2011.

Harakalova M, et al: Dominant missense mutations in *ABCC9* cause Cantú syndrome, *Nat Genet* 44:793, 2012.

Bregje WMVB, et al: Cantú syndrome is caused by mutations in *ABCC9*, *Am J Hum Genet* 90:1094, 2012.

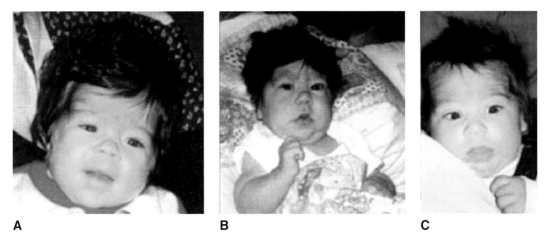

FIGURE 1.   Two 3-month-olds (**A** and **B**) and a 3-week-old (**C**). Note the epicanthic folds; short nose with broad, flat nasal bridge; and long philtrum. (From Scurr I et al: *Am J Med Genet A* 155A:508, 2011, with permission.)

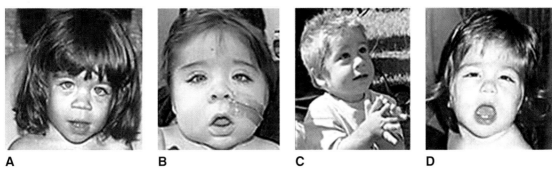

FIGURE 2.   Same patient as in Figure 1A at age 19 months (**A**), a 13-month-old (**B**), same patient as in Figure 1C at age 2 years (**C**), and a 19-month-old (**D**). Note the long palpebral fissures with long, thick eyelashes. (From Scurr I et al: *Am J Med Genet A* 155A:508, 2011, with permission.)

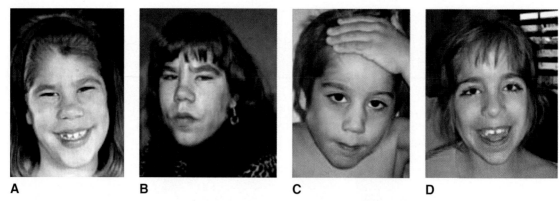

FIGURE 3.   Same patient as in Figure 1B at age 7 years (**A**) and 12 years (**B**), same patient as in Figures 1C and 2C at age 4 years (**C**), and same patient as in Figure 2D at age 8½ years (**D**). Note the tall forehead, long face, prominent chin, and prominent nasal bridge. (From Scurr I et al: *Am J Med Genet A* 155A:508, 2011, with permission.)

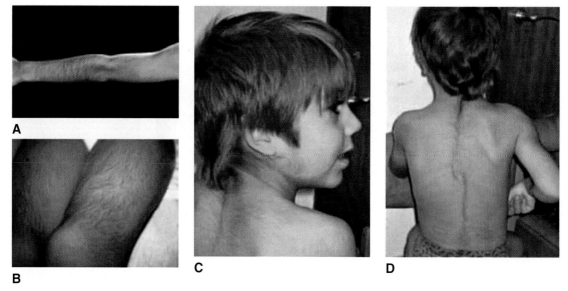

FIGURE 4.   Note the excessive hair growth over the extensor surfaces of the limbs of the same patient as in Figure 1A at age 9 years (**A** and **B**). Note the muscular appearance of the thighs. Same patient as in Figures 1C and 2C at age 4 years (**C** and **D**). Note the pattern of hypertrichosis. (From Scurr I et al: *Am J Med Genet A* 155A:508, 2011, with permission.)

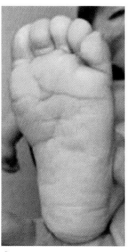

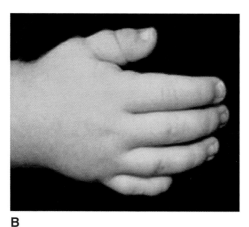

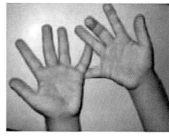

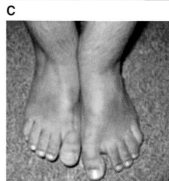

A

B

C

D

FIGURE 5.   Note the broad, puffy hands over the extensor surfaces; the deep-set nails; and prominent plantar creases in a 13-month-old (**A** and **B**). Hands and feet of a 4-year-old. Note the fetal finger pads. (From Scurr I et al: *Am J Med Genet A* 155A:508, 2011, with permission.)

N

LÉRI-WEILL DYSCHONDROSTEOSIS
Short Forearms with Madelung Deformity, with or without Short Lower Leg

Léri and Weill described dyschondrosteosis in 1929. Most patients previously categorized as having Madelung deformity have Léri-Weill dyschondrosteosis (LWD).

ABNORMALITIES

Growth. Variable small stature, adult height from 135 cm to normal; mean adult height −2.2 SD; birth length mildly reduced; height deficit noted by preschool age; reduced arm span and leg length.

Limbs. Short forearm with bowing of radius and distal hypoplasia of the dorsally dislocated ulna leading to a widened gap between radius and ulna, and altered osseous alignment at wrist (Madelung deformity); may have partial dislocation of ulna at wrist, elbow, or both, with limitation of movement; short lower leg; muscular hypertrophy of the calves (one third).

Imaging. Triangular distal radial epiphysis without trapezium; wedge-shaped carpal row; pyramidalization of the carpal row; lucent ulnar side of distal radius.

OCCASIONAL ABNORMALITIES

Short hands and feet with metaphyseal flaring in metacarpal and metatarsal bones, short fourth and fifth metacarpal or metatarsal bones, curvature of tibia, osteophytes from proximal tibia and/or fibula, abnormal femoral neck, coxa valga, abnormal tuberosity of humerus; increased carrying angle of the elbow; scoliosis; micrognathia; high arched palate.

NATURAL HISTORY

The only problems are moderate shortness of stature and limitation of joint mobility at the wrist, elbow, or both. In many children younger than 6 years, there may be no obvious manifestation in spite of a careful clinical evaluation. Because of the dominant inheritance, the examination of the wrists of the parents can give valuable hints in familial cases. Growth hormone therapy is effective with a similar gain in height as in girls with Turner syndrome.

ETIOLOGY

Autosomal dominant, with an excess of affected females in the recorded cases. In approximately 70% of cases, LWD is caused by *SHOX* haploinsufficiency; in the remaining cases, the cause is unknown. Deletions—including *SHOX* or its downstream and, less commonly, upstream enhancers in the pseudoautosomal region 1 (PAR1)—account for approximately 90% of identified mutations. The remaining 10% are missense and nonsense mutations. The PAR1 region is a recombination "hotspot" in male meiosis. Therefore, pseudoautosomal inheritance of Léri-Weill syndrome has been reported, from a male carrying a *SHOX* deletion in the Y chromosome to his daughter. Clinically affected females outnumber males, because the characteristic clinical signs are more frequent and more severe in girls, due to estrogen effects, but also to a higher rate of deletions in PAR1 in the X chromosome than in the Y chromosome.

The clinical spectrum of *SHOX* haploinsufficiency includes idiopathic short stature (ISS), short stature with subtle auxologic and radiologic findings, and the full picture of Léri-Weill dyschondrosteosis. *SHOX* haploinsufficiency has been recognized as the primary cause of ISS in 2% to 15% of patients.

COMMENT

Langer mesomelic dysplasia, first delineated in 1967, is the result of homozygous *SHOX* deficiency. Most cases are homozygous for *SHOX* mutations, but homozygous deletions of the *SHOX* gene and the pseudoautosomal 1 region (PAR1) distal enhancer region have also been seen. Affected individuals have marked disproportionate short stature with a final height of 130 cm and primarily shortening of the middle limb segment (forearms and lower legs). Mandibular hypoplasia and micrognathia are also seen. Radiographically the fibula is rudimentary, the tibia is short with proximal hypoplasia, the ulna is reduced distally, and the radius is bowed and short. Intelligence is normal. Growth hormone treatment has not been of benefit.

References

Léri A, Weill J: Une affection congénitale et symétrique du développement osseux: La dyschondrostéose, *Bull Mem Soc Med Hop (Paris)* 45:1491, 1929.

Langer LO: Mesomelic dwarfism of the hypoplastic ulna, fibula, mandible type, *Radiology* 89:654, 1967.

Espiritu C, et al: Probable homozygosity for the dyschondrosteosis genes, *Am J Dis Child* 129:375, 1975.

Belin V, et al: *SHOX* mutations in dyschondrosteosis (Leri-Weill syndrome), *Nat Genet* 19:67, 1998.

Shears DJ, et al: Mutation and deletion of the pseudoautosomal gene *SHOX* causes Leri-Weill dyschondrosteosis, *Nat Genet* 19:70, 1998.

Zinn AR, et al: Complete *SHOX* deficiency causes Langer mesomelic dysplasia, *Am J Med Genet* 110:158, 2002.

Binder G: Short stature due to *SHOX* deficiency: Genotype, phenotype, and therapy, *Horm Res Paediatr* 75:81, 2011.

N

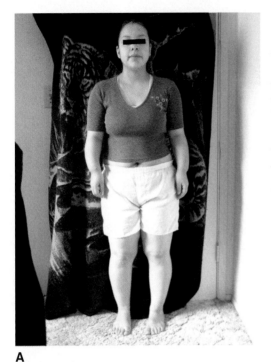

A

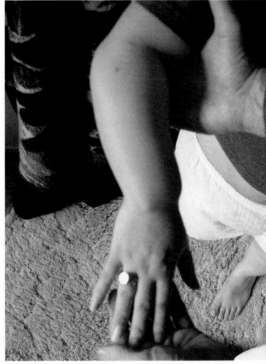

B

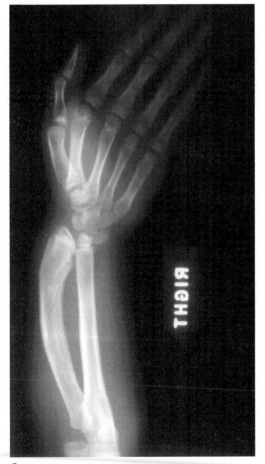

C

FIGURE 1. Léri-Weill dyschondrosteosis. **A–C,** A 20-year-old woman. Note the short forearms with bowing of the radius and distal hypoplasia of the dorsally dislocated ulna.

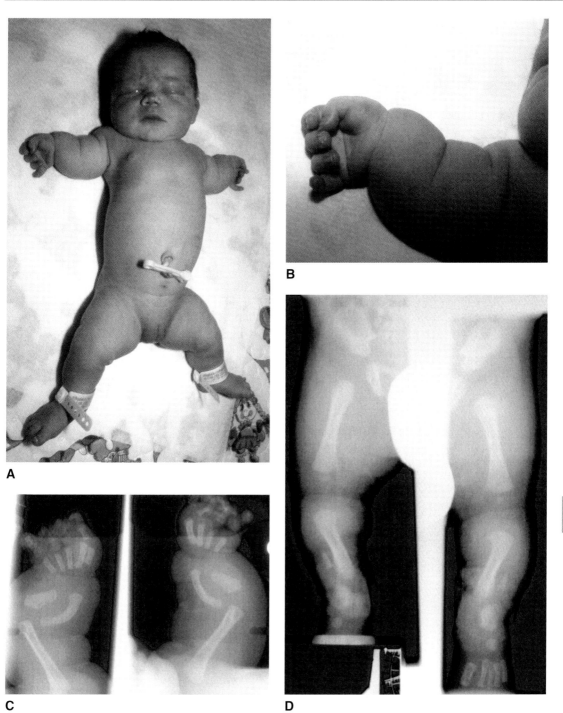

A

B

C

D

N

FIGURE 2.   Langer mesomelic dysplasia. **A–D,** A newborn with unusual shortness of stature with disproportionate smallness of forearms and lower legs, especially the ulnae and fibulae.

ACRODYSOSTOSIS
Short Hands with Peripheral Dysostosis, Small Nose, Intellectual Disability

Maroteaux and Malamut first described this disorder in three patients in 1968, and there are now more than 50 published cases.

ABNORMALITIES

Growth. Mild to moderate prenatal onset of growth deficiency; short stature (55%).

Performance. Intellectual disability in 77%, average IQ of 61 with a range from 24 to 85; hearing deficit (67%).

Craniofacial. Brachycephaly; low nasal bridge; broad and small upturned nose (97%); tendency to hold mouth open; hypoplastic maxilla (100%) with prognathism; increased mandibular angle (68%).

Limbs. Short, especially distally, with progressive deformity in distal humerus, radius, and ulna; hands appear short and broad, with wrinkling of dorsal skin; large great toe.

Genitalia. Hypoplastic genitalia (29%), cryptorchidism (29%), irregular menses (18%), hypogonadism.

Endocrine. Resistance to parathormone, but calcium and phosphorus usually normal; resistance to thyroid-stimulating hormone, occasionally clinical hypothyroidism, usually subclinical; resistance to growth hormone–releasing hormone; gonadotrophin resistance.

Imaging. Cone-shaped epiphyses that fuse prematurely in hands and feet; vertebral defects, including loss of normal caudal widening of the lumbar interpedicular distance (75%), small vertebrae that may collapse, spinal canal stenosis; advanced bone age; epiphyseal stippling noted in neonatal period principally involving the lumbosacral and cervical vertebral bodies, the carpal and tarsal bones, proximal humeri, terminal phalanges, knees, and hips; stippling regresses by 4 months and is almost always gone by 8 months of age.

OCCASIONAL ABNORMALITIES

Hydrocephalus, epicanthal folds (39%), hypertelorism (35%), optic atrophy, hearing loss, dimpled nasal tip, malocclusion of teeth, delayed tooth eruption (23%), hypodontia (3%), calvarial hyperostosis, pigmented nevi, scoliosis, dislocated radial heads, renal anomalies (3%), hypothyroidism.

NATURAL HISTORY

Most patients with this disorder do relatively well except for the problems of intellectual disability and arthritic complaints. Progressive restriction of movement of the hands, elbows, and spine may occur. Decompressive laminectomy for spinal stenosis may be required. Multihormone resistance is more common than previously thought and should be treated. Growth hormone therapy appears to have a favorable impact on growth.

ETIOLOGY

This disorder has an autosomal dominant inheritance pattern. Two genes have been implicated. *PRKAR1A*, the cyclic AMP (cAMP)–dependent regulatory subunit of protein kinase A (PKA) was mutated in three patients with acrodysostosis who also exhibited hormone resistance. Missense mutations in *PDE4D*, the gene encoding cAMP-dependent phosphodiesterase, also cause this phenotype. Mutations in both genes cause reduced cAMP binding and result in reduced PKA activation and, consequently, reduced downstream signaling. No significant differences in the phenotype exist in the few cases with identified mutations in each of the two genes.

COMMENT

Albright hereditary osteodystrophy and acrodysostosis share several clinical features, including metacarpal abnormalities, obesity, cryptorchidism, and resistance to hormones that depend on the generation of cAMP. The skeletal dysplasia is more severe in acrodysostosis. Radiographic features that distinguish this disorder from Albright hereditary osteodystrophy include decreased interpediculate distance and a characteristic metacarpophalangeal pattern profile for the brachydactyly, including metacarpals 2 to 5 that are more severely affected than the corresponding phalanges as well as sparing of the thumbs and halluces. Gs-α (the dysregulated protein in Albright hereditary osteodystrophy), *PDE4D*, and *PRKAR1A* are all components of the cAMP signaling pathway.

References

Maroteaux P, Malamut GL: L'acrodysostose, *Presse Med* 76:2189, 1968.

Graham JM, et al: Radiographic findings and Gs-alpha bioactivity studies and mutation screening in acrodysostosis indicate a different etiology from pseudohypoparathyroidism, *Pediatr Radiol* 31:2, 2001.

Linglart A, et al: Recurrent PRKAR1A mutation in acrodysostosis with hormone resistance, *N Engl J Med* 364:2218, 2011.

Lee H, et al: Exome sequencing identifies *PDE4D* mutations in acrodysostosis, *Am J Hum Genet* 90:746, 2012.

Michot C, et al: Exome sequencing identifies *PDE4D* mutations as another cause of acrodysostosis, *Am J Hum Genet* 90:740, 2012.

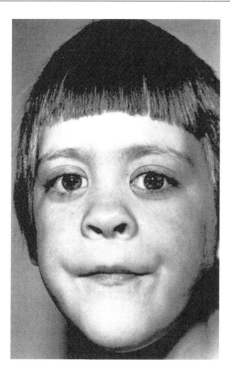

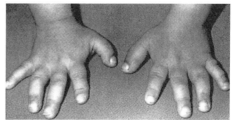

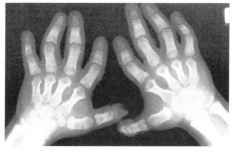

FIGURE 1. Acrodysostosis. A 5-year-old girl. Note the low nasal bridge, epicanthal folds, prominent mandible, short and broad fingers with skin wrinkling, and the broad and short metacarpals and phalanges with cone-shaped epiphyses.

N

ALBRIGHT HEREDITARY OSTEODYSTROPHY
(PSEUDOHYPOPARATHYROIDISM, PSEUDOPSEUDOHYPOPARATHYROIDISM)
Short Metacarpals, Rounded Facies, with or without Hypocalcemia or Heterotopic Calcification

Albright and colleagues described this condition in 1942 and referred to it as pseudohypoparathyroidism (PHP) because of hypocalcemia and hyperphosphatemia that were unresponsive to parathormone. Two variants of Albright hereditary osteodystrophy (AHO) have been described: PHP type-Ia (PHP-Ia), and pseudopseudohypoparathyroidism (PPHP). Individuals with PHP-Ia present with hypocalcemia and hyperphosphatemia, despite elevated serum parathyroid hormone levels. Resistance to thyroid-stimulating hormone and gonadotropins, as well as to growth hormone–releasing hormone and calcitonin, also occurs. Individuals with PPHP have the characteristic features of AHO, but show no evidence of resistance to parathyroid hormone or any other hormone. Both variants result from decreased activity of the alpha subunit of the trimeric Gs (Gs-α) regulatory protein, the function of which is to couple membrane receptors to adenyl cyclase, an action that stimulates cyclic adenosine monophosphate.

ABNORMALITIES

Growth. Small stature; final height, 137 to 152 cm; occasionally normal; moderate obesity; span decreased for height.

Performance. Intellectual disability is variable, IQs of 20 to 99, mean IQ of approximately 60.

Craniofacial. Rounded face; low nasal bridge; cataracts; delayed dental eruption, aplasia, or enamel hypoplasia; short neck.

Limbs. Recessed knuckles, especially the fourth and fifth; short distal phalanx of thumb.

Imaging. Short metacarpals and metatarsals, especially fourth and fifth; cone-shaped epiphyses; osteoporosis; areas of mineralization in subcutaneous tissues, basal ganglia.

Endocrine. Resistance to parathormone, variable alterations of calcium and phosphorus; resistance to thyroid-stimulating hormone, occasionally clinical hypothyroidism; resistance to growth hormone–releasing hormone; gonadotrophin resistance; hypogonadism.

OCCASIONAL ABNORMALITIES

Seizures, peripheral lenticular opacities, nystagmus, unequal size of pupils, blurring of disk margins, tortuosity of vessels, diplopia, microphthalmia, optic atrophy, macular degeneration, hypertelorism, thick calvarium, short ulna, short phalanges, genu valgum, fibrous dysplasia, exostosis, osteitis fibrosa cystica, epiphyseal dysplasia, advanced bone age, clavicular abnormalities, cervical vertebral anomalies with associated spinal cord compression, osteochondroma, pancreatic dysfunction.

NATURAL HISTORY

The shortened metacarpal or phalangeal bones represent early epiphyseal fusion and may not be evident until several years of age. Hypocalcemia, when present, usually becomes evident in childhood, seizures being the most common presenting symptom. Hypocalcemia may also become manifest during periods of increased calcium utilization, as in adolescence or in pregnancy. Treatment with active vitamin D metabolites, particularly calcitriol, with or without oral calcium supplementation, is used to maintain normocalcemia, and may favorably impact growth. Height, growth velocity, body mass index, and pubertal development should be monitored such that appropriate interventions are instituted in a timely fashion. Screening for growth hormone deficiency and hypothyroidism is warranted.

ETIOLOGY

This disorder has an autosomal dominant inheritance pattern. Documentation of more than one affected child born to unaffected parents is an indication of germline mosaicism. A variety of different loss of function mutations in the gene encoding the α subunit of the membrane-bound G-protein (*GNAS*) that stimulates adenyl cyclase activity are responsible for both the PHP-Ia and the PPHP variants. The gene is localized to chromosome 20q13.11. PHP-Ia and PPHP have been reported in the same family, but never in the same sibship, and are dependent on the parent of origin. Inheritance of the altered gene from a father affected by either PHP-Ia or PPHP leads to PPHP, whereas inheritance of the same mutation from the mother with either variant leads to PHP-Ia. This pattern of inheritance is consistent with the known tissue-specific paternal imprinting of *GNAS* and with the evidence that the main protein product Gs-α shows a predominant maternal expression in specific endocrine human tissues. In families in which PHP-Ia and PPHP coexist, mutations in *GNAS* can be detected in all affected members. On the contrary, no mutation in the *GNAS* coding sequence is usually found in families in whom sporadic or familial PPHP is the only clinical manifestation. PHP-Ia and isolated PPHP seem to represent two genetically distinct entities. A subset of patients with PHP-Ia and variable degrees of AHO showed epigenetic defects of *GNAS* without mutation.

COMMENT

PHP-Ic is clinically and biochemically indistinguishable from type Ia. However, PHP-Ic patients show normal Gs activity in peripheral blood cell and lack mutations in *GNAS*. The McCune-Albright syndrome is caused by mosaic gain of function mutations in this same gene.

References

Albright F, et al: Pseudohypoparathyroidism-an example of "Seabright-bantam syndrome": Report of three cases, *Endocrinology* 30:922, 1942.

Levine MA, et al: Genetic deficiency of the alpha subunit of the guanine nucleotide-binding protein Gs as the molecular basis for Albright hereditary osteodystrophy, *Proc Natl Acad Sci U S A* 85:615, 1988.

Patten JL, et al: Mutation in the gene encoding the stimulatory G protein of adenylate cyclase in Albright's hereditary osteodystrophy, *N Engl J Med* 322:1412, 1990.

Mantovani G: Clinical review: Pseudohypoparathyroidism: diagnosis and treatment, *J Clin Endocrinol Metab* 96:3020, 2011.

Izzi B, et al: Methylation defect in imprinted genes detected in patients with an Albright's hereditary osteodystrophy like phenotype and platelet Gs hypofunction, *PLoS One* 7:e38579, 2012.

Mantovani G, et al: GNAS epigenetic defects and pseudohypoparathyroidism: Time for a new classification? *Horm Metab Res* 44:716, 2012.

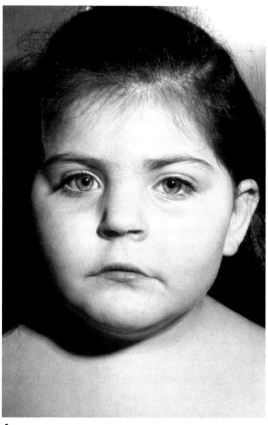

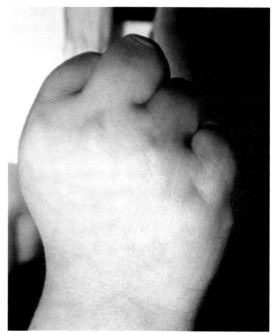

B

A

FIGURE 1.   Albright hereditary osteodystrophy. **A** and **B,** Moderately retarded girl showing rounded face and indications of short fourth and fifth metacarpal bones in fisted hand.

N

YUNIS-VARÓN SYNDROME
Distal Digital Hypoplasia, Hypotrichosis, Delayed Calvarial Maturation

Yunis and Varón reported five patients from three families with this disorder in 1980. A total of 23 cases from 18 families have been reported.

ABNORMALITIES

Growth. Prenatal growth deficiency (approximately 50% of patients); severe failure to thrive postnatally; microcephaly (50%).

Performance. Severe developmental delay in the majority of children who survive the neonatal period.

Craniofacial. Sparse scalp hair, eyebrows, and eyelashes; wide calvarial sutures and enlarged fontanels; prominent eyes; short upslanting palpebral fissures; anteverted nares; labiogingival retraction; short philtrum; tented upper lip; thin vermilion; full cheeks; low-set/dysplastic ears with hypoplastic lobes; stenosis of external auditory canal; broad secondary alveolar ridge; micrognathia; hypodontia; delayed dental eruption; premature loss of deciduous teeth; impacted permanent teeth.

Limbs. Agenesis/hypoplasia of thumbs and great toes; short tapering fingers and toes with nail hypoplasia; agenesis/hypoplasia of distal phalanges of fingers and toes, middle phalanges of fingers, and first metatarsals; simian crease.

Imaging. Absence or hypoplasia of all the phalanges in thumb and first toe, first metacarpals, and first metatarsals; hypoplasia of distal phalanges; hypoplastic clavicles; absent sternal ossification; pelvic dysplasia; abnormal scapula; hypoplasia of inner ear. Prenatal imaging findings have included ventriculomegaly, Dandy-Walker variant, hydrops, and polyhydramnios.

Other. Loose nuchal skin, cardiomegaly, hip dislocation, hypospadias, micropenis, cryptorchidism, fractures.

OCCASIONAL ABNORMALITIES

Hydrops; microphthalmia; sclerocornea; cataracts; mild ocular hypertelorism; cleft lip and palate; bifid uvula; median pseudocleft; cystic dental follicles; glossoptosis; central nervous system malformations, including arrhinencephaly, agenesis of the corpus callosum, abnormality of cerebellar vermis, hydrocephalus, delayed brain maturation; tetralogy of Fallot; ventricular septal defect; cardiomyopathy; primary pulmonary hypertension; arrhythmia; hypertension; atrophy of left lobe of liver and anomalous hepatic vessel; syndactyly of fingers and toes; absent nipples.

NATURAL HISTORY

Eighteen percent of patients have delivered prematurely. Death in the first few months from cardiorespiratory failure has occurred in three quarters of live-born infants. Although intellectual performance was normal in one mildly affected 7-year-old boy, the other survivors have had severe developmental delay. Hearing loss is documented in some survivors. Limb abnormalities are more severe on the radial side.

ETIOLOGY

Homozygous or compound heterozygous mutations in *FIG4* cause this autosomal recessive disorder. *FIG4* encodes a phosphoinositide phosphatase that regulates phosphatidylinositol 3,5-bisphosphate, autophagy and endosomal trafficking. All mutations result in loss of protein function. Genetic heterogeneity has been suggested.

References

Yunis E, Varón H: Cleidocranial dysostosis, severe micrognathism, bilateral absence of thumbs and first metatarsal bones, and distal aphalangia: A new genetic syndrome, *Am J Dis Child* 134:649, 1980.

Ades LD, et al: Congenital heart malformation in Yunis-Varón syndrome, *J Med Genet* 30:788, 1993.

Basel-Vanagaite L, et al: Yunis-Varón syndrome: Further delineation of the phenotype, *Am J Med Genet A* 146A:532, 2008.

Champeau PM, et al: Yunis-Varón syndrome is caused by mutations in *FIG4*, encoding a phosphoinositide phosphatase, *Am J Hum Genet* 92:781, 2013.

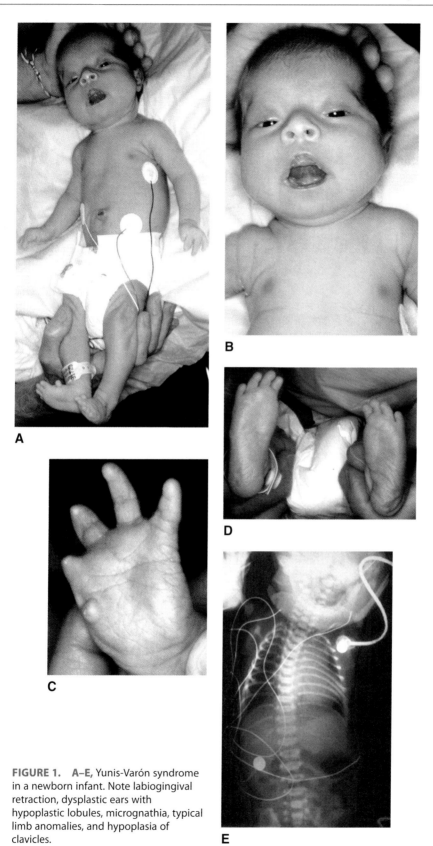

FIGURE 1. **A–E,** Yunis-Varón syndrome in a newborn infant. Note labiogingival retraction, dysplastic ears with hypoplastic lobules, micrognathia, typical limb anomalies, and hypoplasia of clavicles.

N

DESBUQUOIS DYSPLASIA

Midface Hypoplasia, Short Stature with Short Limbs, "Swedish Key" Appearance of Proximal Femur, Advanced Carpal and Tarsal Bone Age

In 1966, Desbuquois and colleagues described two sisters with short stature, dislocation of the joints, glaucoma, cardiac defects, and severe psychomotor retardation. In 1995, Gillessen-Kaesbach et al reviewed more than 20 cases, reporting the major clinical and radiologic findings of this condition. The condition is clinically heterogeneous and classified into two types on the basis of presence (type 1) or absence (type 2) of characteristic radiologic hand anomalies.

ABNORMALITIES

Growth. Markedly short length (−4 SD to −10 SD), with short limbs of prenatal onset. Proportionate and milder short stature in some cases with the Kim variant.

Performance. Both intellectual disability and normal development have been reported.

Craniofacial. Rounded flat face, depressed nasal bridge, midface hypoplasia, proptosis, anteverted nares, long philtrum, cleft palate.

Trunk. Narrow thorax, widely spaced or downplaced nipples, protuberant abdomen.

Limbs. Short extremities with proportionate short long bones. Dislocations and deformities at any joint can occur.

Hands and Feet. Brachydactyly and selective distal phalangeal shortening. Dislocation of the interphalangeal joints may be present. Contractures can result.

Imaging. Five consistent features occurring in greater than 90% of patients: the "Swedish key" appearance of the proximal femur (the femoral neck is short, there is medial metaphysical beaking and an exaggerated lesser trochanter producing a characteristic monkey wrench appearance), flat acetabular roof, elevated greater trochanter, proximal fibular overgrowth, and advanced carpal and tarsal bone age. Only present in type 1, the hand abnormalities include an extra ossification center distal to the second metacarpal, delta phalanx or delta-like phalanx, bifid distal thumb phalanx, and dislocation of the interphalangeal joints. Near-normal hands are present in greater than 50% of patients with type 2. Other typical radiologic manifestations present in more than 50% are wide metaphyses, flat epiphyses, coxa valga, coronal and saggital clefts of the vertebrae, wide anterior rib portions, medial deviation of the foot, and enlarged first metatarsal.

OCCASIONAL ABNORMALITIES

Cardiac defects (ASD, VSD, coarctation of the aorta), pulmonary hypoplasia, glaucoma, hydronephrosis, omphalocele, progressive myopia, coxa vara, short first metacarpals, radioulnar or other long bone dislocations or subluxations, kyphoscoliosis, cervical spine abnormalities.

NATURAL HISTORY

While severe antenatal growth retardation and postnatal lethality primarily related to respiratory compromise occur frequently, significant variability in prognosis and severity of growth failure is the rule. Intellectual disability occurs in less than 50% of patients and does not seem predictable based on the severity of the skeletal findings.

ETIOLOGY

Families with types 1 and 2 and the Kim variant have mutations in the calcium-activated nucleotidase 1 gene (*CANT1*) on chromosome 17q25, which encodes a soluble UDP-preferring nucleotidase belonging to the apyrase family. The specific function of *CANT1* is unknown, but its substrates are involved in several major signaling functions, including calcium release through activation of pyrimidinergic signaling. Inclusion bodies within distended rough endoplasmic reticulum in Desbuquois patient chondrocytes and fibroblasts have been identified. Several families with types 1 and 2 do not show mutations in *CANT1*, indicating genetic heterogeneity. Specific clinical molecular correlations need definition. However, an early death due to cardiorespiratory failure has been observed in children with nonsense mutations.

COMMENT

Recently, a third type—the Kim variant—was identified. Differences in the phenotype relative to types 1 and 2 include lack of an accessory ossification center distal to the second metacarpal and shortness of one or all metacarpals, leading to elongated appearance of the phalanges. This results in near-equal length of the second to fifth fingers. Abnormal proportions of the sizes of the toes are seen. Long-term follow-up showed that severe precocious osteoarthritis of the hand and spine is frequent.

References

Desbuquois G, et al: Nanisme chondrodystrophique avec ossification anarchique et polymalformations chez deux soeurs, *Arch Fr Pediatr* 23:573, 1966.

Gillessen-Kaesbach G, et al: Desbuquois syndrome: Three further cases and review of the literature, *Clin Dysmorphol* 4:136, 1995.

Faivre L, et al: Desbuquois dysplasia, a reevaluation with abnormal and "normal" hands: Radiographic manifestations, *Am J Med Genet A* 124A:48, 2004.

Huber C, et al: Identification of *CANT1* mutations in Desbuquois dysplasia, *Am J Hum Genet* 85:706, 2009.

Faden M, et al: Mutation of *CANT1* causes Desbuquois dysplasia, *Am J Med Genet A* 152A:1157, 2010.

Kim OH, et al: A variant of Desbuquois dysplasia characterized by advanced carpal bone age, short metacarpals, and elongated phalanges: Report of seven cases, *Am J Med Genet A* 152A:875, 2010.

Furuichi T, et al: *CANT1* mutation is also responsible for Desbuquois dysplasia, type 2 and Kim variant, *J Med Genet* 48:32, 2011.

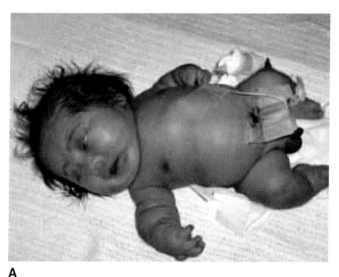

A

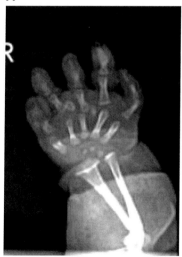

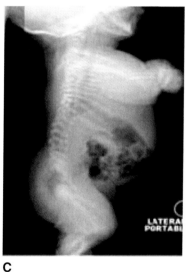

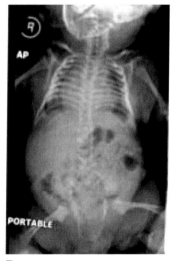

B   C   D

FIGURE 1.   Desbuquois dysplasia. **A,** Note the narrow and short thorax, widely spaced nipples, protuberant abdomen, short limbs with brachydactyly, and bilateral clubfoot deformity. **B,** Hand x-ray showing two extra ossification centers and the dislocation between the middle and proximal phalanges of the fifth finger. **C,** Lateral spine x-ray shows coronal clefts of the vertebrae. **D,** Note the spur in the lesser trochanter on the babygram. (From Faden M et al: *Am J Med Genet* 152A:1157, 2010, with permission.)

LEROY I-CELL SYNDROME (MUCOLIPIDOSIS II)
Early Alveolar Ridge Hypertrophy, Joint Limitation, Thick Tight Skin in Early Infancy

This disorder was recognized by Leroy and DeMars when they noted unusual cytoplasmic inclusions in the cultured fibroblasts of a girl who had been considered to have the Hurler syndrome despite the fact that she did not have cloudy corneas or excessive acid mucopolysaccharide in the urine. Mucolipidosis II (ML II) is a progressive inborn error of metabolism sometimes evident at birth. Fatal outcome occurs most often in early childhood.

ABNORMALITIES

Growth. Birth weight less than 5½ pounds; marked growth deficiency with lack of linear growth after infancy.

Performance. Slow progress from early infancy, reaching a plateau at approximately 18 months with no apparent deterioration subsequently.

Craniofacial. Progressive coarsening of facial features; high, narrow forehead; shallow orbits; thin eyebrows; puffy eyelids; inner epicanthal folds; clear or faintly hazy corneas; low nasal bridge, anteverted nostrils; long philtrum; progressive hypertrophy of alveolar ridges.

Skeletal. Moderate progressive joint limitation in flexion, especially of hips; dorsolumbar kyphosis; thoracic deformity; clubfeet; dislocation of the hip; broadening of wrists and fingers.

Skin. Thick, relatively tight skin during early infancy that becomes less tight as the patients become older, most noticeable in the earlobes; cavernous hemangiomata.

Cardiac. Thickening and insufficiency of the mitral valve and, less frequently, the aortic valve; in rare cases, cardiomyopathy.

Imaging. In the later phases, changes of dysostosis multiplex similar to those seen in children with the Hurler syndrome; in early infancy, periosteal new bone formation leading to a "cloaking" of the long tubular bones, best seen in femora and humeri; in newborns with severe ML II, radiographic abnormalities similar to those of hyperparathyroidism or rickets.

Other. Minimal hepatomegaly, diastasis recti, inguinal hernia, neonatal cholestasis, proximal tubular dysfunction.

NATURAL HISTORY

By 18 months of age, most patients can sit with support, and some stand with support, but walking and functional speech are usually never acquired. However, severe progressive retardation of growth and development occur. Recurrent bouts of bronchitis, pneumonia, and otitis media are frequent during early childhood. Progressive mucosal thickening narrows the airways and gradually stiffens the thoracic cage contributing to respiratory insufficiency and congestive heart failure, the most common cause of death, which usually occurs by 5 years of age.

ETIOLOGY

This disorder has an autosomal recessive inheritance pattern. Activity of nearly all lysosomal hydrolases is 5- to 20-fold higher in plasma and other body fluids than in normal controls, but normal or decreased in leukocytes and fibroblasts because of improper targeting of lysosomal acid hydrolases (β-D-hexosaminidase, β-D-glucuronidase, β-D-galactosidase, α-L-fucosidase) to lysosomes. Urinary excretion of oligosaccharides is excessive and can be used as a screening test. Lysosomal hydrolase N-acetylglucosamine-1-phosphotransferase (GNPTAB) is the deficient enzyme in this disorder as well as in pseudo-Hurler polydystrophy (mucolipidosis IIIA). Mutations in the GlcNAc-phosphotransferase a/b-subunits precursor gene (*GNPTAB*) are the cause. ML II is caused by two severe mutations leading to almost absent enzyme activity, whereas ML IIIA/B occurs when at least one mild mutation can produce some active GlcNAc-phosphotransferase. The prenatal presentation of ML II was previously called Pacman dysplasia. Mutations in *GNPTAB* have also been identified in this severe variant.

Prenatal diagnosis can be based on demonstration of elevated lysosomal enzyme activity in cell-free amniotic fluid as well as vacuolation of chorionic villus cells on electron microscopy; however, molecular testing with prior identification of the mutations in the family is preferable. Molecular testing is necessary to detect carriers, since enzyme levels do not distinguish carriers from non-carriers. Ultrasound findings are not present in all affected fetuses.

COMMENT

Bone marrow transplant, reported in only a few children with I-cell disease, has prevented progressive cardiac and pulmonary disease and allowed the attainment of neurodevelopmental milestones, although at a much slower than normal rate 5 years following transplantation, in one 7-year-old child.

References

Leroy JG, DeMars RI: Mutant enzymatic and cytological phenotypes in cultured human fibroblasts, *Science* 157:804, 1967.

Leroy JG, et al: I-cell disease, a clinical picture, *J Pediatr* 79:360, 1971.

Grewal S, et al: Continued neurocognitive development and prevention of cardiopulmonary complications after successful BMT for I-cell disease: A long-term follow-up report, *Bone Marrow Transplant* 32:957, 2003.

Kudo M, et al: Mucolipidosis II (I-cell disease) and mucolipidosis IIIA (classical pseudo-Hurler polydystrophy) are caused by mutations in the GlcNAc-phosphotransferase alpha/beta-subunits precursor gene, *Am J Hum Genet* 78:451, 2006.

Cathey SS, et al: Phenotype and genotype in mucolipidoses II and III alpha/beta: A study of 61 probands, *J Med Genet* 47:38, 2010.

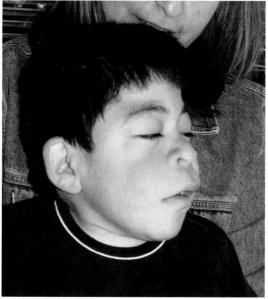

A

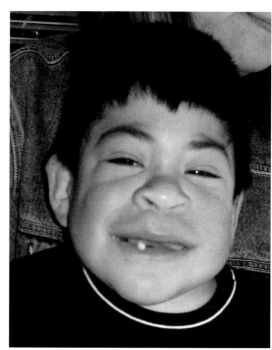

B

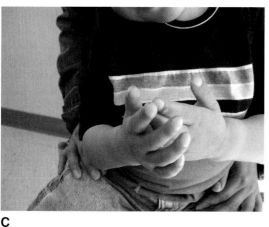

C

FIGURE 1. Leroy I-cell syndrome. **A–C,** A 9-year-old child. Note the high, narrow forehead, puffy eyelids, anteverted nares, long philtrum, hypertrophy of alveolar ridges, and joint contractures. (Courtesy Dr. Lynne M. Bird, Rady Children's Hospital, San Diego.)

MUCOPOLYSACCHARIDOSIS I H, I H/S, 1 S
(HURLER SYNDROME, HURLER-SCHEIE SYNDROME, SCHEIE SYNDROME)
Coarse Facies, Stiff Joints, Intellectual Disability, Cloudy Corneas

Hurler set forth the disorder mucopolysaccharidosis I H (MPS IH) in 1919. Scheie and colleagues described the milder form in 1962 (MPS IS), and Stevenson and colleagues set forth the intermediate form IH/S (MPS IH/S) in 1976. At least 80% of individuals with MPS I fall at the severe or Hurler syndrome end of the spectrum. No significant biochemical differences are seen among the three forms, all caused by deficiency of the lysosomal hydrolase α-L-iduronidase (IDUA). The phenotype of Hurler syndrome is set forth below.

ABNORMALITIES

Growth. Deceleration of growth between 6 and 18 months; maximal stature, 110 cm.

Performance. Significant delay by 6 to 12 months, with developmental plateau by 2 to 5 years.

Craniofacial. Scaphocephalic macrocephaly with frontal prominence; coarse facies with full lips; flared nostrils; low nasal bridge; tendency toward hypertelorism; inner epicanthal folds; corneal clouding (all forms of MPS I); retinal pigmentation and degeneration; optic nerve compression and atrophy; visual cortical damage; open-angle glaucoma; hypertrophied alveolar ridge and gums with small malaligned teeth; enlarged tongue.

Skeletal. Joint limitation results in the clawhand and other joint deformities, with more limitation of extension than flexion; flaring of the rib cage; kyphosis and thoracolumbar gibbus secondary to anterior vertebral wedging: short neck.

Cardiac. Intimal thickening in the coronary vessels or the cardiac valves; valvular dysfunction; cardiomyopathy; sudden death from arrhythmia.

Imaging. Cranial thickening with narrowing of cranial foramina; J-shaped sella turcica; odontoid hypoplasia; diaphyseal broadening of short misshapen bones; widening of medial end of clavicle; dysostosis multiplex.

Other. Hirsutism, hepatosplenomegaly, inguinal hernia, umbilical hernia, dislocation of hip, tracheal stenosis, compression of the spinal cord, chronic mucoid rhinitis, middle ear fluid, cranial nerve compressions, deafness, urinary excretion of dermatan sulfate and heparan sulfate.

OCCASIONAL ABNORMALITIES

Communicating hydrocephalus, presumably a result of thickened meninges; arachnoid cysts; hydrocele; nephrotic syndrome; carpal tunnel syndrome; trigger thumb; hypoplasia of mandibular condyles.

NATURAL HISTORY

Infants appear normal at birth. Growth during the first year may be more rapid than usual, with subsequent slowing. Subtle changes in the facies, macrocephaly, hernias, limited hip motility, noisy breathing, and frequent respiratory tract infections may be evident during the first 6 months. Deceleration of developmental and mental progress is evident during the latter half of the first year. By age 3 years, linear growth ceases. Intellectual disability is progressive and profound. Upper airway obstruction secondary to thickening of the epiglottis and tonsillar and adenoidal tissues, as well as tracheal narrowing caused by mucopolysaccharide accumulation, can lead to sleep apnea and serious airway compromise. Because of the upper airway problems, as well as odontoid hypoplasia with or without C1-C2 subluxation, cervical myelopathy can require intervention and anesthesia is a significant risk. Hearing loss is almost always present. These patients are usually placid, easily manageable, and affectionate. Hypertension frequently occurs and is either centrally mediated or secondary to aortic coarctation. Death usually occurs in childhood secondary to respiratory tract or cardiac complications, and survival past 10 years of age is unusual. In the attenuated forms of the disorder, onset of symptoms will be between 3 and 8 years in MPS I H/S, and survival into the 20s is common, whereas in MPS I S, symptoms will be evident during the second and third decades and life span is normal. Growth is only affected in MPS I H/S, a short trunk being most common. Performance can be mildly impaired in the intermediate form with slow but evident deterioration, but will be normal in MPS I S, where late-onset psychiatric manifestations can occur. Corneal clouding, skeletal deformities, cardiac valvular abnormalities, and hearing impairment will develop by the early to mid teens in MPS I H/S and will cause significant disability. In MPS I S, vision impairment and pain and limitations due to skeletal problems will occur later in life.

ETIOLOGY

This disorder has an autosomal recessive inheritance pattern. The primary defect is an absence of the lysosomal hydrolase α-L-iduronidase (IDUA), which is responsible for the degradation of the glycosaminoglycans, heparan sulfate and dermatan sulfate. The pathologic consequence is an accumulation of mucopolysaccharides in parenchymal and mesenchymal tissues and the storage of lipids within neuronal tissues. The gene encoding IDUA is located on chromosome 4p16.3. Intragenic mutations can all be detected through sequencing; no deletions or other rearrangements have been reported. Up to 70% of mutations are recurrent and thus may be helpful in phenotype prediction. In the remaining 30%, prediction of the severity of the phenotype is not possible

Diagnosis is confirmed by the physical appearance, the excretion of dermatan sulfate and heparan sulfate in the urine, and the absence of α-L-iduronidase in cultured fibroblasts, leukocytes, or plasma. Mutation analysis is the only reliable method for heterozyote detection. Prenatal diagnosis is possible by measuring α-L-iduronidase in cultured amniotic fluid cells or through detection of the previously known familial mutation in chorionic villi or amniotic fluid.

COMMENT

Bone marrow transplantation (BMT) has been effective in the treatment of selected patients with MPS I H before age 2 years. BMT can increase survival by 67%, reduce facial coarseness and hepatosplenomegaly, improve hearing and airway problems, and maintain normal heart function, although valvular abnormalities often progress. Skeletal manifestations and corneal clouding continue to progress. In children with baseline Mental Developmental Index greater than 70, who are engrafted before 24 months, a favorable neurobehavioral outcome has occurred. Enzyme replacement therapy using recombinant human α-L-iduronidase improves liver size, linear growth, joint mobility, breathing, and sleep apnea, and can also be expected to stabilize cardiac dysfunction in persons with attenuated disease (MPS I S and MPS I H/S). However, its lack of central nervous system penetration is a major drawback to its use in patients with α-L-iduronidase deficiency for whom the central nervous system is already severely involved.

References

Hurler G: Ueber einen Typ multipler Abartungen, vorwiegend am Skelettsystem, *Z Kinderheilkd* 24:220, 1919.

Scheie HG, Hambrick GW Jr, Barness LA: A newly recognized forme fruste of Hurler's disease (gargoylism), *Am J Ophthalmol* 53:753, 1962.

Stevenson RE, et al: The iduronidase-deficient mucopolysaccharidoses: Clinical and roentgenographic features, *Pediatrics* 57:111, 1976.

Peters C, et al: Hurler syndrome: II. Outcome of HLA-genotypically identical siblings and HLA-haploidentical related bone marrow transplantation in fifty-four children, *Blood* 91:2601, 1998.

Clarke LA, et al: Long-term efficacy and safety of laronidase in the treatment of mucopolysaccharidosis I, *Pediatrics* 123:229, 2009.

Moore D, et al: The prevalence of and survival in mucopolysaccharidosis I: Hurler, Hurler-Scheie and Scheie syndromes in the UK, *Orphanet J Rare Dis* 3:24, 2008.

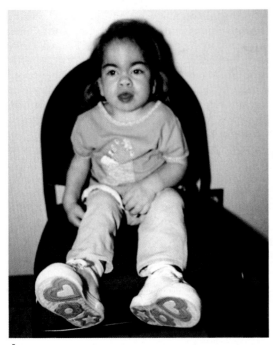

A

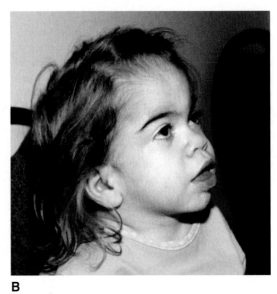

B

FIGURE 1.   Hurler syndrome. **A** and **B,** A 4-year-old girl.

Continued

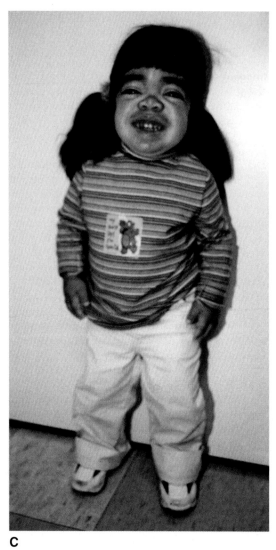

C

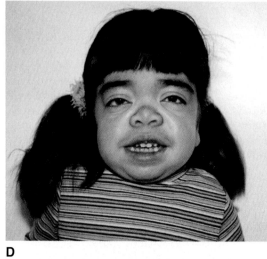

D

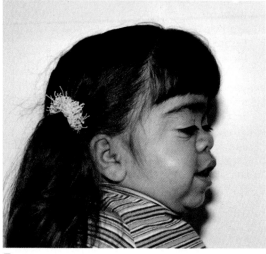

E

FIGURE 1, cont'd.   C–E, A 6-year-old girl. Note the coarse facies and contractures of the hands.

HUNTER SYNDROME (MUCOPOLYSACCHARIDOSIS II)
Coarse Facies, Growth Deficiency, Stiff Joints, Clear Corneas

Hunter described this condition found in two brothers in 1917. A mild and severe type have been delineated, based on the age of onset, degree of central nervous system involvement, and rapidity of deterioration. Both types have the same deficiency of iduronate sulfatase. The severe type is outlined below. Onset is at approximately 2 to 4 years.

ABNORMALITIES

Growth. Deficiency, onset at 1 to 4 years; adult height, 120 to 150 cm.

Performance. Mental and neurologic deterioration at approximately 2 to 5 years of age to the point of severe intellectual disability with aggressive hyperactive behavior and spasticity. Eighteen percent of males have an attenuated form without central nervous system (CNS) involvement.

Craniofacial. Coarsening of facial features, full lips, macrocephaly, macroglossia; delayed tooth eruption.

Joints and Skeletal. Joint contractures, including ankylosis of the temporomandibular joint; carpal tunnel syndrome; spinal stenosis.

Cardiac. Valvular disease (>50%), cardiomyopathy, arrhythmia, hypertension, and coronary disease.

Imaging. Dysostosis multiplex.

Other. Hepatosplenomegaly, hypertrichosis, inguinal hernias, mucoid nasal discharge, progressive deafness, dentigerous cysts, hoarse voice.

OCCASIONAL ABNORMALITIES

Diarrhea, nodular skin lesions over scapular area and on arms, dermal melanocytosis/mongolian spots (excessive), kyphosis, pes cavus, osteoarthritis of head of femur, retinal pigmentation, chronic disk edema, ptosis, hydrocephalus, airway obstruction, seizures, neurogenic bladder secondary to a narrow cervical spinal canal with myelopathy.

IMPORTANT DIFFERENCES IN CONTRAST WITH THE HURLER SYNDROME

(1) Clear corneas, (2) less severe gibbus, (3) more gradual onset of features, (4) nodular skin lesions, and (5) no affected females; on rare occasions carrier females manifest mild findings.

NATURAL HISTORY

Gradual decline in growth rate from 2 to 6 years. Deafness frequently is evident by 2 to 3 years. Severe neurologic complications develop in the late stages. Cardiac complications resulting from valvular, myocardial, and ischemic factors as well as airway obstruction caused by macroglossia, a deformed pharynx, a short thick neck, and gradual

deformation and collapse of the trachea caused by progressive storage along the airway, not uncommonly lead to death before 15 years of age.

In the mild type, maintenance of intelligence occurs into adult life. Survival into the fifth and sixth decades is not unusual. Adult hearing loss is frequent. Carpal tunnel syndrome and joint contractures are common. Somatic involvement occurs in patients with the mild type, but the rate of progression is much less rapid.

ETIOLOGY

The primary defect is a deficiency of iduronate sulfatase (I2S), which can be measured in peripheral white blood cells, fibroblasts, or plasma. Diagnosis of MPS II in a male proband is confirmed if deficient iduronate sulfatase enzyme activity is found in the presence of normal activity of at least one other sulfatase (to rule out multiple sulfatase deficiency). Excess dermatan sulfate and heparan sulfate are found in urine, and can be a useful screening test. The gene for Hunter syndrome, *IDS*, has been mapped to Xq27-q28. Mutations within the gene (82%), exonic and whole-gene deletions (9%), and gross alterations resulting from recombination with the nearby *IDS* pseudogene, *IDS2* (9%), require a combined sequencing and dosage testing approach for diagnosis. The broad variability of expression, which includes the severe and mild types, is due to different mutations in the same gene. Deletions and rearrangements are always associated with severe disease with CNS involvement. Point mutations have been shown to result in variable severity of the disease, even in the same family. Measurement of I2S enzyme activity is not reliable for detection of carrier females. Mutation analysis is preferable. Germline mosaicism has been reported. Prenatal diagnosis can be performed using chorionic villus sampling (CVS) or amniocentesis through assessment of enzyme activity or mutation analysis if the familial mutation is known.

COMMENT

Engraftment following bone marrow transplantation (BMT) has shown less promising results than in Hurler syndrome. Of 10 patients who underwent BMT, 3 survived more than 7 years. A steady progression of disease occurred in two of the survivors, while maintenance of normal intellectual development occurred in one. Enzyme replacement therapy with a recombinant form of human iduronate 2-sulfatase called idursulfase has been shown to improve growth and cardiopulmonary function in older children and adults with the milder form of the disease. No information is yet available in younger children. Severe CNS disease is expected to have no improvement since the enzyme does not reach the brain.

O

References

Hunter C: A rare disease in two brothers, *Proc R Soc Med* 10:104, 1917.

Upadhyaya M, et al: Localization of the gene for Hunter syndrome on the long arm of X chromosome, *Hum Genet* 74:391, 1986.

Vellodi A, et al: Long-term follow-up following bone marrow transplantation for Hunter disease, *J Inherit Metab Dis* 22:638, 1999.

Muenzer J, et al: A phase II/III clinical study of enzyme replacement therapy with idursulfase in mucopolysaccharidosis II (Hunter syndrome), *Genet Med* 8:465, 2006.

Froissart R, Da Silva IM, Maire I: Mucopolysaccharidosis type II: An update on mutation spectrum, *Acta Paediatr Suppl* 96:71, 2007.

Schulze-Frenking G, et al: Effects of enzyme replacement therapy on growth in patients with mucopolysaccharidosis type II, *J Inherit Metab Dis* 34:203, 2011.

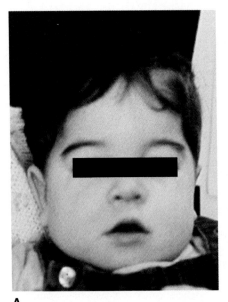

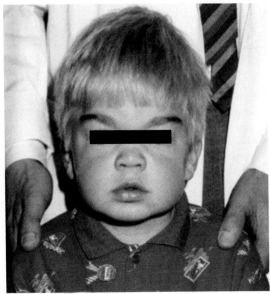

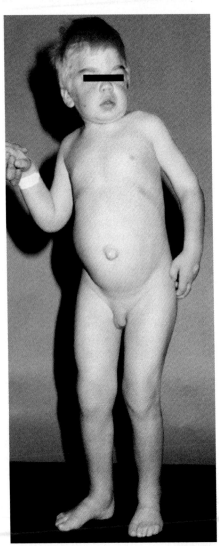

A

B

C

O

FIGURE 1. Hunter syndrome. **A–C,** Three boys with coarsening of the face and evidence of joint contractures who presumably have a mild type of disease. (Courtesy Dr. Jules Leroy, Ghent University Hospital, Ghent, Belgium.)

SANFILIPPO SYNDROME
(MUCOPOLYSACCHARIDOSIS III, TYPES A, B, C, AND D)
Mild Coarse Facies, Mild Stiff Joints, Intellectual Disability

This clinical disorder was recognized by Sanfilippo and colleagues in 1963 and appears to be the most common mucopolysaccharidosis. The excess urinary excretion of MPS is heparan sulfate alone. Four types are recognized, each due to deficiency of a different enzyme involved in degradation of heparan sulfate. Progressive mental deterioration is the main feature of this condition, along with subtle physical findings. Skeletal findings are infrequent and milder than in MPS I and II. These individuals usually have clear corneas. Onset is in early childhood.

ABNORMALITIES

Growth. Normal to accelerated growth for 1 to 3 years, followed by slow growth, usually deficient before the second decade.

Performance. Slowing mental development by 1½ to 3 years, followed by deterioration of gait and speech; severe behavioral issues; hyperactivity; epileptic seizure; hearing impairment.

Craniofacial. Macrocephaly in children, decreasing to normal head size in older patients; mildly coarse facies with prominent broad eyebrows, medial flaring and synophrys; dry coarse hair, upturned upper lip with prominent philtrum, everted and thick lower lip; thickened ear helices; fleshy tip of the nose; obliteration of pulp chambers of teeth by irregular secondary dentin.

Imaging. Dense calvarium, ovoid dysplasia of vertebrae, osteonecrosis of the femoral head.

Other. Variable hepatosplenomegaly, hypertrichosis, arthritis, scoliosis.

OCCASIONAL ABNORMALITIES

Contractures at the elbows or digits, carpal tunnel syndrome, cardiomyopathy, arrhythmias, hernias, diarrhea that responds to loperamide, skin blistering.

NATURAL HISTORY

Early development is typically normal. Sleep disturbances and frequent upper respiratory tract infections may be early evidence of the disorder before the slowing of growth and mental deterioration, particularly loss of speech with a restless, chaotic, destructive, and sometimes aggressive behavior.

Severe dementia will be followed by swallowing difficulties, spasticity, and motor regression, leading to a bedridden vegetative state. Death occurs in the second or third decade. Antipsychotic drugs appear to be the most effective for the treatment of behavioral problems, and melatonin is recommended for regulation of patients' day-night rhythm, which is often reversed.

ETIOLOGY

This disorder has an autosomal recessive inheritance pattern. Sanfilippo A is a deficiency of sulfamidase encoded by the gene *SGSH* at 17q25.3. Sanfilippo B, due to deficiency of α-*N*-acetylglucosaminidase, is caused by mutations in *NAGLU* at 17q21.1. Sanfilippo C, a deficiency of acetyl-CoA:α-glucosaminide-*N*-acetyltransferase, is encoded by *HGSNAT* at 8p11.1. Sanfilippo D, a deficiency of *N*-acetylglucosamine-6-sulfate sulfatase, is due to mutations in *GNS* at 12q14. Excess heparan sulfate is excreted in the urine in all four types, without increased secretion of dermatan sulfate. Assay of specific enzyme activity in leukocytes or cultured fibroblasts will identify the subtype MPS III. The identification of heterozygote carriers requires molecular testing in the proband, because of considerable overlap in enzyme activity between heterozygotes and normals. Prenatal diagnosis can be achieved by direct enzyme assay in CVS or even by analysis of heparan sulfate in amniotic fluid. However, mutation analysis is preferred if the familial mutation is known. The clinical phenotype is similar in each, although MPS IIIA is more severe, with earlier onset of symptoms and shorter survival (15 years in MPS IIIA versus 34 years in MPS IIIC). Type B may be seen more often in older surviving adults. Cardiac disease (in particular, cardiomyopathy and atrial fibrillation), arthritis, skin blistering, hernias, and susceptibility to infections occur in addition to mental deterioration and aberrant behavior.

COMMENT

No effective therapies are yet available. Bone marrow transplantation has not been successful in affecting the course of the disease. Substrate deprivation therapy using a genistein-rich isoflavone extract appears to decrease the synthesis of glycosaminoglycans and may benefit cognitive functions and behavior.

References

Sanfilippo SJ, et al: Mental retardation associated with acid mucopolysacchariduria (heparitin sulfate type), *J Pediatr* 63:837, 1963.

Guerrero JM, et al: Impairment of the melatonin rhythm in children with Sanfilippo syndrome, *J Pineal Res* 40:192, 2006.

Moog U, et al: Is Sanfilippo type B in your mind when you see adults with mental retardation and behavioral problems? *Am J Med Genet C Semin Med Genet* 145C:293, 2007.

Valstar MJ, et al: Sanfilippo syndrome: A mini-review, *J Inherit Metab Dis* 31:240, 2008.

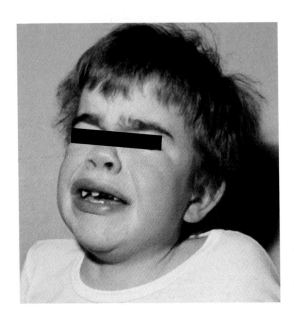

FIGURE 1. Sanfilippo syndrome. An 8-year-old boy whose capabilities have been regressing rapidly. (Courtesy Dr. Jules Leroy, Ghent University Hospital, Ghent, Belgium.)

O

MORQUIO SYNDROME (MUCOPOLYSACCHARIDOSIS IV, TYPES A AND B)
Onset at 1 to 3 Years of Age, Mild Coarse Facies, Severe Kyphosis and Knock-Knees, Cloudy Corneas

Mistakenly interpreted by Osler in 1898, this condition was described by Morquio in 1929; it was recognized as an MPS in 1963. Deficiencies of two different enzymes leading to a more severe form, MPS IVA, and a milder form, MPS IVB, are now recognized. Within both forms, marked clinical heterogeneity has been documented. Patients with MPS IV can usually be distinguished clinically from patients with other mucopolysaccharidoses by preservation of intelligence and a unique progressive spondyloepiphyseal dysplasia with joint laxity.

ABNORMALITIES

Growth. Severe limitation with cessation by later childhood, adult stature 82 to 115 cm.
Craniofacial. Mild coarsening of facial features, with broad mouth; short anteverted nose; cloudy cornea evident by slit lamp examination, usually after 5 to 10 years of age; glaucoma; refraction errors; cataracts; widely spaced teeth with thin enamel that tends to become grayish.
Skeletal. Short neck and trunk; kyphoscoliosis; early flaring of rib cage progressing to bulging sternum/pectus carinatum; short, stubby hands; joint laxity, most evident at wrists and small joints; joint restriction in some of the larger joints, especially the hips.
Imaging. Marked platyspondyly, with vertebrae changing to ovoid with anterior projection, to flattened form, with odontoid hypoplasia; short, curved long bones with irregular tubulation; widened metaphyses; abnormal femoral neck; flattening of femoral head; knock-knee with medial spur of tibial metaphysis; conical bases of widened metacarpals; irregular epiphyseal form; osteoporosis.
Cardiac. Mitral and aortic regurgitation.
Other. Hearing loss, inguinal hernia, hepatomegaly, urinary excretion of keratan sulfate.

Occasional Abnormalities

Macrocephaly, intellectual disability, pigmentary retinal degeneration in older patients, hydrops fetalis.

NATURAL HISTORY
The earliest recognized indications of the disease have been flaring of the lower rib cage, prominent sternum, frequent upper respiratory tract infections (including otitis media), hernias, and growth deficiency, all becoming evident by 18 to 24 months of age. Severe defects of vertebrae may result in cord compression or respiratory insufficiency. Odontoid hypoplasia, in combination with ligamentous laxity and extradural mucopolysaccharide deposition, results in atlantoaxial subluxation and cervical myelopathy. This, in addition to the respiratory or cardiac complications resulting from storage, may result in death before 20 years of age in the most severe cases. In the milder form, longer survival is the rule, dental enamel is normal, and C2-C3 subluxation has been documented in addition to C1-C2 subluxation. Intelligence is usually normal in both the severe and the mild forms, although attention deficits and mild abnormal findings on MRI have been reported. Patients with mild manifestations of MPS IVA or MPS IVB have been reported to survive into the seventh decade of life. Currently, treatment is symptomatic. Bone marrow transplant has not improved the course of the disease in these patients.

ETIOLOGY
Autosomal recessive: In type IVA, the basic defect is a deficiency of N-acetylgalactosamine-6-sulfatase, whereas in type IVB, there is a deficiency of ß-galactosidase. The gene for N-acetylgalactosamine-6-sulfatase (*GALNS*) has been mapped to 16q24.3. The gene for ß-galactosidase (*GLB1*) has been mapped to 3p21.33. Both types of Morquio syndrome have similar phenotypes, although type B tends to have a slower course. Confirmation of the diagnosis is dependent on demonstration of enzyme deficiency in cultured skin fibroblasts or leukocytes or through DNA testing. Heterozygote detection is possible. Prenatal diagnosis has been performed using both amniotic fluid cells and chorionic villi. As in other types of MPS, hydrops fetalis can be an unusual prenatal manifestation of the disorder.

COMMENT
Different mutations in *GLB1* cause generalized gangliosidosis syndrome, type I.

References

Osler W: Sporadic cretinism in America, *Trans Congr Am Phys* 4:169, 1898.
Morquio L: Sur une forme de dystrophie osseuse familiale, *Arch Med Enf* 32:129, 1929.
Morris CP, et al: Morquio A syndrome: Cloning, sequence and structure of the human N-acetylgalactosamine 6-sulfatase (*GALNS*) gene, *Genomics* 22:652, 1994.

Montaño AM, et al: International Morquio A Registry: Clinical manifestation and natural course of Morquio A disease, *J Inherit Metab Dis* 30(2):165, 2007.

Caciotti A, et al: GM1 gangliosidosis and Morquio B disease: An update on genetic alterations and clinical findings, *Biochim Biophys Acta* 1812:782, 2011.

Tomatsu S, et al: Mucopolysaccharidosis type IVA (Morquio A disease): Clinical review and current treatment, *Curr Pharm Biotechnol* 12:931, 2011.

Davison JE, et al: Intellectual and neurological functioning in Morquio syndrome (MPS IVa), *J Inherit Metab Dis* 2012. [Epub ahead of print].

Hendriksz CJ, et al: Clinical overview and treatment options for non-skeletal manifestations of mucopolysaccharidosis type IVA, *J Inherit Metab Dis* 36:309, 2013.

O

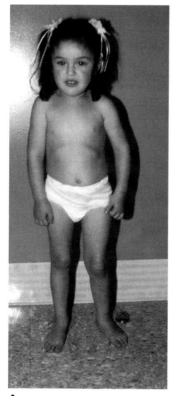

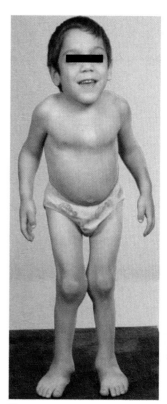

A

B

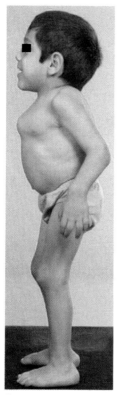

C

FIGURE 1.   Morquio syndrome. **A–C,** Two affected children. Note the joint contractures and prominent sternum. (**B** and **C,** courtesy Dr. Jules Leroy, Ghent University Hospital, Ghent, Belgium.)

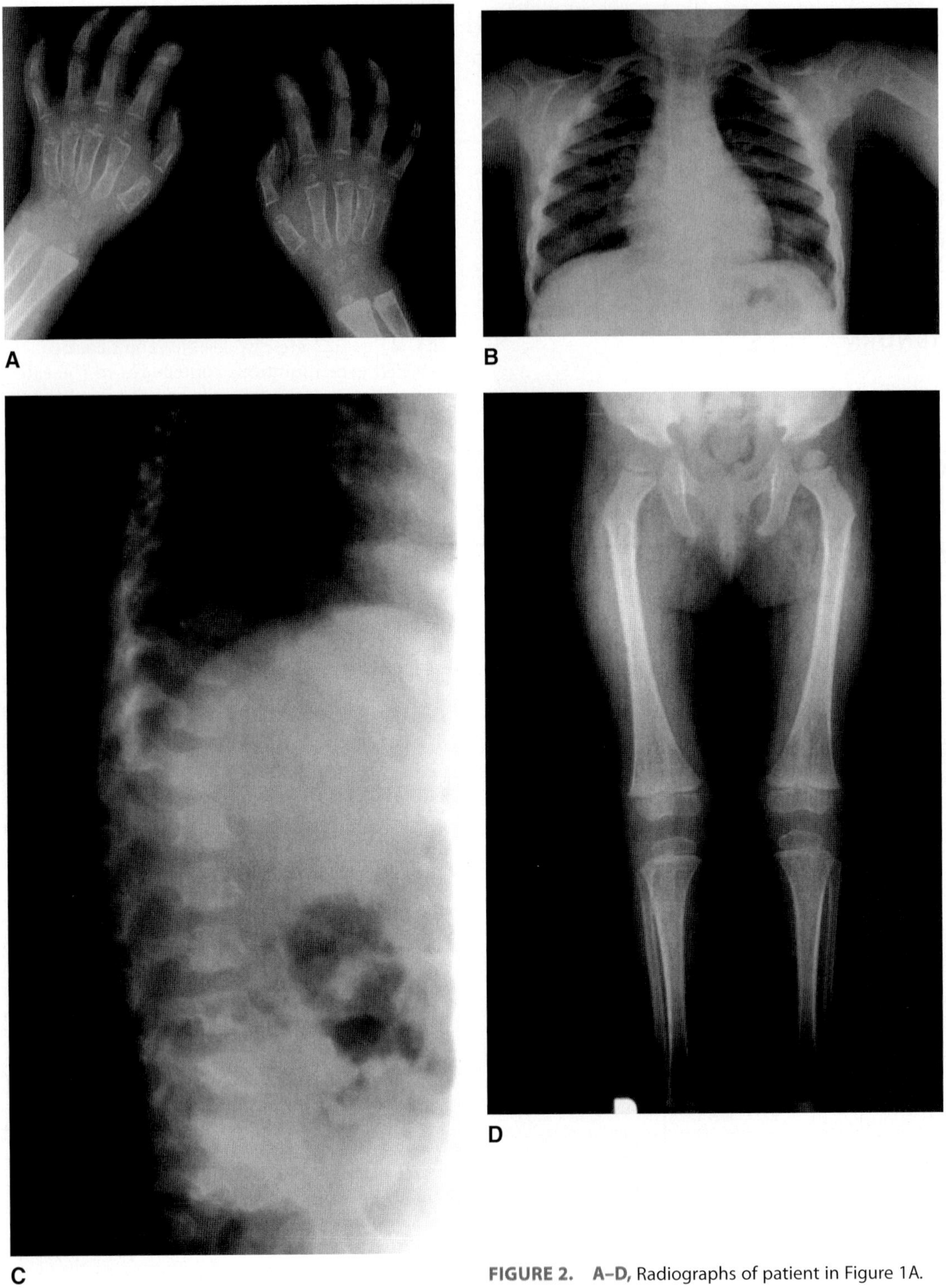

FIGURE 2.   A–D, Radiographs of patient in Figure 1A.

MUCOPOLYSACCHARIDOSIS VII
(SLY SYNDROME, ß-GLUCURONIDASE DEFICIENCY)

Initially described by Sly and colleagues in an infant with short stature, skeletal deformities, hepatosplenomegaly, and intellectual disability, fewer than 75 cases have been reported subsequently. A widely variable clinical phenotype has been noted from severely affected infants to mildly affected adults. The estimated incidence is 0.29 per 10^5 live births.

ABNORMALITIES

Growth. Postnatal growth deficiency.
Performance. Moderately severe intellectual disability.
Craniofacial. Macrocephaly, coarsened facies, corneal clouding in the severe form, optic nerve swelling.
Skeletal. Thoracolumbar gibbus, metatarsus adductus, flaring of lower ribs, prominent sternum.
Imaging. J-shaped sella turcica, acetabular dysplasia, narrow sciatic notches and hypoplastic basilar portions of ilia, widening of ribs, pointed proximal metacarpals.
Other. Inguinal hernia, hepatosplenomegaly.

OCCASIONAL ABNORMALITIES
Joint contractures; hydrocephalus; involvement of heart valves; odontoid hypoplasia; shortening and anterior irregularities of vertebral bodies; wedge deformities of lumbar vertebrae; anterior, inferior beaking of lower thoracic and lumbar vertebrae; hip dysplasia; hydrops fetalis.

NATURAL HISTORY
Unlike the other known mucopolysaccharidoses, MPS VII is sometimes recognizable in the neonatal period, associated with hydrops fetalis and hepatosplenomegaly. For some of these cases, death occurs in the first few months. A milder form, also presenting in the newborn period, is associated with developmental delay, much less rapid deterioration, and survival into adolescence. In addition, there exists at least one additional form of ß-glucuronidase deficiency that presents during the second decade of life and is characterized by mild skeletal abnormalities and normal intelligence. Mortality is usually the result of respiratory compromise and cardiac disease, which may include aortic and mitral valvular disease, left ventricular hypertrophy, and pulmonary hypertension.

ETIOLOGY
This disorder has an autosomal recessive inheritance pattern. The basic defect is a deficiency of ß-glucuronidase, which can be documented in fibroblasts and leukocytes. Mutations in the gene for ß-glucuronidase (*GUSB*) located at chromosome 7q11.21-q11.22 are responsible. The heterogeneity in *GUSB* gene mutations contributes to the extensive clinical variability among patients with MPS VII.

COMMENT
Bone marrow transplantation in one patient, a 12-year-old girl, resulted in improved motor function, decreased respiratory and ear infections, but no improvement in cognition. No enzyme replacement therapy (ERT) is yet available, but studies in mice showed that enzyme therapy at higher doses than are used in conventional ERT trials over a sufficient period of time can deliver enzyme across the blood-brain barrier.

References

Sly WS, et al: Beta glucuronidase deficiency: Report of clinical radiologic, and biochemical features of a new mucopolysaccharidosis, *J Pediatr* 82:249, 1973.

Speleman F, et al: Localization by fluorescence in situ hybridization of the human functional beta-glucuronidase gene (GUSB) to 7q11.21-q11.22 and two pseudogenes to 5p13 and 5q13, *Cytogenet Cell Genet* 72:53, 1996.

Yamada Y, et al: Treatment of MPS VII (Sly syndrome) by allogeneic BMT in a female with a homozygous A619V mutation, *Bone Marrow Transplant* 21:629, 1998.

Ashworth JL, et al: Mucopolysaccharidoses and the eye, *Surv Ophthalmol* 51:1, 2006.

Tomatsu S, et al: Mutations and polymorphisms in GUSB gene in mucopolysaccharidosis VII (Sly Syndrome), *Hum Mutat* 30:511, 2009.

Braunlin EA, et al: Cardiac disease in patients with mucopolysaccharidosis: Presentation, diagnosis and management, *J Inherit Metab Dis* 34:1183, 2011.

Valayannopoulos V, Wijburg FA: Therapy for the mucopolysaccharidoses, *Rheumatology (Oxford)* 50(Suppl 5):v49, 2011.

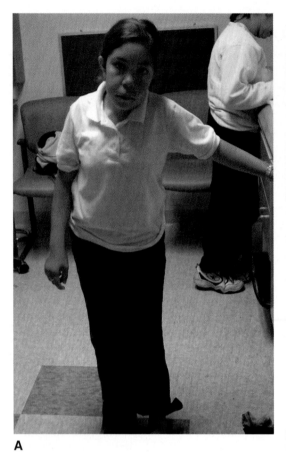

A

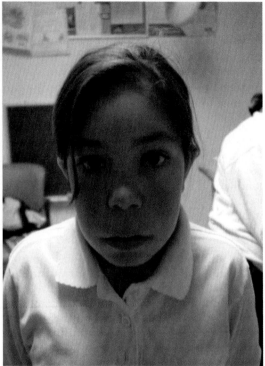

B

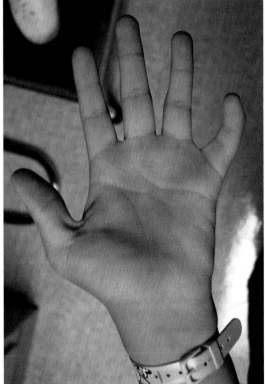

C

FIGURE 1.   Mucopolysaccharidosis VII. **A–C,** A mildly affected adolescent girl. Note the coarse facies and joint contractures. She has a mild degree of intellectual disability.

Connective Tissue Disorders

MARFAN SYNDROME
Arachnodactyly with Hyperextensibility, Lens Subluxation, Aortic Dilatation

Described as dolichostenomelia in the initial report by Marfan, this disorder was extensively studied and recognized as an autosomal dominant connective tissue disorder by McKusick. In 2010 an international expert panel established a revised Ghent nosology, which puts more emphasis on the cardiovascular and ocular manifestations than was the case in the 1996 Ghent criteria. The presence of both aortic root dilatation/aneurysm and ectopia lentis is sufficient for the diagnosis. There are two situations in which only one of the two cardinal features is sufficient for diagnosis; these situations are (1) if a family history or a causal *FBN1* mutation has been identified, and (2) if the combined score of the associated malformations is 7 or higher. (Associated manifestations of the cardiovascular, ocular, and other organ systems contribute to a "systemic score" with a maximum of 20 points; see below.)

ABNORMALITIES

Growth. Tendency toward tall stature with long slim limbs, little subcutaneous fat, and muscle hypotonia; mean birth length and final height 53 cm and 191 cm, respectively, in males and 52.5 cm and 175 cm, respectively, in females; peak growth velocity 2.4 years earlier than normal in boys and 2.7 years earlier in girls; mean age at menarche 11.7 years.

Skeletal. Pectus carinatum; pectus excavatum; decreased upper to lower segment ratio (lower than 0.85 in adults), or span-height ratio greater than 1.05 (both ratios should be compared to normal values for age in younger children); wrist and thumb sign; scoliosis greater than 20 degrees or spondylolisthesis; reduced elbow extension (<170 degrees); pes planus with hindfoot deformity; protrusio acetabuli (protrusion/dislocation of acetabulum); joint laxity is common but nonspecific. The combination of wrist and thumb signs is assigned 3 points in the systemic score. If either of the two signs is absent, only 1 point is assigned. Pectus carinatum, pes planus, and protrusio acetabuli, seen on radiograph, are assigned 2 points each when present. Significant pectus excavatum is assigned 1 point.

Craniofacial. Typical facial characteristics include dolichocephaly, downslanting palpebral fissures, enophthalmos, retrognathia, and malar hypoplasia. When three or more of these characteristics are present, 1 point is added to the systemic score. High palate with dental crowding is frequent.

Ocular. Lens subluxation, usually upward but can occur in every direction, with defect in suspensory ligament, flat cornea, increased axial globe length, hypoplastic iris or ciliary muscle causing decreased miosis. Myopia of more than 3 diopters contributes 1 point to the systemic score.

Cardiovascular. Dilatation of ascending aorta precisely measured at the level of the sinus of Valsalva (z score ≥ 2 in individuals 20 years or older and ≥ 3 in individuals less than 20, always adjusted for age and body size) with or without aortic regurgitation is the vascular hallmark of the condition. Dissection of ascending aorta is commonly seen in previously dilated aortas. Mitral valve prolapse (1 point in the scoring system). Dilated pulmonary artery, calcified mitral annulus, dilatation or dissection of descending thoracic or abdominal aorta.

Pulmonary. Spontaneous pneumothorax (2 points), apical blebs.

Skin and Integument. Lumbosacral dural ectasia on computed tomography or magnetic resonance imaging is assigned 2 points. Skin striae not associated with marked weight changes or present in uncommon locations are assigned 1 point. Recurrent or incisional hernias occur.

Family/Genetic History. A family member firmly diagnosed with Marfan syndrome or a causal mutation in *FBN1* will lead to the diagnosis of Marfan syndrome when combined with ectopia lentis, aortic root dilatation, or a systemic score of 7 or higher.

OCCASIONAL ABNORMALITIES
Large ears, cataracts, retinal detachment, glaucoma, strabismus, refractive errors, diaphragmatic hernia, hemivertebrae, colobomata of iris, cleft palate, incomplete rotation of colon, ventricular dysrhythmias, cardiomyopathy, intracranial aneurysms, sleep apnea, neuropsychologic impairment including learning disability and attention deficit disorder in 42% of 19 individuals (5 to 18 years of age) despite normal IQ, schizophrenia.

NATURAL HISTORY

Aortic root dilatation is usually progressive. Its absence in children or even in adults does not exclude the diagnosis or the need for follow-up. There is good correlation between the z scores of aortic diameters (corrected for age and body surface) and the risk of type A dissection or rupture, which allows for predictive echocardiographic follow-up and well-established medical or surgical intervention guidelines. Patients with a firm diagnosis should undergo yearly echocardiograms. More frequent imaging should be performed if the aortic diameter is approaching a surgical threshold (>4.5 cm in adults; not as well defined in children) or shows rapid change (>0.5 cm/year) or with concerns regarding heart or valve function. Adults with repeatedly normal aortic diameters can be seen every 2 to 3 years. Standard treatment is β-blockade, which should be initiated in children and adults even with diameters less than 40 mm, unless contraindicated, as soon as the diagnosis is made. Mitral valve changes may be the earliest feature, and mitral regurgitation may require surgery even before the aorta is widely dilated.

Antibiotic prophylaxis should be used before any dental procedure. Special consideration should be given to children and adolescents (<20 years old). In sporadic cases, these children may not yet fit a diagnosis of Marfan syndrome. The term *nonspecific connective tissue disorder* until follow-up echocardiographic evaluation shows aortic root dilation (z ≥ 3) has been suggested. In general, patients with MFS should avoid contact sports, exercise to exhaustion, and especially isometric activities involving a Valsalva maneuver. Most patients can and should participate in aerobic activities performed in moderation. The third trimester of pregnancy, labor and delivery, and the first postpartum month represent a particularly vulnerable time for dissection.

During childhood and adolescence, special care should be directed toward detection of scoliosis. Annual ophthalmological evaluation for the detection of ectopia lentis, cataract, glaucoma, and retinal detachment is essential. Early monitoring and aggressive refraction is required for children with Marfan syndrome to prevent amblyopia. For many patients treated prophylactically, life expectancy now approaches normal. Health supervision guidelines for children with Marfan syndrome have been established by the American Academy of Pediatrics, the National Marfan Foundation (http://www.marfan.org), and the American Heart Association/American College of Cardiology task forces.

ETIOLOGY

This disorder has an autosomal dominant inheritance pattern, with wide variability in expression.

Mutations in the very large fibrillin (*FBN1*) gene located on chromosome 15q15-21.3 are responsible.

COMMENT

Severe Marfan syndrome diagnosed in the first 3 months of life is the result of point mutations or small deletions in the middle third of the fibrillin-1 protein. Serious cardiac defects including mitral valve prolapse, valvular regurgitation, and aortic root dilatation occur in approximately 80% of cases, often causing heart failure. Congenital contractures are present in 64%. A very characteristic facies, dolichocephaly, a high-arched palate, micrognathia, hyperextensible joints, arachnodactyly, pes planus, chest deformity, iridodonesis, megalocornea, and lens dislocation are also frequently present. Fourteen percent of affected children die during the first year.

References

Marfan AB: Un cas de déformation congénitales des quatre membres plus prononcée aux extrémities charactérisée par l'allongement des os avec un certain degré d'amincissement, *Bull Mem Soc Med Hop (Paris)* 13:220, 1896.

Pyeritz RE, McKusick VA: The Marfan syndrome: Diagnosis and management, *N Engl J Med* 300:772, 1979.

Hofman KJ, et al: Increased incidence of neuropsychologic impairment in the Marfan syndrome, *Am J Hum Genet* 37:4A, 1985.

Gott VL, et al: Surgical treatment of aneurysms of the ascending aorta in the Marfan syndrome: Results of composite-graft repair in 50 patients, *N Engl J Med* 314:1070, 1986.

Morse RP, et al: Diagnosis and management of infantile Marfan syndrome, *Pediatrics* 86:888, 1990.

Lee B, et al: Linkage of Marfan syndrome and a phenotypically related disorder to two different fibrillin genes, *Nature* 352:330, 1991.

Kainulainen K, et al: Mutations in the fibrillin gene responsible for dominant ectopia lentis and neonatal Marfan syndrome, *Nat Genet* 6:64, 1994.

Rossiter JP, et al: A prospective longitudinal evaluation of pregnancy in the Marfan syndrome, *Am J Obstet Gynecol* 173:1599, 1995.

American Academy of Pediatrics: Health supervision for children with Marfan syndrome, *Pediatrics* 98:978, 1996.

De Paepe A, et al: Revised diagnostic criteria for the Marfan syndrome, *Am J Med Genet* 62:417, 1996.

Pyeritz RE: The Marfan syndrome, *Annu Rev Med* 51:481, 2000.

Dean JCS: Management of Marfan syndrome, *Heart* 88:97, 2002.

Jones EG, et al: Growth and maturation in Marfan syndrome, *Am J Med Genet* 109:100, 2002.

Maron BJ, et al: Recommendations for physical activity and recreational sports participation for young patients with genetic cardiovascular diseases, *Circulation* 109:2807, 2004.

P

Habashi JP, et al: Losartan, an AT1 antagonist, prevents aortic aneurysm in a mouse model of Marfan syndrome, *Science* 312:117, 2006.

Lacro RV, et al: Rationale and design of a randomized clinical trial of beta-blocker therapy (atenolol) versus angiotensin II receptor blocker therapy (losartan) in individuals with Marfan syndrome, *Am Heart J* 154:624, 2007.

Brooke BS, et al: Angiotensin II blockade and aortic-root dilation in Marfan's syndrome, *N Engl J Med* 358:2787, 2008.

Loeys BL, et al: The revised Ghent nosology for the Marfan syndrome, *J Med Genet* 47:476, 2010.

Aalberts JJ, et al: Diagnostic yield in adults screened at the Marfan outpatient clinic using the 1996 and 2010 Ghent nosologies, *Am J Med Genet A* 158A:982, 2012.

Pyeritz RE, et al: Evaluation of the adolescent or adult with some features of Marfan syndrome, *Genet Med* 14:171, 2012.

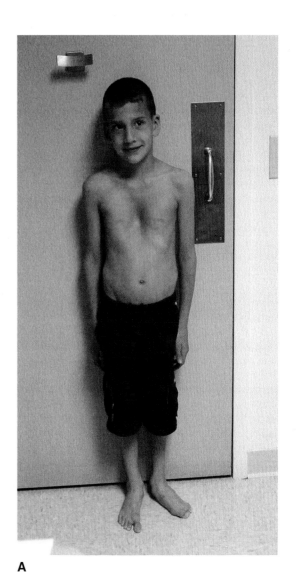

FIGURE 1.   Marfan syndrome. **A–C,** Unrelated 9- and 13-year-old boys. Note the long slim limbs, pectus excavatum, narrow face, and reduced elbow extension.

A

Continued

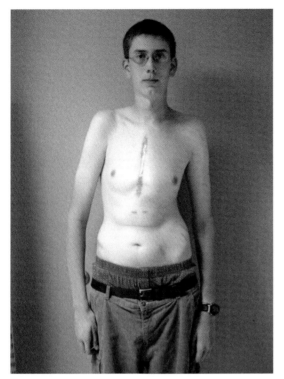

B

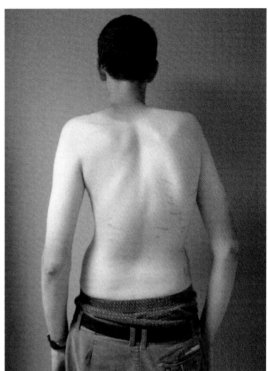

C

FIGURE 1, cont'd

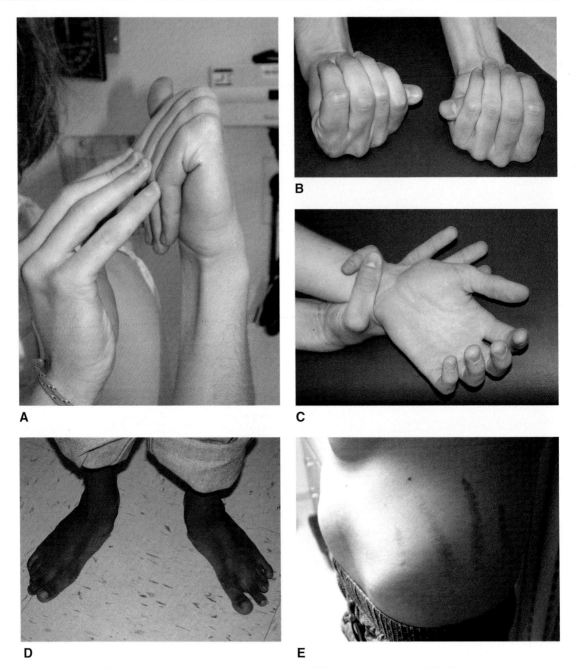

FIGURE 2.   Note the joint laxity **(A)**, Steinberg thumb sign **(B)**, ability to join thumb and fifth finger around the wrist (Walker-Murdoch sign) **(C)**, pes planus **(D)**, and striae over hips and back **(E)**. (A–D, Courtesy Dr. Lynne M. Bird, Rady Children's Hospital, San Diego.)

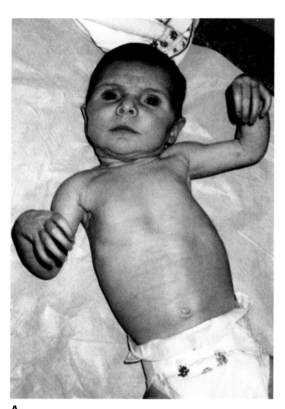
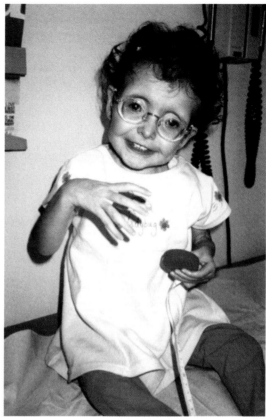

A   **B**

FIGURE 3.   **A** and **B,** Child with neonatal form of Marfan syndrome. (Courtesy Dr. Stephen Braddock, University of Missouri, Columbia.)

BEALS SYNDROME (BEALS CONTRACTURAL ARACHNODACTYLY SYNDROME)
Joint Contractures, Scoliosis, Arachnodactyly, "Crumpled" Ear

Beals and Hecht described this syndrome in 1971. They found 11 probable past reports of the same entity, including the original Marfan report. Over 75 cases have been reported to date, half of which are familial cases. Aortic root dilatation can be present, but appears to be nonprogressive, and the ocular findings of Marfan syndrome are rarely seen.

ABNORMALITIES

Growth. Tall stature (55%), marfanoid habitus.
Limbs. Long slim limbs (dolichostenomelia 40%) with arachnodactyly (81%), camptodactyly (84%), ulnar deviation of fingers; large joint contractures, especially of knees, elbows, and hips (83%).
Other Skeletal. Progressive scoliosis and/or kyphosis (64%), relatively short neck, metatarsus varus, mild talipes equinovarus, generalized muscle weakness (74%), hypoplasia of calf muscles, and shoulder muscles. High arched palate (49%), pectus deformity (43%).
Ears. "Crumpled" appearance with poorly defined conchas and prominent crura from the root of the helix (79%).
Cardiovascular. Aortic root dilatation (12%), mitral valve prolapse (6%), and septum defects (4%). Two patients had an interrupted aortic arch or aortic coarctation, and one had transient cardiomyopathy with noncompaction.

OCCASIONAL ABNORMALITIES
Micrognathia; cleft palate; cranial abnormalities, including scaphocephaly, brachycephaly, dolichocephaly, and frontal bossing; subluxation of patella; iris coloboma; keratoconus; myopia; cataract, coloboma, and glaucoma have been seen in two patients, choroidal neovascularization in one case.

NATURAL HISTORY
Although there tends to be gradual improvement in the joint limitations in the majority of patients, scoliosis and/or kyphosis are progressive in 64% of the cases. The long-term prognosis for aortic root dilatation is unknown, but the risks appear to be much less than in Marfan syndrome.

ETIOLOGY
This disorder has an autosomal dominant inheritance pattern. Mutations in the *FBN2* gene are responsible. However, a detectable mutation in the *FBN2* gene has been documented in only 44% of cases. No apparent phenotypic differences exist between mutation positive and negative patients. High inter- and intrafamilial variability has been demonstrated, including incomplete penetrance.

COMMENT
A severe form of this disorder, lethal in the neonatal period, has been described. In addition to the characteristic features of Beals syndrome, severe cardiac defects occur, including interrupted aortic arch, ventricular septal defect, atrial septal defect, and aortic root dilatation, as well as gastrointestinal anomalies, including duodenal and esophageal atresia and intestinal malrotation.

References

Beals RK, Hecht F: Delineation of another heritable disorder of connective tissue, *J Bone Joint Surg Am* 53:987, 1971.

Hecht F, Beals RK: "New" syndrome of congenital contractural arachnodactyly originally described by Marfan in 1896, *Pediatrics* 49:574, 1972.

Anderson RA, et al: Cardiovascular findings in congenital contractural arachnodactyly: Report of an affected kindred, *Am J Med Genet* 18:265, 1984.

Ramos Arroyo MA, et al: Congenital contractural arachnodactyly. Report of four additional families and review of literature, *Clin Genet* 25:570, 1985.

Lee B, et al: Linkage of Marfan syndrome and a phenotypically related disorder to two different fibrillin genes, *Nature* 352:330, 1991.

Viljoen D: Congenital contractural arachnodactyly (Beals syndrome), *J Med Genet* 31:640, 1994.

Putnam EA, et al: Fibrillin-2 (*FBN2*) mutations result in the Marfan-like disorder, congenital contractural arachnodactyly, *Nat Genet* 11:456, 1995.

Wang M, et al: Familial occurrence of typical and severe lethal contractural arachnodactyly caused by missplicing of exon 34 of fibrillin-2, *Am J Hum Genet* 59:1027, 1996.

Gupta PA, et al: Ten novel *FBN-2* mutations in congenital contractural arachnodactyly: Delineation of the molecular pathogenesis and clinical phenotype, *Hum Mutat* 19:39, 2002.

Gupta PA, et al: *FBN2* mutation associated with manifestations of Marfan syndrome and congenital contractural arachnodactyly, *J Med Genet* 41:334, 2004.

Takaesu-Miyagi S, et al: Ocular findings of Beals syndrome, *Jpn J Ophthalmol* 48:470, 2004.

Matsumoto T, et al: Transient cardiomyopathy in a patient with congenital contractural arachnodactyly (Beals syndrome), *J Nihon Med Sch* 73:285, 2006.

Callewaert BL, et al: Comprehensive clinical and molecular assessment of 32 probands with congenital contractural arachnodactyly: Report of 14 novel mutations and review of the literature, *Hum Mutat* 30:334, 2009.

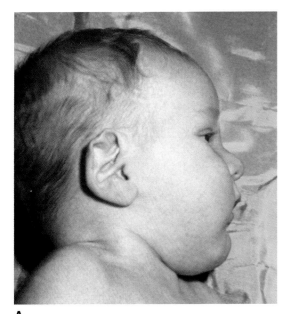

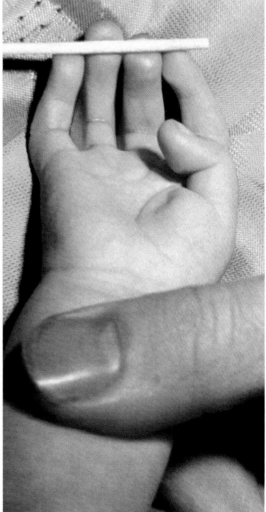

FIGURE 1.   Beals syndrome. **A** and **B,** Young infant showing folded helices of ears and relative arachnodactyly with camptodactyly. Severe scoliosis developed by 2 years of age.

A

B

P

SHPRINTZEN-GOLDBERG SYNDROME
Marfanoid Habitus, Dolichocephaly, Micrognathia, Ocular Proptosis

In 1982, Shprintzen and Goldberg described two unrelated males with craniosynostosis and marfanoid habitus. Robinson and colleagues (2005) provide a good review of 37 cases and suggest a set of craniofacial, skeletal, and radiographic diagnostic features for these patients, who commonly have intellectual disability and only rarely have cardiovascular abnormalities.

ABNORMALITIES

Growth. Birth length tends to be increased; with increasing age, weight frequently drops below the third percentile and is associated with decreased subcutaneous fat.

Performance. Hypotonia, delayed developmental milestones, intellectual disability.

Craniofacial. Craniosynostosis (50%); dolichocephaly; large anterior fontanel; high prominent forehead; ocular proptosis; strabismus; hypertelorism; downslanting palpebral fissures; ptosis; maxillary hypoplasia; broad secondary alveolar ridge; micrognathia; low-set, posteriorly rotated ears.

Skeletal. Arachnodactyly, camptodactyly, genu valgum, genu recurvatum, pectus excavatum, pectus carinatum, hyperextensible joints, joint contractures, metatarsus adductus, talipes equinovarus, scoliosis.

Cardiac. Aortic root dilatation, mitral valve prolapse.

Radiologic. Thin ribs; 13 pairs of ribs; square, box-like vertebral bodies; bowing of femora; hypoplastic hooked clavicles; osteopenia.

Other. Hydrocephalus (40%), myopia, umbilical hernia, cryptorchidism.

OCCASIONAL ABNORMALITIES

Microcephaly; fine sparse hair; hyperelastic skin; ptosis; myopia; hearing loss; upturned nose; Chiari I malformation; C1-C2 abnormality; bifid uvula; cleft palate; choanal atresia/stenosis; vocal cord paralysis; dental malocclusion; prominent/malformed ears; tetralogy of Fallot; subvalvar aortic stenosis; inguinal hernia; joint dislocation; bowing of ribs, ulna, radii, tibiae, or fibulae; fusion of vertebrae; hypospadias; cryptorchidism; growth hormone deficiency.

NATURAL HISTORY

Severe hypotonia with feeding difficulties (often requiring nasogastric tube feeding), stridorous breathing during sleep, cyanosis, and respiratory compromise are frequent in infancy. Obstructive apnea is common and infrequently requires tracheostomy. With advancing age, linear growth rate begins to decrease. Delay in attainment of developmental milestones is usual. Mild to severe degrees of intellectual disability have occurred in most patients. Aortic aneurysm and dissection can be life-threatening and should be closely monitored.

ETIOLOGY

Autosomal dominant transmission seems clear and clinical evidence of germline mosaicism has been reported in two patients. Analysis of the fibrillin-1 (*FBN1*) gene has been carried out in many patients but only two causal familial mutations were found in patients with a somewhat convincing Shprintzen-Goldberg syndrome phenotype. Mutations in *TGFBR2* have been reported in several cases, but developmental delay was usually absent or mild, and the phenotype in those cases was mostly consistent with the Loeys-Dietz syndrome. Recently a variant in the gene *SKI*, involved in the TGF-ß SMAD signaling pathway, has been identified by exome sequencing. Subsequently, heterozygous mutations were identified in 9 of 11 sporadic cases. The Sloan-Kettering Institute (SKI) family of proteins, which also includes the SKI-like protein SKIL, negatively regulate SMAD-dependent TGF-ß signaling. Loss of function mutations in *SKI* lead to an excess of canonical TGF-ß signaling, also caused by *FBN1* mutations (Marfan syndrome) and *TGFBR1* and *TGFBR2* mutations (Loeys-Dietz syndrome).

References

Sugarman G, Vogel MW: Case report 76: Craniofacial and musculoskeletal abnormalities—a questionable connective tissue disease, *Synd Ident* 7:16, 1981.

Shprintzen RJ, Goldberg RB: A recurrent pattern syndrome of craniosynostosis associated with arachnodactyly and abdominal hernias, *J Craniofac Genet Dev Biol* 2:65, 1982.

Adès LC, et al: Distinct skeletal abnormalities in four girls with Shprintzen-Goldberg syndrome, *Am J Med Genet* 57:565, 1995.

Sood S, et al: Mutation in fibrillin-1 and marfanoid-craniosynostosis (Shprintzen-Goldberg) syndrome, *Nat Genet* 12:209, 1996.

Greally MT, et al: Shprintzen-Goldberg syndrome: A clinical analysis, *Am J Med Genet* 76:202, 1998.

Robinson PN, et al: Shprintzen-Goldberg syndrome: Fourteen new patients and a clinical analysis, *Am J Med Genet A* 135:251, 2005.

Kosaki K, et al: Molecular pathology of Shprintzen-Goldberg syndrome, *Am J Med Genet A* 140:104, 2006.

van Steensel MA, et al: Shprintzen-Goldberg syndrome associated with a novel missense mutation in *TGFBR2*, *Exp Dermatol* 17:362, 2008.

Doyle AJ, et al: Mutations in the TGF-ß repressor *SKI* cause Shprintzen-Goldberg syndrome with aortic aneurysm, *Nat Genet* 44:1249, 2012.

Shanske AL: Germline mosaicism in Shprintzen-Goldberg syndrome, *Am J Med Genet A* 158A:1574, 2012.

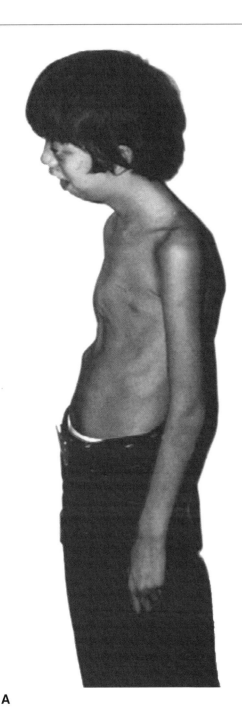

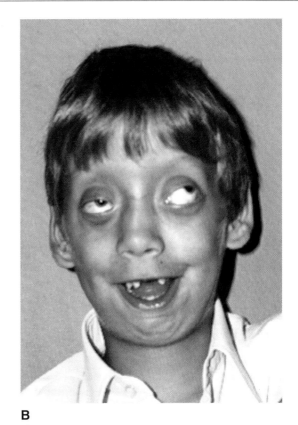

B

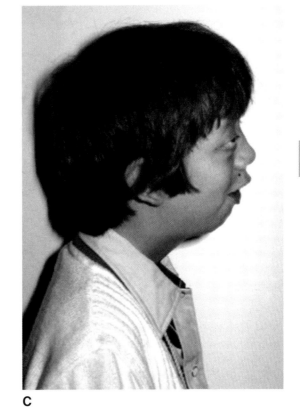

C

FIGURE 1. Shprintzen-Goldberg syndrome. **A–C,** A 4-year-old boy. Note the marked exophthalmos, micrognathia, and pectus carinatum. (**A–C,** From Shprintzen RJ, Goldberg RB: *J Craniofac Genet Dev Biol* 2:65, 1982.)

A

P

Continued

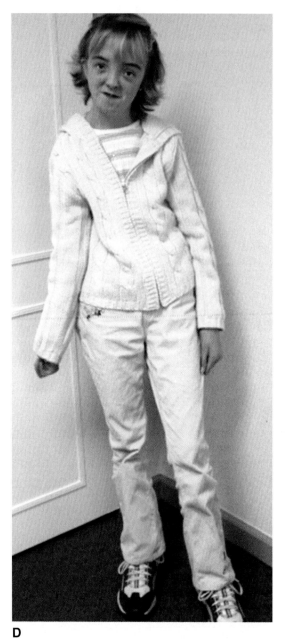

D

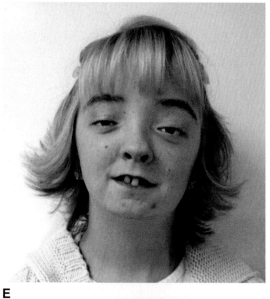

E

F

FIGURE 1, cont'd.   **D–F,** A 7-year-old girl. Note the low-set, posteriorly rotated ears, micrognathia, and downslanting palpebral fissures. (**D–F,** Courtesy Dr. Cynthia Curry, University of California, San Francisco.)

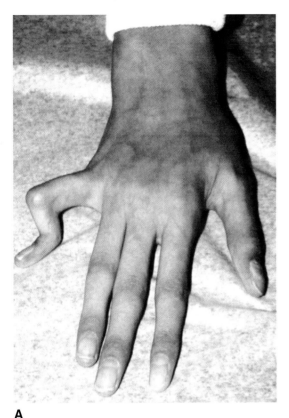

A

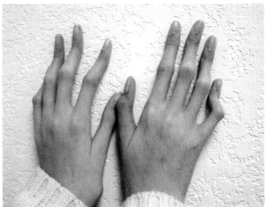

B

FIGURE 2.   **A** and **B,** Note the arachnodactyly and camptodactyly. (**A,** From Shprintzen RJ, Goldberg RB: *J Craniofac Genet Dev Biol* 2:65, 1982.)

EHLERS-DANLOS SYNDROME
Hyperextensibility of Joints, Hyperextensibility of Skin, Poor Wound Healing with Thin Scar

Originally described by Van Meekeren in 1682, this condition was further clarified by Ehlers in 1901 and Danlos in 1908. The possibility has been raised that the celebrated violinist Paganini may have had Ehlers-Danlos syndrome, thus accounting for his unusual dexterity and reach. The Ehlers-Danlos syndrome (EDS) comprises a spectrum of monogenic conditions with variable manifestations affecting the skin, ligaments and joints, blood vessels, and internal organs. An updated classification by De Paepe and Malfait in 2012 includes new clinical and molecular findings. The classic, hypermobile, and vascular subtypes of EDS are common, whereas the kyphoscoliosis, arthrochalasis, and dermatosparaxis types and all newly defined variants are rare conditions. For each of the major subtypes, a set of major and minor diagnostic criteria has been defined. Vascular Ehlers-Danlos (Type IV) is described in detail in the following section.

CLASSIC TYPE (EDS I AND II)

ABNORMALITIES

Diagnostic Criteria

Major: Skin hyperextensibility; widened atrophic scars; joint hypermobility leading to sprains, dislocations/subluxation, pes planus.

Minor: Smooth, velvety skin; molluscous pseudotumors (fleshy lesions associated with scars, frequently found over pressure points); subcutaneous spheroids (small subcutaneous spherical hard bodies, often mobile and palpable on forearms and shins; may calcify and become detectable radiographically); muscle hypotonia; easy bruising; tissue extensibility and fragility manifest by hiatal hernia, anal prolapse, cervical insufficiency; postoperative hernia; mitral valve prolapse; aortic root dilatation, usually non-progressive; premature rupture of amniotic membranes.

Other: Characteristic facial features include epicanthic folds, excess skin over the eyelids, presence of dilated scars on the forehead, and a pale, somewhat prematurely aged appearance of the face.

ETIOLOGY

This disorder has an autosomal dominant inheritance pattern. Genetic heterogeneity has been documented. Mutations in *COL5A1* and *COL5A2* genes coding for the collagen type V fibrils account for the great majority (>90%) of classic EDS cases. Several rare variants, which include the features of classic EDS plus additional features, can be caused by type I collagen alterations. *Vascular-like type Ehlers-Danlos* is associated with arterial rupture in young adulthood and is caused by missense mutations in *COL1A1*. The *cardiac valvular type Ehlers-Danlos* is an autosomal recessive condition caused by total absence of the α2(I) collagen chain due to mutations in *COL1A2*. This condition presents in childhood with mild skin and joint hypermobility, osteopenia, and muscular hypotonia and is complicated in adulthood by the development of severe cardiac valve insufficiency. Autosomal recessive *EDS due to complete deficiency of tenascin-X* is phenotypically distinct from classic EDS. Patients present with skin and joint hypermobility and easy bruising, but they also have generalized muscle weakness and distal contractures. Atrophic scarring is not observed. The diagnosis can be confirmed by the absence of tenascin-X in serum and mutation analysis of the *TNX-B* gene.

COMMENT

The classic type has been separated into type I (gravis) and type II (mitis), which are allelic and best considered the same disorder with variable phenotype.

HYPERMOBILE TYPE (EDS III)

ABNORMALITIES

Diagnostic Criteria

Major: Hyperextensible or smooth velvety skin; generalized joint hypermobility, most frequently involving the shoulder, patella, and temporomandibular joints.

Minor: Recurring joint dislocations, chronic joint/limb pain, positive family history, mitral valve prolapse, aortic root dilatation.

ETIOLOGY

This disorder has an autosomal dominant inheritance pattern. The genetic basis of EDS-hypermobile type (EDS-HT) remains unknown. The striking preponderance of affected women versus men in EDS-HT is also unexplained. Haploinsufficiency for tenascin-X has been documented in a small number of patients.

COMMENT

Patients with EDS-HT have been mistakenly diagnosed with fibromyalgia, chronic fatigue syndrome, or depression. Chronic joint pain can be severe, and mobility can be markedly impaired in older patients.

KYPHOSCOLIOSIS TYPE (EDS VIA AND VIB)

ABNORMALITIES

Diagnostic Criteria

(The presence of three major criteria in infancy is diagnostic.)

Major: Generalized joint laxity, severe muscle hypotonia at birth, progressive scoliosis with onset at birth, scleral fragility, and rupture of ocular globe.
Minor: Tissue fragility, easy bruising, arterial rupture, marfanoid habitus, microcornea, osteopenia.
Ocular: Microcornea, blue sclera, myopia, retinal detachment, and glaucoma.

ETIOLOGY

This disorder has an autosomal recessive inheritance pattern. Two types of EDS VI have been proposed. EDS type VIA is caused by mutations in *PLOD1* causing deficient activity of the enzyme lysyl hydroxylase-1. Type VIB results from mutations in *CHST14,* encoding dermatan-4-sulfotransferase 1, and has a clinical phenotype that is distinct from type VIA with features including characteristic craniofacial abnormalities, joint contractures, wrinkled palms, tapered fingers, and gastrointestinal and genitourinary manifestations.

COMMENT

Loss of ambulation is frequent in EDS VIA and VIB in the second and third decades.

ARTHROCHALASIA TYPE (EDS VIIA AND VIIB)

ABNORMALITIES

Diagnostic Criteria

Major: Severe generalized joint hypermobility with recurrent subluxations, congenital hip dislocation.
Minor: Skin hyperextensibility, tissue fragility, easy bruising, muscle hypotonia, kyphoscoliosis, osteopenia.
Ocular: Xerophthalmia, steep corneas, pathologic myopia, vitreous abnormalities, and lens opacities.

ETIOLOGY

This disorder has an autosomal dominant inheritance pattern. Mutations in the *COL1A1* and *COL1A2* genes that encode the α1 and α2 chains of type I collagen are responsible.

DERMATOSPARAXIS TYPE (EDS VIIC)

ABNORMALITIES

Diagnostic Criteria

Major: Severe skin fragility, sagging redundant skin.
Minor: Soft, doughy skin; easy bruising; premature rupture of amniotic membranes; umbilical and inguinal hernias.
Other: Delayed closure of the fontanels, characteristic facies with edema of the eyelids and blue sclera, umbilical hernia, short stature, and short fingers. Fragility of internal tissues, with spontaneous bladder rupture.

ETIOLOGY

This disorder has an autosomal recessive inheritance pattern. Homozygous or compound heterozygous mutations in the gene *ADAMTS2,* encoding procollagen I N-terminal peptidase are responsible. Electrophoretic demonstration of pNα1(I) and pNα2(I) chains from type I collagen extracted from dermis in the presence of protease inhibitors or obtained from fibroblasts is diagnostic. Wound healing is normal.

OTHER NEW TYPES OF EHLERS-DANLOS SYNDROME

EDS VIII is characterized by joint hypermobility, normal scar formation but eventual scar atrophy (especially over the knees), and severe periodontal disease leading to premature loss of permanent teeth. Nasal bridge is long and narrow with prominent tip. Premature osteoarthritis and scoliosis are common. Linkage to 12p13 was reported in a family but excluded in others, suggesting genetic heterogeneity with no known causal gene.

Spondylocheirodysplastic form of EDS is characterized by hyperextensible, thin skin, easy bruising, hypermobility of the small joints with a tendency to contractures, prominent eyes with bluish sclera, wrinkled palms, atrophy of the thenar muscles, and tapering fingers. Moderate short stature and a mild skeletal dysplasia characterized by platyspondyly, osteopenia, and widened metaphyses are the rule. An intragenic deletion in *SLC39A13,* a zinc transporter involved in the intracellular trafficking of zinc, has been shown to be causative.

In addition, a *brittle cornea syndrome,* caused by mutation in *ZNF469* or *PRDM5,* and an *Ehlers-Danlos/osteogenesis imperfecta overlap syndrome,* caused by mutations in *COL1A1* or *COL1A2,* have been identified.

References

Van Meekeren JA: De dilatabiltate extraordinaria cutis, In *Observations Medicochirogicae,* Amsterdam, 1682.

P

Ehlers E: Cutis laxa, Neigung zu Harmorrhagien in der Haut, Lockerung mehrer Artikulationen, *Dermat Ztschr* 8:173, 1901.

Danlos H: Un cas de cutis laxa avec tumeurs par contusion chronique des coudes et des genoux (xanthome juvenile pseudodiabetique de MM. Hallopeau et Mace de Lepinay), *Bull Soc Fr Dermat Syph* 19:70, 1908.

Barabas AP: Ehlers-Danlos syndrome: Associated with prematurity and premature rupture of foetal membranes; possible increase in incidence, *BMJ* 2:682, 1966.

Leier CV, et al: The spectrum of cardiac defects in Ehlers-Danlos syndrome, types I and III, *Ann Intern Med* 92:171, 1980.

Yeowell HN, Pinnell SR: The Ehlers-Danlos syndrome, *Semin Dermatol* 12:229, 1993.

Schievink WI, et al: Neurovascular manifestations of heritable disorders of connective tissue, *Stroke* 25:889, 1994.

Tilstra DJ, Byers PH: Molecular basis of hereditary disorders of connective tissue, *Annu Rev Med* 45:149, 1994.

Beighton P, et al: Ehlers-Danlos syndrome: Revised nosology, Villefranche, 1997, *Am J Med Genet* 77:31, 1998.

Burrows NP, et al: The molecular genetics of the Ehlers-Danlos syndrome, *Clin Exp Dermatol* 24:99, 1999.

Nuytinck L, et al: Classical Ehlers-Danlos syndrome caused by a mutation in type I collagen, *Am J Hum Genet* 66:1398, 2000.

Pepin M, et al: Clinical and genetic features of Ehlers-Danlos syndrome type IV, the vascular type, *N Engl J Med* 342:673, 2000.

Schalkwijk J, et al: A recessive form of the Ehlers-Danlos syndrome caused by tenascin-X deficiency, *N Engl J Med* 345:1167, 2001.

Malfait F, et al: Total absence of the alpha2(I) chain of collagen type I causes a rare form of Ehlers-Danlos syndrome with hypermobility and propensity to cardiac valvular problems, *J Med Genet* 43:36, 2006.

Cabral WA, et al: Y-position cysteine substitution in type I collagen (alpha1(I) R888C/p.R1066C) is associated with osteogenesis imperfecta/Ehlers-Danlos syndrome phenotype, *Hum Mutat* 28:396, 2007.

Giunta C, et al: Spondylocheiro dysplastic form of the Ehlers-Danlos syndrome—an autosomal-recessive entity caused by mutations in the zinc transporter gene *SLC39A13*, *Am J Hum Genet* 82:1290, 2008.

Malfait F, et al: Clinical and genetic aspects of Ehlers-Danlos syndrome, classic type, *Genet Med* 12:597, 2010.

Reinstein E, et al: Ehlers-Danlos type VIII, periodontitis-type: Further delineation of the syndrome in a four-generation pedigree, *Am J Med Genet Part A* 155:742, 2011.

Reinstein E, et al: Early-onset osteoarthritis in Ehlers-Danlos syndrome type VIII, *Am J Med Genet Part A* 158A:938, 2012.

Mendoza-Londono R, et al: Extracellular matrix and platelet function in patients with musculocontractural Ehlers-Danlos syndrome caused by mutations in the *CHST14* gene, *Am J Med Genet A* 158A:1344, 2012.

De Paepe A, Malfait F: The Ehlers-Danlos syndrome, a disorder with many faces, *Clin Genet* 82:1, 2012.

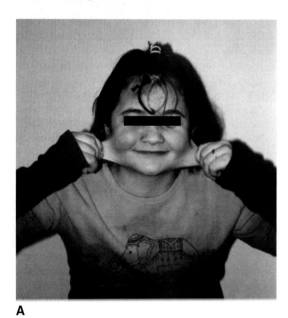

A

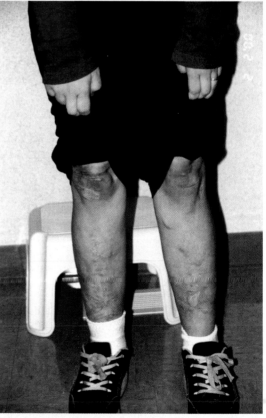

B

FIGURE 1. Ehlers-Danlos syndrome. **A** and **B,** A 12-year-old girl showing hyperelasticity of skin and persistence of scars. (Courtesy Dr. Stephen Braddock, University of Missouri, Columbia.)

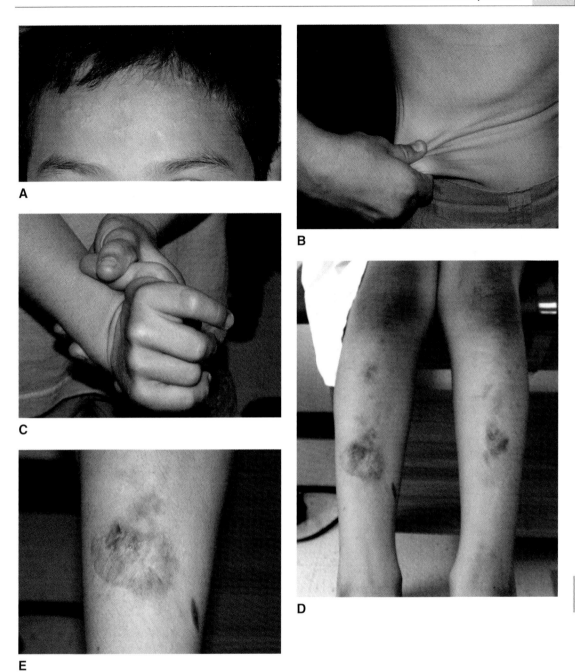

FIGURE 2. Note the persistence of scars over the forehead (A), hyperelasticity of the skin of the abdomen (B), hyperextensibility of the joints (C), and parchment-thin scars (D and E). (Courtesy Dr. Lynne M. Bird, Rady Children's Hospital, San Diego.)

VASCULAR EHLERS-DANLOS SYNDROME (EDS IV)
Skin Translucency, Excessive Bruising, Risk of Arterial and Organ Rupture

This type of Ehlers-Danlos syndrome is associated with significant health risks not present in the other types of EDS. Therefore, an early and precise recognition of this phenotype is essential.

ABNORMALITIES

Diagnostic Criteria

(The presence of two or more major criteria is extremely suggestive.)

Major: Thin translucent skin; arterial/intestinal/uterine fragility or rupture; extensive bruising; characteristic facial appearance, including a thin pinched nose, thin lips, tight skin, hollow cheeks, and prominent eyes secondary to a deficiency of adipose tissue.

Minor: Hypermobility of small joints, tendon and muscle rupture, bladder rupture, talipes equinovarus, varicose veins, arteriovenous and carotid-cavernous sinus fistula, pneumothorax/pneumohemothorax, gingival recession, unusual old-looking skin over hands and feet ("acrogeria"), or positive family history.

Imaging: Multiple vascular abnormalities, including aneurysms, dissection and ectasia involving the visceral arteries, aorta, and head and neck.

NATURAL HISTORY

Propensity to rupture arteries and hollow organs at a young age is common. The skin is not hyperextensible but rather thin and translucent, showing a visible venous pattern over the chest, abdomen and extremities. Excessive bruising is the most common sign and is often the presenting complaint in children, and the facial features can be very suggestive but not always present in young children. Excessive wrinkling and thinness of the skin are present over hands and feet. The vascular abnormalities are progressive. Intense physical activity, scuba diving, and violent sports should be avoided. Various medications, such as acetylsalicylic acid, clopidogrel, and/or antivitamin K agents that interfere with platelet function, should be avoided as should invasive vascular or other endoscopic procedures. Stripping of varicose veins can cause severe complications. However, elective surgical repair of blood vessels at risk of rupture may be safely undertaken. Mortality during pregnancy is about 12%. Early cesarean delivery prior to 37 weeks has been advocated with good results. Recently, a multicenter randomized trial showed that celiprolol, a long-acting ß1 antagonist with partial ß2-agonist properties, decreased by threefold the incidence of arterial rupture or dissection.

ETIOLOGY

This disorder has an autosomal dominant inheritance pattern. Confirmation of a suspected diagnosis of vascular EDS is possible by biochemical demonstration of quantitative or qualitative type III collagen defects, which identify more than 95% of affected individuals. Mutations in *COL3A1* are found in all cases.

References

Germain DP: Ehlers-Danlos syndrome type IV, *Orphanet J Rare Dis* 19:32, 2007.

Erez Y, Ezra Y, Rojansky N: Ehlers-Danlos type IV in pregnancy. A case report and a literature review, *Fetal Diagn Ther* 23:7, 2008.

Brooke BS: Contemporary management of vascular complications associated with Ehlers-Danlos syndrome, *J Vasc Surg* 51:131, 2010.

Lum YW, Brooke BS, Black JH 3rd: Contemporary management of vascular Ehlers-Danlos syndrome, *Curr Opin Cardiol* 26:494, 2011.

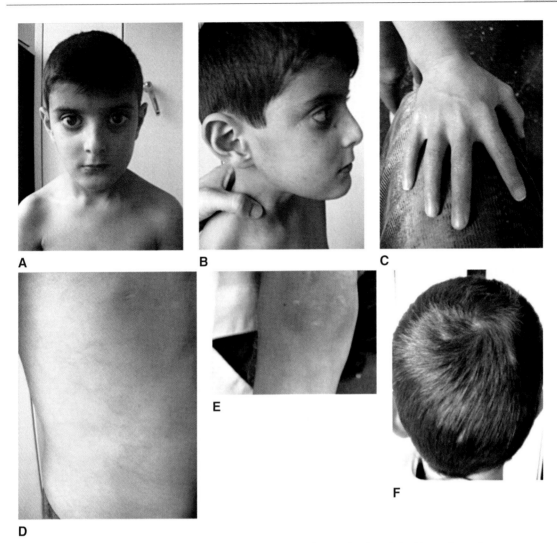

FIGURE 1. Vascular Ehlers-Danlos syndrome. Note a thin pinched nose, thin lips, tight skin, and prominent eyes (**A** and **B**); tight and old-looking skin over the hands (**C**); superficial vessels visible under the thin, translucent skin (**D**); and multiple scars over the knees and scalp after minor trauma, reflecting skin friability (**E** and **F**).

LOEYS-DIETZ SYNDROME

In 2005, Loeys and colleagues described 10 families with a new aortic aneurysm syndrome characterized by hypertelorism, bifid uvula, and/or cleft palate, and generalized arterial tortuosity with ascending aortic aneurysm and dissection. In 2006, the same authors differentiated Loeys-Dietz syndrome (LDS) type 1 when characteristic craniofacial features were present, and the less frequent LDS type 2 when the phenotype resembled vascular Ehlers-Danlos. Both types are caused by mutations in the TGFβ receptors. Although the distinction between types 1 and 2 is widely used, the two types most likely represent two ends of the spectrum of a single disorder with variable expression. More than 300 cases have been reported.

LOEYS-DIETZ TYPE 1
Hypertelorism, Bifid Uvula and/or Cleft Palate, Craniosynostosis

ABNORMALITIES

Growth. Normal stature. Subtle marfanoid habitus.
Performance. Usually normal intelligence, but 15% of patients may show cognitive delays.
Craniofacial. Craniosynostosis, predominantly sagittal, leading to dolichocephaly or scaphocephaly. Hydrocephalus, Arnold-Chiari malformation, hypertelorism, blue sclerae, bifid uvula, cleft palate, high arched palate, malar hypoplasia, retrognathia.
Skeletal. Dolichostenomelia, arachnodactyly, pectus excavatum or carinatum, scoliosis, cervical spine instability, spondylolisthesis, dural ectasia, talipes equinovarus, contractures and camptodactyly, joint laxity and dislocations, protrusio acetabuli, discordance of bone age between carpal bones and phalangeal epiphysis with an advanced carpal age, metaphyseal cupping of the distal ulna, coxa valga, genu valgum, multiple early fractures with osteoporosis.
Skin. Velvety, translucent skin.
Cardiovascular. Aortic root dilatation, aneurysm, dissection or rupture. Arterial tortuosity, often intracranial. Aneurysm of other vessels.

OCCASIONAL ABNORMALITIES
Patent ductus arteriosus, atrial septal defects, bicuspid aortic valve, bicuspid pulmonary valve, mitral valve prolapse, coronary artery aneurysms, submandibular branchial cysts, hip dysplasia.

LOEYS-DIETZ TYPE 2
Vascular Ehlers-Danlos-like Phenotype

ABNORMALITIES

Craniofacial. Subtle features, including dolichocephaly, tall broad forehead, frontal bossing, high anterior hairline, hypoplastic supraorbital margins, a "jowly" double-chinned appearance (particularly in the first 3 years of life), translucent and redundant facial skin, prominent upper central incisors in late childhood/adulthood, an open-mouthed myopathic face, facial asymmetry without obvious craniosynostosis. The adult face appears prematurely aged.
Skin. Velvety, translucent skin, blood vessels visible through the skin, easy bruising, venous varicosities, friable skin with minor trauma, wide and atrophic scars.
Cardiovascular. Aortic root dilatation, aneurysm, dissection, or rupture; easy bruising; arterial tortuosity, often intracranial; aneurysm of other vessels. Rupture of vessels with minor trauma and surgery.
Skeletal. Joint laxity and dislocations, arachnodactyly, contractures, camptodactyly.
Other. Rupture of spleen and bowel. Pregnancy complications with rupture of gravid uterus or the uterine arteries.

OCCASIONAL ABNORMALITIES
Bifid uvula.

NATURAL HISTORY
Arterial aneurysms leading to death, often before diagnosis and usually in the third and fourth decades, is of greatest concern. The phenotype ranges from severe neonatal forms to isolated moderate aortic dilatation in late adulthood. Aortic dilation can occur prenatally. Prominent craniofacial features, hypertelorism, bifid uvula and/or cleft

palate, and craniosynostosis in LDS type 1 can predict an even higher risk of aortic rupture and may speak for earlier intervention in children. In type 2, there is a high incidence of pregnancy-related complications and some risk of organ rupture, but lower surgical risks than in vascular Ehlers-Danlos caused by mutation in *COL3A1*. Magnetic resonance or computed tomographic angiographies (MRAs, CTAs) are indicated at diagnosis and follow-up since more than half of the patients will have aneurysms or extensive arterial tortuosity not detectable by echocardiogram. LDS patients are typically managed medically with beta-blockers and exercise restriction to reduce hemodynamic stress. Given the greater risk for aortic complications, replacement surgery of the aorta is advised at earlier ages and with less dilated aortas than in Marfan syndrome.

ETIOLOGY

Autosomal dominant inheritance with incomplete penetrance and widely variable expression. LDS is caused by genes encoding for receptors 1 and 2 of the transforming growth factor β (*TGFBR1* and *TGFBR2*). Both LDS type 1 and LDS type 2 can be caused by a mutation in either *TGFBR1* or *TGFBR2*. The phenotype of type 1 and 2 is concordant within a family. An increase in the availability of TGFβ, with the subsequent activation of the transcription SMAD cascade appears to underlie the development of abnormally weak histologically distorted connective tissue, which is the hallmark of this disorder.

COMMENT

Almost 20% of patients with aortic aneurysms have an affected first-degree relative but not one of the known genetic syndromes such as Loeys-Dietz syndrome, Marfan syndrome, or vascular Ehlers-Danlos syndrome. These patients have been included in a category referred to as familial thoracic aortic aneurysms and dissection (FTAAD).

References

Loeys BL, et al: A syndrome of altered cardiovascular, craniofacial, neurocognitive and skeletal development caused by mutations in *TGFBR1* or *TGFBR2*, *Nat Genet* 37:275, 2005.

Loeys BL, et al: Aneurysm syndromes caused by mutations in the TGF-beta receptor, *N Engl J Med* 355:788, 2006.

Aalberts JJ, et al: The many faces of aggressive aortic pathology: Loeys-Dietz syndrome, *Neth Heart J* 16(9):299, 2008.

Arslan-Kirchner M, et al: Clinical utility gene card for Loeys-Dietz syndrome (*TGFBR1/2*) and related phenotypes, *Eur J Hum Genet* 19(10), 2011.

Yetman AT, et al: Importance of the clinical recognition of Loeys-Dietz syndrome in the neonatal period, *Pediatrics* 119(5):e1199–e1202, 2007.

Stheneur C, et al: Identification of 23 *TGFBR2* and 6 *TGFBR1* gene mutations and genotype-phenotype investigations in 457 patients with Marfan syndrome type I and II, Loeys-Dietz syndrome and related disorders, *Hum Mutat* 29(11):E284, 2008.

Attias D, et al: Comparison of clinical presentations and outcomes between patients with *TGFBR2* and *FBN1* mutations in Marfan syndrome and related disorders, *Circulation* 120(25):2541, 2009. Epub 2009 Dec 7.

Rodrigues VJ, et al: Neuroradiologic manifestations of Loeys-Dietz syndrome type 1, *AJNR Am J Neuroradiol* 30(8):1614, 2009. Epub 2009 Jun 25.

Van Hemelrijk C, et al: The Loeys-Dietz syndrome: An update for the clinician, *Curr Opin Cardiol* 25:546, 2010.

Sousa SB, et al: Expanding the skeletal phenotype of Loeys-Dietz syndrome, *Am J Med Genet A* 155A(5):1178, 2011. doi: 10.1002/ajmg.a.33813. Epub 2011 Apr 11.

P

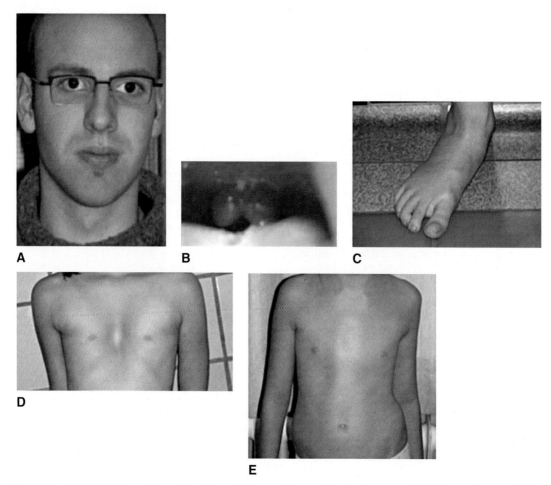

FIGURE 1.   Physical features of several patients with Loeys-Dietz syndrome. Note very subtle hypertelorism and bluish sclerae **(A),** bifid uvula **(B),** long toes **(C),** pectus excavatum **(D),** and pectus carinatum with scoliosis **(E).** (Courtesy Prof. Julie de Backer, Ghent, Belgium.)

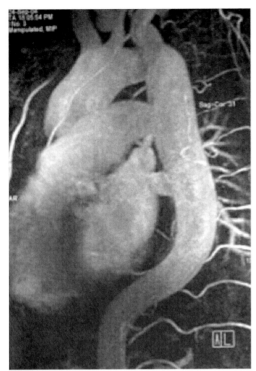

A

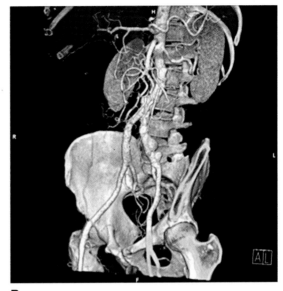

B

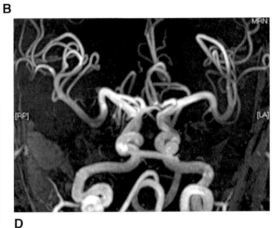

D

FIGURE 2. Imaging techniques showing marked dilatation of the ascending and descending aorta (**A**), several areas of arterial tortuosity and regional dilatation of the aorta and iliac vessels on angio-MRI (**B**), dilatation of the aorta and tortuosity of carotid arteries (**C**), and marked tortuosity of the intracranial vasculature (**D**). (**A**, **B**, and **D**, Courtesy Prof. Julie de Backer, Ghent, Belgium; **C**, courtesy Dr. Gisela Teixidor, Barcelona.)

C

P

OSTEOGENESIS IMPERFECTA SYNDROME, TYPE I
(AUTOSOMAL DOMINANT OSTEOGENESIS IMPERFECTA, LOBSTEIN DISEASE)
Fragile Bone, Blue Sclerae, Hyperextensibility, Presenile Deafness

Osteogenesis imperfecta is defined for all subtypes by the presence of bone fractures and osteopenia. Currently, an expanded version of the original classification Sillence proposed in 1979 is widely used. Differences in the clinical expression of the disorder, as well as different inheritance patterns and the many causal genes involved, define the different types. Thirteen types of osteogenesis imperfecta (OI) are currently recognized. Only types I, II, and III occur frequently. Although approximately 90% of cases are caused by mutations in the *COL1A1/COL1A2* genes, a total of eight genes are involved in causing these phenotypes. Only type I and type II are discussed in detail in this book.

ABNORMALITIES

Growth. Normal or near-normal.

Dentition. Hypoplasia of dentin and pulp with translucency of teeth (which have a yellowish or bluish gray color), and susceptibility to caries, irregular placement, and late eruption.

Sclerae and Skin. The skin and sclerae tend to be thin and translucent; partial visualization of the choroid gives the sclerae a blue appearance; easy bruising (75%).

Skeletal. Postnatal onset of mild limb deformity, primarily anterior or lateral bowing of femora and anterior bowing of tibiae (20%), fractures (92%), scoliosis (mild to moderate in 17%; severe in 3%), kyphosis (mild to moderate in 18%; severe in 2%), hyperextensible joints (100%), wormian bones in cranial sutures, osteopenia.

Hearing. Impairment in 35%, secondary to otosclerosis, and usually first noted in third decade.

Other. Macrocephaly (18%), triangular facial appearance (30%), inguinal or umbilical hernia.

OCCASIONAL ABNORMALITIES

Prenatal growth deficiency (7%), embryotoxon (opacity in the peripheral cornea), keratoconus, megalocornea, syndactyly, aortic or mitral valve disease, aortic root dilatation.

NATURAL HISTORY

Eight percent of patients have first fracture noted at birth, 23% in the first year, 45% in preschool, and 17% during school years. Bowing of the limbs is almost never noted in newborns. After adolescence, the likelihood of fracture diminishes, although inactivity, pregnancy, or lactation can apparently enhance the likelihood of fracture. Scoliosis, usually not diagnosed before the end of the first decade, progresses during puberty and in some cases can be severe in adulthood. Loss of stature secondary to progressive platyspondyly and kyphosis caused by spinal osteoporosis occurs in adults. Hearing impairment is common in adults, who often require hearing aids or surgery for osteosclerosis. Virtually all patients are ambulatory. The cyclic administration of intravenous pamidronate has been effective in decreasing bone pain and increasing mobility as well as in reducing bone resorption and increasing bone density. Treatment is recommended for children born with multiple fractures, long bone deformity, and demineralization on skeletal radiographs. It has been suggested that children with either a total of three fractures or more than two fractures in 1 year, including vertebral fractures, and with decreased bone mineral content (z scores less than 2nd centile for age) undergo treatment.

ETIOLOGY

OI type I has an autosomal dominant inheritance pattern with marked variability in expression. From a molecular standpoint, OI type I results from mutations in *COL1A1* or *COL1A2*, the genes that encode the pro-α-1(I) and pro-α-2(I) chains of type I procollagen. Mutations are typically functional nulls leading to a quantitative decrease in the production of type I collagen.

COMMENT

Major features of types III through VI are summarized below. Type II is described in detail separately.

Type III. Prenatal onset of growth deficiency, macrocephaly with a triangular facial appearance,

Kussmaul MG, et al: Pulmonary and cardiac function in advanced fibrodysplasia ossificans progessiva, *Clin Orthop* 346:104, 1998.

Kitterman JA, et al: Iatrogenic harm caused by diagnostic errors in fibrodysplasia ossificans progressiva, *Pediatrics* 116:654, 2005.

Shore EM, et al: A recurrent mutation in the BMP type I receptor ACVR1 causes inherited and sporadic fibrodysplasia ossificans progressiva, *Nat Genet* 38:525, 2006.

Kaplan FS, et al: Classic and atypical fibrodysplasia ossificans progressiva (FOP) phenotypes are caused by mutations in the bone morphogenetic protein (BMP) type I receptor ACVR1, *Hum Mutat* 30:379, 2009.

Hammond P, et al: The face signature of fibrodysplasia ossificans progressiva, *Am J Med Genet A* 158A:1368, 2012.

P

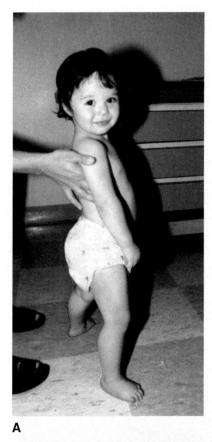

A

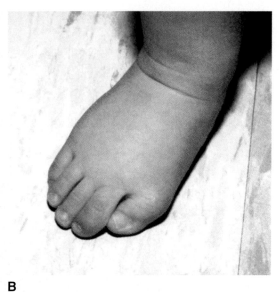

B

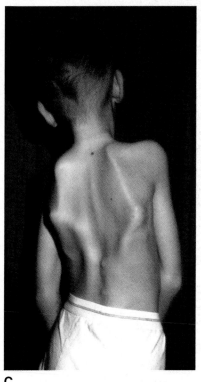

C

D

FIGURE 1. Fibrodysplasia ossificans progressiva syndrome. **A** and **B,** A 15-month-old child. Note the straight back, which is due to early ossification and the short hallux. **C** and **D,** A 13-year-old child showing progressive ossification in back musculature and short valgus hallux.

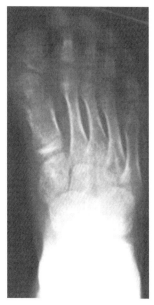

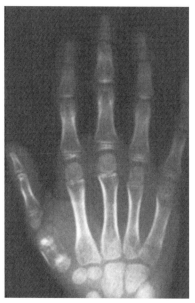

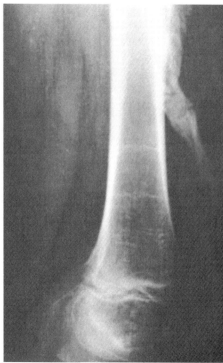

FIGURE 2. Note the short and deformed first metatarsal, hallux, and first metacarpal. Aberrant ossification is evident in the lower thigh. (From Herrmann J, et al: Fibrodysplasia ossificans progressiva and the XXXXY syndrome in the same sibship. *Birth Defects* OAS 5(5):43, 1969. Courtesy Dr. John M. Opitz, University of Utah, Salt Lake City.)

P

Q | Hamartoses

STURGE-WEBER SEQUENCE
Flat Facial Hemangiomata, Meningeal Hemangiomata with Seizures

The association and localization of aberrant vasculature in the facial skin, eyes, and meninges are compatible with a defect arising in a limited part of the cephalic neural crest, cells of which migrate to the supraocular dermis, choroid, and pia mater.

ABNORMALITIES

Performance. Seizures, paresis, intellectual disability.

Craniofacial. Port-wine capillary malformation, most commonly in a trigeminal facial distribution, sometimes involving the choroid of the eye with secondary buphthalmos or glaucoma as well as the conjunctiva or episcleral region; involvement usually unilateral, sometimes bilateral; overgrowth of bony maxilla secondary to the vascular anomaly.

Imaging. Capillary malformation involving arachnoid and pia mater, especially in occipital and temporal areas produces secondary cerebral cortical atrophy, sclerosis, and "double contour" convolutional calcification.

OCCASIONAL ABNORMALITIES
Capillary malformation in nonfacial areas; microgyria; macrocephaly; colobomata of iris, retinal vasculature tortuosity, iris heterochromia, retinal detachment, and strabismus; coarctation of aorta; enlargement of the ear when involved with capillary malformation; macrodactyly.

NATURAL HISTORY
The surface capillary malformations are usually present at birth and seldom progress. Seizures most commonly begin between 2 and 7 months of age and are grand mal in type. The degree of central nervous system (CNS) involvement is variable, with 30% having paresis and approximately 83% having seizures; 39% have normal intelligence. A poor prognosis for cognitive development is predicted by the number of seizures, an early age of onset, a poor response to treatment, bilateral cerebral involvement or severe unilateral lesions. An increased risk for emotional and behavioral problems, including mood disorder, attention deficit hyperactivity disorder, disruptive behavior disorder, and adjustment disorder.

Aggressive control of seizures is recommended. Focal resections may be needed. Stroke-like episodes in children with Sturge-Weber sequence are common. Low-dose aspirin has been proposed to improve long-term cognitive function and overall quality of life.

Glaucoma presents before 2 years of age if tissues destined to form the anterior chamber angle are affected. If only conjunctival and episcleral vascular tissues are involved, glaucoma frequently does not occur until after 5 years of age. Heterochromia iridis with darker iris on the glaucomatous side appears to be a marker for cases that will develop glaucoma.

Cerebral calcification is usually not evident by radiography until later infancy. Vascular magnetic resonance imaging (MRI) or computed tomography (CT) scan often does not detect lesions before 1 year of age. Although pulsed dye laser therapy is the treatment of choice, complete clearance of the port-wine stain rarely occurs.

ETIOLOGY
A recurrent somatic activating mutation in GNAQ (c.548G>A, p.ARG183Gln) has been identified in affected tissue from 88% of evaluated individuals. Mutations have also been found in affected tissue from individuals with non-syndromic port-wine stains suggesting that the extent of the phenotype is determined by the developmental time point at which the mutation occurs.

COMMENT
Port-wine facial nevi occur frequently without eye or brain abnormalities. Only patients with lesions involving the ophthalmic distribution of the trigeminal nerve (dermatome V1, including the upper eyelid) are at risk for neuro-ocular complications. In rare cases, the leptomeninges are involved without the face or choroid.

References

Chaeo DH-C: Congenital neurocutaneous syndromes of childhood. III: Sturge-Weber disease, *J Pediatr* 55:635, 1959.

Kossof EM, et al: Outcome of 32 hemispherectomies for Sturge-Weber syndrome worldwide, *Neurology* 59: 1735, 2002.

Aggarwal NK, et al: Heterochromia iridis and pertinent clinical findings in patients with glaucoma associated with Sturge-Weber syndrome, *J Pediatr Ophthalmol Strabismus* 47:361, 2010.

Turin E, et al: Behavioral and psychiatric features of Sturge-Weber syndrome, *J Nerv Ment Dis* 198:905, 2010.

Shirley MD, et al: Sturge-Weber syndrome and port-wine stains caused by somatic mutation in GNAQ, *N Eng J Med* 368:1971, 2013.

Lo W, et al: Updates and future horizons on the understanding, diagnosis, and treatment of Sturge-Weber syndrome brain involvement. Brain Vascular Malformation Consortium National Sturge-Weber Syndrome Workgroup, *Dev Med Child Neurol* 54:214, 2012.

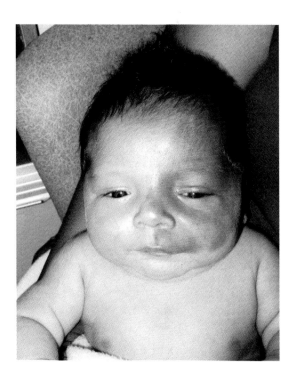

FIGURE 1. Sturge-Weber sequence. Note that the lesion involves the upper eyelid, which includes the ophthalmic distribution of the trigeminal nerve.

Q

NEUROCUTANEOUS MELANOSIS SEQUENCE
Melanosis of Skin and Pia-Arachnoid, Central Nervous System Deterioration

This melanocytic hamartomatosis of the skin and pia-arachnoid was first described in 1861. More than 100 cases have been reported.

ABNORMALITIES

Performance. Liable to development of seizures and deterioration of CNS function; cranial nerve palsies, particularly VI and VII.

Skin. Giant pigmented nevi (66%) usually in a "bathing trunk" or lumbosacral distribution, less frequently in the occipital region or upper back; numerous congenital nevi (at least three) without a prominent large lesion (34%); associated small or medium-sized congenital melanocytic nevi on the scalp, face, or neck occur in association with the larger lesions.

Visceral. Thick and pigmented with nests and sheets of melanotic cells, 88% with cranial involvement and 88% with spinal involvement;

Imaging. Hydrocephalus secondary to blockage of cisternal pathways or obliteration of arachnoid villi by the tumor; involvement of spinal cord and its coverings.

OCCASIONAL ABNORMALITIES

Syringomyelia; Dandy-Walker malformation; psychosis; Meckel diverticulum; urinary tract anomalies, including renal pelvis and ureteral malformations, unilateral renal cysts, rhabdomyosarcoma; leptomeningeal melanoma; extracranial melanoma, probably representing metastases from meningeal melanoma; liposarcoma; malignant peripheral nerve sheath tumor.

NATURAL HISTORY

The cutaneous melanosis is grossly evident at birth. CNS function may be normal initially, but seizures and other signs of increased intracranial pressure often develop before the age of 2 years. Mental deterioration may begin before 1 year of age, apparently related to the melanoblastic involvement of the pia-arachnoid and spinal cord compression. Leptomeningeal melanoma occurs in 40% to 62% of patients with CNS infiltration, and intracranial melanomas are found frequently.

The CNS consequences of the disorder often result in early demise. Three of the initially described patients were stillborn; the majority died before 2 years of age, and only 10% of the patients are known to have survived past the age of 25 years. The interval between the age at initial presentation and death ranges from immediate to 21 years, with more than one half occurring within 3 years of initial diagnosis.

In 25% of patients with neurologically asymptomatic, large congenital melanocytic nevi, focal magnetic resonance signals are present in the leptomeninges or adjacent brain parenchyma. Although the prognosis for these patients is unknown, the vast majority followed for 5 years have not developed symptomatic neurocutaneous melanosis. MRI scans of the brain are recommended in all infants with congenital nevi with a diameter more than 2 cm in the cranial area or over the spine as well as in infants with more than 20 satellite nevi so that involvement of the brain is detected early. Imaging should be repeated at regular intervals to detect progress of intracerebral melanosis or development of hydrocephalus. Patients with satellite nevi are of greatest risk for development of neurocutaneous melanosis. Patients without nevi on the head or neck or the posterior midline rarely develop neurologic complications.

The risk of malignant melanoma degeneration of the cutaneous melanosis is reported as 5% to 15%, with half becoming evident by 5 years of age. Thus, surgery to reduce the skin lesions is indicated in patients in whom careful evaluation has documented a lack of leptomeningeal involvement.

ETIOLOGY

Somatic mutations in codon 61 of NRAS have been documented in the majority of patients studies to date. Moreover, loss of heterozygosity of this gene has been demonstrated in two cases that progressed to melanoma. The sex incidence of this disorder is equal.

References

Rokitansky J: Ein ausgezeichneter Fall von Pigmentmal mit ausgebreiteter Pigmentirung der inneren Hirn- und Rückenmarkshäute, *Allg Wien Med Ztg* 6:113, 1861.

Van Bogaert L: La Mélanose neurocutanée diffuse hérédo-famiale, *Bull Acad R Med Belg (6th series)* 13:397, 1948.

Kinsler VA, et al: Multiple congenital melanocytic nevi and neurocutaneous melanosis are caused by postzygotic mutations in codon 61 of NRAS, *J Invest Derm* doi:10.1038/jid.2013.70

Foster RD, et al: Giant congenital melanocytic nevi: The significance of neurocutaneous melanosis in neurologically asymptomatic children, *Plast Reconstr Surg* 107:933, 2001.

Makkar HS, Frieden IJ: Congenital melanocytic nevi: An update for the pediatrician, *Clin Opin Pediatr* 14:397, 2002.

Livingstone E, et al: Neurocutaneous melanosis: A fatal disease in early childhood, *J Clin Oncol* 27:2290, 2009.

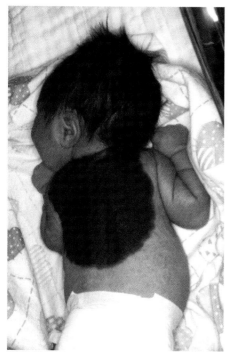

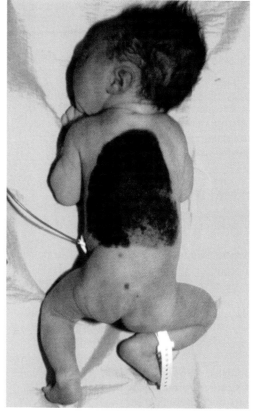

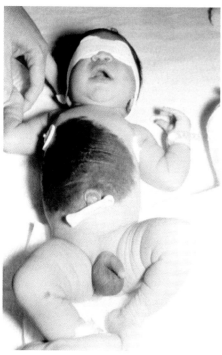

FIGURE 1. Neurocutaneous melanosis sequence.

LINEAR SEBACEOUS NEVUS SEQUENCE
(NEVUS SEBACEUS OF JADASSOHN, EPIDERMAL NEVUS SYNDROME)
Midfacial Nevus Sebaceus, Seizures, Mental Deficiency

Nevus sebaceous of Jadassohn is most commonly found in an otherwise normal individual. However, the association of this type of lesion in the midfacial area with seizures and intellectual disability has been reported in at least 100 cases.

ABNORMALITIES

Growth. Asymmetric overgrowth, advanced bone age.

Performance. Seizures of major motor, focal, or minor motor types; intellectual disability.

Skin. Nevus sebaceous with hyperpigmentation and hyperkeratosis; lesions most commonly in the midfacial area, from the forehead down into the nasal area, tending to be linear in distribution; may also affect trunk and limbs.

OCCASIONAL ABNORMALITIES

Skeletal. Cranial asymmetry or hemimacrocephaly; premature closure of sphenoid frontal sutures, sphenoid bone malformation, and abnormalities of sella turcica; scoliosis, kyphosis, abnormalities of ulna, head of radius, humerus, and fibula; polydactyly, syndactyly; vitamin D–resistant rickets.

Eyes. Esotropia, lipodermoid of conjunctiva, cloudy cornea, colobomata of eyelid, coloboma of iris and choroid, atrophy of optic nerve, subretinal neovascularization, microphthalmia.

Central Nervous System. Micro- and/or macrocephaly, cerebral and cerebellar hypoplasia, arachnoid cysts, hydrocephalus, hemiparesis, cranial nerve palsy, cortical blindness, hypertonia, cerebral vascular changes, intracerebral calcifications, cerebral neoplasia/hamartoma.

Other. Short palpebral fissures, pigmented nevi; spotty alopecia; coarctation of aorta, patent ductus arteriosus, hypoplastic left heart, ventricular septal defect; cardiac arrhythmias; hypoplasia of aortic branches, renal or pulmonary artery; cleft palate; hypoplastic teeth; renal hamartomata, nephroblastoma, double urinary collecting system, horseshoe kidneys; rhabdomyosarcoma; enlarged clitoris; undescended testes, cystic biliary adenoma of liver; dental anomalies; hemihypertrophy.

NATURAL HISTORY

The nevus sebaceous is usually present at birth as a slightly yellow to orange to tan waxy-appearing lesion containing deficiencies or papillomatous excesses of epidermal elements, especially sebaceous glands and immature hair follicles. Pubertal expansion of the lesion commonly involves rapid growth with hormonally driven development of sebaceous glands and maturation of apocrine glands. The lesions tend to become verrucous and unsightly. Tumors can occur in infancy but are more frequent in adult life. Although the risk was initially reported to be 15% to 20%, recent studies suggest 2% to 3% risk for tumor and less than 1% risk for malignancies. Trichoblastomas and other benign tumors may account for 90% of the associated tumors. In rare cases, basal cell carcinomas (the most common malignant lesion), sebaceous carcinomas, squamous cell carcinomas, and keratoacanthomas occur. Early surgical removal should be considered. In the cases with associated CNS features, the onset of seizures has been from 2 months to 2 years, and they are difficult to control. The intellectual disability has been moderate to severe, although an occasional patient may have normal intelligence. The vitamin D–resistant rickets that sometimes occurs is a variant of tumor-induced osteomalacia. The associated ricketic lesions, muscle weakness, and bone pain, as well as the biochemical abnormalities, reverse following surgical removal of the skin lesions.

ETIOLOGY

The *linear sebaceous nevus* sequence and isolated *epidermal nevi* are caused by somatic activating mutations in HRAS or KRAS. A very specific HRAS mutation, c.37G>C (p.Gly13Arg), has been detected in the majority of cases. A mutation in the adjacent paralogous residue of KRAS (p.Gly12Asp or p.Gly12Val) accounts for some cases. The HRAS c.37G>C mutation causes constitutive activation of the MAPK and PI3K-Akt signaling pathways. Other mutations in these genes are rarely identified.

COMMENT

Two unique conditions have recently been described in a few patients with *nevus sebaceous*: 1) *aplasia cutis congenita* and *nevus sebaceous* and 2) SCALP (nevus sebaceus, CNS malformation, aplasia cutis congenita, limbal dermoid, pigmented nevus) syndrome. Although the co-occurrence of two purportedly disparate skin lesions gave rise in the literature to the twin spot hypothesis implicating two homozygous recessive mutations as causal, the recent finding of heterozygous HRAS and KRAS mutations in *phacomatosis pigmentokeratotica* (another such disorder) has disproved this theory.

References

Mehregan AH, Pinkus H: Life history of organoid nevi: Special reference to nevus sebaceus of Jadassohn, *Arch Dermatol* 91:574, 1965.

Marden PM, Venters HD: A new neurocutaneous syndrome, *Am J Dis Child* 112:79, 1966.

Lansky LL, et al: Linear sebaceous nevus syndrome, *Am J Dis Child* 123:587, 1972.

Carey DE, et al: Hypophosphatemic rickets/osteomalacia in linear sebaceous nevus syndrome: A variant of tumor-induced osteomalacia, *J Pediatr* 109:994, 1986.

Lam J, et al: SCALP syndrome: sebaceous nevus syndrome, CNS malformations, aplasia cutis congenita, limbal dermoid, and pigmented nevus (giant congenital melanocytic nevus) with neurocutaneous melanosis: A distinct syndromic entity, *J Am Acad Dermatol* 58: 884, 2008.

Moody MN, et al: Nevus sebaceous revisited, *Pediatr Dermatol* 29:15, 2012.

Groesser L, et al: Postzygotic HRAS and KRAS mutations cause nevus sebaceous and Schimmelpenning syndrome, *Nat Genet* 44:783, 2012.

Groesser L, et al: Phacomatosis pigmentokeratotica is caused by a postzygotic HRAS mutation in a multipotent progenitor cell, *J Invest Derm* doi:10.1038/jid.2013.24

Sun BK, et al: Mosaic activating RAS mutations in nevus sebaceus and nevus sebaceus syndrome, *J Invest Derm* 133:824, 2013.

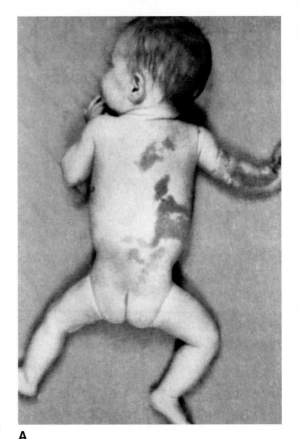

FIGURE 1.   Linear sebaceous nevus sequence. **A,** A
2-week-old infant with facial and extensive body
sebaceous nevi. Intractable seizures began at 5 months,
and the patient died at 9 months with pneumonia.
Necropsy revealed renal nodular nephronoblastomatosis.
(**A,** From Lansky LL et al: *Am J Dis Child* 123:587, 1972, with
permission.)

A

Continued

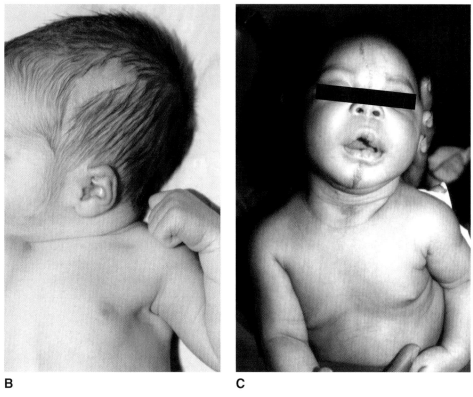

B   **C**

FIGURE 1, cont'd.   Note the orange to tan waxy-appearing lesion (**B**) and verrucous change that developed in older childhood (**C**).

Q

INCONTINENTIA PIGMENTI SYNDROME
(BLOCH-SULZBERGER SYNDROME)
Irregular Pigmented Skin Lesions with or without Dental Anomaly, Patchy Alopecia

Bardach originally described the condition in twin sisters in 1925, and soon thereafter Bloch set forth the term *incontinentia pigmenti* to depict the unusual skin lesions. The preponderance of cases occurs in females.

ABNORMALITIES

Performance. Seizures (20%), infantile encephalopathy, acute disseminated encephalomyelitis, and ischemic stroke. One third have significant intellectual disability.

Craniofacial. Approximately 30% have strabismus, often with refractive errors; abnormalities of the retinal vessels and underlying pigment cells in 40%, leading to retinal ischemia, new vessel proliferation, bleeding, and fibrosis; retinal detachment, uveitis, keratitis, cataract, microphthalmos, and optic atrophy occur infrequently; hypodontia (>50%), delayed eruption, or conical form.

Skin. Blisters, preceded by erythema, develop typically in a linear distribution along the limbs and around the trunk within the first 4 months (bullous stage); as the blisters begin to heal, hyperkeratotic lesions develop on the distal limbs and scalp and rarely on the trunk or face for several months (verrucous stage); hyperpigmentation, most apparent on the trunk distributed along lines of Blaschko, occur in streaks and whorls, usually developing after the blisters have disappeared (hyperpigmentation stage); pale, hairless patches or streaks most evident on the lower legs develop usually at the time the hyperpigmentation disappears (atretic stage).

Hair and Nails. Atrophic patchy alopecia, especially on the posterior scalp at the vertex; lusterless, wiry, coarse hair as well as thin, sparse hair in early childhood; mild ridging or pitting to severe nail dystrophy.

Skeletal. Approximately 20% have hemivertebrae, kyphoscoliosis, extra rib, syndactyly, hemiatrophy, or short arms and legs.

OCCASIONAL ABNORMALITIES

High arched palate, cleft of the lip and palate (1.5%), breast hypoplasia, supernumerary nipple, nipple hypoplasia, dacryostenosis, eczema, short stature, hydrocephalus, subungual keratotic tumors.

NATURAL HISTORY

Bullous skin lesions are generally present in early infancy and tend to progress from inflammatory or vesicular to pigmented and may fade in childhood. General eosinophilia is often present in infancy and the vesicles contain eosinophils. Verrucous lichenoid lesions develop during infancy in approximately one third of cases, especially over the dorsum of the hands and feet. During the period when the blisters are present, the lesions should be kept dry and protected from trauma. The development of the irregular marble cake–like pigmentation may or may not coincide with the sites of bullous or verrucous lesions. The pigmented areas gradually fade in the second to third decades, and the adult may show only slightly atrophic depigmented "achromic stains," especially over the lower legs. Because the retinal vascular changes sometimes progress during the neonatal period, monthly ophthalmologic evaluations are recommended during the first 2 to 3 months of life. In approximately 10% of cases, this process progresses to severe scarring with significant visual loss. The greatest risk for retinal detachment is in infancy and childhood; it almost never occurs after age 6 years. Approximately one half of the patients show other features, the most serious being the CNS abnormalities. Seizures in the neonatal period are reported in 20%, seem to correlate with the degree of cerebrovascular damage, and thus represent an ominous sign relative to future neurologic development. In their absence, prognosis, in most cases, is good. No patients have developed new neurologic symptoms during adolescence or at adult age.

ETIOLOGY

This disorder has an X-linked dominant inheritance pattern with male lethality in the vast majority of cases. *IKBKG*, previously the nuclear factor-kappa B (NF-κB) essential modulator (*NEMO*) gene located at Xq28, is the only gene known to be associated with incontinentia pigmenti (IP). A deletion that removes exons 4 through 10 of *IKBKG* mediated through recombination of direct tandem repeats is present in about 80% of affected individuals. The product of this gene protects against apoptosis. In females with IP, the functionally aberrant cell clone is eliminated by apoptosis, resulting in eradication of defective cells and healing of skin lesions soon after birth as well as detectable skewing of X-inactivation that occurs in 98% of females with IP. Cases of males with IP have been reported.

Survival in a male is mediated through one of three mechanisms: a less deleterious mutation, mainly in exon 10; a 47XXY karyotype; or somatic mosaicism. A female with IP may have inherited the *IKBKG* mutation from her mother or have a de novo mutation (65%). In familial cases, parents may either be clinically affected or unaffected but have germline mosaicism. Molecular testing of the mother is warranted because of the widely variable expressivity of the phenotype in adult women. Affected women have a 50% chance of transmitting the mutant *IKBKG* allele at conception; however, male conceptuses with a loss-of-function mutation of *IKBKG* do not survive.

COMMENT

Three other conditions are caused by mutations in *IKBKG*: X-linked hypohidrotic ectodermal dysplasia and immunodeficiency (HED-ID), HED-ID with osteopetrosis and lymphedema, and X-linked atypical mycobacteriosis, all affecting males exclusively, caused by missense mutations that result in impaired but not absent signaling.

References

Bardach M: Systematisierte Naevusbildungen bei einem eineiigen Zwillingspaar: Ein Beitrag zur Naevusätiologie, *Z Kinderheilkd* 39:542, 1925.

Bloch B: Eigentümliche bisher nicht beschriebene Pigmentaffektion (Incontinentia pigmenti), *Schweiz Med Wochenschr* 56:404, 1926.

International IP Consortium: Genomic rearrangement in NEMO impairs NF-kB activation and is a cause of incontinentia pigmenti, *Nature* 405:466, 2000.

Aradhya S, et al: A recurrent deletion in the ubiquitously expressed NEMO (IKK-gamma) gene accounts for the vast majority of incontinentia pigmenti mutations, *Hum Mol Genet* 10:2171, 2001.

Fusco F, et al: Clinical diagnosis of incontinentia pigmenti in a cohort of male patients, *J Am Acad Dermatol* 56:264, 2007.

Fusco F, et al: Microdeletion/duplication at the Xq28 IP locus causes a de novo IKBKG/NEMO/IKKgamma exon4-10 deletion in families with incontinentia pigmenti, *Hum Mutat* 30:1284, 2009.

Meuwissen ME, Mancini GM: Neurological findings in incontinentia pigmenti: A review, *Eur J Med Genet* 55:323, 2012.

Q

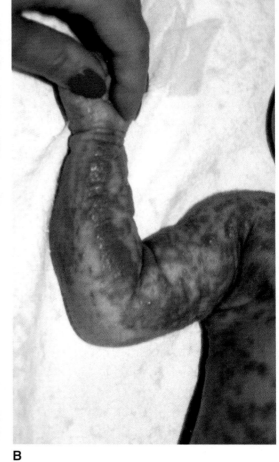

A

B

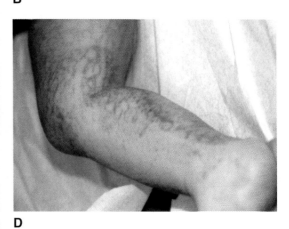

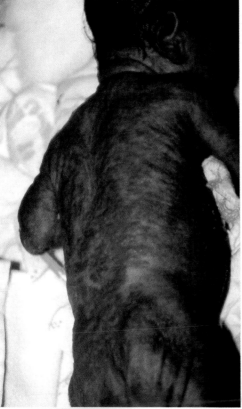

C

D

FIGURE 1.   Incontinentia pigmenti syndrome.
A–D, Progression of lesions from erythema to blisters to hyperkeratosis to hyperpigmentation over the first year of life.

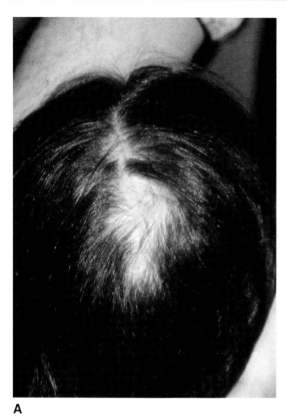

A

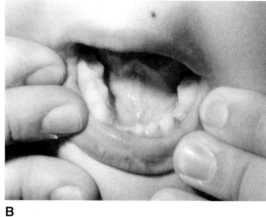

B

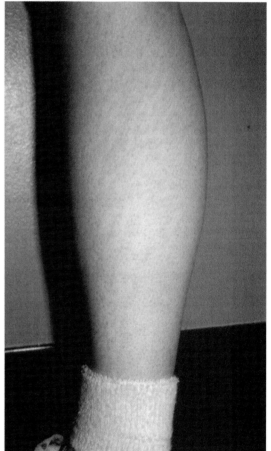

C

FIGURE 2.   A, Atrophic patchy alopecia. **B,** Lack of alveolar ridge indicating anodontia. **C,** Pale hairless streaks on lower leg.

Q

HYPOMELANOSIS OF ITO (INCONTINENTIA PIGMENTOSA ACHROMIANS)

Initially described by Ito in 1952, numerous affected individuals subsequently have been reported. The characteristic skin lesions involve streaked, whorled, or mottled areas of hypopigmentation on limbs or trunk, usually evident in infancy. It is now clear that hypomelanosis of Ito is not a specific disorder but rather an etiologically heterogeneous physical finding that is frequently indicative of chromosomal or genetic mosaicism, also named pigmentary mosaicism of the Ito type. Approximately 70% of reported cases have associated anomalies. With the exception of intellectual disability, seizures, and cerebral atrophy, all other associated abnormalities have occurred in a small number of patients.

ABNORMALITIES

Performance. Variable intellectual disability in 30% to 50%; autistic behavior; seizures, including generalized tonic-clonic seizures, partial seizures, myoclonic seizures, and infantile spasms.

Craniofacial. Macrocephaly; coarse facies; hypertelorism; epicanthal folds; thick lips; cleft lip/palate; malformed auricles; iridial heterochromia; coloboma of iris; abnormal retinal pigmentation (most often hypopigmented); strabismus; nystagmus; myopia; dacryostenosis; corneal asymmetry; pannus; cataract and pinpoint pupils; microphthalmia; small optic nerve; optic atrophy.

Other. Central precocious puberty; café au lait spots; cutis marmorata; angiomatous nevi; nevus of Ota; mongolian blue spots; abnormal sweating; ichthyosis; morphea; hypertrichosis; diffuse alopecia; variations in hair color and texture; ridging, dystrophy, or occasional absence of nails; dysplasia of teeth, abnormal number and shape, enamel defects, irregularly spaced teeth; clinodactyly, syndactyly, ectrodactyly, polydactyly, triphalangeal thumb, genu valga; asymmetry of length or size of limbs and body parts, joint contractures, particularly talipes; kyphoscoliosis/lordosis, pectus excavatum, and carinatum; short stature.

NATURAL HISTORY

The skin lesions, which are best appreciated by a Wood's lamp examination, do not go through a prodrome phase as in incontinentia pigmenti. The skin lesions are often not detected in the newborn period but become apparent within the first months of life (80%). In some cases, they may remain unrecognized until some other symptoms appear or until the child is first exposed to the sun. Seizures commonly appear early within the first years of life. Autistic behavior, severe intellectual disability, and drug-resistant epilepsy may occur. There are a limited number of reported cases of hypomelanosis of Ito associated with tumors.

ETIOLOGY

Hypomelanosis of Ito is etiologically heterogeneous. Karyotyping of characteristic skin findings to rule out chromosomal mosaicism when developmental delay or structural anomalies are also present is indicated. Although only a small number of cases of smaller chromosomal rearrangements detected by chromosomal arrays have been reported in association with hypomelanosis of Ito, it is likely that new cases will be identified. Recurrence risk is low, except in those chromosomally abnormal individuals in whom a balanced parental translocation is present. A single-gene basis for hypomelanosis of Ito probably does not exist.

References

Ito M: Studies on melanin XI: Incontinentia pigmenti; achromians, *Tohoku J Exp Med* 55(Suppl):57, 1952.

Küster W, Künig A: Hypomelanosis of Ito: No entity, but a cutaneous sign of mosaicism, *Am J Med Genet* 85:346, 1999.

Taibjee SM, et al: Abnormal pigmentation in hypomelanosis of Ito and pigmentary mosaicism: The role of pigmentary genes, *Br J Dermatol* 151:269, 2004.

Assogba K, et al: Heterogeneous seizure manifestations in Hypomelanosis of Ito: Report of four new cases and review of the literature, *Neurol Sci* 31:9, 2010.

Park JM, et al: Sexual precocity in hypomelanosis of Ito: Mosaicism-associated case report and literature review, *Int J Dermatol* 50:168, 2011.

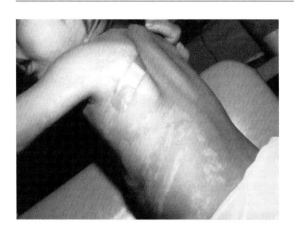

FIGURE 1. Hypomelanosis of Ito. A 14-month-old with developmental delay, hypotonia, and seizures. Note the irregular, streaky distribution of hypopigmentation.

Q

TUBEROUS SCLEROSIS SYNDROME
Hamartomatous Skin Nodules, Seizures, Phakomata, Bone Lesions

Von Recklinghausen is said to have described this disease, but Bourneville is usually given credit for its recognition in 1880. Hamartomatous lesions develop in many tissues, especially the skin and brain. Diagnostic criteria were set forth by the National Tuberous Sclerosis Association in 1992 and modified in 2004. Two major features or one major feature plus two minor features are diagnostic of tuberous sclerosis complex (TSC). The incidence of TSC has been estimated to be 1 in 5800 live births.

ABNORMALITIES

Performance. Seizures (80%), intellectual disability (50%), autism spectrum disorder (40%).

Craniofacial. Major ocular feature: multiple retinal nodular hamartomas, most often bilateral; minor ocular feature: retinal achromic patches; minor feature: multiple randomly distributed pits in dental enamel, most evident by close inspection of labial premolar surfaces; gingival fibroma.

Skin. Major features: facial angiofibromas (varying in color from flesh to pink to yellow to brown in the nasolabial fold, cheeks, and elsewhere), nontraumatic ungual or periungual fibromas, shagreen patch (connective tissue nevus with a goose flesh–like appearance), hypomelanotic macules (three or more may be "thumb-print" macules, "lance-ovate" macules [one end rounded, the other with a sharp tip] or ash leaf macule); minor feature: confetti macules (tiny 1- to 3-mm macules). Some type of hypomelanotic macules can be found in virtually all patients. The other skin lesions occur in approximately half.

Imaging. Major CNS features: subependymal nodules, cortical tubers (both in more than 70% of cases), subependymal giant cell astrocytoma; minor feature: cerebral white matter radial migration lines; minor feature: bone cysts occurring mainly in phalanges (66%) with areas of periosteal thickening yielding radiologic evidence of "sclerosis."

Visceral. Major feature: multiple renal angiomyolipomas (greater than 50%), usually benign; minor feature: renal epithelial cysts, including tubular enlargement and cyst formation with hyperplasia of tubular cells; major feature: single or multiple cardiac rhabdomyomas; arrhythmias; major feature: pulmonary lymphangiomyomatosis (40% of women of childbearing age).

Other minor features. Hamartomatous rectal polyps, nonrenal hamartoma (liver and pancreas and other).

OCCASIONAL ABNORMALITIES
Other hamartomas, lipomas, angiomas, nevi, angiomas of heart, hepatic angiomyolipomas, hypothyroidism; thyroid adenomas; sexual precocity; lymphedema; hypertension; neuroendocrine tumors, including pituitary adenomas, parathyroid adenomas and hyperplasia, and pancreatic adenomas (insulinoma and islet cell neoplasm); oncocytoma (benign adenomatous hamartoma); malignant angiomyolipoma; renal cell carcinoma.

NATURAL HISTORY
Hamartomatous lesions usually become evident in early childhood and may increase at adolescence. Facial nodular lesions are present in 50% of children by 5 years, whereas white macules are present at birth or in early infancy in almost all patients, and are visualized easily with a Wood's lamp. Brain tumors develop in approximately 10% of patients. These giant cell astrocytomas may enlarge, causing pressure and obstruction and resulting in significant morbidity and mortality. However, malignant transformation of the periventricular nodules is rare. The seizures, which tend to develop in early childhood, may initially be myoclonic and later grand mal in type and are difficult to control. Electroencephalographic abnormality is found in 87% of patients and may be of the grossly disorganized hypsarrhythmic pattern. The seizures, the severity of intellectual disability, and autistic behavior seem to be related to the extent of hamartomatous change in the brain. Mental deterioration is unusual, except in relation to frequent seizures of status epilepticus. None of the skin lesions results in serious medical problems, but facial angiofibromas can be a cosmetic problem. Eye lesions are usually asymptomatic but retinal astrocytic hamartomas can cause retinal detachment and neovascular glaucoma. At least 80% of children will have some renal finding by age 10 years.

Renal angiomyolipomas can cause pain from hemorrhage into the tumor. Those larger than 3.5 to 4.0 cm should be considered for prophylactic renal arterial embolization or renal sparing surgery.

An unknown percentage of patients die before 20 years of age as the consequence of status epilepticus, general debility, pneumonia, or tumor. However, there is marked variability. Seizures and/or mental deficiency do not develop in all patients with skin lesions, and the above noted pattern of abnormality is biased toward the more severe cases.

It is not infrequent to diagnose an asymptomatic parent of a severely affected child. Females tend to have milder disease than males.

ETIOLOGY

This disorder has an autosomal dominant inheritance pattern. Approximately two thirds of cases represent fresh mutations. Mutations in *TSC1,* located at 9q34 and of *TSC2* located at 16p13, encoding proteins referred to as hamartin and tuberin, respectively, are responsible. Both are tumor suppressor genes. Molecular genetic testing of *TSC1* and *TSC2* will identify a mutation in approximately 85% of individuals. The frequency of somatic mosaicism for large deletions and duplications of *TSC1* and *TSC2* in patients with normal sequencing analysis may be as high as 5%. Thus, careful parental evaluation is strongly recommended before genetic counseling. *TSC1* mutations have milder disease manifested by fewer seizures and less severe intellectual disability and autism, fewer subependymal nodules and cortical tubers, less severe kidney involvement, no retinal hamartomas, and less severe facial angiofibromas. Individuals with large deletions of *TSC2,* which also include *PKD1,* are at risk of developing the complications of autosomal dominant polycystic kidney disease,

COMMENT

Cardiac rhabdomyomas are the most frequent early prenatal finding in 30% to 50% of fetuses with TSC. When rhabdomyomas are identified on fetal ultrasound examination, the risk of TSC is 50% to 80%, and much greater if the lesions are multiple. Third-trimester MRI of the brain may identify lesions consistent with TSC in up to 80% of cases.

References

Bourneville D: Scléreuse tubéreuse des circonvolutions cérébrales: Idiote et epilepsie hémiplégique, *Arch Neurol (Paris)* 1:81, 1880.

Roach ES, et al: Diagnostic criteria: Tuberous sclerosis complex. Report of the diagnostic criteria committee of the National Tuberous Sclerosis Association, *J Clin Neurol* 7:221, 1992.

Dabora SL, et al: Mutational analysis in a cohort of 224 tuberous sclerosis patients indicates increased severity of TSC2, compared to TSC1 disease, in multiple organs, *Am J Hum Genet* 68:64, 2001.

Roach ES, Sparagana SP: Diagnosis of tuberous sclerosis complex, *J Child Neurol* 19:643, 2004.

Au KS, et al: Genotype/phenotype correlation in 325 individuals referred for a diagnosis of tuberous sclerosis complex in the United States, *Genet Med* 9:88, 2007.

Kozlowski P, et al: Identification of 54 large deletions/duplications in *TSC1* and *TSC2* using MLPA, and genotype-phenotype correlations, *Hum Genet* 121:389, 2007.

Saada J, et al: Prenatal diagnosis of cardiac rhabdomyomas: Incidence of associated cerebral lesions of tuberous sclerosis complex, *Ultrasound Obstet Gynecol* 34: 155, 2009.

Numis AL, et al: Identification of risk factors for autism spectrum disorders in tuberous sclerosis complex, *Neurology* 76:981, 2011.

Q

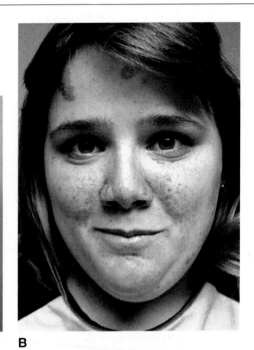

A

B

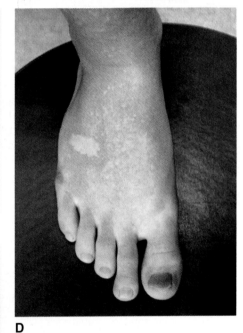

C

D

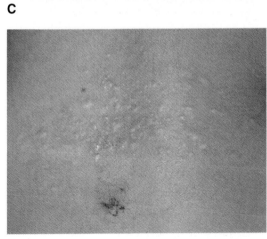

E

FIGURE 1. Tuberous sclerosis syndrome. **A** and **B,** Two teenagers with fibrous-angiomatous lesions in the nasolabial folds and cheeks. **C** and **D,** White macules over the tibia and foot. **E,** Shagreen patches over the lower back. (**C** and **E,** Courtesy of Dr. John Kanegaye, Rady Children's Hospital, San Diego.)

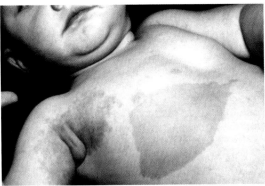

A

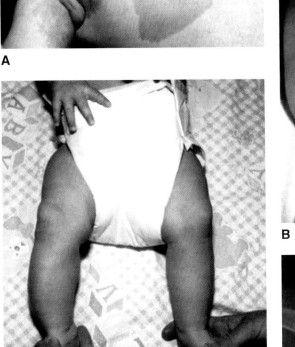

C

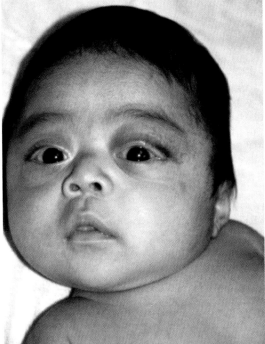

B

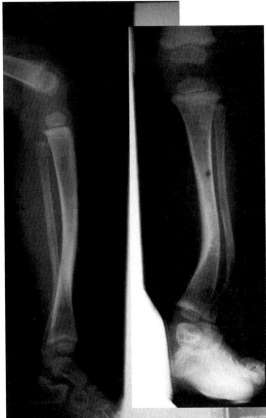

Q

D

FIGURE 2.   **A** and **B,** Plexiform neurofibromas on the upper trunk and orbit. **C** and **D,** Pseudoarthrosis of distal tibia.

MCCUNE-ALBRIGHT SYNDROME
Polyostotic Fibrous Dysplasia, Irregular Skin Pigmentation, Sexual Precocity

McCune and Albright and colleagues described this condition in 1936 and 1937, respectively. The relative frequency of diagnosis in females versus males is 3 to 2. Monostotic (MFD) or polyostotic fibrous dysplasia (PFD) can occur without other manifestations. Fibrous dysplasia of the bone and either "café au lait" macules or a hyperfunctioning endocrinopathy is enough to establish a diagnosis.

ABNORMALITIES

Skeletal. Multiple areas of fibrous dysplasia, usually unilateral, most commonly in long bones and pelvis; may also include cranium, facial bones (causing macrocephaly and facial asymmetry), ribs, and occasionally the spine; may result in deformity, pain, fractures, scoliosis.

Imaging. Expansile lesions with endosteal scalloping and thinning of the cortex; intramedullary "ground glass" appearance; involved metaphyses and diaphyses with sparing of the epiphyses; increased thickness of bone; "shepherd's crook" deformity of proximal femur.

Skin. Irregular brown pigmentation, referred to as café au lait spots with "coast of Maine" borders, most commonly over sacrum, buttocks, nape of the neck, and upper spine; unilateral in approximately 50% of patients; the pattern of the pigmentary changes often follows the Blaschko lines.

Endocrine. Precocious puberty, hyperthyroidism, hyperparathyroidism, pituitary adenomas secreting growth hormone (GH), acromegaly, Cushing syndrome, hyperprolactinemia; concentrations of tropic hormones are initially normal or reduced. Renal phosphate wasting with or without rickets/osteomalacia in 50% of patients.

OCCASIONAL ABNORMALITIES

Gastrointestinal reflux or polyps, pancreatitis, sudden death, tachycardia, high-output heart failure, aortic root dilatation, platelet dysfunction, chondroblastosarcoma, clear cell carcinoma of the thyroid, breast cancer, learning and speech disorders, global developmental delay, tall stature, acromegalic features.

NATURAL HISTORY

The pigmentation is usually evident in infancy. The bone dysplasia may progress during childhood, resulting in pain, deformity, and/or fracture most commonly in the upper femur. Craniofacial lesions develop before 5 years of age and may lead to cranial nerve compression with serious consequences such as blindness or deafness. Any bone can be involved, but the skull base and the proximal femur are most commonly involved. Bisphosphonates reduce bone pain but have no effect on the natural history of the disease. Malignant transformation into chondroblastic sarcoma occurs in less than 2%. There may be a greater tendency for malignant transformation in patients with GH excess. The sexual precocity in the female is often unusual in character, with menstruation before development of breasts, often with no pubic hair. In boys, bilateral or unilateral testicular enlargement (Leydig cell hyperplasia) with penile enlargement, and secondary sexual characteristics develop. The accelerated maturation coincident with sexual precocity may result in early attainment of full stature, so that adult height can be relatively short. GH and prolactin excess are common. GH excess can aggravate craniofacial bone disease. Cushing syndrome, if present, develops before age 1. Thyrotoxicosis occurs frequently, and postoperative thyroid storm has occurred on rare occasions. Thyroid cancer and testicular cancer are rare. Renal phosphate wasting, as part of a proximal tubulopathy, is common and is likely due to elaboration of the phosphaturic factor, fibroblast growth factor-23 (FGF23), by affected tissue.

ETIOLOGY

A somatic activating mutation of the gene (GNAS1) encoding the alpha-subunit of the G protein is responsible for this disorder. G proteins are involved in signal transduction pathways that affect the production of cyclic adenosine monophosphate (cAMP). All published cases of McCune-Albright syndrome have the same activating mutation in GNAS1 at the R201 position. Mutations at position Q227 and V224 have been identified in isolated fibrous dysplasia. No vertical transmission has occurred. All patients are somatic mosaics. An overactive cAMP pathway stimulates the growth and function of the gonads, adrenal cortex, specific pituitary-cell populations, osteoblasts, and melanocytes. This explains the observation that the endocrinologic abnormalities in McCune-Albright syndrome are the result of autonomous hyperfunction of the endocrine glands rather than being centrally mediated, although puberty may become central secondarily. The variable clinical expression is determined by the relative number of mutant cells as well as by the tissues and areas of the body involved.

COMMENT

Loss-of-function mutations in this same gene lead to Albright hereditary osteodystrophy, a distinct entity encompassing pseudohypoparathyroidism, learning disabilities, growth deficiency, and dysmorphic features.

References

McCune DJ: Osteitis fibrosa cystica, *Am J Dis Child* 52:745, 1936.

Albright F, et al: Syndrome characterized by osteitis fibrosa disseminata, area of pigmentation and endocrine dysfunction, with precocious puberty in females: Report of five cases, *N Engl J Med* 216:727, 1937.

Weinstein LS, et al: Activating mutations of the stimulatory G protein in the McCune-Albright syndrome, *N Engl J Med* 325:1688, 1991.

Schwindinger WF, et al: Identification of a mutation in the gene encoding the a subunit of the stimulatory G protein of adenyl cyclase in McCune-Albright syndrome, *Proc Natl Acad Sci U S A* 89:5152, 1992.

Collins MT: Spectrum and natural history of fibrous dysplasia of bone, *J Bone Miner Res* 21(Suppl 2):P99, 2006.

Hart ES, et al: Onset, progression, and plateau of skeletal lesions in fibrous dysplasia and the relationship to functional outcome, *J Bone Miner Res* 22:1468, 2007.

Collins MT, et al: McCune-Albright syndrome and the extraskeletal manifestations of fibrous dysplasia, *Orphanet J Rare Dis* 7(Suppl 1):S4, 2012.

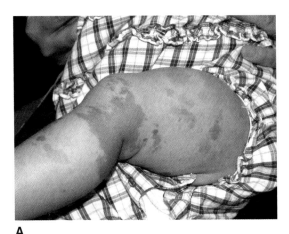

A

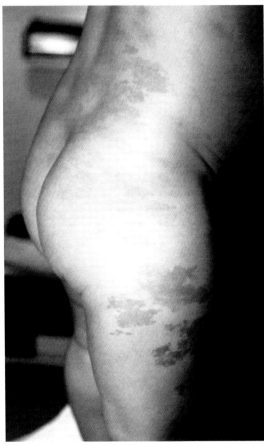

B

FIGURE 1.   McCune-Albright syndrome. **A** and **B,** Irregular café au lait pigmentation over lower back and leg. (**A,** Courtesy of Dr. Lynne M. Bird, Rady Children's Hospital, San Diego.)

Q

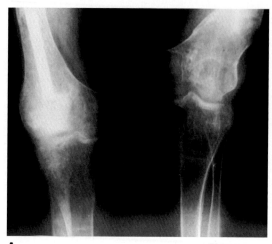

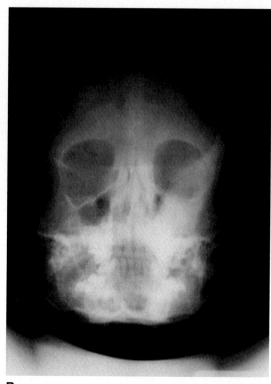

A

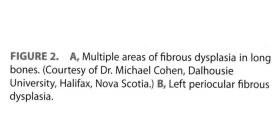

FIGURE 2.   A, Multiple areas of fibrous dysplasia in long bones. (Courtesy of Dr. Michael Cohen, Dalhousie University, Halifax, Nova Scotia.) **B,** Left periocular fibrous dysplasia.

B

Continued

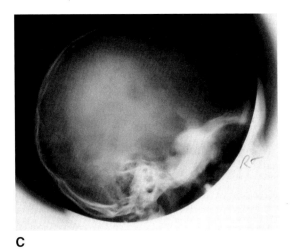

C

FIGURE 2, cont'd.   C, Dense thick bone at base of skull.

Q

KLIPPEL-TRENAUNAY SYNDROME
Asymmetric Limb Hypertrophy, Vascular Malformation, Varicosities

This entity was originally reported by Klippel and Trenaunay in 1900. It has been confused with Park-Weber syndrome, in which significant arteriovenous fistulas are a feature.

ABNORMALITIES

Skeletal. Congenital or early childhood hypertrophy of usually one, but occasionally more than one, limb; the lower limb is involved in 95% of cases, the upper limb in 5%, and both are involved in 15%.

Skin. Slow-flow vascular malformations of the capillary, venous, and lymphatic types occurring in any area, but more commonly on the legs, buttocks, abdomen, and lower trunk; unilateral distribution predominates, but bilateral involvement is not uncommon; varicosities of unusual distribution, particularly the lateral venous anomaly, which begins as a plexus of veins on the dorsum and lateral side of the foot and extends superiorly for various distances.

OCCASIONAL ABNORMALITIES

Craniofacial. Asymmetric facial hypertrophy; microcephaly; macrocephaly caused by a large brain; intracranial calcifications; eye abnormalities such as glaucoma, cataracts, heterochromia, and a Marcus Gunn pupil.

Skeletal. Macrodactyly, disproportionate growth of the digits whether large or small; syndactyly; polydactyly; oligodactyly; congenital hip dislocation, atrophy.

Skin. Hyperpigmented nevi and streaks, neonatal and childhood ulcers and vesicles, cutis marmorata, telangiectasia.

Viscera. Visceromegaly; capillary malformation of the intestinal tract, urinary system, mesentery, and pleura; aberrant major blood vessel; lymphectasia; insignificant arteriovenous fistula.

Imaging. Hemimegalencephaly, hydrocephalus, choroid plexus abnormalities, atrophy, calcifications, leptomeningeal enhancement, cortical dysplasia.

Other. Seizures, enlargement of the genitalia, intravascular clotting problems, lipodystrophy, absence of inferior vena cava, hematochezia, hematuria, esophageal variceal bleeding, hemorrhage, infarction, venous malformation, arteriovenous malformations, cavernoma, aneurysm.

NATURAL HISTORY

The usual patient with this syndrome does relatively well without any treatment or with elastic compression only. There may be disproportionate growth, which requires epiphyseal fusion or removal of the appropriate phalanx. Joint discomfort is not uncommon, and arthritic-type problems may develop. Leg swelling can be bothersome, and ulcers and other chronic skin difficulties may occur. Clinically significant arteriovenous shunting never occurs. Surgical intervention is almost never needed. However, in the rare situation in which the extremity reaches gigantic proportions or secondary clotting difficulties occur, amputation is necessary. Vascular malformations of the viscera, brain, eyes, urinary and gastrointestinal tracts, and other areas should always be looked for in this extremely variable disorder. Magnetic resonance imaging is the best noninvasive imaging technique to evaluate patients with vascular malformations.

ETIOLOGY

The cause of this disorder is unknown; it has a sporadic occurrence, although some reports mention several families with autosomal dominant transmission.

COMMENT

Mutations in the *RASA1* gene, encoding for a Ras GTPase, have been shown to be associated with the autosomal dominant co-occurrence of capillary malformation and arteriovenous malformations (CM/AVM syndrome), At least one of the patients had a phenotype consistent with the Klippel-Trenaunay syndrome. In addition, a chromosomal translocation apparently involving the *RASA1* locus was previously reported in a patient with Klippel-Trenaunay syndrome.

References

Klippel M, Trenaunay P: Du naevus variqueux osteohypertrophique, *Arch Gen Med* 185:641, 1900.

Gloviczki P, et al: Klippel-Trenaunay syndrome: The risks and benefits of vascular interventions, *Surgery* 110:469, 1991.

Whelan AJ, et al: Klippel-Trenaunay-Weber syndrome associated with a 5:11 balanced translocation, *Am J Med Genet* 59:492, 1995.

Cohen MM: Some neoplasms and some hamartomatous syndromes: Genetic considerations, *Int J Oral Maxillofac Surg* 27:363, 1998.

Cohen MM: Klippel-Trenaunay syndrome, *Am J Med Genet* 93:171, 2000.

Capraro PA, et al: Klippel-Trenaunay syndrome, *Plast Reconst Surg* 109:2052, 2002.

Hershkovitz D, et al: A novel mutation in *RASA1* causes capillary malformation and limb enlargement, *Arch Dermatol Res* 300:385, 2008.

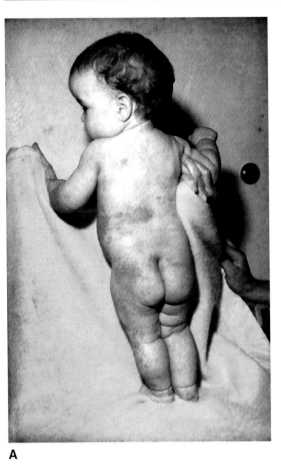

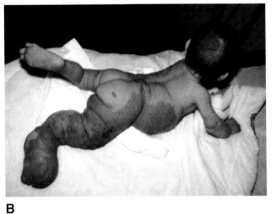

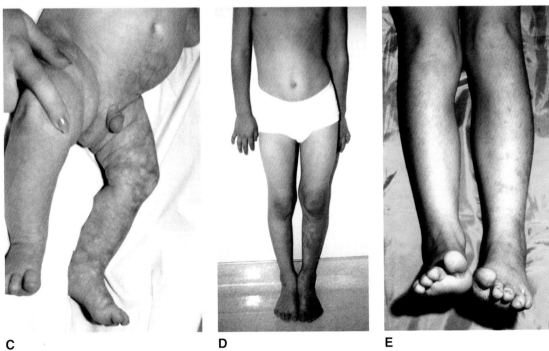

FIGURE 1.   Klippel-Trenaunay. **A,** Mentally normal girl with macrocephaly and hemangiomata in left trunk and lower limb. **B,** Child with severe involvement of right leg and trunk. (**B,** From Bird LM, et al: *Pediatrics* 97:739, 1996. Reproduced with permission from *Pediatrics*, vol. 97, pp. 739–741, copyright © 1996 by the AAP.) **C,** Less severely affected newborn boy. **D** and **E,** A 14-year-old child showing asymmetric hypertrophy of legs with abnormal vasculature.

Q

MACROCEPHALY-CAPILLARY MALFORMATION SYNDROME
(MACROCEPHALY-CUTIS MARMORATA TELANGIECTASIA CONGENITA, MEGALENCEPHALY POLYMICROGYRIA-POLYDACTYLY HYDROCEPHALUS [MPPH] SYNDROME)

This disorder was first recognized as a distinct syndrome in two independent publications in 1997 (Clayton-Smith et al and Moore et al). In retrospect, cases of this distinct disorder had been included in several series describing findings associated with cutis marmorata telangiectasia congenita. The phenotype of MPPH was described in the neurology literature as a separate entity; however, the description of three cases with remarkable overlap (Gripp et al) suggested that the two conditions are likely the same disorder.

ABNORMALITIES

Growth. Prenatal onset overgrowth with slow subsequent linear growth. Progressive macrocephaly typically not secondary to hydrocephalus.

Performance. Hypotonia, intellectual disability (mild to severe) not associated with regression.

Craniofacial. Macrocephaly, frontal bossing, large fontanel, dolichocephaly, deep-set eyes, full cheeks, facial asymmetry.

Eye. Anisocoria, strabismus, optic atrophy, poor visual responsiveness.

Limbs. Joint laxity, asymmetry (mostly of the lower extremities), postaxial polydactyly, syndactyly.

Skin. Nevus flammeus of midface (nose and philtrum); cutis marmorata; dilated veins of head, neck, and trunk; cavernous hemangiomas; loose, velvety, stretchable skin; thick, doughy subcutaneous tissue.

Imaging. Ventriculomegaly, hemimegalencephaly, perisylvian and insular polymicrogyria, cortical dysplasia, progressive cerebellar tonsillar herniation associated with rapid brain growth in infancy, Chiari I malformation, cavum septum pellucidum or vergae, hydrocephalus, white matter irregularities (increased signal on T2-weighted images), dilated dural venous sinuses, prominent Virchow-Robin spaces, lumbar syrinx, advanced bone age.

OCCASIONAL ABNORMALITIES
Seizures, ischemic stroke, craniosynostosis, macrodactyly, nail hypoplasia, cardiac defect, arrhythmia, inguinal and umbilical hernia, leukemia, meningioma (two cases), Wilms tumor, retinoblastoma.

NATURAL HISTORY
Affected infants are typically large at birth. The progressive increase in head size in the absence of hydrocephalus is quite striking and continues even after associated hydrocephalus has been treated. Capillary malformations, typically present at birth, may fade with time and be unnoticed in the older child. Most patients have mild asymmetry. A few cases have presented prenatally with macrocephaly, ventriculomegaly, and brain migrational anomalies.

Although the vascular skin lesions were originally felt to represent cutis marmorata telangiectasia congenita (CMTC), the skin findings are not the serpiginous, depressed, and often ulcerating lesions of CMTC. The lesions in this condition are patchy, reticular stains, which often fade but never ulcerate and are best understood as capillary malformations.

ETIOLOGY
Unknown. All cases have been sporadic.

References

Clayton-Smith J, et al: Macrocephaly with cutis marmorata, hemangioma and syndactyly: A distinctive overgrowth syndrome, *Clin Dysmorphol* 6:291, 1997.

Moore CA, et al: Macrocephaly-cutis marmorata telangiectasia congenita: A distinctive disorder with developmental delay and connective tissue abnormalities, *Am J Med Genet* 70:67, 1997.

Lapunzina P, et al: Macrocephaly-cutis marmorata telangiectasia congenita: Report of six new patients and a review, *Am J Med Genet A* 130A:45, 2004.

Mirzaa GM, et al: Megalencephaly-capillary malformation (MCAP) and megalencephaly-polydactyly-polymicrogyria-hydrocephalus (MPPH) syndromes: two closely related disorders of brain overgrowth and abnormal brain and body morphogenesis, *Am J Med Genet A* 158A:269, 2012.

Conway RL, et al: Neuroimaging findings in macrocephaly-capillary malformation: A longitudinal study of 17 patients, *Am J Med Genet A* 143A:2981, 2007.

Toriello HV, Mulliken JB: Accurately renaming macrocephaly-cutis marmorata telangiectatica congenita (M-CMTC) as macrocephaly-capillary malformation (M-MC), *Am J Med Genet A* 143A:3009, 2007.

Gripp KW, et al: Significant overlap and possible identity of macrocephaly capillary malformation and megalencephaly polymicrogyria-polydactyly hydrocephalus syndromes, *Am J Med Genet A* 149A:868, 2009.

Q

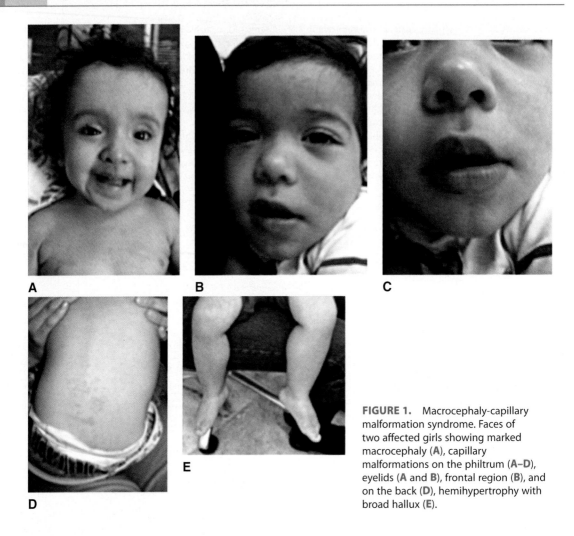

FIGURE 1. Macrocephaly-capillary malformation syndrome. Faces of two affected girls showing marked macrocephaly (**A**), capillary malformations on the philtrum (**A–D**), eyelids (**A** and **B**), frontal region (**B**), and on the back (**D**), hemihypertrophy with broad hallux (**E**).

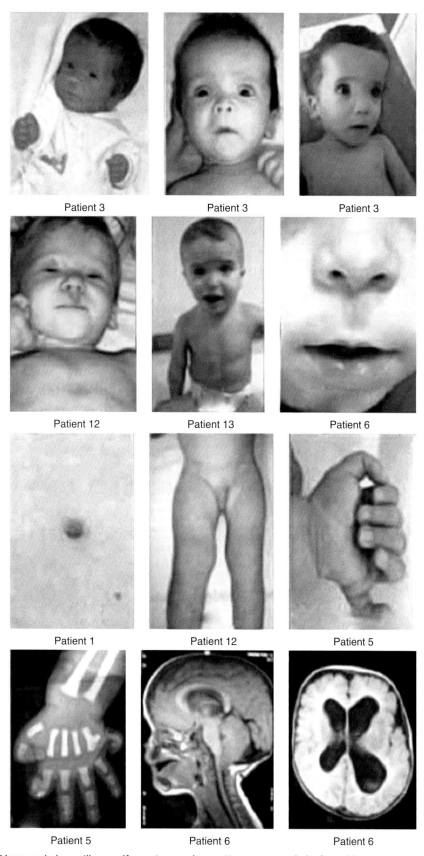

Patient 3   Patient 3   Patient 3

Patient 12   Patient 13   Patient 6

Patient 1   Patient 12   Patient 5

Patient 5   Patient 6   Patient 6

FIGURE 2. Macrocephaly-capillary malformation syndrome. Note macrocephaly; frontal bossing; overgrowth/asymmetry; capillary malformations on philtrum/upper lip, limbs, and trunk/abdominal area; polydactyly; tonsillar herniation; and hemimegalencephaly. (Reprinted from Martínez-Glez V et al: *Am J Med Genet A* 152A:3101, 2010.)

PROTEUS SYNDROME
Hemihypertrophy, Subcutaneous Tumors, Macrodactyly

Initially described in 1979 by Cohen and Hayden, this disorder was set forth as a clinical entity in 1983 by Wiedemann, who used the term *proteus* (after the Greek god Proteus, the polymorphous) to characterize the variable and changing phenotype of this condition. The consensus criteria developed by Biesecker and colleagues in 1999, including mosaic distribution of lesions, progressive course, and connective tissue nevi, have been proven to have strong diagnostic specificity. It has been suggested by Dr. Michael Cohen, Dalhousie University, Halifax, Nova Scotia, that John Merrick, the elephant man, most likely had Proteus syndrome.

ABNORMALITIES

Growth. Asymmetric and disproportionate overgrowth of body parts, normal somatic growth during adolescence and normal final height attainment, tissue overgrowth plateaus after adolescence, macrocephaly.

Skin and Subcutaneous Tissue. Generalized thickening; epidermal nevi of the flat nonorganoid type; lipomas; asymmetrical subcutaneous fat overgrowth, usually seen over the torso; regional absence of fat; vascular malformations of the venous, capillary, and lymphatic types with a predilection for the thorax and upper abdomen.

Skeletal. Hemihypertrophy, scoliosis; kyphosis; hip dislocation; angulation defects of knees; valgus deformities of halluces and feet; macrodactyly; clinodactyly, cerebriform connective tissue nevus involving the soles of the feet, palms, or another part of the body with deep grooves and gyration.

Visceral. Splenomegaly with or without cystic changes; nephromegaly; hydronephrosis; renal calculi and hemangiomas; gastromegaly; colonic polyps; pancreatic lipomatosis; uterine leiomyomatas; hypoplastic uterus, cervical uterine cysts; enlarged ovaries; hypertrophic cardiomyopathy and cardiac conduction defects; pulmonary emphysema, lung cysts and scarring; enlarged thymus.

Imaging. Hyperostosis of skull; abnormal vertebral bodies (asymmetric vertebral body overgrowth, posterior scalloping), segmentation defects, premature degenerative changes; coarse ribs and scapula; abnormal gray-white matter differentiation.

OCCASIONAL ABNORMALITIES

Cerebral arteriovenous malformations; CNS tumors; hydrocephalus; schizencephaly; spinal lipomatosis; perineural cysts; elongation of neck and trunk; craniosynostosis; broad, depressed nasal bridge; gyriform hyperplasia over side of nose or in other locations; ptosis; strabismus; epibulbar dermoid; enlarged eyes; microphthalmia; myopia; cataracts; nystagmus; submucous cleft palate; pectus excavatum; elbow ankylosis; intellectual disability; seizures; cyst-like alterations of lungs; muscle atrophy; abdominal and pelvic lipomatosis; café au lait spots; hyperostosis of external auditory canals, on alveolar ridges, and of nasal bridge; fibrocystic disease of breast; adenoma of parotid gland; ovarian cystadenoma; yolk sac tumor and other tumors of the testes; papillary adenoma of the epididymis; goiter; enlarged penis; macro-orchidism.

NATURAL HISTORY

Although infants are usually normal at birth, the characteristic features become obvious over the first year of life. Progressive postnatal overgrowth proceeds at a rapid, frequently alarming, rate. Growth of the hamartomas and the generalized hypertrophy usually cease after puberty. Moderate intellectual disability in 20% of cases. Morbidity is significant. Deep vein thrombosis leading to pulmonary embolism is the most common cause of death. Spinal stenosis and neurologic sequelae may develop as a result of vertebral anomalies or tumor infiltration. Cystic emphysematous pulmonary disease, CNS tumors, and abscesses are also associated with premature death. Affected individuals should be carefully monitored for the development of all types of neoplasms, because the full spectrum of this disorder is not known.

ETIOLOGY

All cases have been sporadic events in otherwise normal families. A specific somatic activating mutation (c.49G>A, p.Glu17Lys) in the oncogene *AKT1*, encoding an enzyme known to mediate cell proliferation and apoptosis, accounts for the majority of cases.

COMMENT

Germline mutations in *PTEN,* the gene responsible for Cowden and Bannayan-Riley-Ruvalcaba syndromes, also cause a Proteus-like syndrome with tumors and overgrowth developing as a result of a second mutation in affected tissues. Somatic *PTEN* mutations are found in SOLAMEN syndrome (segmental overgrowth, lipomatosis, arteriovenous malformation, and epidermal nevus). AKT1 is activated by loss-of-function mutations in *PTEN,* which explains the overlapping phenotypes. Patients with *PTEN* mutations need longitudinal follow-up for the development of *PTEN*-related malignancies.

References

Cohen MM, Hayden PW: A newly recognized hamartomatous syndrome, *Birth Defects* 15(5B):291, 1979.

Wiedemann HR, et al: The proteus syndrome: Partial gigantism of the hands and/or feet, nevi, hemihypertrophy, subcutaneous tumors, macrocephaly or other skull anomalies and possible accelerated growth and visceral affections, *Eur J Pediatr* 140:5, 1983.

Biesecker LG, et al: Proteus syndrome: Diagnostic criteria, differential diagnosis and patient evaluation, *Am J Med Genet* 84:389, 1999.

Caux F, et al: Segmental overgrowth, lipomatosis, arteriovenous malformation and epidermal nevus (SOLAMEN) syndrome is related to mosaic *PTEN* nullizygosity, *Eur J Hum Genet* 15:767, 2007.

Orloff MS, Eng C: Genetic and phenotypic heterogeneity in the *PTEN* hamartoma tumour syndrome, *Oncogene* 27:5387, 2008.

Lindhurst MJ, et al: A mosaic activating mutation in *AKT1* associated with the proteus syndrome, *N Engl J Med* 365:611, 2011.

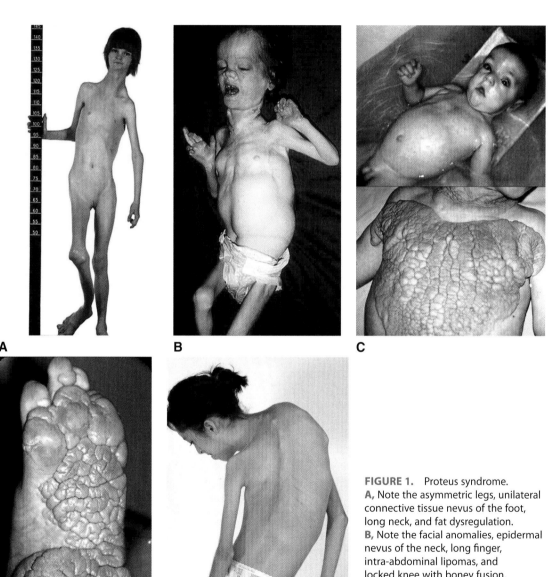

FIGURE 1.   Proteus syndrome. **A,** Note the asymmetric legs, unilateral connective tissue nevus of the foot, long neck, and fat dysregulation. **B,** Note the facial anomalies, epidermal nevus of the neck, long finger, intra-abdominal lipomas, and locked knee with boney fusion. **C,** Development and progression of connective tissue nevus in child with Proteus syndrome. **D,** Sole of foot of child with Proteus syndrome. **E,** Severe kyphoscoliosis developing over a 3-year period in a child with Proteus syndrome. (**A–E,** Courtesy of M. Michael Cohen Jr., Halifax, Nova Scotia.)

ENCEPHALOCRANIOCUTANEOUS LIPOMATOSIS
Unilateral Craniofacial Lipomas, Ipsilateral Cerebral Atrophy, Focal Areas of Alopecia

This disorder was initially described by Haberland and Perou in 1970. Subsequently, more than 54 cases have been reported, and Moog (2009) provides an excellent review.

ABNORMALITIES

Performance. Marked developmental delay, intellectual disability (30%), seizures (50%) can be refractory to treatment, spasticity.

Craniofacial. Hairless fatty tissue nevus of the scalp (nevus psiloliparus) with overlying alopecia, most commonly in the frontotemporal or zygomatic areas, usually unilateral; alopecia without fatty nevus; focal aplastic skin defects; asymmetry of the skull and face; small nodular skin tags on the eyelids or in the area between outer canthus and tragus, which histologically represent fibromas, lipomas, fibrolipomas, or choristomas; unilateral lipomatous involvement of the dermis of the skin covering the face on the same side as the brain defect; ipsilateral skin tags; hard pedunculated outgrowths attached to margin of upper lid made up of connective tissue; unilateral epibulbar or limbal choristoma (dermolipomas and lipodermoids); corneal and scleral abnormalities; ocular and palpebral colobomas; aniridia; microphthalmia; calcification of the eyeglobe; irregular disrupted eyebrows.

Imaging. Intracranial lipomas, most often in the cerebello-pontine angle; spinal lipomas that can extend over the entire spinal cord; arachnoid cysts; unilateral porencephalic cysts; cortical atrophy and calcification of the cerebral cortex overlying the cyst; ventricular dilatation; hemisphere atrophy; defective lamination of the cerebrum; micropolygyri; lipomas in the meninges covering the affected cerebral hemisphere; leptomeningeal angiomatosis.

OCCASIONAL ABNORMALITIES

Macrocephaly, subcutaneous lipomas outside the craniofacial areas, café au lait spots, hyperpigmentation following the lines of Blaschko, limb asymmetry, lipomas of the heart, jaw tumors (osteomas, odontogenic tumor, or ossifying fibromas), bone lytic lesions, coarctation of the aorta, hypospadias, hydronephrosis, pelvic kidney.

NATURAL HISTORY
Seizures can develop during childhood in about 50% of cases. Although motor delay is frequent, the degree of intellectual disability is variable and two thirds of the patients are intellectually normal. There is no correlation between intracranial or ocular findings and performance. Prognoses thus cannot be based on neuroimaging findings. Except for skeletal cysts and jaw tumors, the features of this condition are present at birth and are nonprogressive.

ETIOLOGY
Unknown. All affected patients have been sporadic. It is most likely that this disorder is the result of a somatic mutation that is lethal when occurring in the nonmosaic state.

COMMENT
Low-grade astroglioma in three pediatric patients and one case of papillary neuroglial tumor have been reported. Whether this condition predisposes to intracranial tumors needs to be confirmed.

References

Haberland C, Perou M: Encephalocranio-cutaneous lipomatosis, *Arch Neurol* 22:144, 1970.

Parazzini C, et al: Encephalocraniocutaneous lipomatosis: Complete neuroradiologic evaluation and follow-up of two cases, *Am J Neuroradiol* 20:173, 1999.

Hauber K, et al: Encephalocraniocutaneous lipomatosis: A case with unilateral odontomas and review of the literature, *Eur J Pediatr* 162:589, 2003.

Moog U: Encephalocraniocutaneous lipomatosis, *J Med Genet* 46:721, 2009.

Valera ET, et al: Are patients with encephalocraniocutaneous lipomatosis at increased risk of developing low-grade gliomas? *Childs Nerv Syst* 28:19, 2012.

Svoronos A, et al: Imaging findings in encephalocraniocutaneous lipomatosis, *Neurology* 77:694, 2011.

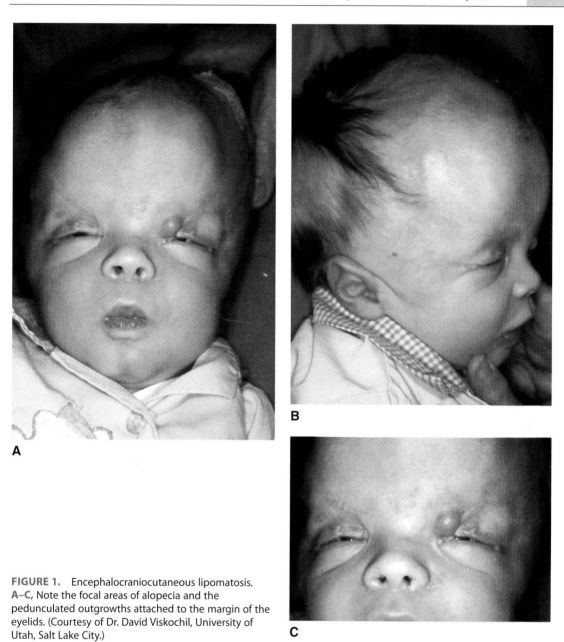

FIGURE 1. Encephalocraniocutaneous lipomatosis. **A–C,** Note the focal areas of alopecia and the pedunculated outgrowths attached to the margin of the eyelids. (Courtesy of Dr. David Viskochil, University of Utah, Salt Lake City.)

Q

MAFFUCCI SYNDROME
Enchondromatosis, Vascular Malformations

Enchondromas appear as radiolucent defects that originate in the metaphyses, grow slowly, and remain centered within the bone of origin. Multiple enchondromas are found in Ollier disease and in combination with vascular malformations in a condition reported first by Maffucci in 1881. More than 200 cases have been recorded subsequently. Onset is from the neonatal period to adolescence. After puberty, gradual ossification of the enchondromas occurs, resulting in solid deformed bones.

ABNORMALITIES

Skeletal. Variable early bowing of the long bones, with asymmetric retarded growth; enchondromas (40% unilateral), primarily in the hands, feet, and tubular long bones. Involvement of spine and skull is rare.

Vascular. Vascular malformations, most frequently located in the dermis and subcutaneous fat adjacent to the areas of enchondromatosis, but may occur anywhere; types of vascular malformations are capillary, venous, and especially phlebectasia, which often have a grape-like appearance; thrombosis of the dilated blood vessels with phlebolith formation occurs in 43% of cases.

OCCASIONAL ABNORMALITIES

Lymphangiectasis; lymphangiomas; vascular malformations of the mucous membranes and gastrointestinal tract; other tumors, both malignant and benign and of mesodermal and nonmesodermal origin (approximately 15%), including intracranial tumors, goiter, parathyroid adenoma, pituitary adenoma, hemangioepithelioma, adrenal tumor, ovarian tumor, chondrosarcoma, breast cancer, and astrocytoma.

NATURAL HISTORY

The patients usually appear normal at birth, but within the first 4 years, vascular malformations become obvious, 25% during the first year.

Subsequent formation of enchondromas is noted before adolescence. The disorder can be mild, but it is often severe enough to require multiple surgical procedures and occasionally amputation. Approximately 26% have fractures related to enchondromata. The risk of chondrosarcomatous change is approximately 15%. There is an increased incidence of CNS tumors.

ETIOLOGY

Three disorders—Ollier disease, Maffucci syndrome, and the rare metaphyseal chondromatosis with 2-hydroxyglutaric aciduria (MC-HGA)—have recently been connected to specific somatic mutations in the genes coding the cytoplasmic and mitochondrial isoforms of isocitrate dehydrogenase, *IDH1* (affecting arginine 132) and *IDH2* (affecting arginine 172). These mutations have been identified in primarily enchondromas and vascular affected areas, but also in blood and other tissues in a mosaic state. The phenotypic differences between these three conditions are determined by the proportion of cells carrying the mutations and by their tissue distribution. The precise mechanisms leading to enchondroma formation is not elucidated. Demonstration of organic aciduria is an important adjunct to diagnosis, but not a requisite.

References

Maffucci A: Di un caso di encondroma ed angioma multiplo: Contribuzione alla genesi embrionale dei tumor, *Movimento Med Chir* 3:399, 1881.

Kaplan RP, et al: Maffucci's syndrome: Two case reports with a literature review, *J Am Acad Dermatol* 29:894, 1994.

Amary MF, et al: Ollier disease and Maffucci syndrome are caused by somatic mosaic mutations of *IDH1* and *IDH2*, *Nat Genet* 43:1262, 2011.

Pansuriya TC, et al: Somatic mosaic *IDH1* and *IDH2* mutations are associated with enchondroma and spindle cell hemangioma in Ollier disease and Maffucci syndrome, *Nat Genet* 43:1256, 2011.

Superti-Furga A, et al: Enchondromatosis revisited: New classification with molecular basis, *Am J Med Genet Part C Semin Med Genet* 160C:154, 2012.

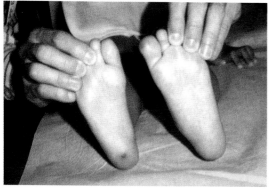

A

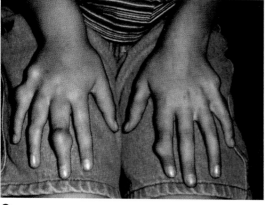

C

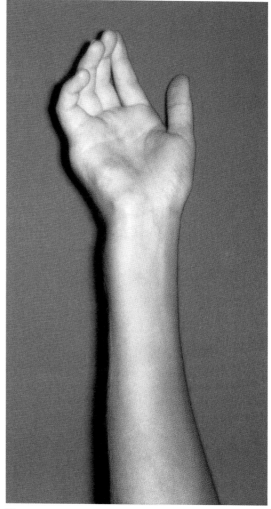

B

FIGURE 1. Maffucci syndrome. Note the vascular lesions on both feet (**A**), the evidence of enchondromas over the outer aspect of the hand (**B**), and the multiple enchondromas of the hands in a child who had multiple hemangiomata elsewhere (**C**).

Q

PEUTZ-JEGHERS SYNDROME
Mucocutaneous Pigmentation, Intestinal Polyposis

In 1896, Hutchinson described the pigmentary changes in an individual who later died of intussusception. Peutz clearly set forth the disease in 1921, and Jeghers and colleagues further established this disease entity in 1949. Many cases have been documented.

ABNORMALITIES

Skin. Vertical bands of epidermal pigment presenting as blue-gray or brownish spots on lips, buccal mucous membrane, perioral area, around the eyes, nostrils, and the perianal area, the digits and elsewhere.

Visceral. Hamartomatous polyps most frequently in small bowel (jejunum and duodenum more frequently than ileum), stomach and colon, and occasionally in nasopharynx, renal pelvis and urinary bladder, biliary tract, and bronchial mucosa; polyps are usually multiple; adenomatous and malignant changes in the polyps as well as in any area of gastrointestinal tract lined by columnar epithelium have been documented. The polyps have mucosa with interdigitating smooth muscle bundles in a characteristic branching tree appearance.

Other. Approximately 35% of patients have extraintestinal malignancies, including bronchogenic carcinoma; benign and malignant neoplasms of the thyroid, gallbladder, and biliary tract; breast cancer, usually ductal; pancreatic cancer; malignant tumors of the reproductive tract, including malignant adenoma of the cervix and ovarian and Fallopian mucinous tumors; unique ovarian sex cord tumors with annular tubules (small and benign) that cause heavy menstrual periods and lead to isosexual precocity; and testicular sex cord and Sertoli cell tumors, leading to sexual precocity and gynecomastia.

NATURAL HISTORY

The pigmentary spots, rarely present at birth, appear from infancy through early childhood and tend to fade in the adult. Seventy percent of patients have some gastrointestinal problem by age 20 years, most commonly colicky abdominal pain (60%), intestinal bleeding (25%), or both. Obstruction and intussusception are the most serious complications. Rectal prolapse can occur. Iron deficiency anemia may result from chronic blood loss, and protein-losing enteropathy has been reported. Natural history of complications from polyps in a family may be a predictor of severity for offspring. Routine endoscopy and polypectomy appear to reduce the frequency of emergency laparotomy for intussusception.

An intestinal or extraintestinal cancer develops in approximately 40% to 80% of affected patients. Almost one half of the patients with malignancy are younger than 30 years. The relative risk for cancer is highest for gastrointestinal cancer and breast cancer. Screening of affected patients as well as potentially affected family members should include colonoscopy, an upper gastrointestinal endoscopy plus small bowel examination, breast examination, mammography and pelvic ultrasonography in females older than 20, and careful examination of testicles in males. Clubbing of the fingers may occasionally occur in this disease.

ETIOLOGY

This disorder has an autosomal dominant inheritance pattern. Mutations in the serine/threonine kinase gene (*LKB1/STK11*) on chromosome 19p13.3, which functions as a tumor suppressor gene, are responsible. About 50% of cases are familial. *LBK1/STK11* mutations have been identified in 100% of familial cases and over 90% of clinically identified sporadic cases.

COMMENT

Individuals with Peutz-Jeghers syndrome also develop many other polyps, including adenomatous polyps in the colon. This may cause confusion with familial adenomatous polyposis.

References

Hutchinson J: Pigmentation of the lips and mouth, *Arch Surg* 7:290, 1896.

Peutz JLA: Very remarkable case of familial polyposis of mucous membrane of intestinal tract and nasopharynx accompanied by peculiar pigmentation of skin and mucous membrane, *Ned Maanschr Geneesk* 10:134, 1921.

Jeghers H, et al: Generalized intestinal polyposis and melanin spots of the oral mucosa, lips, and digits: A syndrome of diagnostic significance, *N Engl J Med* 241:993, 1949.

Hemminki A, et al: A serine/threonine kinase gene defective in Peutz-Jeghers syndrome, *Nature* 391:184, 1998.

Aretz S, et al: High proportion of large genomic *STK11* deletions in Peutz-Jeghers syndrome, *Hum Mutat* 26:513, 2005.

Beggs AD, et al: Peutz-Jeghers syndrome: A systematic review and recommendations for management, *Gut* 59:975, 2010.

De Rosa M, et al: Alu-mediated genomic deletion of the serine/threonine protein kinase 11 (*STK11*) gene in Peutz-Jeghers syndrome, *Gastroenterology* 138:2558, 2010.

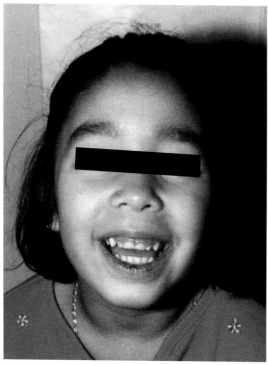

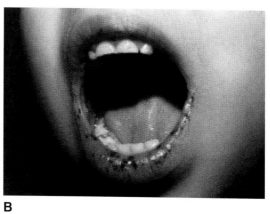

FIGURE 1. Peutz-Jeghers syndrome. **A** and **B,** Spotty pigmentation of lips and buccal mucous membrane in a 4-year-old girl.

A

B

Q

BANNAYAN-RILEY-RUVALCABA SYNDROME

(RUVALCABA-MYHRE SYNDROME, RILEY-SMITH SYNDROME, BANNAYAN SYNDROME)

Macrocephaly, Polyposis of Colon, Lipomas, Pigmentary Changes of the Penis

In 1986, Saul and Stevenson proposed that Bannayan syndrome and Ruvalcaba-Myhre syndrome were the same disorder. Subsequently, Dvir and colleagues added Riley-Smith syndrome and suggested that all three of these conditions represent one etiologic entity, which Cohen referred to as Bannayan-Riley-Ruvalcaba syndrome.

ABNORMALITIES

Growth. Birth weight greater than 4 kg and birth length greater than 97th percentile, normal adult stature.

Performance. Hypotonia, gross motor and speech delay (50%), mild-to-severe mental deficiency (15% to 20%), seizures (25%), autism spectrum disorders.

Craniofacial. Macrocephaly with ventricles of normal size (mean occipital frontal circumference +4.89 standard deviations); downslanting palpebral fissures (60%); high arched palate; strabismus or amblyopia (15%); prominent Schwalbe lines and prominent corneal nerves (35%).

Visceral. Ileal and colonic hamartomatous polyps (45%).

Neoplasms. Hamartomas that are lipomas (75%); vascular malformations, most commonly fast flow arteriovenous malformation (10%); and mixed type (20%). Most are subcutaneous, although they can be cranial (20%) or osseous (10%).

Other. Tan, nonelevated spots on the glans penis and shaft not always present at birth; myopathic process in proximal muscles (60%); cutaneous angiolipomas (50%), encapsulated or diffusely infiltrating; joint hyperextensibility; pectus excavatum; scoliosis (50%).

OCCASIONAL ABNORMALITIES

Frontal bossing, pseudopapilledema, diabetes, Hashimoto thyroiditis, acanthosis nigricans, lymphangiomyomas, angiokeratomas, verruca vulgaris–type facial skin changes, oral papillomas, trichilemmomas, café au lait spots, tongue polyps, supernumerary nipples, enlarged testes, enlarged penis, broad thumbs/great toes, hypoglycemia, multiple neurocutaneous neuromas.

NATURAL HISTORY

Although overgrowth is usually present in the newborn period, final adult height is within the normal range. The ileal and colonic polyps often present in childhood with intussusception, rectal prolapse, and rectal bleeding; sometimes they do not become evident until middle age. Lipomas can be extremely large. Speckling of the penis more likely becomes evident in later childhood. Delays in performance frequently improve with age. Rapamycin has been used in a patient with extensive arteriovenous malformation with good response.

ETIOLOGY

This disorder has an autosomal dominant inheritance pattern. Mutations in the tumor suppressor gene *PTEN* (phosphatase and tensin homologue deleted from chromosome 10), located at 10q23.3, are responsible and have been found in approximately 70% or more of cases. At least 10% are caused by intragenic or large deletions, which makes necessary a combined sequencing and dosage testing approach. Macrocephaly appears to be a constant finding in mutation-positive patients.

COMMENT

Cowden syndrome—characterized by trichilemmomas (small benign hair follicle tumors), oral papillomas, intestinal polyps, and an increased frequency of breast and thyroid cancer—is also caused by mutations in *PTEN*. Cowden syndrome and Bannayan-Riley-Ruvalcaba syndrome (BRRS) are allelic. For this reason, individuals with *PTEN*-positive BRRS should be monitored for malignant tumors using a similar protocol as is used for Cowden syndrome. In addition, *PTEN* mutations have been found in pediatric patients presenting with autistic spectrum disorders that do not fulfill criteria for either Cowden syndrome or BRRS. Severe progressive macrocephaly appears to be a good predictor of a *PTEN* mutation in this subgroup of patients, and penile freckles should always be looked for. This complex spectrum of conditions is frequently referred to as the PTEN hamartoma tumor syndrome (PHTS).

References

Riley HD, Smith WR: Macrocephaly, pseudopapilledema, and multiple hemangiomata, *Pediatrics* 26:293, 1960.

Bannayan GA: Lipomatosis, angiomatosis and macrocephaly: A previously undescribed congenital syndrome, *Arch Pathol* 92:1, 1971.

Ruvalcaba RHA, et al: A syndrome with macrencephaly, intestinal polyposis and pigmentary penile lesions, *Clin Genet* 18:413, 1980.

Marsh DJ, et al: *PTEN* mutation spectrum and genotype-phenotype correlations in Bannayan-Riley-Ruvalcaba syndrome suggest a single entity with Cowden syndrome, *Hum Mol Genet* 8:1461, 1999.

Hendriks YMC, et al: Bannayan-Riley-Ruvalcaba syndrome: Further delineation and management of *PTEN* mutation-positive cases, *Familial Cancer* 2:79, 2003.

Butler MG, et al: Subset of individuals with autism spectrum disorders and extreme macrocephaly associated with germline *PTEN* tumour suppressor gene mutations, *J Med Genet* 42:318, 2005.

Rodríguez-Escudero I, et al: A comprehensive functional analysis of *PTEN* mutations: Implications in tumor- and autism-related syndromes, *Hum Mol Genet* 20:4132, 2011.

Tan MH, et al: A clinical scoring system for selection of patients for *PTEN* mutation testing is proposed on the basis of a prospective study of 3042 probands, *Am J Hum Genet* 88:42, 2011.

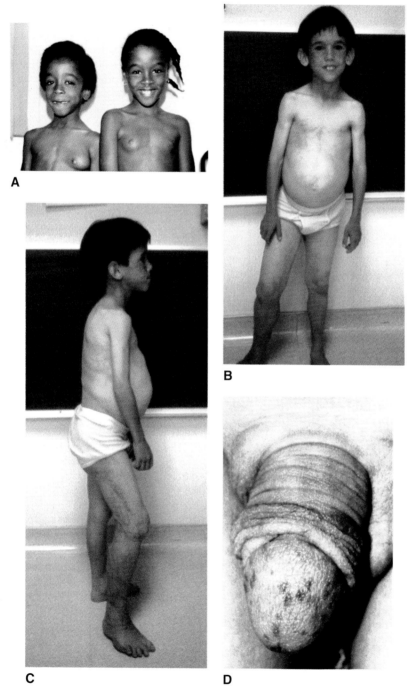

FIGURE 1. Bannayan-Riley-Ruvalcaba syndrome. **A,** Brother and sister with macrocephaly and lipomata. The boy has intellectual disability. (From Higginbottom MC et al: *Pediatrics* 69:632, 1982, with permission.) **B** and **C,** A boy with multiple subcutaneous hamartomas. The child had recurrent rectal prolapse. **D,** Pigmented spots on the penis. (**D,** Courtesy of Dr. Michael Cohen, Dalhousie University, Halifax, Nova Scotia.)

HEREDITARY HEMORRHAGIC TELANGIECTASIA
(OSLER HEMORRHAGIC TELANGIECTASIA)
Epistaxis, Multiple Telangiectases

This entity was set forth in 1901 by Osler. Hereditary hemorrhagic telangiectasia (HHT) is characterized by the presence of multiple arteriovenous malformations (AVMs) that lack intervening capillaries and result in direct connections between arteries and veins. Small AVMs are called telangiectases, which contain dilated vessels having only an endothelial wall with no elastic tissue. Many affected families have been reported, and the incidence is approximately 1 in 50,000.

ABNORMALITIES

Vascular anomalies. Pinpoint, spider, or nodular telangiectases most commonly on tongue, mucosa of lips, face, conjunctiva, ears, fingertips, nail beds, and nasal mucous membrane; occasionally in gastrointestinal tract, bladder, vagina, uterus, lungs, liver, or brain; cutaneous telangiectases (in second or third decade); arteriovenous fistulas in lungs (30%) and liver; mucosal and submucosal AVMs of the gastrointestinal tract; arterial aneurysms; venous varicosities; arteriovenous fistulas of celiac and mesenteric vessels; vascular anomalies in brain (10%) and spinal cord.

OCCASIONAL ABNORMALITIES
Cirrhosis of liver, cavernous angiomas, port-wine stain, duodenal ulcer.

NATURAL HISTORY
Three or more of the following lead to a definite diagnosis of HHT; two indicate possible or suspected HHT: (1) nosebleeds (epistaxis), spontaneous and recurrent; (2) mucocutaneous telangiectasts; (3) visceral AVM (pulmonary, cerebral, hepatic, spinal, gastrointestinal, pancreatic); and (4) a first-degree relative with a diagnosis of HHT. Epistaxis, which often occurs in late childhood (mean age of onset 12 years, 90% by age 21), spontaneous and recurrent, is the most common form of bleeding, followed by gastrointestinal, genitourinary, pulmonary, and intracerebral, all of which tend to occur in adults. Transillumination of the digits is helpful for detecting vascular lesions not evident on the skin. Intraocular hemorrhage is rare. Ten percent of patients never bleed, whereas approximately one third require hospitalization for bleeding. Neurologic complications occur at any age, with a peak incidence in the third decade, and result from

pulmonary arteriovenous fistula (60%), vascular malformation of the brain (28%) and spinal cord (8%), and portosystemic encephalopathy (3%). Of major concern is the potential for brain abscess, cerebral embolism, and hypoxemia secondary to the pulmonary arteriovenous fistulas. Hepatic arteriovenous fistula can cause hepatomegaly, right upper quadrant pain, pulsatile mass, a thrill, or bruit. Left to right shunting through the fistula can lead to high-output congestive heart failure. Bleeding is generally aggravated by pregnancy. Fewer than 10% of patients die of associated complications. Specific guidelines have been developed for management of the vascular findings in these patients. Examinations for pulmonary arteriovenous fistulas and for retinal telangiectases should be performed periodically. Oral iron supplementation is almost always necessary. Oral estrogen and septal dermoplasty have been used to successfully manage the epistaxis in some cases. Because of the high associated risks, any pulmonary AVM with a feeding vessel that exceeds 1.0 mm in diameter requires consideration of occlusion before any symptoms have occurred. Cerebral AVMs should be treated, when indicated by location or symptoms.

ETIOLOGY
This disorder has an autosomal dominant inheritance pattern. HHT is caused by mutations in a number of genes involved in the TGF-ß/BMP signaling cascade: *ENG* (causing HHT1), the gene encoding the cell surface co-receptor endoglin, and *ACVRL1/ALK1* (HHT2), member of the serine-threonine kinase receptor family expressed in endothelium. Mutations in either of those two genes can be found in 90% of patients with a definite diagnosis. *SMAD4*, a gene encoding an intracellular signaling molecule, can cause a combined syndrome of juvenile polyposis syndrome and HHT and is mutated in 1% to 2% of cases. Linkage studies suggest at least two other as-yet unidentified genes. A higher frequency of pulmonary AVMs has been associated with *ENG* mutations.

References

Osler W: On a family form of recurring epistaxis, associated with multiple telangiectases of skin and mucous membrane, *Bull Hopkins Hosp* 12:333, 1901.
McAllister KA, et al: Endoglin, a TGF-b binding protein of endothelial cells is the gene for hereditary haemorrhagic telangiectasia type 1, *Nat Genet* 8:345, 1994.

Johnson DW, et al: Mutations in the activin receptor-like kinase 1 gene in hereditary haemorrhagic telangiectasia type 2, *Nat Genet* 13:189, 1996.

Shovlin CL, et al: Diagnostic criteria for hereditary hemorrhagic telangiectasia (Rendu-Osler-Weber syndrome), *Am J Med Genet* 91:66, 2000.

Bayrak-Toydemir P, et al: Hereditary hemorrhagic telangiectasia: An overview of diagnosis and management in the molecular era for clinicians, *Genet Med* 6:175, 2004.

Mohler ER III, et al: Transillumination of the fingers for vascular anomalies: A novel method for evaluating hereditary hemorrhagic telangiectasia, *Genet Med* 11:356, 2009.

Faughnan ME, et al: International guidelines for the diagnosis and management of hereditary haemorrhagic telangiectasia, *J Med Genet* 48:73, 2011.

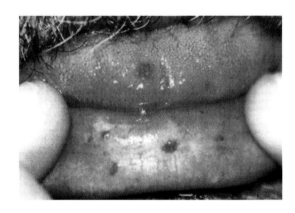

FIGURE 1.   Osler hemorrhagic telangiectasia syndrome. Small telangiectases on mucosa of the lips. (Courtesy of Eric Rosenthal, University of California, San Diego.)

Q

MULTIPLE ENDOCRINE NEOPLASIA, TYPE 2B
(MULTIPLE NEUROMA SYNDROME)
Multiple Neuromata of Tongue, Lips with or without Medullary Thyroid Carcinoma, with or without Pheochromocytoma

This disorder represents one of the three different forms of multiple endocrine neoplasia type 2 (MEN2). The other two forms, MEN2A and medullary thyroid cancer (MTC)–only, are associated with normal physical appearance. MEN2A is characterized by medullary thyroid carcinoma, parathyroid hyperplasia, and pheochromocytoma, while MTC syndrome represents familial medullary thyroid carcinoma without other components of MEN2A. MEN2B is the only one of these three disorders associated with a pattern of malformation and it accounts for only 2% of cases of MEN2.

ABNORMALITIES

Craniofacial. Prominent lips; nodular tongue; involvement of nasal, laryngeal, and intestinal mucous membranes; thickened, anteverted eyelids caused by neuromatous involvement of the mucosal surface; tendency toward coarse-appearing facies.

Visceral. Ganglioneuromatosis extending from lips to rectum; medullary thyroid carcinoma; pheochromocytoma.

Skeletal. Marfanoid habitus; pes cavus; slipped femoral capital epiphyses; pectus excavatum; kyphosis; lordosis, scoliosis; increased joint laxity; weakness of proximal extremity muscles.

OCCASIONAL ABNORMALITIES

Slit-lamp examination may reveal prominent medullated nerve fibers in the cornea; subconjunctival neuromas, cutaneous neuromata, or neurofibromata; parathyroid hyperplasia; hypotonia; developmental delay; deficient lacrimation.

NATURAL HISTORY

Oral neuromata are usually evident in infancy or early childhood and should immediately suggest the diagnosis of MEN2B. Affected individuals have a 100% lifetime risk of MTC, which may present in early childhood. Pheochromocytoma will affect 50% of patients, usually after 8 years of age. MTC can be suspected in the presence of an elevated plasma calcitonin concentration, a specific and sensitive marker. Prophylactic thyroidectomy is indicated as soon as the diagnosis is made. Individuals with MEN2B who do not undergo thyroidectomy before 1 year of age are likely to develop metastatic MTC. Prior to intervention with early prophylactic thyroidectomy, the average age of death in individuals with MEN2B was 21 years. Pheochromocytoma is suspected when biochemical screening reveals elevated excretion of catecholamines and catecholamine metabolites. Annual biochemical screening is recommended for early detection of pheochromocytoma beginning at 8 years of age. When a tumor is detected, a thorough exploration should be accomplished, since it is often bilateral and may also be extra-adrenal. Constipation with megacolon often severe enough to suggest Hirschsprung disease or diarrhea frequently develops. This is usually the result of gastrointestinal ganglioneuromatosis resulting in thickening of the myenteric plexi and hypertrophy of ganglion cells.

ETIOLOGY

This disorder has an autosomal dominant inheritance pattern. Point mutations in the *RET* proto-oncogene leading to gain of function are the cause of MEN2B and MEN2A and are detected in 98% of cases. Screening for common recurrent mutations is suggested prior to full sequencing.

COMMENT

About 50% of familial cases and 35% of sporadic cases of Hirschsprung disease are caused by germline loss-of-function mutations in the *RET* proto-oncogene.

References

Gorlin RJ, et al: Multiple mucosal neuromas, pheochromocytoma and medullary carcinoma of the thyroid–a syndrome, *Cancer* 22:293, 1968.

Schimke RN, et al: Syndrome of bilateral pheochromocytoma, medullary thyroid carcinoma and multiple neuromas, *N Engl J Med* 279:1, 1968.

Hofstra RMW, et al: A mutation in the *RET* proto-oncogene associated with multiple endocrine neoplasia type 2B and sporadic medullary thyroid carcinoma, *Nature* 367:375, 1994.

Torre M, et al: Diagnostic and therapeutic approach to multiple endocrine neoplasia type 2B in pediatric patients, *Pediatr Surg Int* 18:378, 2002.

Kouvaraki MA, et al: RET proto-oncogene: A review and update of genotype-phenotype correlations in hereditary medullary thyroid cancer and associated endocrine tumors, *Thyroid* 15:531, 2005.

American Thyroid Association Guidelines Task Force: Medullary thyroid cancer: Management guidelines of the American Thyroid Association, *Thyroid* 19:565, 2009.

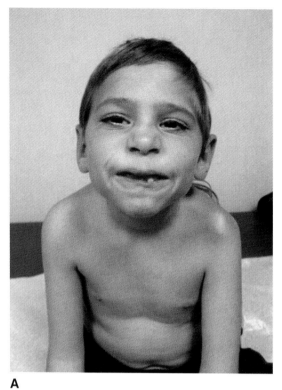

A

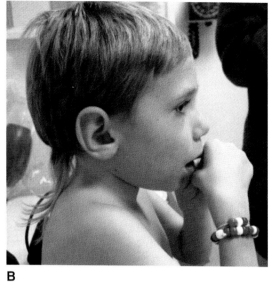

B

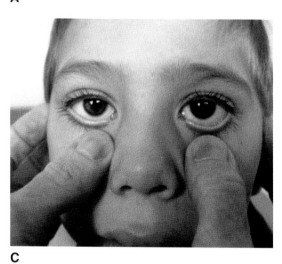

C

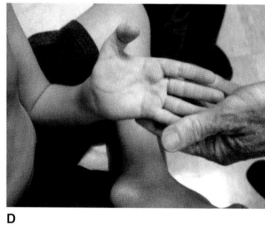

D

FIGURE 1.   Multiple endocrine neoplasia type 2B. **A–D,** Note the multiple neuromata involving the conjunctiva and contributing to the prominent lips.

Q

GORLIN SYNDROME (NEVOID BASAL CELL CARCINOMA SYNDROME)
Basal Cell Carcinomas, Broad Facies, Rib Anomalies

Although this condition had been described, it was Gorlin and Goltz who recognized the full extent of this pattern of malformation in 1960. Its prevalence is approximately 1 in 60,000.

ABNORMALITIES

Craniofacial. Macrocephaly (80%); frontoparietal bossing (66%); broad nasal bridge (59%); well-developed supraorbital ridges; heavy, often fused eyebrows; mild hypertelorism; prognathism (33%); hyperpneumatization of paranasal sinuses; bony bridging of sella turcica (60%–80%); odontogenic keratocysts of jaws (75%); misshapen or carious teeth.

Skeletal. Scoliosis; sloping, narrow shoulders (41%); short metacarpals, especially the fourth (29%).

Skin. Nevoid basal cell carcinomas over neck, upper arms, trunk, and face; epidermal cysts; punctate dyskeratotic pits on palms (65%), soles (68%), or both (58%); milia, especially facial (52%).

Visceral. Calcified ovarian fibromata (14%).

Imaging. Bifid, synostotic, or partially missing ribs (60%); thoracic or cervical vertebral anomalies (40%); ectopic calcification in falx cerebri (85%); falx cerebelli (40%); petroclinoid ligament (20%); dura, pia, and choroid plexi.

OCCASIONAL ABNORMALITIES

Intellectual disability, agenesis of corpus callosum, vermian dysgenesis, anosmia, hydrocephalus, hypertelorism, telecanthus, epicanthal folds, highly arched eyebrows, cataract, coloboma of iris, prominent medullated retinal nerve fibers, retinal atrophy, orbital cyst, microphthalmia, glaucoma, chalazion, strabismus, cleft lip with or without cleft palate, mandibular coronoid process hyperplasia, low-pitched female voice, pectus excavatum/carinatum, Sprengel deformity, "marfanoid" build, arachnodactyly, pre- or postaxial polydactyly, immobile thumbs, pseudocystic lytic lesions of bones, lumbarization of sacrum, hypogonadism in males, subcutaneous calcifications of skin, renal anomalies, other neoplasms including medulloblastoma, meningioma, fibromata, lipomata, melanoma, neurofibromas of skin, cardiac fibromas, eyelid carcinomas, breast cancer, lung cancer, chronic lymphoid leukemia, non-Hodgkin lymphoma, ovarian dermoid, ameloblastoma, lymphomesenteric cysts that tend to calcify, and hepatic mesenchymal tumor.

NATURAL HISTORY

Although nevoid basal cell carcinomas have occurred in 2-year-old children, they usually appear between puberty and 35 years of age with a mean age of about 20 years. Before puberty, the lesions are harmless. Thereafter, concern should be raised when the lesions begin to grow, ulcerate, bleed, or crust.

The jaw cysts enlarge, especially in later childhood, and may recur following curettage. Mean age of onset is about 15 years. A constant vigil must be maintained to detect other tumors that are a common feature of this syndrome. In particular, medulloblastoma occurs in 5% to 10% of children with the condition in early infancy (mean age 2 years) and should be excluded with routine MRI up to 8 years of age. Treatment with X-irradiation results in large numbers of invasive basal cell carcinomas appearing in the radiation field and should therefore be avoided. Excessive sun exposure should also be avoided. A protocol for surveillance of children and adults with Gorlin syndrome has been recently proposed by an expert consensus group.

Palmar pitting can be made more obvious by immersion of the hands in water for 15 minutes.

ETIOLOGY

This disorder has an autosomal dominant inheritance pattern. Mutations in *PCTH1*, a tumor suppressor gene that maps to 9q22.3-q31, are responsible. *PCTH1* is a human homologue of the *Drosophila* segment polarity gene, *patch*. The PTCH protein is a receptor for sonic hedgehog, a secreted molecule that is important in formation of embryonic structures and tumorigenesis. More than two thirds of cases are familial; the rest are de novo mutations. In some de novo cases, somatic mosaicism may be present, and testing should be performed in at least two different tumors if the mutation is not found in blood. Partial or whole gene deletions account for 6% of cases. When severe developmental delay, short stature, and other dysmorphic features that go beyond the typical findings in Gorlin syndrome are present, diagnosis of a 9q22.3 microdeletion syndrome should be considered.

COMMENT

Gain-of-function mutations in *PTCH1* have been reported in holoprosencephaly, presumably through repression of the hedgehog signaling pathway. By contrast, mutations and deletions of the gene leading to Gorlin syndrome allow for excessive activation of the hedgehog signaling pathway.

References

Binkley GW, Johnson HH Jr: Epithelioma adenoides cysticum: Basal cell nevi, agenesis of the corpus callosum and dental cysts: A clinical and autopsy study, *Arch Dermatol* 63:73, 1951.

Gorlin RJ, Goltz RW: Multiple nevoid basal-cell epithelioma, jaw cysts, and bifid ribs: A syndrome, *N Engl J Med* 262:908, 1960.

Hahn H, et al: Mutations of the human homologue of *Drosophila* patched in the nevoid basal cell carcinoma syndrome, *Cell* 85:841, 1996.

Amlashi SF, et al: Nevoid basal cell carcinoma syndrome: Relation with desmoplastic medulloblastoma in infancy. A population-based study and review of the literature, *Cancer* 98:618, 2003.

Bree AF, Shah MR, BCNS Colloquium Group: Consensus statement from the first international colloquium on basal cell nevus syndrome (BCNS), *Am J Med Genet A* 155A:2091, 2011.

Muller EA, et al: Microdeletion 9q22.3 syndrome includes metopic craniosynostosis, hydrocephalus, macrosomia, and developmental delay, *Am J Med Genet A* 158A:391, 2012.

Q

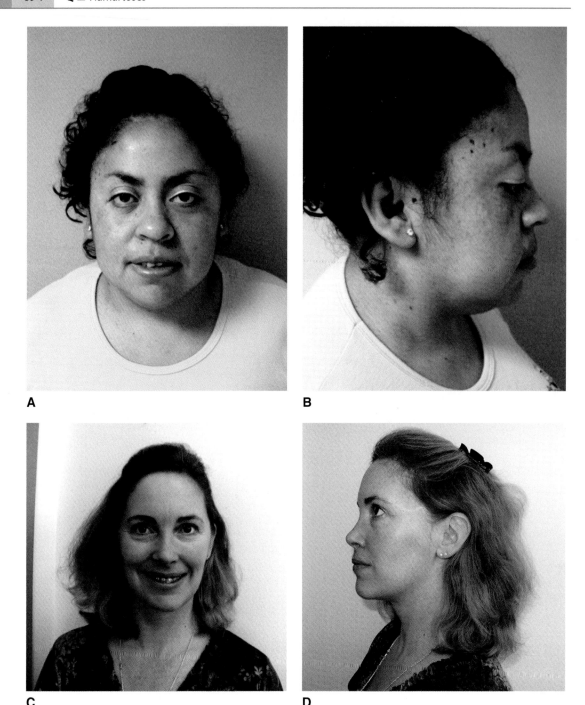

FIGURE 1.   Gorlin syndrome. **A–D,** Two adults. Note the frontoparietal bossing, well-developed supraorbital ridges, prognathism, and pigmented nevi. (**C** and **D,** Courtesy of Dr. Virginia Kimonis, Harvard Medical School, Boston.)

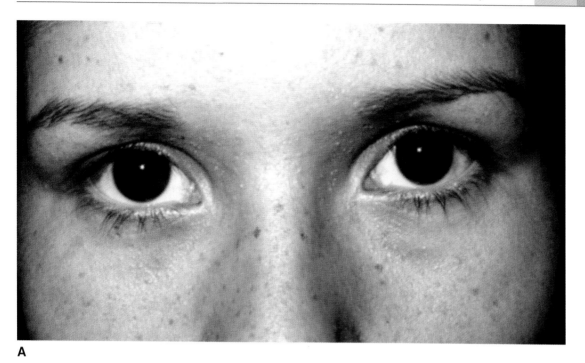

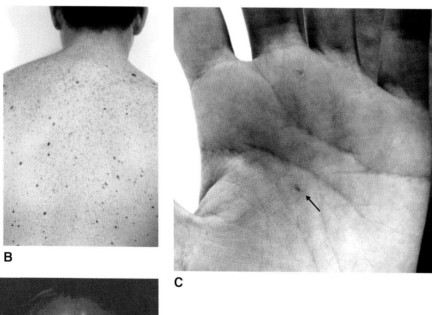

FIGURE 2. **A,** A 15-year-old girl with milia over the face. **B,** Multiple basal cell nevi. **C,** Palmar pits. **D,** Mineralization in falx cerebri. (**B** and **D,** From Ferrier PE, Hinrichs WL: *Am J Dis Child* 113:538, 1967, with permission.)

MULTIPLE LENTIGINES SYNDROME (LEOPARD SYNDROME)
Multiple Lentigines, Pulmonic Stenosis, Mild Hypertelorism, Deafness

Gorlin and colleagues recognized the multiple defect nature of this disorder and utilized the acronym LEOPARD to denote the *l*entigines, *E*KG abnormalities, *o*cular hypertelorism, *p*ulmonic stenosis, *a*bnormalities of genitalia, *r*etardation of growth, and *d*eafness. More than 80 cases have been described.

ABNORMALITIES

Craniofacial. Mild ocular hypertelorism; downslanting palpebral fissures; broad, flat nose; low-set, posteriorly rotated ears with thickened helices; short neck, excess nuchal skin, low posterior hairline.

Skin. Multiple 1- to 5-mm dark lentigines, especially on neck and trunk, but can be present on palms, soles, face, scalp, and external genitalia, with sparing of the mucosa; café au lait spots.

Cardiac. Mild pulmonic stenosis (40%), most commonly a dysplastic pulmonary valve; hypertrophic obstructive cardiomyopathy (70%); electrocardiographic changes of prolonged P-R and QRS, abnormal P waves.

Other. Mild growth deficiency with short stature in less than 50%; mild intellectual disability in 30%; mild-to-moderate sensorineural deafness (15%–25%); winged scapulae; pectus excavatum or carinatum; late adolescence; cryptorchidism; hypospadias; urinary tract defects.

OCCASIONAL ABNORMALITIES

Electroencephalograph abnormalities, cleft palate, mandibular prognathism, axillary freckling, localized areas of hypopigmentation, unilateral gonadal agenesis or hypoplasia, hypogonadism, hyposmia, subaortic stenosis, kyphoscoliosis, joint hypermobility.

NATURAL HISTORY

Lentigines differ from freckles in being darker and not related to sunlight exposure. They are rarely present at birth, usually develop during childhood, increase in number into the thousands until puberty, and darken with age. Café au lait spots can be present in 70% of patients before lentigines

appear. Many of the other features of the disorder are not readily apparent and require investigation; examples are deafness and cardiac findings. Hypertrophic obstructive cardiomyopathy can be a major problem. It may be progressive and often involves the intraventricular septum. Hypogonadism may be secondary to hypogonadotropism; hence, these individuals should be observed closely at adolescence to determine whether sex hormone replacement therapy is indicated.

ETIOLOGY

This disease has an autosomal dominant inheritance pattern with wide variability in expression, including lack of lentigines in an occasional patient. Mutations in *PTPN11*, *RAF1*, or *BRAF* cause this condition. Molecular genetic testing of the three genes identifies mutations in about 95% of affected individuals. Specific mutations in these genes are associated with the LEOPARD phenotype, and targeted sequencing is the best approach to molecular diagnosis.

COMMENT

These three genes are implicated in the RAS/ERK/MAPK pathway, altering cell proliferation, and are also responsible for Noonan syndrome. *BRAF* is the most common gene causing cardiofaciocutaneous syndrome.

References

Gorlin RJ, et al: Multiple lentigines syndrome, *Am J Dis Child* 117:652, 1969.

Digilio MC, et al: Grouping of multiple lentigines/ LEOPARD and Noonan syndromes on the *PTPN11* gene, *Am J Hum Genet* 71:389, 2002.

Digilio MC, et al: LEOPARD syndrome: Clinical diagnosis in the first year of life, *Am J Med Genet A* 140A:740, 2006.

Pandit B, et al: Gain-of-function *RAF1* mutations cause Noonan and LEOPARD syndromes with hypertrophic cardiomyopathy, *Nat Genet* 39:1007, 2007.

Sarkozy A, et al: Germline *BRAF* mutations in Noonan, LEOPARD, and cardiofaciocutaneous syndromes: Molecular diversity and associated phenotypic spectrum, *Hum Mutat* 30:695, 2009.

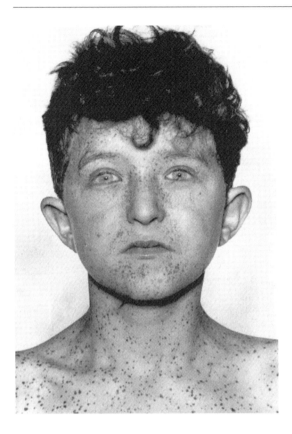

FIGURE 1.   Multiple lentigines syndrome. Adolescent boy showing lentigines, prominent ears, and mild ocular hypertelorism. (From Gorlin RJ et al: *Am J Dis Child* 117:652, 1969, with permission.)

Q

GOLTZ SYNDROME
Poikiloderma with Focal Dermal Hypoplasia, Syndactyly, Dental Anomalies

This mesoectodermal disorder was recognized as a distinct entity by Goltz and colleagues in 1962, although well-described cases had been reported prior to that time. More than 175 cases have been documented.

ABNORMALITIES

Craniofacial. Asymmetry with mild hemihypertrophy; narrow nasal bridge and broad tip sometimes with unilateral notch of ala nasi; thin, protruding, simple low-set ears; pointed chin; strabismus; coloboma of the iris and aniridia; microphthalmos; anophthalmos; microcornea; chorioretinal coloboma; lacrimal duct abnormalities; hypoplasia of teeth, anodontia, enamel hypoplasia, late eruption, irregular placement, malocclusion, or notched incisors.

Skin. Pink or red, atrophic macules that may be slightly raised or depressed and have a linear and asymmetric distribution following the lines of Blaschko; mainly on thighs, forearm, and cheeks; telangiectasis; lipomatous nodules projecting through localized areas of skin atrophy; angiofibromatous nodules around lips, in vulval and perianal areas, around the eyes, the ears (on pinnae and in middle ear), the fingers and toes, the groin and umbilicus, inside the mouth, the larynx, and esophagus; skin scarring.

Nails and Hair. Dystrophic nails, narrow or hypoplastic; sparse and brittle hair, localized areas of alopecia in head and pubic region.

Skeletal. Asymmetric involvement of hands and feet in 60%, including syndactyly, absence or hypoplasia of digits, ectrodactyly, polydactyly, and absence of an extremity; scoliosis (20%); longitudinal striations in the metaphyses of long bones; fibrous dysplasia of bone; spina bifida occulta; clavicular dysplasia; failure of pubic bone fusion; skeletal asymmetry.

OCCASIONAL ABNORMALITIES

Moderate short stature; microcephaly; aplasia cutis congenita; joint hypermotility; split sternum; vertebral and rib anomalies; scoliosis; mental retardation (15%); hearing impairment; bulbar angiofibroma of eye; optic atrophy; ocular hypertelorism; alveolar irregularity; CNS malformation; congenital heart defects; expansile, tumor-like bone lesions; horseshoe kidney; cystic dysplasia of kidney; umbilical, inguinal, diaphragmatic, hiatus, or epigastric herniae; omphalocele; intestinal malrotation.

NATURAL HISTORY

The skin lesions are usually present at birth, although the skin lipomata and the lip and anal papillomata may develop later. In rare cases, esophageal or laryngeal papillomas can cause obstruction or gastroesophageal reflux. No effective therapy is known except plastic surgery for the syndactyly and removal of the papillomas when indicated. However, the latter may recur. Despite serious structural anomalies of the eyes, acuity may be surprisingly good. Development is usually normal, but cognitive impairment has been reported.

ETIOLOGY

PORCN, a regulator of Wnt signaling, is the causal gene for this condition. The vast majority of cases have been sporadic, mediated by de novo mutations (95%), and female (90%). X-linked dominant inheritance with lethality in hemizygous males is the mode of inheritance. All affected males have been mosaic and generally more mildly affected than females. An affected female will have an expected sex ratio of offspring of 33% unaffected females, 33% affected females, 33% unaffected males. Large deletions account for 15% of the mutations and usually cause extreme skewing of X-inactivation in females.

References

Jessner M: Falldemonstration Breslauer dermatologische Vereinigung, *Arch Dermatol Syph (Berlin)* 133:48, 1921.

Wodniansky P: Über die Formen der congenitalen Poikilodermie, *Arch Klin Exp Dermatol* 205:331, 1957.

Goltz RW, et al: Focal dermal hypoplasia, *Arch Dermatol* 86:708, 1962.

Temple IK, et al: Focal dermal hypoplasia (Goltz syndrome), *J Med Genet* 27:180, 1990.

Grzeschik KH, et al: Deficiency of *PORCN*, a regulator of Wnt signaling, is associated with focal dermal hypoplasia, *Nat Genet* 39:833, 2007.

Wang X, et al: Mutations in X-linked *PORCN*, a putative regulator of Wnt signaling, cause focal dermal hypoplasia, *Nat Genet* 39:836, 2007.

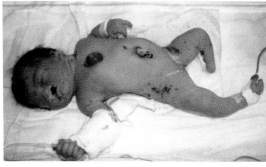

A

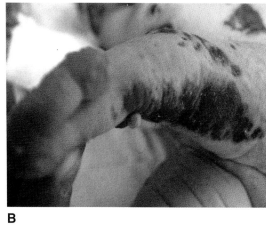

B

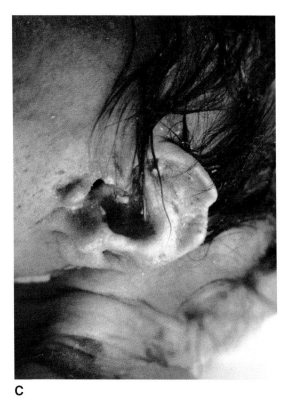

C

FIGURE 1.   Goltz syndrome. A newborn girl. Red atrophic macules are depressed in **A** and raised in **B. C,** Note the angiofibromatous nodules around the ears. (From Loguercio Leite JC et al: *Clin Dysmorphol* 14:37, 2005, with permission.)

Q

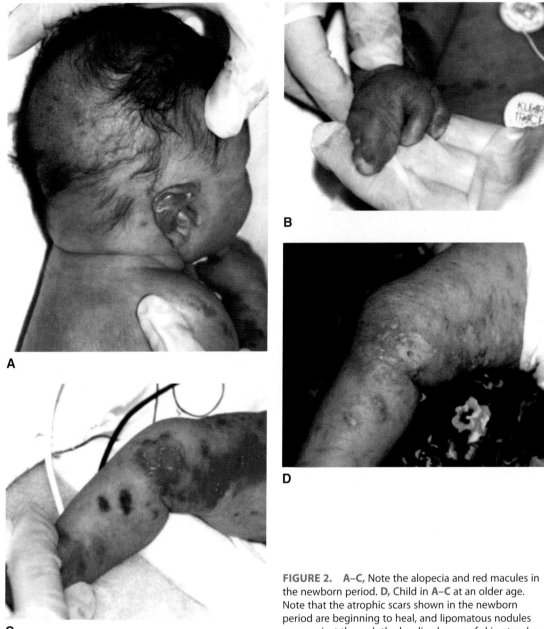

A

B

C

D

FIGURE 2. **A–C,** Note the alopecia and red macules in the newborn period. **D,** Child in **A–C** at an older age. Note that the atrophic scars shown in the newborn period are beginning to heal, and lipomatous nodules now project through the localized areas of skin atrophy.

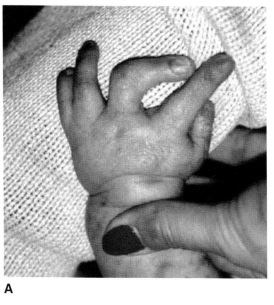

A

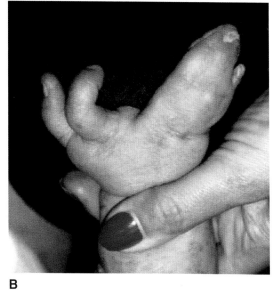

B

C

FIGURE 3.   A–C, Note the severe defects of the hands and feet including syndactyly, ectrodactyly, and nail dystrophy.

Q

MICROPHTHALMIA–LINEAR SKIN DEFECTS SYNDROME
(MIDAS SYNDROME)
Microphthalmia, Dermal Aplasia, Sclerocornea

Al-Gazali and colleagues described two females with this disorder in 1988. MIDAS (*m*icrophthalmia, *d*ermal *a*plasia, and *s*clerocornea) has been suggested as a mnemonic designation. Approximately 42 cases have been reported.

ABNORMALITIES

Craniofacial. Microphthalmia, sclerocornea.
Skin. Dermal aplasia—without herniation of fatty tissue and usually involving face, scalp, and neck but occasionally upper part of the thorax—that heals, leaving hyperpigmented areas.

OCCASIONAL ABNORMALITIES
Microcephaly; CNS defects, including agenesis of corpus callosum, absence of septum pellucidum, anencephaly, hydrocephalus, and ventriculomegaly; mild-to-severe intellectual disability (24%); infantile seizures; additional eye abnormalities, including anterior chamber defects such as corneal leukoma, iridocorneal adhesion (Peters anomaly), congenital glaucoma with total/peripheral anterior synechiae, aniridia, cataracts, iris coloboma, pigmentary retinopathy, and orbital cysts; preauricular pits and hearing loss; structural cardiac defects (atrial septal defect, ventricular septal defect, overriding aorta); cardiac conduction defects; hypertrophic cardiomyopathy; oncocytic cardiomyopathy; diaphragmatic hernia; nail dystrophy; rib/vertebral defects; anterior or imperforate anus; bicornuate uterus; ambiguous genitalia.

NATURAL HISTORY
Developmental milestones are reached at an appropriate age in the majority of cases when the severe visual handicap is taken into consideration. Death occurred in the first year of life in two children, presumably secondary to cardiac arrhythmias.

ETIOLOGY
The vast majority of patients have been females, indicative of an X-linked mutation lethal in males. Eighty percent have had a gross deletion or a translocation involving the short arm of the X chromosome, resulting in monosomy for Xp22.3. Three genes from this critical region have been implicated in the phenotype, including *MID1*, *HCCS*, and *ARHGAP6*; however, sequencing has not yet identified the causal gene. Several males with MIDAS syndrome and an XX karyotype with detectable Y-chromosome material resulting from an X/Y translocation have been described.

References

Al-Gazali LI, et al: An XX male and two t (X;Y) females with linear skin defects and congenital microphthalmia: A new syndrome at Xp22.3, *J Med Genet* 25:638, 1988.

Happle R, et al: MIDAS syndrome (microphthalmia, dermal aplasia, and sclerocornea): An X-linked phenotype distinct from Goltz syndrome, *Am J Med Genet* 47:710, 1993.

Prakash SK, et al: Loss of holocytochrome c-type synthetase causes the male lethality of X-linked dominant microphthalmia with linear skin defects (MLS) syndrome, *Hum Mol Genet* 11:3237, 2002.

Morleo M, et al: Microphthalmia with linear skin defects (MLS) syndrome: Clinical, cytogenetic, and molecular characterization of 11 cases, *Am J Med Genet A* 137A:190, 2005.

Kapur R, et al: Corneal pathology in microphthalmia with linear skin defects syndrome, *Cornea* 27:734, 2008.

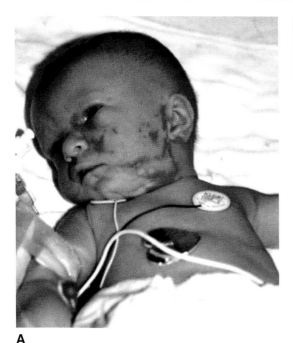

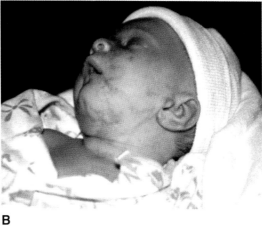

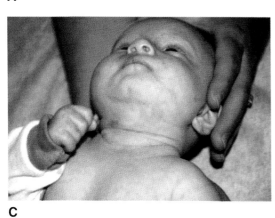

A

B

C

FIGURE 1.   Microphthalmia-linear skin defects syndrome. Female infant: newborn (**A**), at 2 weeks (**B**), and at 2 months (**C**). Note the irregular areas of skin hypoplasia that have healed significantly by 2 months of age. (From Bird LM et al: *Am J Med Genet* 53:141, 1994. Copyright © 1994. Reprinted with permission of Wiley-Liss, Inc., a subsidiary of John Wiley & Sons, Inc.)

Q

HYPOHIDROTIC ECTODERMAL DYSPLASIA
Defect in Sweating, Alopecia, Hypodontia

There are a number of ectodermal dysplasia syndromes, only a few of which are represented in this text. The division into hypohidrotic and hidrotic categories based on the extent of the deficit of sweat glands is in no way absolute. Just as there is variable hypoplasia of hair follicles, there is variable hypoplasia of sweat glands.

Thurman described this entity in 1848. In 1875, Charles Darwin set forth the following concise commentary about this disease: "I may give an analogous case, communicated to me by Mr. W. Wedderhorn of a Hindoo family in Scinde, in which ten men, in the course of four generations, were furnished, in both jaws taken together, with only four small and weak incisor teeth and with eight posterior molars. The men thus affected have very little hair on the body, and became bald early in life. They also suffer much during hot weather from excessive dryness of the skin. It is remarkable that no instance has occurred of a daughter being thus affected." In 1929, Weech clearly separated this condition from other clinical problems having ectodermal dysplasia as a feature. However, there is significant genetic and clinical heterogeneity. At least 1 in 17,000 newborns is affected.

ABNORMALITIES

Skin. Thin and hypoplastic, with decreased pigment and tendency toward papular changes on face; periorbital wrinkling and hyperpigmentation; scaling or peeling of skin in immediate newborn period.

Skin Appendages. Hair: fine, dry, and hypochromic; sparse to absent scalp and body hair, secondary sexual hair near normal; sweat glands: hypoplasia to absence of eccrine glands; apocrine glands more normally represented; sebaceous glands: hypoplasia to absence. Lack of dermal ridges.

Mucous Membranes. Hypoplasia, with absence of mucous glands in oral and nasal membranes; mucous glands may also be absent from bronchial mucosa.

Dentition. Hypodontia to anodontia, with an average of nine permanent teeth, most commonly canines and first molars, resulting in deficient alveolar ridge; anterior teeth tend to be conical in shape. Retruded appearance of the midface.

Craniofacial. Low nasal bridge, small nose with hypoplastic alae nasi, full forehead, prominent supraorbital ridges, prominent lips.

OCCASIONAL ABNORMALITIES
Hoarse voice, hypoplasia to absence of mammary glands or nipples, deficient milk production during nursing, absence of tears, failure to develop nasal turbinates, mild-to-moderate nail dystrophy, eczematous change in skin, asthmatic symptoms.

NATURAL HISTORY
Neonates with hypohidrotic ectodermal dysplasia (HED) may be diagnosed because of peeling skin, similar to that of "post-mature" babies, and periorbital hyperpigmentation. In infancy, irritability may occur because of heat intolerance. Hyperthermia as a consequence of inadequate sweating not only is a serious threat to life but may be the cause of intellectual disability, which is an occasional feature of this disorder. Living in a cool climate and cooling by water when overheated are important measures. The hypoplasia of mucous membranes plus thin nares may require frequent irrigation of the nares to limit the severity of mucous clots and purulent rhinitis. Otitis media and lung infection may also be consequences of the mucous membrane defect. Mucous glands are hypoplastic to absent not only in the respiratory tract but in esophageal and colonic mucosa as well. Although the patient is often hairless at birth, some hair may develop. Short stature is not considered a feature of this disorder. Therefore, affected males with growth deficiency should be evaluated for other causes of short stature, such as endocrine deficiencies.

ETIOLOGY
This disorder has an X-linked recessive inheritance pattern. The gene (*ED1*) has been localized within the region Xq12-q13.1. It encodes a protein, ectodysplasin, which is important for normal development of ectodermal appendages. This gene accounts for approximately 60% of the forms of hypohidrotic ectodermal dysplasia. Deletions and duplications have been reported. Dosage studies must follow sequencing if negative. It has been estimated that 90% of female carriers can be identified by dental examination and sweat testing. Approximately 95% of patients with HED have the X-linked form of disease.

COMMENT

A clinically identical autosomal recessive form (autosomal recessive HED) and a milder autosomal dominant form (autosomal dominant HED) have been described. Mutations in the ectodysplasin anhidrotic receptor (*EDAR*) gene located at 2q11-q13 (15%–20%), as well as mutations in the ectodysplasin anhidrotic receptor–associated death domain (*EDARADD*) gene located at 1q42.2-q43 (1%–2%), are responsible for the autosomal dominant and recessive form.

Loss-of-function and missense mutations in the *WNT10A* gene, located on chromosome 2q35, have been reported to cause odonto-onycho-dermal dysplasia, a rare form of ectodermal dysplasia. The phenotype may not be distinguished from classic HED, except for generalized microdontia, but may be milder and account for 15% of cases. HED phenotypes can be classified as both classic and mild. Those affected by the X-linked form (males) and the autosomal recessive forms will have the classic, more severe phenotype. Those affected by the autosomal dominant form and female carriers of the X-linked form have the mild, more variable phenotype.

References

Thurman J: Two cases in which the skin, hair and teeth were very imperfectly developed, *Medico-Chir Trans* 31:71, 1848.

Darwin C: *The Variations of Animals and Plants under Domestication*, ed 2, London, 1875, John Murray.

Weech AA: Hereditary ectodermal dysplasia (congenital ectodermal defect): A report of two cases, *Am J Dis Child* 37:766, 1929.

Passarge E, Nuzum CT, Schubert WK: Anhidrotic ectodermal dysplasia as autosomal recessive trait in an inbred kindred, *Humangenetik* 3:181, 1966.

Gorlin RJ, Old T, Anderson VE: Hypohidrotic ectodermal dysplasia in females: A critical analysis and argument for genetic heterogeneity, *Z Kinderheilkd* 108:1, 1970.

Clarke A: Hypohidrotic ectodermal dysplasia, *J Med Genet* 24:659, 1987.

Clarke A, Burn J: Sweat testing to identify female carriers of X-linked hypohidrotic ectodermal dysplasia, *J Med Genet* 28:330, 1991.

Crawford PJM, et al: Clinical and radiographic dental findings in X-linked hypohidrotic ectodermal dysplasia, *J Med Genet* 28:181, 1991.

Zonana J, et al: Detection of de novo mutations and analysis of their origin in families with X-linked hypohidrotic ectodermal dysplasia, *J Med Genet* 31:287, 1994.

Munoz F, et al: Definitive evidence for an autosomal recessive form of hypohidrotic ectodermal dysplasia clinically indistinguishable from the more common X-linked disorder, *Am J Hum Genet* 61:94, 1997.

Ho L, et al: A gene for autosomal dominant hypohidrotic ectodermal dysplasia (*EDA3*) maps to chromosome 2q11-q13, *Am J Hum Genet* 62:1102, 1998.

Monreal AW, et al: Identification of a new splice form of the *EDA1* gene permits detection of nearly all X-linked hypohidrotic ectodermal dysplasia mutations, *Am J Hum Genet* 63:380, 1998.

Headon DJ, et al: Gene defect in ectodermal dysplasia implicates a death domain adapter in development, *Nature* 414:913, 2001.

Cluzeau C, et al: Only four genes (*EDA1, EDAR, EDARADD, and WNT10A*) account for 90% of hypohidrotic/anhidrotic ectodermal dysplasia cases, *Hum Mutat* 32:70, 2011.

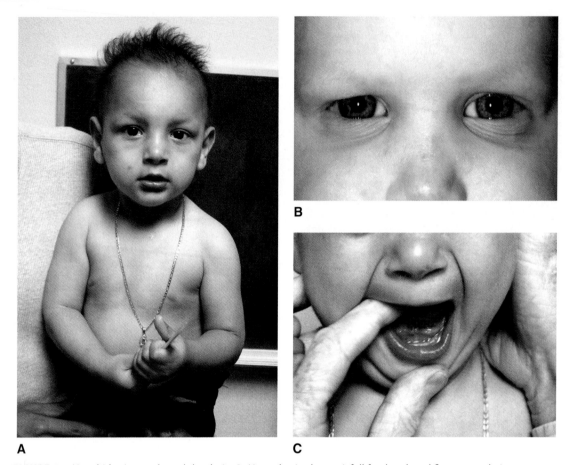

FIGURE 1.   Hypohidrotic ectodermal dysplasia. **A,** Hypoplastic alae nasi; full forehead; and fine, sparse hair.
B, Periorbital skin wrinkling and sparse eyelashes and eyebrows. **C,** Hypoplasia of alveolar ridge in a 2-year-old child.

Continued

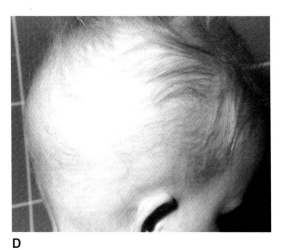

D

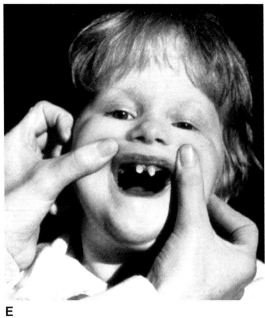

FIGURE 1, cont'd. D, Fine, dry, hypochromic hair.
E, Partial expression in a girl.

E

R

RAPP-HODGKIN ECTODERMAL DYSPLASIA
Hypohidrosis, Oral Clefts, Dysplastic Nails

Rapp and Hodgkin reported three affected individuals in 1968, and Summitt and Hiatt added one additional case. More than 40 cases have been reported.

ABNORMALITIES

Skin. Thin, with decreased number of sweat pores; congenital erythroderma; skin erosions, mostly in scalp; scarring and reticulated hyperpigmentation on the neck and intertriginous areas.

Hair. Sparse, fine wiry hair; pili canaliculi.

Nails. Small. Characteristic nail dystrophy with small, thick, hyperconvex nails or anonychia.

Dentition. Hypodontia with small, conical teeth; mean of permanent teeth is five.

Face. Low nasal bridge, narrow nose with hypoplastic ala nasi, maxillary hypoplasia, short philtrum, high forehead.

Mouth. Small mouth, cleft lip with or without cleft palate, cleft palate alone, cleft uvula, velopharyngeal incompetence, trismus.

Genitalia. Hypospadias.

OCCASIONAL ABNORMALITIES

Short stature, ptosis, atretic ear canals, hearing loss, absent lacrimal puncta with obstruction, labial anomalies, absent lingual frenulum and sublingual caruncles, glossy tongue, hypothelia, supernumerary nipples, palmoplantar keratoderma with erosions, syndactyly, camptodactyly.

NATURAL HISTORY

Hyperthermia occurs, in rare cases, in early childhood. Thereafter, although reduced sweating is described subjectively, heat intolerance is not usually a problem, and sweat studies may be normal. Superficial skin erosions vary from limited to severe full-body involvement. The erosions most typically affect the scalp at birth and during infancy. Severe scalp erosions often lead to scarring alopecia and hypotrichosis.

There is frequent occurrence of purulent conjunctivitis and otitis media, the latter presumably related to palatal incompetence. Feeding and speech difficulties are common. Whereas the clefting seen in most genetic syndromes is consistent (i.e., either cleft lip with or without cleft palate [CLP] or cleft palate alone [CPA]), mixed clefting (the occurrence of CLP and CPA in the same family) occurs in this disorder. Deficient mucous coating of vocal cords can affect vocal quality.

ETIOLOGY

This disorder has an autosomal dominant inheritance pattern. Mutations of the *p63* gene located on 3q27 are responsible. More than 80% of documented mutations are found in the sterile alpha motif (SAM) domain with the remaining 20% occurring in the transactivation inhibitory (TI) domain. Targeted studies of exons 13 and 14 can be done prior to whole gene sequencing. Marked intrafamilial variability in expression is often seen. Somatic and germline mosaicism has been reported.

COMMENT

Mutations of the *p63* gene have been identified in other autosomal dominant disorders with some overlapping features including ectrodactyly-ectodermal dysplasia–clefting syndrome (EEC syndrome) type 3, Hay-Wells syndrome or ankyloblepharon–ectodermal dysplasia–clefting syndrome (AEC syndrome), dermato-ungual-lacrimal-tooth syndrome (ADULT syndrome), limb-mammary syndrome (LMS), and in some cases of nonsyndromic split-hand/foot syndrome (SHFM) type 4. Allelic heterogeneity for the same condition and marked clinical variability for single mutations are the rule within the wide spectrum of P63-associated disorders. Hay-Wells (AEC) syndrome and Rapp-Hodgkin syndrome are now thought to be the same condition with variable presence of ankyloblepharon.

References

Rapp RS, Hodgkin WE: Anhidrotic ectodermal dysplasia: Autosomal dominant inheritance with palate and lip anomalies, *J Med Genet* 5:269, 1968.

Summitt RL, Hiatt RL: Hypohidrotic ectodermal dysplasia with multiple associated anomalies, *Birth Defects* 7(8):121, 1971.

Wannarachue N, Hall BD, Smith DW: Ectodermal dysplasia and multiple defects (Rapp-Hodgkin type), *J Pediatr* 81:1217, 1972.

Schroeder HW, Sybert VP: Rapp-Hodgkin ectodermal dysplasia, *J Pediatr* 110:72, 1987.

Salinas CF, Montes GM: Rapp-Hodgkin syndrome: Observations on ten cases and characteristic hair changes (pili canaliculi), *Birth Defects* 24:149, 1988.

O'Donnell BP, James WD: Rapp-Hodgkin ectodermal dysplasia, *J Am Acad Dermatol* 27:323, 1992.

Cambiaghi S, et al: Rapp-Hodgkin syndrome and AEC syndrome: Are they the same entity? *Br J Dermatol* 130:97, 1994.

McGrath JA, et al: Hay-Wells syndrome is caused by heterozygous missense mutations in the SAM domain of P63, *Hum Mol Genet* 10:221, 2001.

Neilson DE, et al: Mixed clefting type in Rapp-Hodgkin syndrome, *Am J Med Genet* 108:281, 2002.

Bougeard G, et al: The Rapp-Hodgkin syndrome results from mutations of the *TP63* gene, *Eur J Hum Genet* 11:700, 2003.

Siegfried E, et al: Skin erosions and wound healing in ankyloblepharon-ectodermal defect-cleft lip and/or palate, *Arch Dermatol* 141:1591, 2005.

Rinne T, Brunner HG, van Bokhoven H: p63-associated disorders, *Cell Cycle* 6:262, 2007.

Prontera P, et al: An intermediate phenotype between Hay-Wells and Rapp-Hodgkin syndromes in a patient with a novel P63 mutation: Confirmation of a variable phenotypic spectrum with a common aetiology, *Genet Couns* 19:397, 2008.

Farrington F, Lausten L: Oral findings in ankyloblepharon-ectodermal dysplasia-cleft lip/palate (AEC) syndrome, *Am J Med Genet A* 149A:1907, 2009.

Julapalli ME, et al: Dermatologic findings of ankyloblepharon-ectodermal defects-cleft lip/palate (AEC) syndrome, *Am J Med Genet A* 149A:1900, 2009.

Clements SE, et al: Rapp-Hodgkin and Hay-Wells ectodermal dysplasia syndromes represent a variable spectrum of the same genetic disorder, *Br J Dermatol* 163:624, 2010.

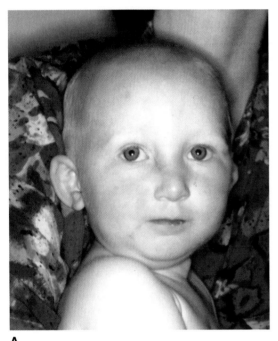

A

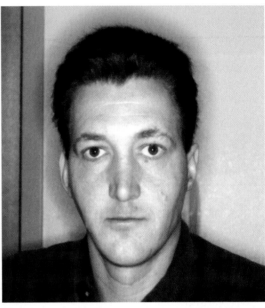

B

FIGURE 1.   Rapp-Hodgkin ectodermal dysplasia. **A–C,** Affected father and son. Note the narrow nose with hypoplastic ala nasi, small mouth, and hypoplastic fingernails.

C

R

TRICHO-DENTO-OSSEOUS SYNDROME (TDO SYNDROME)
Kinky Hair, Enamel Hypoplasia, Sclerotic Bone

Lichtenstein and colleagues defined this disorder in 107 individuals from one large kindred in 1972. Robinson and colleagues had previously described an autosomal dominant disorder with curly hair and enamel hypoplasia, with or without nail hypoplasia.

ABNORMALITIES

Hair. Kinky/curly present at birth.

Dentition. Small, widely spaced, pitted teeth with poor enamel and increased pulp chamber size (taurodontism); both primary and permanent dentition are affected. Markedly delayed or advanced dental maturity. Filling of tooth pulps with amorphous denticle-like material.

Facies. Frontal bossing, dolichocephaly, square jaw with retruded maxilla and relative prognathism.

Bone. Mild-to-moderate increased bone density and thickness, most evident in calvarium, which is thick, lacks visible pneumatization of the mastoid process or visible obliteration of the cranial diploë; obtuse mandibular angles; short mandibular; increased height of the mandibular ramus; long bones and spine also can be affected.

Nails. Brittle, with superficial peeling (approximately 50%).

Other. Delayed bone age.

OCCASIONAL ABNORMALITIES

Partial craniosynostosis, congenitally missing teeth. Severe atopic dermatitis (one case).

NATURAL HISTORY

The hair sometimes straightens with age but can remain coarse and unmanageable in adults. The teeth become eroded and discolored, are prone to periapical abscesses, and are lost by the second to third decade. The sclerotic bone appears to be secondary to closely compacted lamellae and is rarely associated with any clinical symptomatology.

ETIOLOGY

This disorder has an autosomal dominant inheritance pattern. A four-nucleotide deletion in the human *DLX3* gene, a member of the distal-less homeobox gene family, located at 17q21 has been identified in affected members of six families and appears to be the most common mutation. A second mutation, a 2-bp deletion in the end of the homeobox, causes an attenuated clinical phenotype. Additional missense mutations in the homeobox have been identified in individual families. Functional studies suggest haploinsufficiency of *DLX3* as the mechanism underlying tooth and bone altered development. Murine studies have indicated the important role of *DLX* genes in the development of hair, teeth, and bone.

References

Robinson GC, Miller JR, Worth HM: Hereditary enamel hypoplasia, its association with characteristic hair structure, *Pediatrics* 37:489, 1966.

Lichtenstein J, et al: The tricho-dento-osseous (TDO) syndrome, *Am J Hum Genet* 24:569, 1972.

Shapiro SD, et al: Tricho-dento-osseous syndrome, *Am J Med Genet* 16:225, 1983.

Wright JR, et al: Tricho-dento-osseous syndrome: Features of the hair and teeth, *Oral Surg Oral Med Oral Pathol* 77:487, 1994.

Wright JR, et al: Analysis of the tricho-dento-osseous syndrome genotype and phenotype, *Am J Med Genet* 72:197, 1997.

Price JA, et al: Identification of a mutation in *DLX3* associated with tricho-dento-osseous (TDO) syndrome, *Hum Mol Genet* 7:563, 1998.

Nieminen P, et al: *DLX3* homeodomain mutations cause tricho-dento-osseous syndrome with novel phenotypes, *Cells Tissues Organs* 194:49, 2011.

Nguyen T, et al: Craniofacial variations in the tricho-dento-osseous syndrome, *Clin Genet* 2012 [Epub ahead of print].

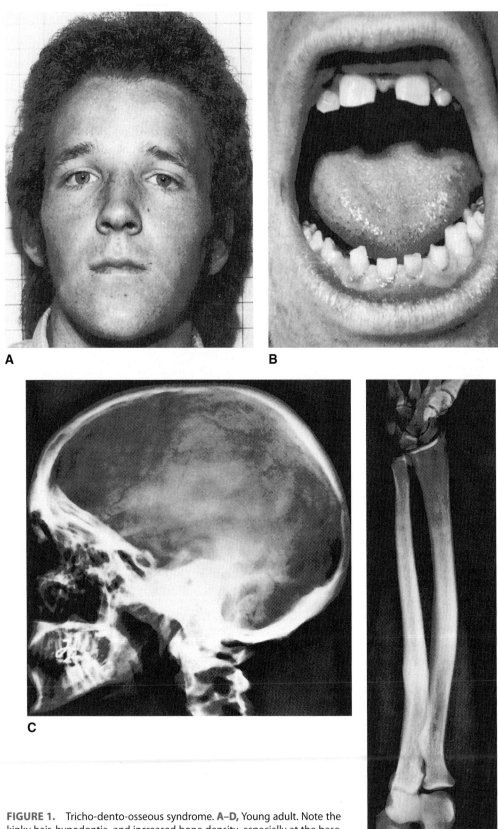

FIGURE 1.   Tricho-dento-osseous syndrome. **A–D,** Young adult. Note the kinky hair, hypodontia, and increased bone density, especially at the base of the skull. (From Lichtenstein JR, et al: *Am J Hum Genet* 24:569, 1972, with permission.)

R

CLOUSTON SYNDROME
Nail Dystrophy, Dyskeratotic Palms and Soles, Hair Hypoplasia , Hidrotic Ectodermal Dysplasia 2

Clouston in 1939 reported 119 individuals in a French-Canadian family. Rajagopalan and Tay described an affected Chinese pedigree in 1977. More than 200 cases have been described. The condition is also known as hidrotic ectodermal dysplasia 2 (HED2).

ABNORMALITIES

Skin. Thick dyskeratotic palms and soles; hyperpigmentation over knuckles, elbows, axillae, areolae, and pubic area. Abnormal sweat glands, sebaceous glands, and teeth.

Hair. Hypoplasia with sparse, pale, fine hair to alopecia (61%); deficiency of eyelashes and eyebrows, pubic and axillary hair.

Nails. Hypoplasia to aplasia; dysplasia with thickening.

Eyes. Strabismus.

OCCASIONAL ABNORMALITIES

Cataract, photophobia, hearing loss, dull mentality, short stature, thickened skull, tufting of terminal phalanges.

NATURAL HISTORY

In infancy, scalp hair is wiry, brittle, patchy, and pale and may progressively fall out, leading to total alopecia by puberty. The nails may be milky white in early childhood; later they thicken and separate from the nail bed. Palmoplantar keratoderma increases in severity with age.

ETIOLOGY

This disorder has an autosomal dominant inheritance pattern with marked variability in expression. Mutations in the *GJB6* gene located at chromosome 13q11-12.1, which encodes the gap junction protein connexin 30, are responsible.

Connexin 30 is expressed in the epidermis, brain, and inner ear. Connexins are membrane proteins that are present in virtually all mammalian cells. Each connexin binds another connexin in an adjacent cell to form an intracellular communication channel known as a gap junction, which functions to allow rapid exchange of information between cells.

COMMENT

Mutations in *GJB6* also cause nonsyndromic deafness and some cases of keratitis-ichthyosis-deafness (KID) syndrome, commonly caused by mutations in *GJB2*.

References

Joachim H: Hereditary dystrophy of the hair and nails in six generations, *Ann Intern Med* 10:400, 1936.

Clouston HR: The major forms of hereditary ectodermal dysplasia (with an autopsy and biopsies on the anhidrotic type), *Can Med Assoc J* 40:1, 1939.

Wilkey WD, Stevenson GH: A family with inherited ectodermal dystrophy, *Can Med Assoc J* 53:226, 1945.

Gold RJM, Scriver CR: Properties of hair keratin in an autosomal dominant form of ectodermal dysplasia, *Am J Hum Genet* 24:549, 1972.

Rajagopalan KV, Tay CH: Hidrotic ectodermal dysplasia: Study of a large Chinese pedigree, *Arch Dermatol* 113:481, 1977.

Kibar Z, et al: The gene responsible for Clouston hidrotic ectodermal dysplasia maps to the pericentromeric region of chromosome 13q, *Hum Mol Genet* 5:543, 1996.

Lamartine J, et al: Mutations in *GJB6* cause hidrotic ectodermal dysplasia, *Nat Genet* 26:142, 2000.

Smith FJ, Morley SM, McLean WH: A novel connexin 30 mutation in Clouston syndrome, *J Invest Dermatol* 118:530, 2002.

Zhang XJ, et al: A mutation in the connexin 30 gene in Chinese Han patients with hidrotic ectodermal dysplasia, *J Dermatol Sci* 32:11, 2003.

Jan AY, et al: Genetic heterogeneity of KID syndrome: Identification of a Cx30 gene (*GJB6*) mutation in a patient with KID syndrome and congenital atrichia, *J Invest Dermatol* 122:1108, 2004.

Baris HN, et al: A novel *GJB6* missense mutation in hidrotic ectodermal dysplasia 2 (Clouston syndrome) broadens its genotypic basis, *Br J Dermatol* 159:1373, 2008.

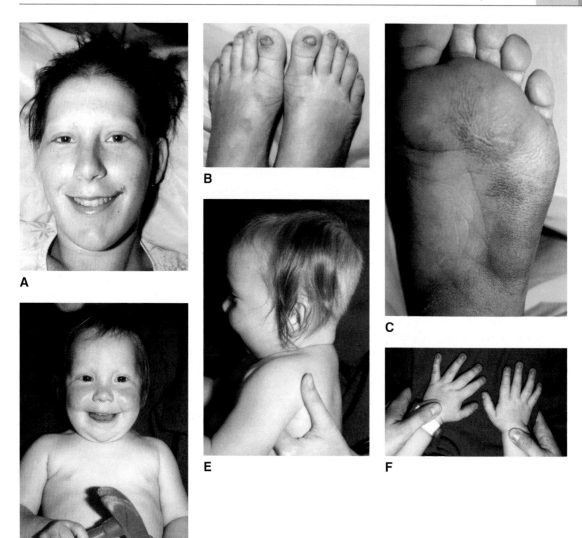

FIGURE 1.   Clouston syndrome. **A–F,** A 19-year-old mother and her 22-month-old daughter. Note the sparse hair, dysplastic nails, and dyskeratotic soles.

R

CRANIOECTODERMAL DYSPLASIA (SENSENBRENNER SYNDROME)
Sagittal Suture Synostosis, Ectodermal Dysplasia, Skeletal Defects

Initially described by Sensenbrenner et al in 1975 in a brother and a sister, this disorder has subsequently been reported in more than 40 cases. It has been categorized within the group of ciliopathies, which include Jeune thoracic dystrophy, Ellis–van Creveld syndrome, and short rib–polydactyly types I, II, III and IV, as well as Weyers acrofacial dysostosis.

ABNORMALITIES

Growth. Postnatal onset short stature.

Craniofacial. Sagittal craniosynostosis, dolichocephaly, frontal bossing, low-set simple ears, everted lower lip, micrognathia.

Thorax. Narrow thorax, pectus excavatum.

Ectodermal Defects. Fine sparse hair, widely spaced teeth with decreased enamel, hypodontia, taurodontism and malformations of cusps, short nails, lax skin.

Limbs. Brachydactyly, finger syndactyly, joint laxity.

Skeletal. Shortening of ribs and long bones, particularly the humeri and fibulae, flattened epiphyses of long bones, delayed ossification of capital femoral epiphysis, convex upper and lower surfaces of vertebral bodies, pedicles of vertebral bodies in lumbar region are short with less than normal widening of the interpedicular distance.

Other. Interstitial fibrosis of the kidneys with atrophic tubules and thickening of the tubular basement membrane indicative of nephronophthisis; liver cystic disease.

OCCASIONAL ABNORMALITIES

Cleft palate, downslanting palpebral fissures, epicanthal folds, hypertelorism, hyperopia, myopia nystagmus, retinal dystrophy, full cheeks, anteverted nares, cardiac defect, clinodactyly, syndactyly of the second and third fingers, single palmar crease, pes planus, broad metacarpals, postaxial polydactyly, triphalangeal thumbs hypotonia, enlarged cisterna magnum, posterior fossa cyst, hypospadias, skin and soft tissue laxity.

NATURAL HISTORY

Head circumference, of normal size at birth, increases disproportionally, whereas the rate of growth with respect to length decreases. Intellectual development is usually normal. Renal failure is the most common cause of death and patients should be monitored carefully. Liver cystic disease occurs less commonly than with Jeune thoracic dystrophy, one of the other ciliopathies.

ETIOLOGY

Cranioectodermal dysplasia (CED) has an autosomal recessive mode of inheritance. Mutations in four different genes, *IFT122, WDR35, WDR19,* and *IFT43,* the products of each of which are part of the intraflagellar transport complex A (IFT-A), are responsible. IFT-A is required for retrograde flagellar transport in cilia.

References

Sensenbrenner JA, et al: New syndrome of skeletal, dental and hair anomalies, *Birth Defects* 11:372, 1975.

Levin LS, et al: A heritable syndrome of craniosynostosis, short thin hair, dental abnormalities and short limbs: Cranioectodermal dysplasia, *J Pediatr* 90:55, 1977.

Young ID: Cranioectodermal dysplasia (Sensenbrenner's syndrome), *J Med Genet* 26:393, 1989.

Zaffanello M, et al: Sensenbrenner syndrome: A new member of the hepatorenal fibrocystic family, *Am J Med Genet* 140:2336, 2006.

Gikissen C, et al: Exome sequencing identifies *WDR35* variants involved in Sensenbrenner syndrome, *Am J Hum Genet* 87:418, 2010.

Walczak-Sztulpa J, et al: Cranioectodermal dysplasia, Sensenbrenner syndrome, is a ciliopathy caused by mutations in the *IFT122* gene, *Am J Hum Genet* 86:949, 2010.

Arts HH, et al: C140RF179 encoding IFT43 is mutated in Sensenbrenner syndrome, *J Med Genet* 48:390, 2011.

Bredrup CB, et al: Ciliopathies with skeletal anomalies and renal insufficiency due to mutations in the IFT-A gene *WDR19, Am J Hum Genet* 89:634, 2012.

Lin A, et al: Cranioectodermal dysplasia: Comparison to Jeune syndrome and other ciliopathies, 2012, David W. Smith Workshop on Malformations and Morphogenesis.

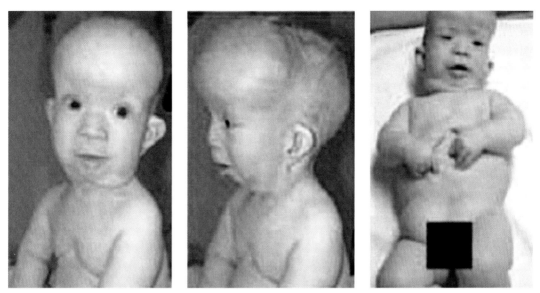

FIGURE 1.   Child at 12 months with sagittal craniosynostosis, frontal bossing, sparse hair, low-set cupped ears, epicanthic folds, redundant skin folds and inguinal hernias. (From Fry AE, et al: *Am J Med Genet Part A* 149A:2212, 2009, with permission.)

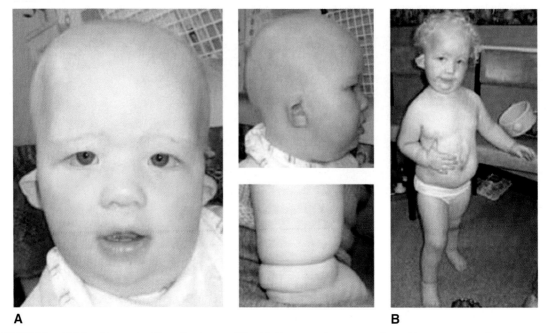

A   B

FIGURE 2.   Child at 20 months **(A)** and at 3 years **(B),** with bitemporal narrowing, frontal bossing, sparse hair, low-set cupped ears, epicanthic folds, short stature, redundant skin folds around ankles, and a repaired periumbilical incisional hernia. (From Fry AE, et al: *Am J Med Genet Part A* 149A:2212, 2009, with permission.)

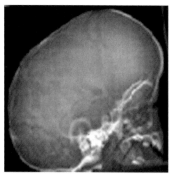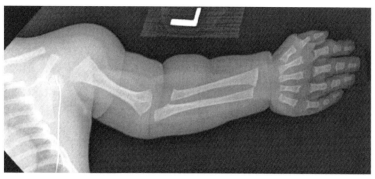

FIGURE 3.   Radiographs of the arm showing shortening of humerus, brachydactyly, and diffuse metaphyseal flaring (contributed by Angela E. Lin, MD) and of the lateral skull showing dolichocephaly and frontal bossing secondary to craniosynostosis of the sagittal suture. (From Fry AE, et al: *Am J Med Genet Part A* 149A:2212, 2009, with permission.)

GAPO SYNDROME
Growth Deficiency, Alopecia, Pseudoanodontia, Optic Atrophy

Initially reported in a Danish patient in 1947, this disorder was referred to as GAPO (growth deficiency, alopecia, pseudoanodontia, optic atrophy) syndrome by Tipton and Gorlin in 1984. Ocular manifestations rather than optic atrophy is a more appropriate designation in that the latter has occurred in only one third of the patients. More than 30 patients have been reported.

ABNORMALITIES

Growth. Mildly decreased birth length; significant postnatal growth deficiency becomes obvious between 6 months and 1 year; delayed bone age.

Craniofacial. Frontal bossing; high forehead, prominent occiput; enlarged anterior fontanel with delayed closure; prominent scalp veins; periorbital swelling; drooping forehead skin; flat nasal bridge; anteverted nares; long philtrum, thick lips; large ears; micrognathia.

Ocular. Progressive optic atrophy; cataracts; exophthalmos; keratoconus; keratitis; glaucoma; horizontal nystagmus.

Hair. Diminished scalp hair beginning between 2 and 3 months with total alopecia by 2 to 3 years; sparse eyelashes and eyebrows; extent of body and facial hair variable.

Teeth. Failure of tooth eruption (pseudoanodontia) involving primary and permanent dentition.

Other. Mild skin laxity, umbilical hernia; hyperconvex nails; brachydactyly.

OCCASIONAL ABNORMALITIES

Mild intellectual disability, ptosis, alopecia at birth, craniosynostosis, absent pneumatization of maxillary sinuses, abnormal electroencephalograph, altered cerebral circulation with tortuosity of arteries and dilatation of basilar vertebral arteries and slow circulation time in one patient and occluded or absent right transverse and sigmoid sinus in another, intracranial venous malformations, visible dilated scalp veins, hypoplastic middle and distal phalanges, wrinkled palms, scythe-like ribs, delayed menarche, dilated cardiomyopathy, pulmonary hypertension, ankyloglossia, prognathism, hypogonadism, breast hypoplasia, early menopause, oligozoospermia, hypospadias, hepatomegaly, polycystic kidney, nephrocalcinosis.

NATURAL HISTORY

Most patients are normal at birth with progressive changes beginning at approximately 6 months, including loss of hair, skin laxity, and optic atrophy. A regular ophthalmologic follow-up is recommended even in the patients who do not show significant changes in the initial work-up. The patients with GAPO syndrome are reported to have reduced life span, and most of them die in their third or fourth decade of life. Autopsy specimens have shown interstitial fibrosis as well as atherosclerotic changes in multiple organs.

ETIOLOGY

This disorder has an autosomal recessive inheritance pattern. Skin biopsies have shown severe atrophy in the epidermis with deposition of a hyaline material in the upper dermis, and hair follicle atrophy. An abnormal breakdown of extracellular components caused by decreased activity of an unknown enzyme appears to underlie the pathogenesis of this condition.

References

Anderson TH, et al: Et tilfaelde at total "pseudo-anodonti" i forbindelse med kraniedeformitet, dvaergvaekst og ektodermal displasi, *Odont T* 55:484, 1947.

Tipton RE, Gorlin RJ: Growth retardation, alopecia, pseudo-anodontia, and optic atrophy—the GAPO syndrome: Report of a patient and review of the literature, *Am J Med Genet* 19:209, 1984.

Wajntal A, et al: GAPO syndrome (McKusick 23074)—a connective tissue disorder: Report on two affected sibs and on the pathologic findings in the older, *Am J Med Genet* 37:213, 1990.

Bacon W, et al: GAPO syndrome: A new case of this rare syndrome and a review of the relative importance of different phenotypic features in diagnosis, *J Craniofac Genet Dev Biol* 19:189, 1999.

Kocabay G, Mert M: GAPO syndrome associated with dilated cardiomyopathy: An unreported association, *Am J Med Genet A* 149A:415, 2009.

Demirgünes EF, Ersoy-Evans S, Karaduman A: GAPO syndrome with the novel features of pulmonary hypertension, ankyloglossia, and prognathism, *Am J Med Genet A* 149A:802, 2009.

Castrillon-Oberndorfer G, et al: GAPO syndrome associated with craniofacial vascular malformation, *Am J Med Genet A* 152A:225, 2010.

Nanda A, et al: GAPO syndrome: A report of two siblings and a review of literature, *Pediatr Dermatol* 27:156, 2010.

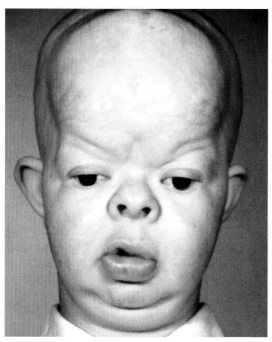

A

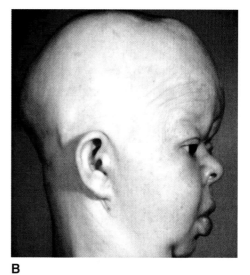

B

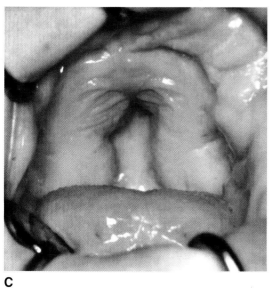

C

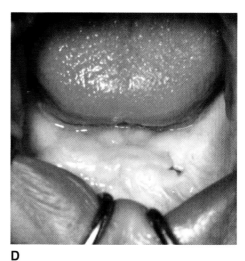

D

FIGURE 1.   GAPO syndrome. A 26-year-old woman. Note the alopecia, high forehead, frontal bossing, periorbital swelling, drooping forehead skin, thick lips, large ears, and micrognathia (**A** and **B**); the failure of tooth eruption (**C** and **D**); and the unerupted teeth (**E**). (From Tipton RE, Gorlin RJ: *Am J Med Genet* 19:209, 1984, with permission.)

E

R

PACHYONYCHIA CONGENITA SYNDROME
Thick Nails, Hyperkeratosis, Foot Blisters

Pachyonychia congenita is an ectodermal dysplasia described by Jadassohn and Lewandowsky, in which there is hypertrophic dystrophy of the distal nails.

ABNORMALITIES

Nails. Progressive thickening, yellow-brown discoloration, pinched margins, and an upward angulation of distal tips; the nails may eventually be hypoplastic or even absent.

Skin. Patchy to complete hyperkeratosis of palms and soles, callosities of feet, palmar and plantar bullae formation in areas of pressure that are often painful; keratosis pilaris with tiny cutaneous horny excrescences, particularly on the extensor surfaces of the arms and legs and on the buttocks; pilosebaceous cysts, including steatocystoma and vellus hair cysts, epidermal cysts filled with loose keratin on face, neck, and upper chest; verrucous lesions on the elbows, knees, and lower legs; hyperhidrosis, particularly of palms and soles (50%).

Mucous Membranes. Leukokeratosis of mouth and tongue, especially in positions of increased trauma; scalloped tongue edge.

Dentition. Erupted teeth at birth, lost by 4 to 6 months; early eruption of primary teeth and early loss of secondary teeth as a result of severe caries.

OCCASIONAL ABNORMALITIES

Intellectual disability; corneal thickening, cataracts; excessive production of waxy material in the ears, severe and unexplained ear pain, thickening of tympanic membrane; dry and sparse hair; osteomas of frontal bones; intestinal diverticula; large joint arthritis; bushy eyebrows; hoarseness secondary to laryngeal leukokeratosis in infancy; malformed teeth and twinning of the incisors.

NATURAL HISTORY

Clinical manifestations are present at birth or by 6 months of age in approximately 80% of patients. Usually the nails are grossly thickened by 1 year of age. Complete surgical removal of the nails is sometimes merited, although any matrix left behind will reform abnormal nails. Blisters develop beneath the keratoderma resulting in intense pain, particularly on the soles, the major cause of disability in these patients. Pain can be reduced by limiting the friction and trauma to the feet. Severe recurrent upper respiratory obstructive symptoms have occurred in those with severe laryngeal involvement with leukokeratosis. Oral leukokeratosis can be misdiagnosed as candida albicans and may cause difficulty in sucking.

ETIOLOGY

This disorder has an autosomal dominant inheritance pattern. Mutations in four different keratin genes are responsible in 90% of cases. *KRT6A,* the gene encoding for keratin, type II cytoskeletal 6A is the most common gene (52%). *KRT16* encoding for keratin, type I cytoskeletal 16 (28%), *KRT17* encoding for keratin, type I cytoskeletal 17, and *KRT6B* encoding for keratin, type II cytoskeletal 6B occur in 3% of cases.

Two of the causal genes have been shown to cause distinct phenotypes. Steatocystoma multiplex (SM), is caused by mutations in *KRT17* and results in widespread pilosebaceous cysts, including both steatocystomas and villus hair cysts that develop primarily on the face and trunk at puberty with little or no nail involvement or palmoplantar keratoderma. Focal non-epidermolytic palmoplantar keratoderma (FNEPPK), also with none-to-very-mild nail dystrophy, but mild-to-severe focal plantar keratoderma, is caused by mutations in *KRT16*.

COMMENT

Formerly, two clinical types were distinguished, the Jadassohn-Lewandowsky form and the Jackson-Lawler form. Phenotype and genotype heterogeneity have shown this classification not to be particularly useful in predicting the phenotype or the associated causal gene, and currently a more rational and useful classification, based on the mutated gene, is widely used.

References

Jadassohn J, Lewandowsky F: Pachyonychia congenita, keratosis disseminata circumscripta (folliculosis): Tylomata; leukokeratosis linguae, *Ikonographia Dermatologica Tab* 629, 1906.

Soderquist NA, Reed WB: Pachyonychia congenita with epidermal cysts and other congenital dyskeratoses, *Arch Dermatol* 97:31, 1968.

Young LL, Lenox JA: Pachyonychia congenita: A long-term evaluation, *Oral Surg* 36:663, 1973.

Stieglitz JB, Centerwall WR: Pachyonychia congenita (Jadassohn-Lewandowsky syndrome): A seventeen-member, four-generation pedigree with unusual respiratory and dental involvement, *Am J Med Genet* 14:21, 1983.

Rohold AE, Brandrup F: Pachyonychia congenita: Therapeutic and immunologic aspects, *Pediatr Dermatol* 7:307, 1990.

Su WPD, et al: Pachyonychia congenita: A clinical study of 12 cases and review of the literature, *Pediatr Dermatol* 7:32, 1990.

McLean WHI, et al: Keratin 16 and keratin 17 mutations cause pachyonychia congenita, *Nat Genet* 9:273, 1995.

Liao H, et al: A spectrum of mutations in keratins K6a, K16 and K17 causing pachyonychia congenita, *J Dermatol Sci* 48:199, 2007.

Wilson NJ, et al: A large mutational study in pachyonychia congenita, *J Invest Dermatol* 131:1018, 2011.

McLean WHI, et al: The phenotypic and molecular genetic features of pachyonychia congenita, *J Invest Dermatol* 131:1015, 2011.

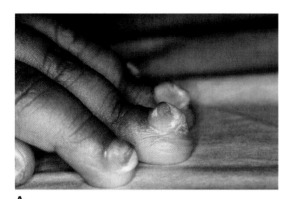

A

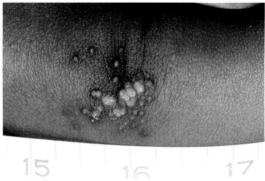

B

C

FIGURE 1.   Pachyonychia congenita syndrome. **A–C,** Child showing altered nails, cutaneous hyperkeratoses at knee, and leukokeratotic lesions on tongue and lateral palate.

R

XERODERMA PIGMENTOSA SYNDROME
Undue Sunlight Sensitivity, Atrophic and Pigmentary Skin Changes, Actinic Skin Tumors

Xeroderma pigmentosa occurs in approximately 1 in 250,000 individuals. Nearly 1000 cases have been reported.

ABNORMALITIES

Skin. Sunlight sensitivity with first exposure; freckling; progressive skin atrophy with irregular pigmentation; cutaneous telangiectasia; angiomata; keratoses; development of basal cell and squamous cell carcinoma, and less often keratoacanthoma, adenocarcinoma, melanoma, neuroma, sarcoma, and angiosarcoma.

Eyes. Photophobia; recurrent conjunctival injection; corneal abnormalities consisting of exposure keratitis leading to corneal clouding or vascularization; neoplasms involving conjunctiva, cornea, and eyelids.

Oral. Atrophic skin of mouth sometimes leading to difficulty opening mouth; squamous cell carcinoma of tongue tip, gingiva, or palate.

Neurologic. Slowly progressive neurologic abnormalities sometimes associated with mental deterioration; microcephaly; cerebral atrophy; choreoathetosis, ataxia, and spasticity; impaired hearing; abnormal speech; abnormal electroencephalography.

OCCASIONAL ABNORMALITIES

Primary internal neoplasms, including brain tumors, lung tumors, and leukemia; immune abnormalities; frequent infections.

NATURAL HISTORY

Cutaneous symptoms have onset at median age of between 1 and 2 years. The mean age of first nonmelanoma skin cancer is 8 years. Ninety-seven percent of squamous cell and basal cell cancers occur on face, head, or neck, indicating the important role that sun exposure has in the induction of these neoplasms. Four percent of squamous cell carcinomas metastasize. Seventy percent probability of survival has been documented at age 40 years. Thirty-three percent of deaths are due to cancer and 11% to infection.

ETIOLOGY

This disorder has an autosomal recessive inheritance pattern. The majority of affected patients have a defect in the excision repair of ultraviolet radiation–induced DNA damage. XP patients fall into one of ten complementation groups (A through I plus a variant). XPA, the gene for which is located on chromosome 9q34.1; XPC, the gene for which is located on chromosome 3p25.1; and XPD, the gene for which is located on chromosome 19q13.2, are most common. Neurologic problems are generally found in group A and D patients, who show the lowest level of DNA repair, whereas group C patients, who show the highest level of repair, are usually without overt neurologic disorders and have a longer life span. The severity of the skin and eye lesions relates more to the degree of sun exposure. The defect can be identified in cultured fibroblasts from amniocentesis.

COMMENT

The De Sanctis-Cacchione syndrome is a subgroup of xeroderma pigmentosa with neurologic involvement that includes xeroderma pigmentosa, progressive mental deterioration, growth deficiency, microcephaly, and hypogonadism probably secondary to hypothalamic insufficiency. Natural history includes slow developmental progress and growth, with variable neurologic dysfunction, including seizures from early childhood, spasticity, ataxia, peripheral neuropathy, and sometimes sensorineural deafness. Progressive skin deterioration occurs, especially related to exposure to the sun. Shortened life expectancy as a result of central nervous system deterioration or malignancy has been documented. The disorder is the result of a pair of autosomal recessive genes. Patients with De Sanctis-Cacchione syndrome usually belong to complementation group A or D.

References

De Sanctis C, Cacchione A: L'idiozia xerodermia, *Riv Spec Freniatr* 56:269, 1932.

Rook A, Wilkinson DS, Ebling FJG, editors: *Textbook of Dermatology,* Oxford, 1968, Blackwell Scientific Publications.

Regan JD, et al: Xeroderma pigmentosa: A rapid sensitive method for prenatal diagnosis, *Science* 174:147, 1971.

Pawsey SA, et al: Clinical, genetic and DNA repair studies on a consecutive series of patients with xeroderma pigmentosa, *Q J Med* 48:179, 1979.

Kraemer KH, et al: Xeroderma pigmentosa: Cutaneous, ocular and neurologic abnormalities in 830 published cases, *Arch Dermatol* 123:241, 1987.

Greenhaw GA, et al: Xeroderma pigmentosum and Cockayne syndrome: Overlapping clinical and bio-chemical phenotypes, *Am J Hum Genet* 50:677, 1992.

Cleaver JE, et al: A summary of mutations in the UV-sensitive disorders: Xeroderma pigmentosum, Cockayne syndrome, and trichothiodystrophy, *Hum Mutat* 14:9, 1999.

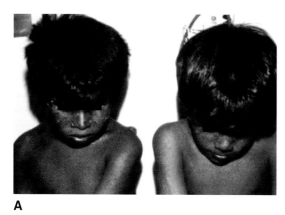

A

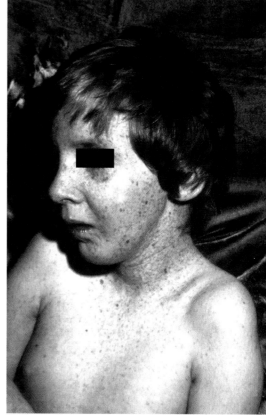

B

FIGURE 1. Xeroderma pigmentosa. **A,** Siblings with normal intelligence and light-sensitive xeroderma pigmentosa. **B,** Child with De Sanctis-Cacchione syndrome.

R

SENTER-KID SYNDROME
Ichthyosiform Erythroderma, Sensorineural Deafness

Initially reported by Burns in 1915, this disorder was further delineated by Senter and colleagues, who reported an affected child in 1978 and recognized 12 similar patients from the literature. Skinner and colleagues introduced the acronym KID (*k*eratitis, *i*chthyosis, *d*eafness) syndrome to highlight the principal features. Controversy exists as to whether ichthyosis is actually a feature of this disorder.

ABNORMALITIES

Hearing. Sensorineural deafness with onset documented from birth to 7 years, often profound.

Skin. Changes occurring at birth in the majority of cases described variably as dry, red, rough skin, erythematous and scaly skin, erythrodermia, and most commonly as erythrokeratodermia; within the first 3 months, the skin becomes thicker with a leathery appearance; well-demarcated, erythrokeratodermic, nonscaling plaques with an erythematous border develop in 89% of cases, predominantly located on the face, scalp, ears, elbows and knees; follicular keratosis commonly occurring over extensor surface of arms, scalp, and nose; spiky hyperkeratosis (hystrix-like ichthyosis) in some cases, palmoplantar hyperkeratosis.

Nails, Hair, Teeth. Variable nail dystrophy; variable malformations of teeth; sparse, fine hair involving scalp, eyebrows, and eyelashes.

Eyes. Corneal dystrophy manifested by progressive vascularization with photophobia and tearing leading to corneal destruction with the development of keratodermia (also called congenital ectodermal vascularizing keratitis, with a pannus of vascular or fibrotic tissue) progressing to occlusion of vision.

Other. Cryptorchidism; variable flexion contractures; oral abnormalities, including leukokeratosis, erythematous lesions, and scrotal tongue.

OCCASIONAL ABNORMALITIES
Ichthyosis secondary to hyperkeratotic plaques, porokeratotic eccrine duct and hair follicle nevus, squamous cell carcinoma of skin and tongue (10%), sebaceous carcinoma, deep furrows around the mouth, congenital alopecia, Hirschsprung disease, intellectual disability, tight heel cords, growth deficiency, decreased sweating, breast hypoplasia,

cochleosaccular abnormality of temporal bone, Dandy-Walker malformation.

NATURAL HISTORY

The corneal dystrophy, which occurs in 83% of patients, is the most serious aspect because it can lead to blindness. Lifelong ophthalmologic examinations are indicated. Corneal allografts are often followed by recurrence of the lesions. Early evaluation of hearing is necessary. Cochlear implants may be necessary. The combined vision and hearing loss may lead to severe intellectual disability. Retinoic acid derivatives have been used to improve the skin manifestations with some success. Mycotic and bacterial skin infections, as well as otitis media, conjunctivitis, and visceral infections (pneumonia, gastroenteritis, and sepsis), occur frequently. Rare fatal cases of severe recurrent infections with septicemia have been reported. These patients should undergo regular surveillance for mucosal carcinomas. MRI may also be indicated to detect cerebellar anomalies, although the reported cases have been associated with mild ataxia only.

ETIOLOGY

This disorder has an autosomal dominant inheritance pattern. Mutations in the *GJB2* gene that encodes the gap junction protein connexin 26 are responsible. Most cases are sporadic and thus represent a fresh gene mutation. A few cases of KID syndrome caused by parental germline mosaicism for the *GJB2* gene have also been described. Connexins are membrane proteins that are present in virtually all mammalian cells. Each connexin binds another connexin in an adjacent cell to form an intracellular communication channel known as a gap junction, which functions to allow rapid exchange of information between cells.

References

Burns FS: A case of generalized congenital erythroderma, *J Cutan Dis* 33:255, 1915.

Senter TP, et al: Atypical ichthyosiform erythroderma and congenital sensorineural deafness—a distinct syndrome, *J Pediatr* 92:68, 1978.

Cram DL, Resneck JS, Jackson WB: A congenital ichthyosiform syndrome with deafness and keratitis, *Arch Dermatol* 115:467, 1979.

Skinner BA, et al: The keratitis, ichthyosis, and deafness (KID) syndrome, *Arch Dermatol* 117:285, 1981.

Langer K, et al: Keratitis, ichthyosis and deafness (KID) syndrome: Report of three cases and a review of the literature, *Br J Dermatol* 122:689, 1990.

Nazzaro V, et al: Familial occurrence of KID (keratitis, ichthyosis, deafness) syndrome, *J Am Acad Dermatol* 23:385, 1990.

Caceres-Rios H, et al: Keratitis, ichthyosis, and deafness (KID syndrome): Review of the literature and proposal of a new terminology, *Pediatr Derm* 13:105, 1996.

R

van Steensel MA, et al: A novel connexin 26 mutation in a patient diagnosed with keratitis-ichthyosis-deafness syndrome, *J Invest Dermatol* 118:724, 2002.

Todt I, et al: Dandy-Walker malformation in patients with KID syndrome associated with a heterozygote mutation (p.Asp50Asn) in the *GJB2* gene encoding connexin 26, *Clin Genet* 76:404, 2009.

Haruna K, et al: Severe form of keratitis-ichthyosis-deafness (KID) syndrome associated with septic complications, *J Dermatol* 37:680, 2010.

Kaku Y, et al: Sebaceous carcinoma arising at a chronic candidiasis skin lesion of a patient with keratitis-ichthyosis-deafness (KID) syndrome, *Br J Dermatol* 166:222, 2012.

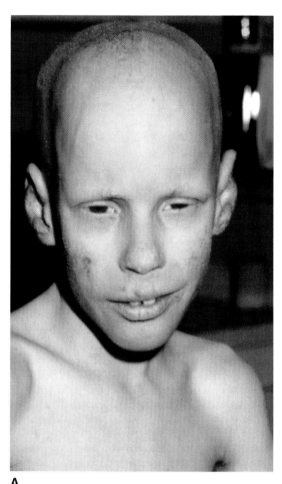

A

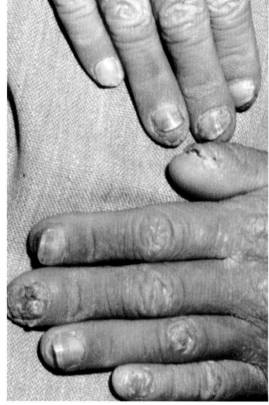

B

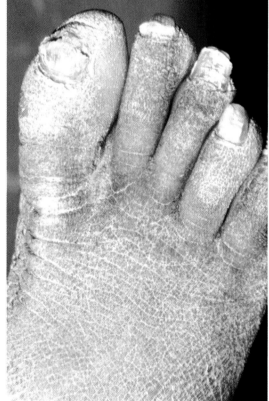

FIGURE 1. Senter syndrome. **A–C,** An 8-year-old child with alopecia, nail dystrophy, and lamellar ichthyosis. (From Senter TP, et al: *J Pediatr* 92:68, 1978, with permission.)

C

R

FETAL ALCOHOL SYNDROME
Prenatal Onset of Growth Deficiency, Microcephaly, Short Palpebral Fissures

In 1968, Lemoine of Nantes, France, recognized the multiple effects that alcohol can have on the developing fetus. Lemoine's report was not well accepted, and the disorder was independently rediscovered in 1973 by Jones et al and was referred to as fetal alcohol syndrome (FAS). In 1996, the Institute of Medicine (IOM) report suggested that prenatal alcohol exposure results in a spectrum of defects with FAS at the severe end followed by partial fetal alcohol syndrome (PFAS), alcohol-related birth defects (ARBD), and alcohol-related neurodevelopmental disorder (ARND) at the mildest end of the spectrum. To facilitate the practical applications of the criteria, Hoyme et al set forth a clarification of the IOM report in 2005, and in 2010 Jones et al extended the range of structural defects in order to provide a better appreciation of the total spectrum. The term *fetal alcohol spectrum disorders* (FASD) is now used to refer to that total spectrum of defects. Alcohol is now appreciated as the most common teratogen to which the fetus is liable to be exposed. Hence, it is of major public health concern as a teratogen.

ABNORMALITIES

Variable features from among the following:

Growth. Prenatal and postnatal onset of growth deficiency.

Performance. Average IQ of 65 with a range of 20 to 120; fine motor dysfunction manifested by weak grasp, poor eye-hand coordination, or tremulousness; irritability in infancy, hyperactivity in childhood. Problems with executive function, working memory, and spatial processing; poor impulse control, problems in social perception, deficits in higher level of receptive and expressive language.

Craniofacial. Mild-to-moderate microcephaly, short palpebral fissures, maxillary hypoplasia. Short nose, smooth philtrum with thin and smooth upper lip.

Skeletal. Joint anomalies, including abnormal position or function, altered palmar crease patterns, small distal phalanges, small fifth fingernails.

Cardiac. Heart murmur, frequently disappearing by 1 year of age; ventricular septal defect most common, followed by atrial septal defect.

OCCASIONAL ABNORMALITIES

Ptosis of eyelid, frank microphthalmia, cleft lip with or without cleft palate, micrognathia, protruding auricles, prominent ear crus extending from the root of the helix across the concha, mildly webbed neck, short neck, cervical vertebral malformations (10%–20%), rib anomalies, tetralogy of Fallot, coarctation of the aorta, strawberry hemangiomata, hypoplastic labia majora, short fourth and fifth metacarpal bones, decreased elbow pronation/supination, incomplete extension of one or more fingers. Other joint contractures, hockey stick palmar crease, meningomyelocele, hydrocephalus. Characteristic neuropathologic features, including abnormalities of the corpus callosum, volume reduction of the cranial, cerebral, and cerebellar vaults, particularly the parietal lobe, portions of the frontal lobe and the basal ganglia, although only the caudate is disproportionally reduced.

NATURAL HISTORY

There may be tremulousness in the early neonatal period. Postnatal linear growth tends to remain retarded, and the adipose tissue is thin. This often creates an appearance of "failure to thrive." These individuals tend to be irritable as young infants, hyperactive as children, and more social as young adults. Problems with dental malalignment and malocclusion, eustachian tube dysfunction, and myopia develop with time. Specific abnormalities have been documented on tests of language, verbal learning and memory, academic skills, fine-motor speed, and visual-motor integration. Poor school performance is the rule even in children with IQ scores within the normal range.

ETIOLOGY

The cause of this disorder is prenatal exposure to ethanol. The least significant effect recognized at two drinks per day has been slightly smaller birth size (approximately 160 g smaller than average). It is not until four to six drinks per day are consumed that additional subtle clinical features are evident. Most of the children believed to have fetal alcohol syndrome have been born to frankly alcoholic women whose intake is eight to ten drinks or more per day. The risk of a serious problem in the offspring of a chronically alcoholic woman has been estimated to be 30% to 50%, the greatest risk being for varying degrees of intellectual disability.

COMMENT

The most serious consequence of prenatal alcohol exposure is the problem of brain development and function. Although the severity of the maternal alcoholism and the extent and severity of the pattern of malformation seem to be most predictive of ultimate prognosis, typical neurobehavioral abnormalities are often seen in children prenatally exposed to alcohol with completely normal physical examinations.

References

Lemoine P, et al: Les enfants de parents alcooliques, *Ovest Med* 21:476, 1968.

Jones KL, et al: Pattern of malformation in offspring of chronic alcoholic mothers, *Lancet* 1:1267, 1973.

Jones KL, Smith DW: Recognition of the fetal alcohol syndrome in early infancy, *Lancet* 2:999, 1973.

Jones KL, et al: Outcome in offspring of chronic alcoholic women, *Lancet* 1:1076, 1974.

Clarren SK, Smith DW: The fetal alcohol syndrome: A review of the world literature, *N Engl J Med* 198:1063, 1978.

Streissguth AP, et al: Fetal alcohol syndrome in adolescents and adults, *JAMA* 265:1961, 1991.

Stratton KR, et al, editors: *Fetal alcohol syndrome: Diagnosis, epidemiology, prevention and treatment*, Washington DC, 1996, National Academy Press.

Jones KL: From recognition to responsibility: Josef Warkany, David Smith, and the fetal alcohol syndrome in the 21st century, *Birth Defects Res A Clin Mol Teratol* 67:13, 2003.

Hoyme HE, et al: A practical approach to diagnosis of fetal alcohol spectrum disorders: Clarification of the 1996 Institute of Medicine criteria, *Pediatrics* 115:39, 2005.

Guerri C, et al: Foetal alcohol spectrum disorders and alterations in brain development, *Alcohol and Alcoholism* 44:108, 2009.

Jones KL, et al: Fetal alcohol spectrum disorders: Extending the spectrum of structural defects, *Am J Med Genet* 152:2731, 2010.

S

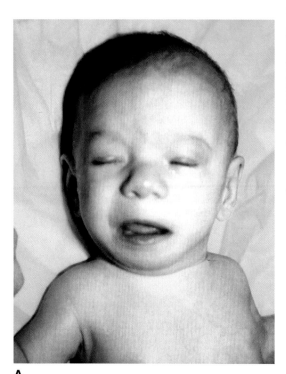

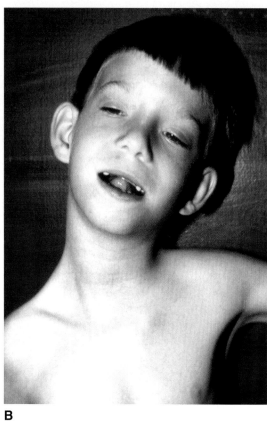

A   **B**

FIGURE 1.   Fetal alcohol syndrome. Affected children of women with chronic alcoholism. **A** and **B,** Same child at 4 months and 8 years of age. (**A** and **B,** From Jones KL: *Birth Defects Res A Clin Mol Teratol* 67:13, 2003, with permission.)

Continued

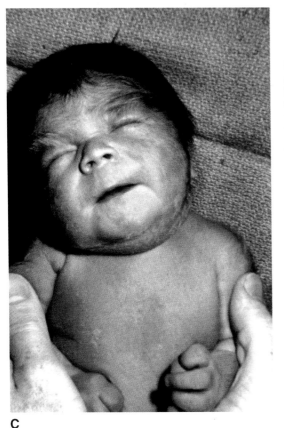

C

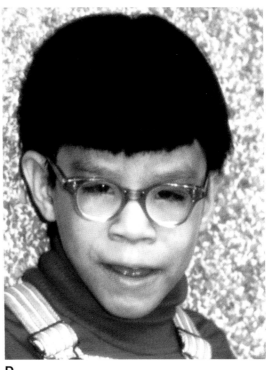

D

FIGURE 1, cont'd.   C and **D,** Same child at birth and at 4 years of age. Note the short palpebral fissures; long, smooth philtrum with smooth vermilion border; and hirsutism in the newborn. (**C** and **D,** From Jones KL, Smith DW: *Lancet* 2:999, 1973.)

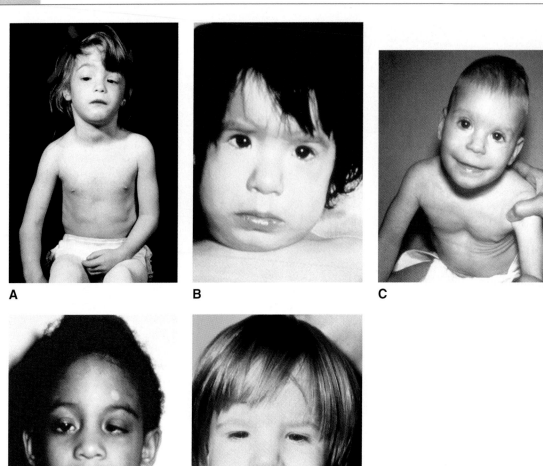

A   B   C

D   E

FIGURE 2. **A–E,** Note the short palpebral fissures; long, smooth philtrum; thin vermilion border; maxillary hypoplasia; and ptosis. (**A** and **C,** From Jones KL: *Birth Defects Res A Clin Mol Teratol* 67:13, 2003, with permission; **B, D,** and **E,** from Jones KL, Smith DW: *Lancet* 2:999, 1973.)

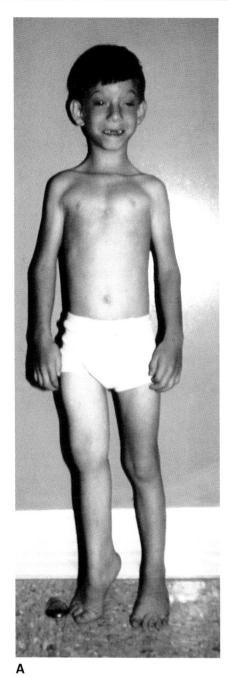

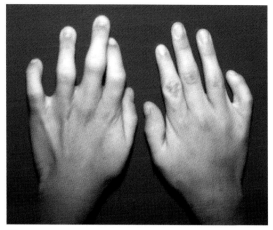

FIGURE 3.   **A,** Short right leg secondary to congenital hip dislocation. (From Jones KL: *Birth Defects Res A Clin Mol Teratol* 67:13, 2003.) **B,** Camptodactyly.

S

FETAL HYDANTOIN SYNDROME (FETAL DILANTIN SYNDROME)

Although data suggesting the possible teratogenic effects of anticonvulsants were first presented by Meadow in 1968, convincing epidemiologic evidence of the association between hydantoins and congenital abnormalities awaited the studies of Fedrick and of Monson and colleagues. Further studies by Speidel and Meadow and by Hill and colleagues revealed a pattern of malformation that may include digit and nail hypoplasia, unusual facies, and growth and mental deficiencies.

ABNORMALITIES

Varying combinations of the following, with the fetal hydantoin syndrome representing the broader, more severe end of the spectrum.

Growth. Mild-to-moderate growth deficiency, usually of prenatal onset, but may be accentuated in the early postnatal months.

Performance. Occasional borderline to mild intellectual disability; performance in childhood may be better than that anticipated from progress in early infancy.

Craniofacial. Wide anterior fontanel; metopic ridging; ocular hypertelorism; broad, depressed nasal bridge; short nose with bowed upper lip; broad alveolar ridge; cleft lip and palate.

Limbs. Stiff, tapered fingers; hypoplasia of distal phalanges with small nails, especially postaxial digits; low-arch dermal ridge patterning of hypoplastic fingertips; digitalized thumb; shortened distal phalanges and metacarpals and cone-shaped epiphyses; dislocation of hip.

Other. Short neck, rib anomalies, widely spaced small nipples, umbilical and inguinal hernias, pilonidal sinus, coarse profuse scalp hair, hirsutism, low-set hairline, abnormal palmar crease, strabismus.

OCCASIONAL ABNORMALITIES

Microcephaly, brachycephaly, positional foot deformities, strabismus, coloboma, ptosis, slanted palpebral fissures, webbed neck, pulmonary or aortic valvular stenosis, coarctation of aorta, patent ductus arteriosus, cardiac septal defects, single umbilical artery, pyloric stenosis, duodenal atresia, anal atresia, renal malformation, hypospadias, micropenis, ambiguous genitalia, cryptorchidism, symphalangism, syndactyly, terminal transverse limb defect, cleft hand, holoprosencephaly.

NATURAL HISTORY

It is not uncommon for infants to have relative failure to thrive during the early months; the reasons for this are unknown. Intellectual disability is of greatest concern and, for the most part, is borderline. In a group of 48 three-year-olds who had been prenatally exposed to hydantoin, mean IQ was 99 with a range from 94 to 104. Verbal abilities were lower than nonverbal abilities. However, no dose-response effect was noted.

ETIOLOGY

The cause of this disorder is prenatal exposure to phenytoin (Dilantin) or one of its metabolites. The risk of a hydantoin-exposed fetus having fetal hydantoin syndrome is approximately 10%. No dose-response curve has been demonstrated, and no "safe" dose has been found below which there is no increased teratogenic risk.

COMMENT

Similar craniofacial features referred to as the "anticonvulsant facies" are associated with prenatal exposure to carbamazepine, hydantoin, primidone, and phenobarbital. In addition, a 1% risk for meningomyelocele has been associated with prenatal exposure to carbamazepine. There is good evidence that exposure to a combination of the anticonvulsants (polytherapy) may increase the risk to the fetus. It has been suggested that the teratogenicity of these agents is associated with cardiac rhythm disturbances secondary to their propensity to inhibit a specific ion current (IKr) and subsequent hypoxic damage. IKr is critical for embryonic cardiac repolarization and rhythm regulation. Studies in early mouse embryo culture suggest that there is a greater risk for malformation in association with polytherapy than monotherapy and that the risk is linked to disturbances in cardiac rhythm.

References

Meadow SR: Anticonvulsant drugs and congenital abnormalities, *Lancet* 2:1296, 1968.

Aase JM: Anticonvulsant drugs and congenital abnormalities, *Am J Dis Child* 127:758, 1970.

Speidel BD, Meadow SR: Maternal epilepsy and abnormalities of the fetus and newborn, *Lancet* 2:839, 1972.

Fedrick J: Epilepsy and pregnancy: A report from the Oxford Record Linkage Study, *BMJ* 2:442, 1973.

Monson RR, et al: Diphenylhydantoin and selected congenital malformations, *N Engl J Med* 289:1049, 1973.

Hill RM, et al: Infants exposed in utero to antiepileptic drugs, *Am J Dis Child* 127:645, 1974.

Hanson JW, Smith DW: The fetal hydantoin syndrome, *J Pediatr* 87:285, 1975.

Hanson JW, et al: Risks to the offspring of women treated with hydantoin anticonvulsant, with emphasis on the fetal hydantoin syndrome, *J Pediatr* 89:662, 1976.

Phelen MC, et al: Discordant expression of fetal hydantoin syndrome in heteropaternal dizygotic twins, *N Engl J Med* 307:99, 1982.

Finnell RH, Chernoff GF: Editorial comment. Genetic background: The elusive component in the fetal hydantoin syndrome, *Am J Med Genet* 19:459, 1984.

Strickler SM, et al: Genetic predisposition to phenytoin-induced birth defects, *Lancet* 2:746, 1985.

Jones KL, et al: Pattern of malformation in the children of women treated with carbamazepine during pregnancy, *N Engl J Med* 320:1661, 1989.

Holmes LB, et al: The teratogenicity of anticonvulsant drugs, *N Engl J Med* 344:1132, 2001.

Holmes LB: The teratogenicity of anticonvulsant drugs: A progress report, *J Med Genet* 39:245, 2002.

Holmes LB, et al: The correlation of deficits in IQ with midface and digit hypoplasia in children exposed in utero to anticonvulsant drugs, *J Pediatr* 146:118, 2005.

Danielsson C, et al: Polytherapy with hERG-blocking antiepileptic drugs: Increased risk for embryonic cardiac arrhythmia and teratogenicity, *Birth Defects Res A Clin Mol Teratol* 79:595, 2007.

Meador KJ, et al: Cognitive function at 3 years of age after fetal exposure to antiepileptic drugs, *N Eng J Med* 360:1597, 2009.

Meador KJ, et al: Foetal antiepileptic drug exposure and verbal versus non-verbal abilities at three years of age, *Brain* 134:396, 2011.

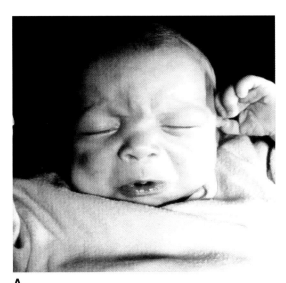

A

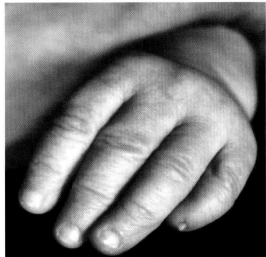

B

FIGURE 1.   Fetal hydantoin syndrome. **A** and **B,** A 3-month-old infant with growth and mental deficiencies whose mother took diphenylhydantoin throughout pregnancy. Note the hypoplastic nails and phalanges, and the relatively low and broad nasal bridge.

S

FETAL VALPROATE SYNDROME

Concern was raised regarding prenatal valproic acid exposure in 1982 by Robert and Guiband, who documented an association between maternal ingestion of valproic acid and meningomyelocele in the offspring. DiLiberti and colleagues and Hanson and colleagues set forth a broader pattern of malformation in 1984.

ABNORMALITIES

Performance. Delayed development. At 3 years of age, poor cognitive development; verbal abilities lower than nonverbal abilities.

Craniofacial. Narrow bifrontal diameter; high forehead; epicanthal folds connecting with an infraorbital crease or groove; telecanthus; broad, low nasal bridge with short nose and anteverted nostrils; midface hypoplasia; long philtrum with a thin vermilion border; relatively small mouth; micrognathia.

Cardiovascular. Aortic coarctation, hypoplastic left heart, aortic valve stenosis, interrupted aortic arch, secundum type atrial septal defect, pulmonary atresia without ventricular septal defect, perimembranous ventricular septal defect.

Limbs. Long, thin fingers and toes; small joint contractures; hyperconvex fingernails.

Other. Lumbosacral spina bifida, myopia.

OCCASIONAL ABNORMALITIES

Growth delay, brain atrophy, cyst of septum pellucidum, septo-optic dysplasia, esotropia, nystagmus, tear duct anomalies, microphthalmia, iris defects, cataracts, corneal opacities, cleft palate, hearing loss, supernumerary nipples, hemangiomas, pigmentary abnormalities, hypospadias, inguinal and umbilical hernias, omphalocele, broad chest, bifid rib, postaxial polydactyly, radial ray reduction defects, nail hypoplasia, preaxial defects of feet, triphalangeal thumbs, tracheomalacia, lung hypoplasia, laryngeal hypoplasia, renal hypoplasia.

NATURAL HISTORY

Increasing concern exists regarding the long-term cognitive effects of prenatal valproate exposure. A significant performance decline in motor functioning, adaptive functioning (as measured by parental ratings), and social skills, as well as an increased risk for attention-deficit disorders, has been documented. Behavioral problems are common, and many of the affected children require educational support. Monotherapy with valproate has been associated with significantly lower IQ than following monotherapy with other antiepileptic drugs. Polytherapy that includes valproate is associated with significantly lower cognitive abilities and greater risk for structural malformations.

ETIOLOGY

The cause of this disorder is prenatal valproic acid exposure.

References

Robert E, Guiband P: Maternal valproic acid and congenital neural tube defects, *Lancet* 2:934, 1982.

DiLiberti JH, et al: The fetal valproate syndrome, *Am J Med Genet* 19:473, 1984.

Hanson JW, et al: Effects of valproic acid on the fetus, *Pediatr Res* 18:306A, 1984.

Ardinger HH, et al: *Cardiac malformations associated with fetal valproic acid exposure*, Proc Greenwood Genet Center 5:162, 1986.

Jager-Roman E, et al: Fetal growth, major malformations, and minor anomalies in infants born to women receiving valproic acid, *J Pediatr* 108:997, 1986.

Sharony R, et al: Preaxial ray reduction defects as part of valproic acid embryofetopathy, *Prenat Diagn* 13:909, 1991.

Omtzigt JGC, et al: The risk of spina bifida aperta after first-trimester exposure to valproate in a prenatal cohort, *Neurology* 42(Suppl 5):119, 1992.

Kozma C, et al: Valproic acid embryopathy: Report of two siblings with further expansion of the phenotypic abnormalities and a review of the literature, *Am J Med Genet* 98:168, 2001.

Viinikainen K, et al: The effects of valproate exposure in utero on behavior and the need for educational support in school-aged children, *Epilepsy Behav* 9:636, 2006.

Meador KJ, et al: Cognitive function at 3 years of age after fetal exposure to antiepileptic drugs, *N Eng J Med* 360:1597, 2009.

Cohen MJ, et al: Fetal antiepileptic drug exposure: Motor, adaptive, and emotional/behavioral functioning at age 3 years, *Epilepsy Behav* 22:240, 2011.

Meador KJ, et al: Foetal antiepileptic drug exposure and verbal versus non-verbal abilities at three years of age, *Brain* 134:396, 2011.

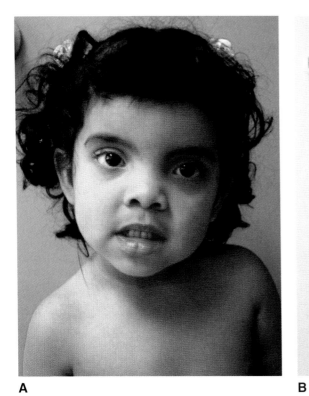
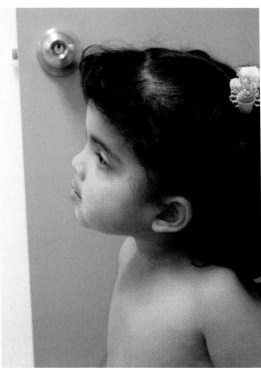

A   **B**

FIGURE 1.   Fetal valproate syndrome. **A** and **B,** A 3-year-old girl with high forehead, broad nasal bridge, short nose, anteverted nares, and long philtrum.

S

FETAL WARFARIN SYNDROME
(WARFARIN EMBRYOPATHY, FETAL COUMARIN SYNDROME)
Nasal Hypoplasia, Stippled Epiphyses, Coumarin Derivative Exposure in First Trimester

Isolated reports of infants who, in retrospect, were affected by warfarin were followed in 1975 by simultaneous recognition of this association in five infants. A number of infants are known to have been affected.

ABNORMALITIES

FOLLOWING PRENATAL EXPOSURE FROM 6 TO 9 WEEKS

Facies. Nasal hypoplasia and depressed nasal bridge, often with a deep groove between the alae nasi and nasal tip.

Skeletal. Stippling of uncalcified epiphyses, particularly of axial skeleton (vertebrae and pelvis), at the proximal femora and in the calcanei; stippling disappears after the first year.

Limbs. Hypoplastic distal phalanges that are shaped like inverted triangles with the apices pointing proximally.

Growth. Low birth weight; most demonstrate catch-up growth.

OCCASIONAL ABNORMALITIES

Choanal atresia, cleft lip and palate, lung hypoplasia, severe rhizomelia; scoliosis; congenital heart defect; vertebral anomalies, asplenia, renal agenesis, hypospadias. Structural defects of brain development.

NATURAL HISTORY

Infants often present with upper airway obstruction, which is relieved by the placement of an oral airway. Cervical spine abnormalities with resultant instability have led to severe neurologic dysfunction and even sudden death in some cases. The majority of affected children have done well with normal cognitive development except for persistent cosmetic malformation of the nose. The stippling is incorporated into the calcifying epiphyses and has resulted in few problems.

FOLLOWING PRENATAL EXPOSURE FROM 14 TO 20 WEEKS

Central Nervous System (CNS). Microcephaly, hydrocephalus, Dandy-Walker malformation, agenesis of corpus callosum, midline cerebellar atrophy, seizures and spasticity, intellectual disability, speech difficulties.

Eye. Optic atrophy, cataracts, microphthalmia, Peters anomaly.

Other. Intrauterine growth retardation, scoliosis, tethered skin in the sacrococcygeal region.

ETIOLOGY

This disorder is caused by prenatal exposure to the vitamin K antagonist warfarin (Coumarin, Coumadin). The critical period of exposure relative to the classic facial and skeletal features of the warfarin embryopathy is between 6 and 9 weeks' gestation. Since vitamin K–dependent clotting factors are absent at that time, another mechanism most likely related is the effect of coumadin on connective tissue proteins. In the majority of cases, CNS abnormalities and intellectual disability are associated with exposure limited to the second and third trimester likely as a consequence of disruption secondary to fetal hemorrhage (Judith G. Hall, personal communication). In addition, warfarin can lead to structural defects in CNS development following first-trimester exposure implying that it has a direct effect on CNS structural development as well. The incidence of warfarin-induced fetal complications has been estimated to be 6.4% of live births.

COMMENT

Two additional disorders with similar clinical features have been associated with disturbances of vitamin K metabolism. Both pseudo-warfarin embryopathy as the result of a defect of vitamin K epoxide reductase and severe maternal malabsorption resulting in fetal vitamin K deficiency are associated with a similar phenotype. In addition, identical clinical features are seen in X-linked recessive chondrodysplasia punctata (CDPX). In vitro studies have shown that warfarin inhibits arylsulfatase E (ARSE) activity, a deficiency of which is responsible for the clinical phenotype of X-linked recessive chondrodysplasia punctata, thus explaining the phenotypic similarity.

References

DiSaia PJ: Pregnancy and delivery of a patient with a Starr-Edwards mitral valve prosthesis: Report of a case, *Obstet Gynecol* 28:469, 1966.

Kerber IJ, Warr OS, Richardson C: Pregnancy in a patient with a prosthetic mitral valve, *JAMA* 203:223, 1968.

Becker MH, et al: Chondrodysplasia punctata: Is maternal warfarin a factor? *Am J Dis Child* 129:356, 1975.

Pettifor JM, Benson R: Congenital malformations associated with the administration of oral anticoagulants during pregnancy, *J Pediatr* 86:459, 1975.

Shaul WL, et al: Chondrodysplasia punctata and maternal warfarin use during pregnancy, *Am J Dis Child* 129:360, 1975.

Hall JG, et al: Maternal and fetal sequelae of anticoagulation during pregnancy, *Am J Med* 68:122, 1980.

Kaplan LC: Congenital Dandy Walker malformation associated with first trimester warfarin: A case report and literature review, *Teratology* 32:333, 1985.

Iturbe-Alessio I, et al: Risks of anticoagulant therapy in women with artificial heart valves, *N Engl J Med* 315:1390, 1986.

Francho B, et al: A cluster of sulfatase genes on Xp22.3: Mutations in chondrodysplasia punctata (CDPX) and implications for warfarin embryopathy, *Cell* 81:15, 1995.

Howe AM, et al: Severe cervical dysplasia and nasal cartilage calcification following prenatal warfarin exposure, *Am J Med Genet* 71:391, 1997.

Menger H, et al: Vitamin K deficiency embryopathy: A phenocopy of the warfarin embryopathy due to a disorder of embryonic vitamin K metabolism, *Am J Med Genet* 72:129, 1997.

Van Driel D, et al: Teratogen update: Fetal effects after in utero exposure to coumarins, overview of cases, follow-up findings, and pathogenesis, *Teratology* 66:127, 2002.

Raghav S, Reutens D: Neurological sequelae of intrauterine warfarin exposure, *J Clin Neuroscience* 14:99, 2007.

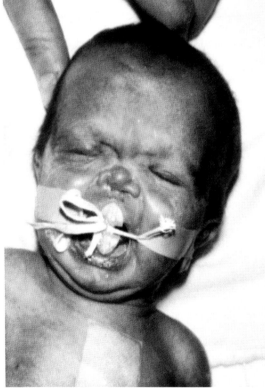

A

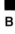

B

FIGURE 1.   Fetal warfarin syndrome. Patient at 5 days of age. **A,** Note hypoplastic nose with low nasal bridge and broad, flat face. **B,** Radiograph at 1 day of age showing stippling along the vertebral column, in the sacral area, and in the proximal femurs. Stippling was also noted in the cervical vertebrae, acromion process, and tarsal bones. (**A** and **B,** From Shaul WL, Emery H, Hall JG: *Am J Dis Child* 129:360, 1975, with permission.)

S

FETAL AMINOPTERIN/METHOTREXATE SYNDROME
Cranial Dysplasia, Broad Nasal Bridge, Low-Set Ears

The folic acid antagonist aminopterin has occasionally been used as an abortifacient during the first trimester of pregnancy. Thiersch first noted abnormal morphogenesis in three abortuses and one full-term offspring of mothers who received aminopterin from 4 to 9 weeks following the presumed time of conception. Subsequently, other cases have been published, including an account of teratogenicity secondary to methotrexate, the methyl derivative of aminopterin that is used for the treatment of rheumatoid arthritis and psoriasis and as an abortifacient. Methotrexate is commonly used for the treatment of ectopic pregnancy.

ABNORMALITIES

Growth. Prenatal onset of growth deficiency, microcephaly.

Craniofacial. Severe hypoplasia of frontal bone, parietal bones, temporal or occipital bones, wide fontanels, and synostosis of lambdoid or coronal sutures; upsweep of frontal scalp hair; broad nasal bridge, shallow supraorbital ridges, prominent eyes, micrognathia, low-set ears, maxillary hypoplasia, epicanthal folds.

Limbs. Relative shortness, especially of forearm (mesomelia), talipes equinovarus, hypodactyly, syndactyly.

OCCASIONAL ABNORMALITIES

Cleft palate, neural tube closure defect, intellectual disability, dislocation of hip, retarded ossification of pubis and ischium, rib anomalies, short thumbs, single crease on fifth finger, dextroposition of the heart, multicystic dysplastic kidney, hydronephrosis, vesicourethral reflux, congenital penile curvature, intestinal malrotation, hypotonia.

NATURAL HISTORY

Although fetal or early postnatal death does occur, a number of patients have survived beyond the first year of age. Postnatal growth deficiency occurs frequently. However, mental and motor performance, in most cases, has been described as normal.

ETIOLOGY

The cause of this disorder is prenatal exposure to aminopterin or methotrexate, its methyl derivative. Both are folic acid antagonists that inhibit dihydrofolate reductase, resulting in decreased production of purines and interference with normal DNA methylation. It has been suggested that a critical period for exposure exists at 6 through 8 weeks after conception and that a maternal methotrexate dose higher than 10 mg/week is necessary to produce defects in the fetus.

COMMENT

It has been suggested that high-dose methotrexate used prior to 6 weeks' gestation (4 post-conception weeks) for a misdiagnosis of ectopic pregnancy may be associated with a distinct syndrome, tetralogy of Fallot, and possibly other neural crest–related defects may be features of that pattern of malformation.

References

Thiersch JB: Therapeutic abortions with a folic acid antagonist, 4-aminopteroylglutamic acid (4-amino P.G.A.) administered by the oral route, *Am J Obstet Gynecol* 63:1298, 1952.

Milunsky A, et al: Methotrexate induced congenital malformations with a review of the literature, *J Pediatr* 72:790, 1968.

Shaw EB, Steinbach HL: Aminopterin-induced fetal malformation, *Am J Dis Child* 115:477, 1968.

Feldkamp M, Carey JC: Clinical teratology counseling and consultation case report: Low dose methotrexate exposure in the early weeks of pregnancy, *Teratology* 47:533, 1993.

Del Campo M, et al: Developmental delay in fetal aminopterin/methotrexate syndrome, *Teratology* 60:10, 1999.

Hyoun SC, et al: Teratogen update: Methotrexate, *Birth Defects Res A Clin Mol Teratol* 94:187, 2012.

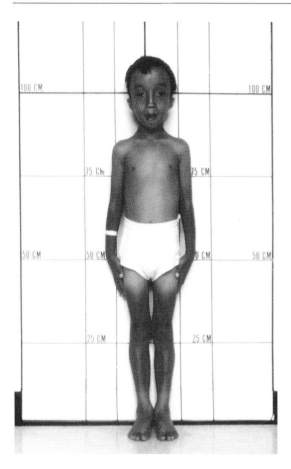

FIGURE 1. Fetal aminopterin syndrome. Note short stature, frontal bossing and prominent eyes secondary to flat supraorbital rim and maxillary hypoplasia.

RETINOIC ACID EMBRYOPATHY (ACCUTANE EMBRYOPATHY)
Central Nervous System Defects, Microtia, Cardiac Defects

First licensed in the United States in September 1982, with the brand name Accutane, isotretinoin (13-cis-retinoic acid) was initially recognized to be a human teratogen 1 year later. In 1985, Lammer and colleagues set forth the spectrum of structural defects. Of 21 affected infants, 17 had defects of the craniofacial area, 12 had cardiac defects, 18 had altered morphogenesis of the CNS, and 7 had anomalies of thymic development.

ABNORMALITIES

Craniofacial. Mild facial asymmetry, bilateral microtia or anotia with stenosis of the external ear canal, posterior helical pits, facial nerve paralysis ipsilateral to malformed ear, accessory parietal sutures, narrow sloping forehead, micrognathia, hair pattern abnormalities, flat depressed nasal bridge and ocular hypertelorism, abnormal mottling of teeth.

Cardiovascular. Conotruncal malformations, including transposition of the great vessels, tetralogy of Fallot, double-outlet right ventricle, truncus arteriosus communis, and supracristal ventricular septal defect; aortic arch interruption (type B); retroesophageal right subclavian artery; aortic arch hypoplasia; hypoplastic left ventricle.

Central Nervous System. Hydrocephalus; microcephaly; structural errors of cortical and cerebellar neuronal migration and gross malformations of posterior fossa structures, including cerebellar hypoplasia, agenesis of the vermis, cerebellar microdysgenesis, and megacisterna.

Performance. Subnormal range of intelligence.

Other. Thymic and parathyroid abnormalities.

OCCASIONAL ABNORMALITIES

Cleft palate, vestibular dysfunction, congenital oculomotor nerve synkinesis, cholesteatoma of the external auditory canal.

NATURAL HISTORY

Among the 21 affected infants evaluated by Lammer and colleagues, 3 were stillborn and 9 were liveborn infants who died secondary to cardiac defects, brain malformations, or combinations of the two. Information regarding the 9 affected infants who survived the neonatal period is unknown. However, in a study designed to determine natural history, 19% of 31 prospectively ascertained 5-year-old children prenatally exposed to isotretinoin had a full-scale IQ less than 70, and an additional 28% had IQs between 71 and 85. Although each of the 5 patients whose IQ was less than 70 had major malformations, 6 of the 10 patients with an IQ in the borderline range did not have major malformations, indicating that the lack of major structural abnormalities does not necessarily predict normal intellectual performance. Of further potential significance, when evaluated at 10 years of age, reduced general mental ability remained, with the effect more pronounced in males than females.

ETIOLOGY

The cause of this disorder is prenatal exposure to isotretinoin (Accutane). A 35% risk for the isotretinoin embryopathy exists in the offspring of women who continue to take isotretinoin beyond the fifteenth day following conception. There have been no affected babies born to women who stopped taking isotretinoin before the fifteenth day following conception. Furthermore, there is no evidence to suggest that maternal use of the drug before conception is teratogenic. Daily dosage of isotretinoin from 0.5 to 1.5 mg/kg of maternal body weight is thought to be teratogenic.

COMMENT

Despite programs to prevent pregnancy in females of childbearing potential taking isotretinoin—such as the iPLEDGE program mandated by the FDA—no evidence is available indicating their effectiveness.

References

Rosa FW: Teratogenicity of isotretinoin, *Lancet* 2:513, 1983.

Fernoff PM, Lammer EJ: Craniofacial features of isotretinoin embryopathy, *J Pediatr* 105:595, 1984.

Lott IT, et al: Fetal hydrocephalus and ear anomalies associated with maternal use of isotretinoin, *J Pediatr* 105:597, 1984.

Lammer EJ, et al: Retinoic acid embryopathy, *N Engl J Med* 313:837, 1985.

Lammer EJ, et al: Risk for major malformations among human fetuses exposed to isotretinoin (13-cis-retinoic acid), *Teratology* 35:68A, 1987.

Teratology Society: Recommendations for isotretinoin use in women of childbearing potential, *Teratology* 44:1, 1991.

Adams J, Lammer EJ: Neurobehavioral teratology of isotretinoins, *Reprod Toxicol* 7:175, 1993.

Adams J, et al: Neuropsychological characteristics of children embryologically exposed to isotretinoin (Accutane): Outcome at age 10, *Neurotoxicol Teratol* 23:297, 2001.

McCaffery PJ, et al: Too much of a good thing: Retinoic acid as an endogenous regulator of neural differentiation and exogenous teratogen, *Eur J Neurosci* 18:457, 2003.

Morrison DG, et al: Congenital oculomotor nerve synkinesis associated with fetal retinoid syndrome, *J AAPOS* 9:166, 2005.

Van Abel M, et al: Development of canal cholesteatoma in a patient with prenatal isotretinoin exposure, *Int J Pediatr Otorhinolaryngol* 74:1082, 2010

Shi J, et al: The impact of the iPLEDGE program on isotretinoin fetal exposure in an integrated health care system, *J Am Acad Dermatol* 65:1117, 2011.

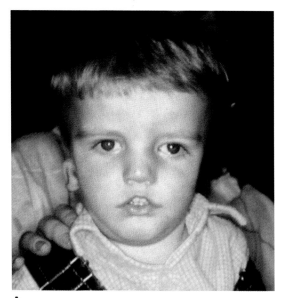

A

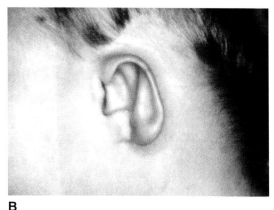

B

FIGURE 1. Retinoic acid embryopathy. **A** and **B,** A 2½-year-old boy showing triangular facies, ocular hypertelorism, downslanting palpebral fissures, and malformed external ear. (**A** and **B,** Courtesy of Dr. Edward Lammer, Children's Hospital, Oakland, Calif.) **C,** More severely affected neonate with hydrocephalus and microtia. (**C,** Courtesy of Dr. Cynthia Curry, University of California, San Francisco.)

C

S

METHIMAZOLE/CARBIMAZOLE EMBRYOPATHY

In 1972, Milham and Elledge first raised concern regarding the teratogenicity of methimazole based on the observation that 2 of 11 newborns with midline scalp defects ascertained in Washington State by birth certificate report and physician questionnaire were born to women treated with methimazole (MMI) for the treatment of hyperthyroidism during pregnancy. Subsequently Clementi et al suggested that prenatal MMI exposure was associated with a recognizable pattern of malformations. Identical features have been associated with prenatal exposure to carbimazole (CBZ) which is converted to MMI after absorption.

ABNORMALITIES

Performance. Developmental delay in 60%.
Craniofacial. Large anterior fontanel; short upslanting palpebral fissures; epicanthal folds; sparse, arched eyebrows; broad nasal bridge; hypoplastic alae nasi; overfolded helices of small ears.
Cardiac. Ventricular septal defect, overriding aorta.
Gastrointestinal. Esophageal atresia, tracheoesophageal fistula.
Other. Aplasia cutis congenita of scalp, iris/retinal coloboma, choanal atresia. athelia/hypothelia.

OCCASIONAL ABNORMALITIES

Macrocephaly, anisocoria, mild sensorineural hearing loss, cleft palate, bifid uvula, prominent columella and nasal tip, short nasal tip, renal pelvis ectasia, persistent vitelline duct, omphalocele, imperforate anus, absent gall bladder, nail hypoplasia.

NATURAL HISTORY

Death occurred in four cases at, or prior to, 3 months of age. These included three neonates who died following surgery for tracheoesophageal fistula and esophageal atresia and one 3-month-old who died of apparent Sudden Infant Death Syndrome (SIDS). Although developmental delay is a feature of the embryopathy, normal intellectual performance has been noted in children who were prenatally exposed to MMI or CBZ but who lacked the physical features of the MMI/CBZ embryopathy.

ETIOLOGY

The cause of MMI/CBZ embryopathy is first-trimester exposure to MMI or CBZ. It has been suggested that the critical window for exposure is between the third and the ninth gestational week. A prospective study of pregnancy outcome in 241 prenatally ascertained women with first-trimester exposure to MMI or CBZ has been reported. There was no increase in the overall rate of malformations. However, there was one case of choanal atresia and one case of esophageal atresia confirming the increased risk for these structural defects following prenatal exposure to these drugs.

References

Milham S, Elledge W: Maternal methimazole and congenital defects in children, *Teratology* 5:125, 1972.

Clementi M, et al: Methimazole embryopathy: Delineation of the phenotype, *Am J Med Genet* 83:43, 1999.

Di Gianantonio E, et al: Adverse effects of prenatal methimazole exposure, *Teratology* 64:262, 2001.

Clementi M, et al: Treatment of hyperthyroidism in pregnancy and birth defects, *J Clin Endocrinol Metab* 95:E337, 2010.

Gripp KW, et al: Grade 1 microtia, wide anterior fontanel and novel type tracheo-esophageal fistula in methimazole embryopathy, *Am J Med Genet* 155:526, 2011.

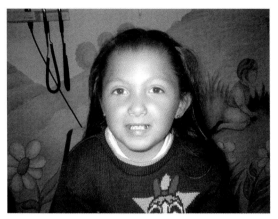

FIGURE 1. Methimazole embryopathy. Note macrocephaly, sparse eyebrows, prominent columella, and nasal tip.

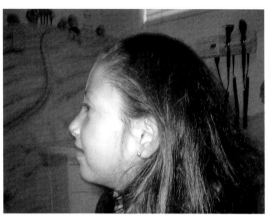

FIGURE 2. Note short nose, prominent columella, hypoplastic alae nasi, and overfolded ears.

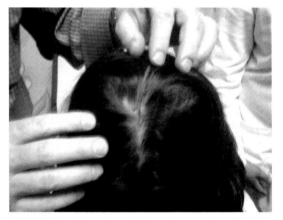

FIGURE 3. Note the aplasia cutis congenita of scalp.

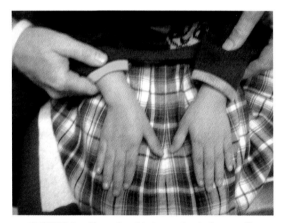

FIGURE 4. Note the thin hypoplastic fingernails.

S

MYCOPHENOLATE MOFETIL EMBRYOPATHY

Initial concern regarding the teratogenicity of mycophenolate mofetil (MMF) in humans was raised by Sifontis et al in 2006 based on data from the National Transplantation Pregnancy Registry. Pérez-Aytés et al first suggested that prenatal exposure to this drug was associated with a recognizable pattern of malformations. Nineteen cases of this disorder have been published.

ABNORMALITIES

Facies. Cleft lip with or without cleft palate; thick, everted lower lip; microtia with aural atresia; micrognathia; ocular hypertelorism; arched eyebrows.

Limbs. Hypoplastic finger and toenails, bilateral shortened fifth fingers.

Cardiac. Conotruncal defects, aortic arch defects.

OCCASIONAL ABNORMALITIES

Agenesis of corpus callosum, developmental delay, colobomatous orbital cyst with microphthalmia, iris and/or retinal coloboma, ptosis, bifid nose, pre-auricular skin tags, cleft palate, brachydactyly, polydactyly, hemivertebrae, scoliosis, hypoplastic scapula, tracheoesophageal fistula, pelvic kidney, renal agenesis, diaphragmatic hernia, pulmonary artery sling, ventricular septal defect with anterior aorta, intestinal malformation, single umbilical artery.

NATURAL HISTORY

Although spontaneous abortion is increased and prematurity has occurred in the majority of liveborn cases, it is unclear if either relates to the underlying disease or to prenatal MMF exposure. Most affected children have had normal development. Hearing impairment is the rule.

ETIOLOGY

Prenatal exposure to MMF, an immunosuppressant used to prevent rejection after organ transplantation as well as for treatment of autoimmune disease. It is a reversible inhibitor of inosine monophosphate dehydrogenase, which blocks purine synthesis in T- and B-cell lymphocytes. A study including 57 prospectively ascertained first-trimester cases of prenatal exposure to MMF has recently been published which raises serious concern regarding the prevalence of this disorder in prenatally exposed offspring. There were 16 spontaneous abortions, 12 elective abortions (2 of which had multiple malformations consistent with the MMF embryopathy), and 29 liveborn infants. Six of the 29 liveborn infants had major malformations, including 2 with external auditory canal atresia, 1 with tracheo-esophageal fistula, one with hydronephrosis, 1 with an atrial septal defect, and 1 with an occipital meningocele.

References

Sifontis NM, et al: Pregnancy outcomes in solid organ transplant recipients with exposure to mycophenolate mofetil or sirolimus, *Transplantation* 82:1698, 2006.

Pérez-Aytés A, et al: In utero exposure to mycophenolate mofetil: A characteristic phenotype? *Am J Med Genet A* 146A:1, 2008.

Jackson P, et al: Intrauterine exposure to mycophenolate mofetil and multiple congenital anomalies in a newborn: Possible teratogenic effect, *Am J Med Genet A* 149A:1231, 2009.

Lin AE, et al: An additional patient with mycophenolate mofetil embryopathy: Cardiac and facial analysis, *Am J Med Genet A* 155A:748, 2011.

Hoeltzenbein M, et al: Teratogenicity of mycophenolate confirmed in a prospective study of the European Network of Teratology Information Services, *Am J Med Genet A* 158A:588, 2012.

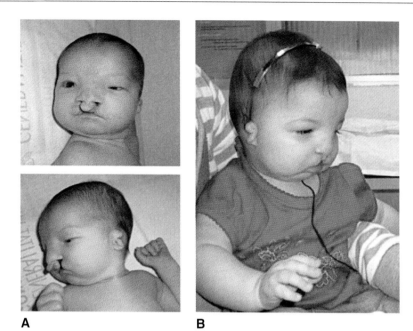

A   **B**

FIGURE 1. **A,** Newborn with hypertelorism, ptosis of the left eyelid, upper bilateral cleft lip, micrognathia, microtia and absence of the external auditory canal. **B,** Infant at 9 months of age. The cleft lip has been surgically repaired. (From Pérez-Aytés A, *Am J Med Genet A* 146A:1, 2008, with permission).

FETAL VARICELLA SYNDROME
Cicatricial Skin, Limb Hypoplasia, Intellectual Disability with Seizures

LaForet and Lynch first described defects in the child of a woman who had varicella during early gestation. Strabstein and colleagues summarized five cases. Many additional cases have been reported.

ABNORMALITIES

Performance. Intellectual disability with or without seizures, autonomic instability.
Growth. Variable prenatal growth deficiency, microcephaly.
Eyes. Chorioretinitis.
Limbs. Hypoplasia with or without rudimentary digits, with or without paralysis, and atrophy of limb; clubfoot.
Skin. Cutaneous scars, cicatricial lesions, hypopigmentation.

OCCASIONAL ABNORMALITIES

Cataracts; microphthalmia; atrophy and hypoplasia of optic disk; anisocoria; nystagmus; Horner syndrome; cardiovascular defects; underdeveloped clavicle, scapula, and rib; scoliosis; hydronephrosis.

NATURAL HISTORY

Fifty percent of affected babies have died in early infancy. Although it has previously been suggested that the majority of the survivors have had intellectual disability with seizures, prospective studies indicate that a wide spectrum of severity exists for this disorder. One of the two affected patients reported by Jones and colleagues had mild cutaneous scars on the face, arms, and legs, a left Horner syndrome, a retinal scar, and normal IQ. Autonomic dysfunction including neurogenic bladder, hydroureter, and esophageal dilatation and reflux leading to pneumonia, and anal/vesicle sphincter dysfunction.

ETIOLOGY

Most cases have occurred in the wake of maternal varicella during the period of 13 to 20 weeks' gestation. The incidence of problems in the offspring of women infected with varicella before the twentieth week of pregnancy is between 1% and 2%. The occurrence of the fetal varicella syndrome following maternal infection from 20 to 28 weeks has only rarely been reported.

COMMENT

Children born to women infected with varicella-zoster virus during pregnancy and who do not have the structural features characteristic of the fetal varicella syndrome are not neurodevelopmentally different from unexposed, uninfected control children.

References

LaForet EG, Lynch CL Jr: Multiple congenital defects following maternal varicella, *N Engl J Med* 236:534, 1947.

Strabstein JC, et al: Is there a congenital varicella syndrome? *J Pediatr* 64:239, 1974.

Higa K, et al: Varicella-zoster virus infections during pregnancy: Hypothesis concerning the mechanisms of congenital malformations, *Obstet Gynecol* 69:214, 1987.

Lambert SR, et al: Ocular manifestations of the congenital varicella syndrome, *Arch Ophthalmol* 107:52, 1989.

Jones KL, et al: Offspring of women infected with varicella during pregnancy: A prospective study, *Teratology* 49:29, 1994.

Mouly F, et al: Prenatal diagnosis of fetal varicella-zoster virus infection with polymerase chain reaction of amniotic fluid in 107 cases, *Am J Obstet Gynecol* 177:894, 1997.

Mattson SN, et al: Neurodevelopmental follow-up of children of women infected with varicella during pregnancy: A prospective study, *Pediatr Infect Dis J* 22:819, 2003.

Tan MP, Koren G: Chickenpox in pregnancy: Revisited, *Reprod Toxicol* 21:419, 2006.

Smith CK, Arvin AM: Varicella in the fetus and newborn, *Reprod Toxicol* 14:209, 2009.

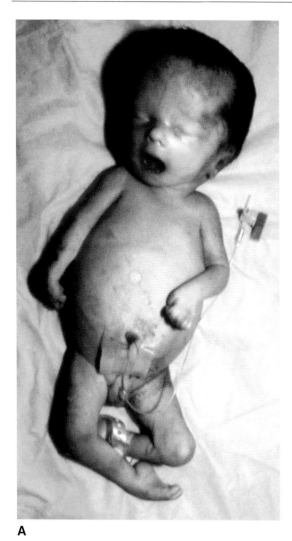

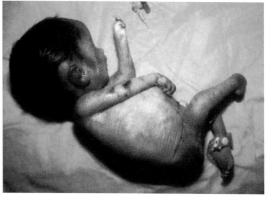

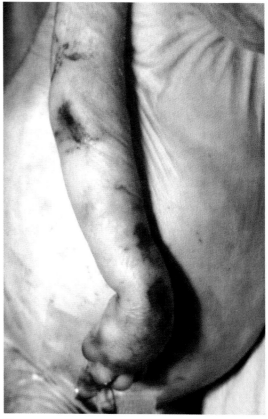

FIGURE 1. Fetal varicella syndrome. **A–C,** Note the hydrocephalus, short limbs with severe neurologic compromise, and cicatricial skin changes in limbs.

S

HYPERTHERMIA-INDUCED SPECTRUM OF DEFECTS

A number of animal studies, the most extensive of which have been those of Edwards on the guinea pig, have shown that severe maternal hyperthermia during the first one third to one half of gestation is teratogenic.

Although studies in the human are limited, problems of growth, development, and dysfunction of the brain similar to those seen in the animal studies have been documented. The nature of the defects relates to the timing and extent of the hyperthermia rather than to its cause. Most of the relevant cases have been tentatively related to febrile illness, with the patient having a temperature of 38.9°C or higher, most commonly 40°C or above. The duration of the high fever has been 1 day or more, usually several days, which is unusual in the first third of gestation. The illness has varied, with influenza, pyelonephritis, and streptococcal pharyngitis being the most common. Two cases were considered secondary to severe hyperthermia induced by prolonged sauna bathing (30–45 minutes), and one case was thought to be related to very prolonged hot tub bathing. It has been recommended that women of reproductive age who have a possibility of being pregnant limit hot tub exposure to less than 15 minutes in 39°C water and less than 10 minutes in 40°C water.

Retrospective human studies of more than 170 cases of neural tube defect, including anencephaly, meningomyelocele, and occipital encephalocele, have disclosed an overall history of maternal hyperthermia during the week of neural tube closure (21–28 days) in approximately 10% of the cases, whereas no such history was determined in the controls. These findings are compatible with the hypothesis that hyperthermia is one cause for neural tube defects in the human.

A 14% incidence of "febrile" illness during early pregnancy in the mothers of 113 embryos with neural tube defects who were aborted therapeutically was documented. The embryos were obtained through the Congenital Anomaly Research Center of Kyoto University. The history of maternal fever was documented before or immediately after the fetal loss, before the neural tube defect was documented.

In addition, a number of craniofacial anomalies, including microcephaly, small midface, microphthalmia, micrognathia, and occasionally cleft lip with or without palate, cleft palate alone, conotruncal heart defects, and ear anomalies, as well as intellectual disabilities, autism, and hypotonia have been reported. Of importance, the fever-associated autism risk was decreased among mothers who took antipyretics.

A single prospective study involving 115 pregnant women who reported a fever of 38.9°C or higher lasting for at least 24 hours (group 1), 147 pregnant women who reported fever of either less than 38.9°C or lasting less than 24 hours (group 2), and 289 pregnant women who reported no fever (group 3) has been reported. The combined prevalence of all major structural malformations was increased but not significantly so in those women in group 1. However, 2 of 34, or 5.9%, of women in group 1 who had a high fever during the critical period for neural tube closure carried fetuses with anencephaly, compared to none in groups 2 and 3. In addition, the specific craniofacial anomalies previously documented in retrospective studies were found more frequently in the offspring of pregnant women in group 1. Reports of Moebius sequence, oromandibular-limb hypogenesis syndrome, and amyoplasia congenita disruption sequence in association with maternal hyperthermia in the second trimester of pregnancy point to a vascular etiology for some hyperthermia-related defects and suggest that not all adverse outcomes are limited to first-trimester exposure.

In addition to potential dysmorphogenesis in early gestation, maternal hyperthermia has been associated with an increase in spontaneous abortion, stillbirth, and prematurity.

References

Edwards MJ: Congenital defects in guinea pigs following induced hyperthermia during gestation, *Arch Pathol* 84:42, 1967.

Edwards MJ: Congenital defects in guinea pigs: Prenatal retardation of brain growth of guinea pigs following hyperthermia during gestation, *Teratology* 2:239, 1969.

Edwards MJ: The experimental production of arthrogryposis multiplex congenita in guinea pigs by maternal hyperthermia during gestation, *J Pathol* 104:221, 1971.

Chance PI, Smith DW: Hyperthermia and meningomyelocele and anencephaly, *Lancet* 1:769, 1978.

Halperin LR, Wilroy RS: Maternal hyperthermia and neural tube defects, *Lancet* 2:212, 1978.

Miller P, et al: Maternal hyperthermia as a possible cause of anencephaly, *Lancet* 1:519, 1978.

Smith DW, et al: Hyperthermia as a possible teratogenic agent, *J Pediatr* 92:878, 1978.

Clarren SK, et al: Hyperthermia—a prospective evaluation of a possible teratogenic agent in man, *J Pediatr* 95:81, 1979.

Shiota K: Neural tube defects and maternal hyperthermia in early pregnancy: Epidemiology in a human embryo population, *Am J Med Genet* 12:281, 1982.

Milunsky A, et al: Maternal heat exposure and neural tube defects, *JAMA* 268:882, 1992.

Lynberg MC: Maternal flu, fever and the risk of neural tube defects: A population based case-control study, *Am J Epidemiol* 140:244, 1994.

Graham JM, et al: Teratogen update: Gestational effects of maternal hyperthermia due to febrile illnesses and resultant patterns of defects in humans, *Teratology* 58:209, 1998.

Chambers CD, et al: Maternal fever and birth outcome: A prospective study, *Teratology* 58:251, 1998.

Shaw GM, et al: Maternal periconceptional vitamins: Interactions with selected factors and congenital anomalies? *Epidemiology* 13:625, 2002.

Chambers CD: Risks of hyperthermia associated with hot tub or spa use by pregnant women, *Birth Defects Res A Clin Mol Teratol* 76:569, 2006.

Zerbo O, et al: Is maternal influenza or fever during pregnancy associated with autism or developmental delays? Results from the CHARGE (CHildhood Autism Risks from Genetics and Environment) study, *J Autism Dev Disord* 43:25, 2013.

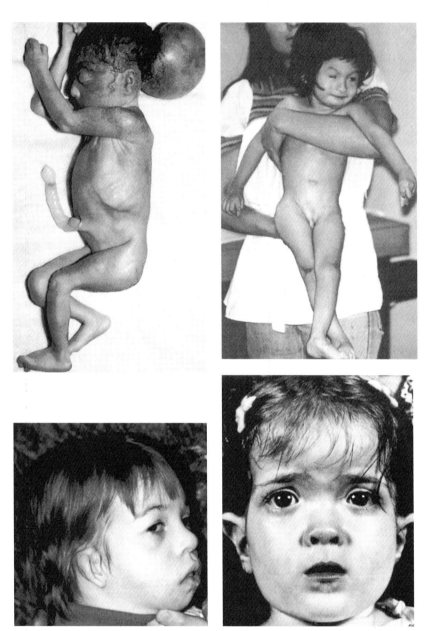

FIGURE 1. Hyperthermia-induced defects. *Upper left,* Encephalocele; maternal history of high fever between days 23 and 25 of gestation. *Upper right,* An 18-month-old severely retarded boy with hypotonic diplegia, micropenis, unilateral microphthalmia, cleft palate, and micrognathia. Maternal fever of 40°C to 41°C between the fourth and fifth weeks of gestation. *Lower left,* A 12-year-old severely retarded girl with hypotonic diplegia, midface hypoplasia, micrognathia, incomplete ear morphogenesis, and a cardiac defect. Maternal "flu" with high fever between the sixth and eighth weeks of gestation. *Lower right,* A 14-month-old infant with moderate hypotonic diplegia and developmental deficiency, who has a hypoplastic midface with mild ocular hypertelorism, low nasal bridge, and prominent auricles. Maternal fever of 40°C between the seventh and eighth weeks of gestation. (*Lower right,* from Pleet H, Graham JM Jr, Smith DW: *J Pediatr* 67:785, 1981, with permission.)

S

Miscellaneous Syndromes

COFFIN-SIRIS SYNDROME
Hypoplastic to Absent Fifth Finger and Toenails, Coarse Facies

Coffin and Siris reported three patients with this disorder in 1970, and Weiswasser and colleagues reported an additional case in 1973. Also, several of the patients described by Senior might represent examples of this syndrome. More than 100 cases have been reported.

ABNORMALITIES

Growth. Prenatal onset of mild-to-moderate growth deficiency, delayed bone age.

Performance. Moderate-to-severe intellectual disability, severe speech impairment, moderate-to-severe hypotonia, seizures, autistic features.

Craniofacial. Mild microcephaly, coarse facies, a wide mouth with full lips, flat nasal bridge, broad nasal tip, anteverted nares, long philtrum, abnormal ears, bushy eyebrows, long eyelashes, periorbital fullness, ptosis, high palate.

Limbs. Hypoplastic to absent fifth finger and toenails, with lesser hypoplasia in other digits; absence of terminal phalanges (particularly of the fifth digit); lax joints with radial dislocation at elbow; coxa valga; small patellae.

Hair. Hypertrichosis with tendency to have sparse scalp hair, low posterior hairline.

Other. Visual problems, hearing loss, abnormal/delayed dentition, congenital heart defects (patent ductus arteriosus, ventricular septal defect, atrial septal defect, tetralogy of Fallot, patent foramen ovale with aberrant pulmonary vein), recurrent infections.

OCCASIONAL ABNORMALITIES

Ptosis of eyelids, hypotelorism, macroglossia, absent tear ducts, preauricular skin tag, choanal atresia, cleft palate, hemangioma, cryptorchidism, umbilical or inguinal hernias, short sternum, gastrointestinal anomalies (gastric and duodenal ulcer, neonatal intussusception, intestinal malrotation, gastric outlet obstruction secondary to redundant gastric mucosa), short forearm, vertebral anomalies, kyphosis, scoliosis, diaphragmatic hernia, Dandy-Walker anomaly of brain, hypoplasia or partial agenesis of corpus callosum, small cerebellum, simplified gyral pattern, and in one patient abnormal olivae and arcuate nuclei and cerebellar heterotopias, renal anomalies (hydronephrosis, microureters with stenosis of the vesicoureteral junction, ectopic kidney), genital anomalies, including cryptorchidism, hypospadias, and absent uterus, hypoglycemia, premature thelarche.

NATURAL HISTORY

The degree of facial dysmorphism is variable, with some patients exhibiting obvious coarseness and others with only mild facial features. Feeding problems and recurrent upper and lower respiratory tract infections are frequent during early life. Onset of speech is severely delayed. The coarse facies may not be present at birth. The sparse scalp hair improves with age.

ETIOLOGY

De novo heterozygous mutations in *ARID1B* mapping to 6q25 as well as *SMARCB1* mapping to 22q11 have been identified in several individuals with Coffin-Siris syndrome (CSS) by exome sequencing. These genes encode subunits of the switch/sucrose nonfermenting (SWI/SNF) complex, which acts as an epigenetic modifier by altering chromatin structure, thereby facilitating the access of transcription factors to DNA. The study of these and other genes encoding for other subunits of this complex in a larger group of patients led to the identification of mutations in one of six SWI/SNF subunit genes, which are *SMARCB1, SMARCA4, SMARCA2, SMARCE1, ARID1A,* and *ARID1B,* in 20 out of 23 individuals (87%) with CSS. Interestingly, some of the patients lacked some typical CSS abnormalities, such as hypoplastic or absent fingernails or toenails. Deletions in *ARID1B* detected by array comparative genomic hybridization have also been reported in individuals with corpus callosum agenesis, developmental delay with severe speech impairment, autism, and only incomplete phenotypic features of CSS. This marked clinical variability and its correlation with specific genotypes needs to be further investigated. All mutations identified to date follow an autosomal dominant inheritance pattern, although autosomal recessive inheritance remains suspected, based on several sibling pairs born to unaffected parents.

COMMENT

Nicolaides-Baraitser syndrome (see Figure 1E), first described in 1993, includes sparse hair, facial features similar to those seen in CSS short stature, microcephaly, brachydactyly, interphalangeal joint, swellings, epilepsy, and intellectual disability with marked language impairment. This condition has marked phenotypic similarities to the Coffin-Siris syndrome, and the two conditions have been proven allelic. Mutations in *SMARCA2* have been found in more than 80% of patients with Nicolaides-Baraitser syndrome; the type and location of the mutations most likely do not impair the SWI/SNF complex assembly but may be associated with disrupted ATPase activity.

References

Coffin GS, Siris E: Mental retardation with absent fifth fingernail and terminal phalanx, *Am J Dis Child* 119:433, 1970.

Senior B: Impaired growth and onychodysplasia: Short children with tiny toenails, *Am J Dis Child* 122:7, 1971.

Carey JC, Hall BD: The Coffin-Siris syndrome, *Am J Dis Child* 132:667, 1978.

DeBassio WA, Kemper TL, Knoefel JE: Coffin-Siris syndrome: Neuropathologic findings, *Arch Neurol* 42:350, 1985.

Bodurtha J, et al: Distinctive gastrointestinal anomaly associated with Coffin-Siris syndrome, *J Pediatr* 109:1015, 1986.

Levy P, Baraitser M: Coffin-Siris syndrome, *J Med Genet* 28:338, 1991.

T

Swillen A, et al: The Coffin-Siris syndrome: Data on mental development, language, behavior and social skills in 12 children, *Clin Genet* 48:177, 1995.

McGhee EM, et al: Candidate region for Coffin-Siris syndrome at 7q32-34, *Am J Med Genet* 93:241, 2000.

Fleck BJ, et al: Coffin-Siris syndrome: Review and presentation of new cases from a questionnaire study, *Am J Med Genet* 99:1, 2001.

Coulibaly B, et al: Coffin-Siris syndrome with multiple congenital malformations and intrauterine death: Towards a better delineation of the severe end of the spectrum, *Eur J Med Genet* 53:318, 2010.

Schrier SA, et al: The Coffin-Siris syndrome: A proposed diagnostic approach and assessment of 15 overlapping cases, *Am J Med Genet A* 158A:1865, 2012.

Santen GW, et al: Mutations in SWI/SNF chromatin remodeling complex gene *ARID1B* cause Coffin-Siris syndrome, *Nat Genet* 44:379, 2012.

Tsurusaki Y, et al: Mutations affecting components of the SWI/SNF complex cause Coffin-Siris syndrome, *Nat Genet* 44:376, 2012.

Van Houdt JK, et al: Heterozygous missense mutations in *SMARCA2* cause Nicolaides-Baraitser syndrome, *Nat Genet* 44:445, 2012.

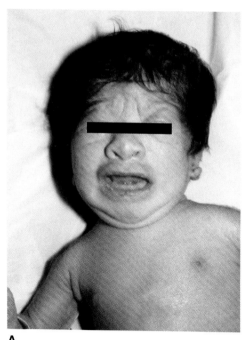

A

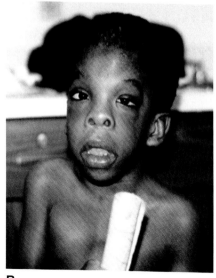

B

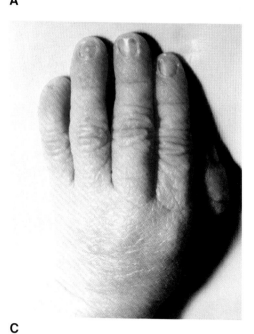

C

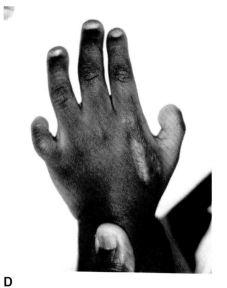

D

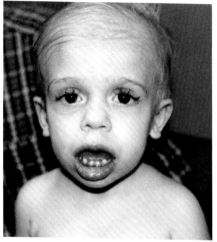

E

FIGURE 1. Coffin-Siris syndrome. **A–D,** Note the coarse face, wide mouth with full lips, long eyelashes, and hypoplastic fifth fingernails. **E,** Nicolaides-Baraitser syndrome. Note the marked similarities to Coffin-Siris syndrome including the sparse hair, coarse face, wide mouth with full lips and long eyelashes.. (**B, D,** and **E,** Courtesy Dr. D. Bryan Hall, University of Kentucky, Lexington.)

BÖRJESON-FORSSMAN-LEHMANN SYNDROME
Large Ears, Hypogonadism, Severe Mental Deficiency

In 1961, Börjeson and colleagues described an entity of X-linked intellectual disability, epilepsy, hypogonadism, obesity, and dysmorphic facies seen in three related males and three of their less severely affected female relatives.

ABNORMALITIES

Growth. Height usually less than 50th percentile, rarely below 3rd percentile. Moderate obesity beginning in adolescence, may decrease in later life,

Performance. Moderate-to-severe intellectual disability, with an IQ of 10 to 40, but milder cases have been reported; supraspinal hypotonia; markedly abnormal electroencephalograph, with very poor alpha rhythms; seizures may be present.

Craniofacial. Head circumference is usually normal, but macrocephaly or microcephaly can occur. Coarse facies with prominent supraorbital ridges and deep-set eyes, large (7.5–9 cm) but normally formed ears.

Eyes. Nystagmus, ptosis, and poor vision, with a variety of retinal or optic nerve abnormalities.

Genitalia. Small penis with small and soft or undescended testes and delayed secondary sexual characteristics; hypogonadism appears to be hypogonadotropic.

Skeletal. Thick calvarium, small cervical spinal canal, mild scoliosis, kyphosis, Scheuermann-like vertebral changes, metaphyseal widening of the long bones and hands, hypoplastic distal and middle phalanges, thin cortices.

Other. Central nervous system (CNS) anomalies due to a primary abnormality of neuronal migration, soft and fleshy hands with tapering fingers, broad feet with short and/or flexed toes, gynecomastia/lipomastia, panhypopituitarism.

NATURAL HISTORY

From birth, these patients are hypotonic, with severe developmental delay. Walking may begin as late as 4 to 6 years and remains awkward. Speech is limited to a few phrases at most. Behavior is usually friendly but can be challenging and aggressive. The characteristic facial appearance becomes apparent in late childhood, concomitant with the onset of obesity. There is no known unusual susceptibility to health problems, although bronchopneumonia was responsible for the demise of two of the original patients at the ages of 20 and 44 years. Life span is presumed to be normal. A sheltered environment is necessary because of severe limitations of neurodevelopmental performance.

ETIOLOGY

This disorder has an X-linked recessive inheritance pattern. Mutations of plant homeodomain (PHD)-like finger gene (*PHF6*) located at Xq26-27 are responsible. *PHF6* is a zinc-finger gene of unknown function, but a role of the protein in chromatin remodeling has been suggested. Heterozygote females fall into a spectrum of those without any observable features to those with the abnormalities of growth and craniofacial, ocular, and skeletal features characteristic of this syndrome. Performance ranges from moderate intellectual disability (IQ 56–70) to above-average intelligence in heterozygous females. The degree of skewing of X-inactivation is not correlated with the severity of the phenotype. Large deletions have been seen only in females.

References

Börjeson M, Forssman H, Lehmann O: An X-linked, recessively inherited syndrome characterized by grave mental deficiency, epilepsy, and endocrine disorder, *Acta Med Scand* 171:13, 1962.

Börjeson M, Forssman H, Lehmann O: *Combination of idiocy, epilepsy, hypogonadism, dwarfism, hypometabolism, and morphologic peculiarities inherited as an X-linked recessive syndrome. Proceedings of the Second International Congress on Mental Retardation, Vienna (1961), Part I*, Basel, 1963, Karger Publishers, p 188.

Brun A, Börjeson M, Forssman H: An inherited syndrome with mental deficiency and endocrine disorder: A patho-anatomical study, *J Ment Defic Res* 18:317, 1974.

Robinson LK, et al: The Börjeson-Forssman-Lehmann syndrome, *Am J Med Genet* 15:457, 1983.

Ardinger HH, Hanson JW, Zellweger HU: Börjeson-Forssman-Lehmann syndrome: Further delineation in five cases, *Am J Med Genet* 19:653, 1984.

Lower KM, et al: Mutations in *PHF6* are associated with Börjeson-Forssman-Lehmann syndrome, *Nat Genet* 32:661, 2002.

Turner G, et al: The clinical picture of the Börjeson-Forssman-Lehmann syndrome in males and heterozygous females with *PHF6* mutations, *Clin Genet* 65:226, 2004.

Visootsak J, et al: Clinical and behavioral features of patients with Börjeson-Forssman-Lehmann syndrome with mutations in *PHF6*, *J Pediatr* 145:819, 2004.

de Winter CF, et al: Behavioural phenotype in Börjeson-Forssman-Lehmann syndrome, *J Intellect Disabil Res* 53:319, 2009.

Carter MT, et al: Further clinical delineation of the Börjeson-Forssman-Lehmann syndrome in patients with *PHF6* mutations, *Am J Med Genet A* 149A:246, 2009.

Berland S, et al: *PHF6* deletions may cause Börjeson-Forssman-Lehmann syndrome in females, *Mol Syndromol* 1:294, 2011.

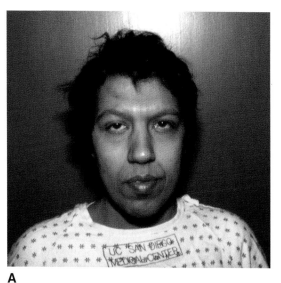
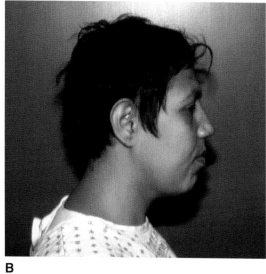

A   **B**

FIGURE 1.   Börjeson-Forssman-Lehmann syndrome. **A** and **B,** A man with coarse face, prominent supraorbital ridges, ptosis, and large ears. (From Robinson LK, et al: *Am J Med Genet* 15:487, 1983.)

ALAGILLE SYNDROME (ARTERIOHEPATIC DYSPLASIA)
Cholestasis, Peripheral Pulmonic Stenosis, Peculiar Facies

Initially described by Alagille and colleagues in 1969, this disorder was more completely delineated in 1973 by Watson and Miller, who reported five families with 21 affected individuals. Since then, hundreds of cases have been described. Males and females are affected equally.

ABNORMALITIES

General. Growth retardation (50%).

Craniofacial. Typical facies (95%) consisting of deep-set eyes, broad forehead, long straight nose with flattened tip, prominent pointed chin, small, low-set or malformed ears.

Eyes. Posterior embryotoxon (abnormal prominence of the Schwalbe line, the line formed by the junction of the Descemet membrane with the uvea at the anterior chamber angle causing the margin of the cornea to be opaque) in 88%, Axenfeld anomaly (iris strands).

Cardiac. Right-sided defects or pulmonary circulation defects; 67% have peripheral pulmonary artery stenosis with or without associated complex cardiovascular abnormalities, particularly tetralogy of Fallot.

Skeletal. Butterfly-like vertebral arch defects (87%); other vertebral defects, including hemivertebrae and spina bifida occulta; rib anomalies.

Hepatic. Paucity of intrahepatic interlobular bile ducts (85%), chronic cholestasis (96%), hypercholesterolemia.

OCCASIONAL ABNORMALITIES

General. Mild intellectual disability (16%).

Eyes. Retinal degeneration, including chorioretinal involvement and pigmentary clumping, strabismus, ectopic pupils, choroidal folds, anomalous optic disk or vessels, and refractive errors.

Cardiac. Atrial septal defect, ventricular septal defect, patent ductus arteriosus, coarctation of the aorta.

Vascular. Neurovascular accidents (15%); anomalies of the basilar, carotid, and middle cerebral arteries; and Moyamoya syndrome. Renovascular anomalies, middle aortic syndrome, hypertension.

Hands. Short distal phalanges, fifth-finger clinodactyly.

Liver. Extrahepatic biliary duct involvement (20%), primary hepatocellular cancer.

Renal. Structural abnormalities (39%), including renal dysplasia, small hyperechoic kidney, ureteropelvic obstruction, renal cysts. Functional abnormalities (74%), including renal tubular acidosis, decreased creatinine clearance, increased blood urea nitrogen, histologic abnormalities consisting of mesangiolipidosis.

Genitalia. Hypogonadism.

Endocrine. Decreased growth hormone, increased testosterone, hypothyroidism, delayed puberty.

Other. Cleft palate, shortened ulna, spina bifida occulta, lack of normal increase in interpedicular distance from L1–L5, abnormalities of inner ear structures, clubfeet, craniosynostosis, increased risk of pathologic early fractures (particularly of lower limbs), thyroid cancer, high-pitched voice, hypodontia, palatal and gingival xanthomas, radioulnar synostosis, pancreatic insufficiency.

NATURAL HISTORY

Most patients present with neonatal jaundice. Cholestasis (elevated serum bile acids), which develops within the first 3 months in 44% and between 4 months and 3 years in the remainder, is manifested by pruritus, acholic stools, xanthomata, or hepatomegaly. Intrahepatic bile duct paucity is often progressive but may not be evident in newborns. Progression to cirrhosis and liver failure occurs in many. Transplantation is required in 15%. Long-term prognosis depends on severity and duration of early cholestasis, severity of cardiovascular defects, liver status as it relates to liver failure or portal hypertension, and occurrence of intracranial bleed. The 20-year predicted life expectancy is 75% for all patients, 80% for those not requiring liver transplantation, and 60% for those who require liver transplantation.

ETIOLOGY

This disorder has an autosomal dominant inheritance pattern with highly variable expressivity. Mutations in JAG1 located within chromosome band 20p12 are responsible in 89% of cases. Less than 7% have a deletion of the entire JAG1 gene. More than half are de novo mutations. Less than 1% have mutations in a second gene, NOTCH2; no clear phenotypic differences are known to be clearly related to the gene involved. Classic diagnostic criteria combine the presence of bile duct paucity with at least three of five systems affected: liver, heart, skeleton, eye, and dysmorphic facies. However, mutations in JAG1 are found in one third of patients presenting with only one or two clinical features, especially if the heart (2% tetralogy of Fallot, 4% peripheral pulmonic stenosis) or liver is affected. JAG1 encodes for a cell surface protein that is a ligand for the Notch transmembrane receptor. JAG1 and Notch are parts of the Notch signaling pathway, which is critical for the regulation of cell fate decisions.

References

Alagille D, et al: L'atrésie des voies biliaires intrahépatiques avec voies biliaires extrahépatiques perméables chez l'enfant, *J Par Pediatr* 301, 1969.

Watson GH, Miller V: Arteriohepatic dysplasia: Familial pulmonary arterial stenosis with neonatal liver disease, *Arch Dis Child* 48:459, 1973.

Alagille D, et al: Hepatic ductular hypoplasia associated with characteristic facies, vertebral malformations, retarded physical, mental and sexual development, and cardiac murmur, *J Pediatr* 86:63, 1975.

Byrne JL, et al: Del(20p) with manifestations of arteriohepatic dysplasia, *Am J Med Genet* 24:673, 1986.

Alagille D, et al: Syndromic paucity of interlobular bile ducts (Alagille syndrome or arteriohepatic dysplasia): Review of 80 cases, *J Pediatr* 110:195, 1987.

Spinner NB, et al: Cytogenetically balanced t(2;20) in a two-generation family with Alagille syndrome: Cytogenetic and molecular studies, *Am J Hum Genet* 55:238, 1994.

Emerick KM, et al: Features of Alagille syndrome in 92 patients: Frequency and relation to prognosis, *Hepatology* 29:822, 1999.

Krantz I, et al: Clinical and molecular genetics of Alagille syndrome, *Curr Opin Pediatr* 11:558, 1999.

Kamath BM, et al: Vascular anomalies in Alagille syndrome: A significant cause of morbidity and mortality, *Circulation* 109:1354, 2004.

Bales CB, et al: Pathologic lower extremity fractures in children with Alagille syndrome, *J Pediatr Gastroenterol Nutr* 51:66, 2010.

Kamath BM, et al: *NOTCH2* mutations in Alagille syndrome, *J Med Genet* 49:138, 2012.

Guegan K, et al: *JAG1* mutations are found in approximately one third of patients presenting with only one or two clinical features of Alagille syndrome, *Clin Genet* 82:33, 2012.

T

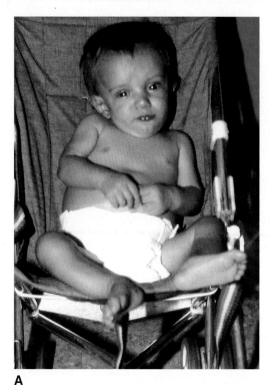

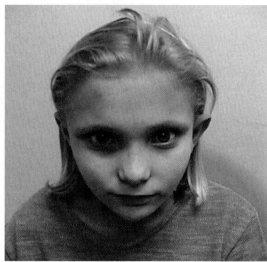

B

A

FIGURE 1.   Alagille syndrome. **A,** A 1½-year-old with broad forehead and prominent chin. **B–E,** Note the deep-set eyes; broad forehead; long, straight nose with flattened tip and prominent chin.

Continued

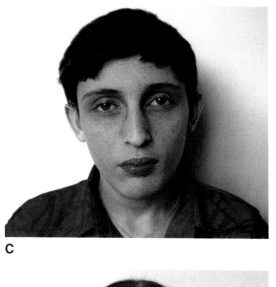

C

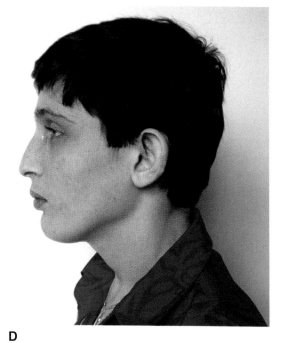

D

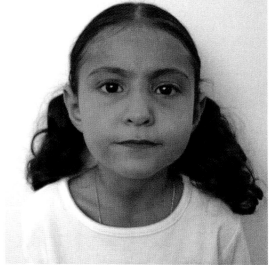

E

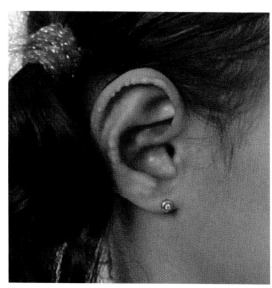

F

FIGURE 1, cont'd. F, Note the xanthomas over the ear. (B–F, Courtesy Dr. Ian Krantz, University of Pennsylvania.)

T

MELNICK-NEEDLES SYNDROME
Prominent Eyes, Bowing of Long Bones, Ribbon-Like Ribs

This disorder was reported by Melnick and Needles in 1966, and subsequently more than 50 cases have been documented.

ABNORMALITIES

Growth. Short stature, with some exceptions.

Craniofacial. Small facies with prominent hirsute forehead with apparent craniofacial disproportion, exophthalmos, prominent lateral margins of the supraorbital ridges, mild hypertelorism, full cheeks, small mandible with an obtuse angle and hypoplastic coronoid process, late closure of fontanels, thickening of calvarium and dense base of skull, lag in paranasal sinus development, micrognathia, malaligned teeth, oligohypodontia.

Limbs. Short upper arms, long fingers and toes.

Imaging. Relatively small thoracic cage with irregular ribbon-like ribs and short clavicles with wide medial ends and narrow shoulders; bowing of humerus, radius, ulna, and tibia; diaphyseal cortical irregularity; metaphyseal flaring of long bones; coxa valga; genu valgum; mild distal phalangeal hypoplasia and cone-shaped epiphyses; undermodeling of the phalanges, metacarpals, and metatarsals; short scapulae; and pectus excavatum; tall vertebrae with anterior concavity in thoracic and lumbar regions; pelvic hypoplasia with supra-acetabular constriction; iliac flaring; kyphoscoliosis; joint subluxations.

OCCASIONAL ABNORMALITIES

Sensorineural or conductive deafness with ossicular or cochlear malformation; strabismus, coarse hair, cleft palate, large ears, hoarse voice, ureteral stenosis leading to hydronephrosis, hip dislocation, clubfeet, pes planus, delayed motor development, short stature, muscle hypotonia, limitations of elbow extension, acro-osteolysis, mitral and tricuspid valve prolapse, hyperlaxity of skin in males.

NATURAL HISTORY

Small face with prominent and hyperteloric-appearing eyes. Abnormal gait and bowing may be the first evident signs of the disorder. Dental malocclusion is frequent, and with time, osteoarthritis of the back or hip may become a problem. A contracted pelvis in the female may make vaginal delivery difficult. Some affected females die in the second or third decade from respiratory failure, and frequent respiratory infections occur, due to the small thoracic cage. Pulmonary hypertension has occurred.

ETIOLOGY

This disorder has an X-linked dominant inheritance pattern. The vast majority of cases have been female with variable expression even within families. Mutations in the gene *FLNA*, which encodes filamin A, a protein that regulates reorganization of the actin cytoskeleton, are responsible. The majority of patients have had one of the three most common mutations found within exon 22. All mutations causing the disorder are presumed to cause a gain of function of the gene product, by increasing the affinity of filamin A for actin. Early lethality and a much more severe phenotype have been documented in males that were born to affected mothers. Characteristic features in males include widely spaced, prominent eyes; severe micrognathia; omphalocele; hypoplastic kidneys; positional deformities of the hands and feet; cervicothoracic kyphosis; thoracolumbar lordosis; bowing of the long bones; and pseudoarthrosis of the clavicles. Severe respiratory failure leads to death prenatally or shortly after birth.

COMMENT

In addition to Melnick-Needles syndrome, gain-of-function mutations in *FLNA* are responsible for oto-palato-digital syndrome, types I (OPDI) and II (OPDII) and frontometaphyseal dysplasia, disorders with overlapping clinical phenotypes, which have been referred to as the OPD spectrum disorders.

References

Melnick JC, Needles CF: An undiagnosed bone dysplasia, *Am J Roentgenol Radium Ther Nucl Med* 97:39, 1966.

Coste F, Maroteaux P, Chouraki L: Osteoplasty (Melnick-Needles syndrome), *Ann Rheum Dis* 27:360, 1968.

von Oeyen P, et al: Omphalocele and multiple severe congenital anomalies associated with osteodysplasty (Melnick-Needles syndrome), *Am J Med Genet* 13:453, 1982.

Krajewska-Walasek M, et al: Melnick-Needles syndrome in males, *Am J Med Genet* 27:153, 1987.

Eggli K, et al: Melnick-Needles syndrome: Four new cases, *Pediatr Radiol* 22:257, 1992.

Robertson S, et al: Are Melnick-Needles syndrome and oto-palato-digital syndrome type II allelic? Observations in a four-generation kindred, *Am J Med Genet* 71:341, 1997.

Verloes A, et al: Fronto-otopalatodigital osteodysplasia: Clinical evidence for a single entity encompassing Melnick-Needles syndrome, otopalatodigital syndrome types 1 and 2, and frontometaphyseal dysplasia, *Am J Med Genet* 90:407, 2000.

Kristiansen M, et al: Phenotypic variation in Melnick-Needles syndrome is not reflected in X inactivation patterns from blood or buccal smear, *Am J Med Genet* 108:120, 2002.

Robertson SP, et al: Localized mutations in the gene encoding the cytoskeletal protein filamin A cause diverse malformations in humans, *Nat Genet* 33:487, 2003.

Robertson SP: Otopalatodigital syndrome spectrum disorders: Otopalatodigital syndrome types 1 and 2, frontometaphyseal dysplasia and Melnick-Needles syndrome, *Eur J Hum Genet* 15:3, 2007.

Foley C, et al: Expansion of the spectrum of *FLNA* mutations associated with Melnick-Needles syndrome, *Mol Syndromol* 1:121, 2010.

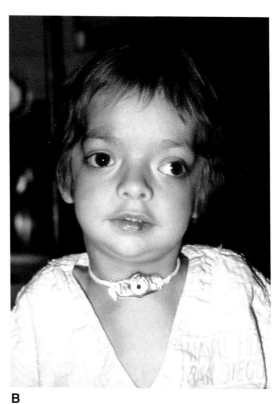

B

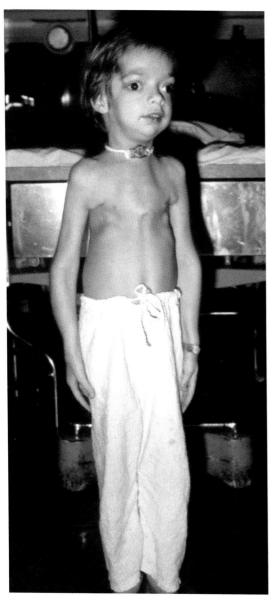

A

FIGURE 1.   Melnick-Needles syndrome. **A** and **B,** Note the exophthalmos, hypertelorism, full cheeks, small mandible, and relatively small thorax. (Courtesy Dr. William Nyhan, University of California, San Diego.)

BARDET-BIEDL SYNDROME
Retinal Pigmentation, Obesity, Polydactyly

The variable manifestations of this syndrome were initially described by Bardet and Biedl in the 1920s. Subsequently, more than 500 cases have been reported. This disorder is clearly different from the condition described in 1865 by Laurence and Moon, although it was referred to as the Laurence-Moon-Biedl syndrome in the third edition of this book.

ABNORMALITIES

Growth. Obesity (83%) with the majority below the 50th percentile for height.

Performance. Slow development of expressive speech, poor articulation. Intellectual disability with verbal IQ of 79 or below in 77% and performance IQ of 79 or below in 44%; IQ correlates with visual handicap. Ataxia, poor coordination. Mental illness or significantly altered behavior and shallow affect are common.

Craniofacial. Macrocephaly, bitemporal narrowing, large ears, short and narrow palpebral fissures, long philtrum, low nasal bridge, short nose, midfacial hypoplasia, and mild retrognathia.

Ocular. Retinal rod-cone dystrophy (100%), myopia (75%), astigmatism (63%), nystagmus (52%), glaucoma (22%), posterior capsular cataracts (44%), mature cataracts or aphakia (30%), typical retinitis pigmentosa (8%).

Limbs. Postaxial polydactyly (58%) of hands, feet, or both, unilateral or bilateral; syndactyly; brachydactyly of hands (50%); broad, short feet.

Kidney. Nephronophthisis, including abnormal calyces (95%), communicating cysts or diverticula (62%), fetal lobulations (95%), diffuse cortical loss (29%), focal scarring (24%).

Genitalia. In males, small penis and testes (88%), hypospadias, chordee, cryptorchidism. In females, partial and complete vaginal atresia; septate vagina; duplex uterus; hydrometrocolpos; vesicovaginal fistula; hypoplastic fallopian tubes, uterus, and ovaries.

OCCASIONAL ABNORMALITIES

Cardiac defects, dental anomalies, unilateral renal agenesis and urologic anomalies, imperforate anus, esophageal atresia with tracheoesophageal fistula, diabetes mellitus, diabetes insipidus, clinodactyly of the fifth finger, cystic dilatation of the intrahepatic and common bile ducts, hepatic fibrosis, hirsutism, hearing loss, Hirschsprung disease.

NATURAL HISTORY

The average age at diagnosis is 9 years. Obesity begins to develop at approximately 2 to 3 years of age. The intellectual disability is usually mild to moderate. However, significant behavioral problems occur in 33%, including immaturity, frustration, disinhibition, and poor concentration/hyperactivity. Schizophrenia has been described in some cases. Ataxia, poor coordination, and imbalance are common. The retinal dystrophy is atypical in that the macula is affected early and generally results in problems with night vision during childhood, constricted visual fields, abnormalities of color vision, and extinguished or minimal rod-and-cone responses on electroretinography. Visual acuity deteriorates with age. Approximately 15% of patients show an atypical retinal pigmentation by 5 to 10 years of age. However, by age 20, 73% of patients are blind. Most patients have mild problems in renal function with partial defects in urine concentration and renal tubular acidosis. Renal failure occurs, requiring transplant in only 4%. Hypertension is present in 60%. The hypogonadism has been described as primary germinal hypoplasia and as hypogonadotropic in type. Although only two males have fathered children, females have often given birth to children. Normal development of secondary sexual characteristics is the rule in women, but vaginal and uterine malformations may be present. Irregular menstrual periods are common. Asthma has occurred in 25% of cases. An increased prevalence of renal malformations and renal cell carcinoma has been described in unaffected relatives of affected individuals.

ETIOLOGY

Mutations in 17 independent Bardet-Biedl syndrome (BBS) genes have been identified. The known genes account for 80% of cases. Targeted high-throughput sequencing of all causal genes is an efficient method for molecular testing due to the high genetic heterogeneity. Bardet-Biedl syndrome results primarily from ciliary dysfunction during development. The previously held concept that Bardet-Biedl syndrome is a Mendelian recessive disorder may be too simplistic because, in at least some cases (<10%), two mutations in one BBS gene and a third mutation in another BBS gene are required for manifestation of the clinical phenotype (oligogenic triallelic inheritance). From a practical standpoint, recurrence risk for unaffected parents who have had one affected child is 25%.

COMMENT

The gene for BBS6 (*MKKS*), located on chromosome 20p12, encodes chaperonins and is also responsible for McKusick-Kaufman syndrome, a disorder strikingly similar to Bardet-Biedl syndrome with overlapping features including vaginal atresia, cardiac defects, and postaxial polydactyly but lacking intellectual disability, obesity, retinal dystrophy, and deterioration of renal function. Significant difficulty exists differentiating between the two disorders prior to 3 to 5 years of age. At that age, obesity, retinal dystrophy, and intellectual disability begin to manifest in Bardet-Biedl syndrome. Mutations in several BBS genes are also responsible for Meckel-Gruber syndrome, Joubert syndrome, Senior-Loken syndrome, and Leber congenital amaurosis. All of these conditions are considered disorders of ciliary function and are referred to as ciliopathies.

References

Bardet G: Sur un syndrome d'obésité infantile avec polydactylie et rétinite pigmentaire. (Contribution à l'étude des formes cliniques de l'obésité hypophysaire.) *Faculté de Medicine de Paris, Thesis* 470, 1920.

Biedl A: Ein Geschwisterpaar mit adiposo-genitaler Dystrophie, *Dtsch Med Wochenschr* 48:1630, 1922.

McKusick VA, et al: Hydrometrocolpos as a simply inherited malformation, *JAMA* 189:813, 1964.

Kaufman RL, et al: Family studies in congenital heart disease II: A syndrome of hydrometrocolpos, postaxial polydactyly and congenital heart disease, *Birth Defects Orig Artic Ser* 8(5):85, 1972.

Hurley RM, et al: The renal lesion of the Laurence-Moon-Biedl syndrome, *J Pediatr* 87:206, 1975.

Green JS, et al: The cardinal manifestations of Bardet-Biedl syndrome: A form of Laurence-Moon-Biedl syndrome, *N Engl J Med* 321:1002, 1989.

Elbedour K, et al: Cardiac abnormalities in the Bardet-Biedl syndrome: Echocardiographic studies of 22 patients, *Am J Med Genet* 52:164, 1994.

Beales PL, et al: New criteria for improved diagnosis of Bardet-Biedl syndrome: Results of a population survey, *J Med Genet* 36:437, 1999.

Slavotinek AM, et al: Mutations in *MKKS* cause Bardet-Biedl syndrome, *Nat Genet* 26:15, 2000.

Slavotinek AM, Biesecker LG: Phenotypic overlap of McKusick-Kaufman syndrome with Bardet-Biedl syndrome: A literature review, *Am J Med Genet* 95:208, 2000.

T

Beales PL, et al: Genetic interaction of *BBS1* mutations with other alleles at other BBS loci can result in non-mendelian Bardet-Biedl syndrome, *Am J Hum Genet* 72:1187, 2003.

Mykytyn K, et al: Evaluation of complex inheritance involving the most common Bardet-Biedl syndrome locus (*BBS1*), *Am J Hum Genet* 72:429, 2003.

Fan Y, et al: Mutations in a member of the Ras superfamily of small GTP-binding proteins causes Bardet-Biedl syndrome, *Nat Genet* 36:989, 2004.

Moore SJ, et al: Clinical and genetic epidemiology of Bardet-Biedl syndrome in Newfoundland: A 22-year prospective, population-based, cohort study, *Am J Med Genet A* 132:352, 2005.

Leitch CC, et al: Hypomorphic mutations in syndromic encephalocele genes are associated with Bardet-Biedl syndrome, *Nat Genet* 40:443, 2008.

Schaefer E, et al: Molecular diagnosis reveals genetic heterogeneity for the overlapping MKKS and BBS phenotypes, *Eur J Med Genet* 54:157, 2011.

Redin C, et al: Targeted high-throughput sequencing for diagnosis of genetically heterogeneous diseases: efficient mutation detection in Bardet-Biedl and Alstrom syndromes, *J Med Genet* 2012 Jul 7. [Epub ahead of print]

Marion V, et al: Exome sequencing identifies mutations in *LZTFL1*, a BBSome and smoothened trafficking regulator, in a family with Bardet-Biedl syndrome with situs inversus and insertional polydactyly, *J Med Genet* 49:317, 2012.

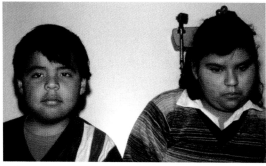

A

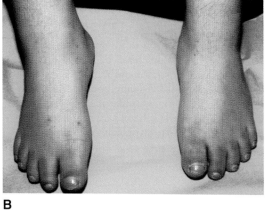

B

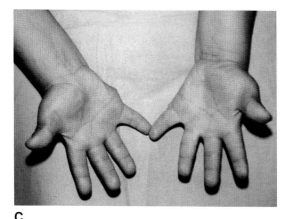

C

FIGURE 1.   Bardet-Biedl syndrome. **A,** Male and female siblings with retinal pigmentation and renal insufficiency. **B** and **C,** Note the short, broad feet and postaxial polydactyly of the hands.

T

AXENFELD-RIEGER SYNDROME
Iris Dysplasia, Hypodontia

The entity was first described by Axenfeld in 1920 in patients with posterior embryotoxon and corectopia. Rieger reported the same condition in a series of individuals with mesodermal dysgenesis of cornea and iris. Although anterior segment dysgenesis can occur in isolation, it is often associated with systemic anomalies such as in the Axenfeld-Rieger syndrome (ARS).

ABNORMALITIES

Ocular. Dysplasia of the iris (goniodysgenesis), including iris hypoplasia, strands of tissue connecting the iris to the posterior cornea (iridocorneal adhesions), prominent Schwalbe line (posterior embryotoxon), abnormal placement of pupil (corectopia), polycoria, glaucoma.

Dentition. Hypodontia or oligodontia, most commonly of maxillary deciduous and permanent incisors and second premolars, conical or peg-shaped crowns of anterior teeth, shortened roots, reduced gingival attachments, hypoplastic enamel, thickened frenulum.

Craniofacial. Midface hypoplasia, broad flat nasal bridge, short philtrum, thin upper lip and larger everted lower lip, prognathic appearance.

Other. Failure of involution of the periumbilical skin (>50%),

OCCASIONAL ABNORMALITIES

Short stature or failure to thrive (13%); developmental delay (21%); congenital heart defects (8%), including truncus arteriosus, mitral valve defects with ruptured chordae, tricuspid valve defects, pulmonic valve stenosis, bicuspid aortic valve, aortic valve stenosis, tetralogy of Fallot, and atrial septal defects; Meckel diverticulum (13%); omphalocele (4%); imperforate or anteriorly-placed anus (8%); hypospadias (4%); hearing loss (4%); cleft palate; abnormal sella turcica; growth hormone deficiency.

NATURAL HISTORY

In spite of the complex anterior segment anomalies, vision can be almost normal, but a 50% to 60% risk for glaucoma exists, usually in the second or third decades but is occasionally congenital. The development of glaucoma is likely to be related to an arrest late in development, causing reduced intertrabecular spaces and a more compressed trabecular meshwork, a mechanism similar to primary infantile glaucoma. Periodic eye exams should start at birth. Significant dental health problems can occur. Intellectual disability is unusual and commonly related to vision and hearing deficits, but it may be severe due to large contiguous gene deletions.

ETIOLOGY

This disorder has an autosomal dominant inheritance pattern with marked clinical and genetic heterogeneity. Two main loci at 4q25 and 6p25 have been identified. *PITX2* encodes a homeodomain transcription factor mapped to 4q25. Loss-of-function mutations, whole gene deletions, and deletions of an upstream regulatory region outside the coding region are responsible for 40% to 55% of cases and in almost 80% of cases in which dental or umbilical defects are present. *FOXC1,* a forkhead transcription factor located at 6p25, harbors mutations in 8% to 25% of ARS including missense, nonsense, and frameshift mutations, whole gene deletions, and, occasionally, duplications. Patients with *FOXC1* duplications are more likely to develop severe glaucoma. Mutations in *FOXC1* are associated with heart and/or hearing defects.

In addition, mutations or deletions of either of these two genes underlie 5% to 10% of cases of isolated anterior segment dysgenesis.

COMMENT

Large deletions including one of the two causal genes can cause more complex and severe phenotypes. The 6p25 recurrent subtelomeric deletion syndrome including *FOXC1* causes anterior segment dysgenesis, hearing loss, congenital heart disease, CNS malformations and hydrocephalus, developmental delay, and a characteristic facial appearance with hypertelorism and downslanting palpebral fissures, in addition to features typical of ARS. In addition, a condition termed De Hauwere syndrome, with similar features and femoral head anomalies, may represent a smaller deletion in this same region.

References

Rieger H: Beiträge zur Kenntnis seltener Missbildungen der Iris, *Arch Ophthalmol* 133:602, 1935.

Fitch N, Kaback M: The Axenfeld syndrome and the Rieger syndrome, *J Med Genet* 15:30, 1978.

Jorgensen RJ, et al: The Rieger syndrome, *Am J Med Genet* 2:307, 1978.

Shields MB, et al: Axenfeld-Rieger syndrome: A spectrum of developmental disorders, *Ophthalmology* 29:387, 1985.

Semina EV, et al: Cloning and characterization of a novel bicoid-related homeobox gene, *RIEG,* involved in Rieger syndrome, *Nat Genet* 14:392, 1996.

Craig JE, Mackey DA: Glaucoma genetics: Where are we? Where will we go? *Curr Opin Ophthalmol* 10:126, 1999.

Amendt BA, et al: Rieger syndrome: A clinical, molecular, and biochemical analysis, *Cell Mol Life Sci* 57:1652, 2000.

Espinoza HM, et al: A molecular basis for differential developmental anomalies in Axenfeld-Rieger syndrome, *Hum Mol Genet* 11:743, 2002.

Tonoki H, et al: Axenfeld-Rieger anomaly and Axenfeld-Rieger syndrome: Clinical, molecular-cytogenetic, and DNA array analyses of three patients with chromosomal defects at 6p25, *Am J Med Genet A* 155A:2925, 2011.

Chang TC, et al: Axenfeld-Rieger syndrome: New perspectives, *Br J Ophthalmol* 318, 2012.

Reis LM, et al: PITX2 and FOXC1 spectrum of mutations in ocular syndromes, *Eur J Hum Genet* 2012 May 9. [Epub ahead of print]

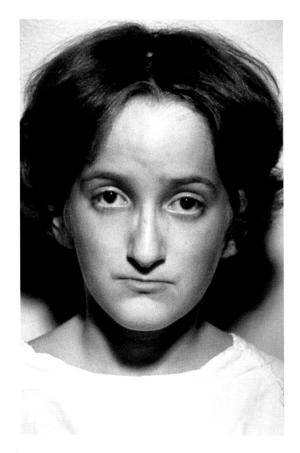

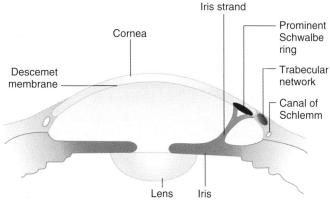

FIGURE 1. Axenfeld-Rieger syndrome. This female patient has irregular pupils, hypodontia, maxillary hypoplasia with malocclusion, and a short philtrum. The diagram depicts the transverse section of the ocular anterior chamber with a normal angle on the left and the Rieger eye malformation on the right. Note the hypoplasia of the iris and the iris strands.

PETERS'-PLUS SYNDROME
Peters Anomaly, Short Limb Dwarfism, Mental Retardation

This disorder was initially set forth in 1984 by Van Schooneveld, who described 11 affected individuals and introduced the term *Peters'-plus syndrome*. More than 50 cases have now been reported.

ABNORMALITIES

Performance. Intellectual disability (83%) varying from mild (34%) to moderate (20%) to severe (26%). Autism spectrum disorders.

Growth. Prenatal onset of growth deficiency; birth length less than 3rd percentile for gestational age in 82%; postnatal short limb growth deficiency in 100%, with adult height in females ranging from 128 to 151 cm and in males ranging from 141 to 155 cm.

Craniofacial. Round face in childhood; prominent forehead; hypertelorism; long philtrum; cupid-bow shape of upper lip; thin vermilion border; small, mildly malformed ears; preauricular pits; micrognathia; broad neck; cleft lip (45%), cleft palate (33%).

Eyes. Peters anomaly or other anterior chamber cleavage disorder, narrow palpebral fissures, nystagmus, cataracts, glaucoma. Eye involvement is frequently bilateral.

Limb. Short limbs, primarily rhizomelic; decreased range of motion at elbows; hypermobility of other joints; broad, short hands and feet; fifth-finger clinodactyly.

Other. Cardiac defects (<30%), including atrial and ventricular septal defects and pulmonary stenosis, subvalvular aortic stenosis, and bicuspid pulmonary valve; hydronephrosis; duplication of kidneys; cryptorchidism.

OCCASIONAL ABNORMALITIES

Short lingular frenulum, microcephaly, macrocephaly, agenesis/hypoplasia of corpus callosum, cerebellar hypoplasia, dilated lateral ventricles, hydrocephalus, myelomeningocele, abnormal ossification of the skull, upslanting palpebral fissures, iris coloboma, mild cutaneous syndactyly, simian crease, pes cavus, seizures, spastic diplegia, multicystic dysplastic kidneys, hypoplastic labia majora, hypoplastic clitoris, hypospadias, abnormal foreskin, vertebral anomaly, pectus excavatum, congenital hypothyroidism.

NATURAL HISTORY

Prenatal lethality is suspected based on the fact that 37% of couples with a child with Peters'-plus syndrome have recurrent miscarriages and/or stillbirths. Polyhydramnios occurs in 20%. Feeding problems in infancy, often requiring prolonged gavage, are common. Good response to human growth hormone has been reported in some cases. All patients learn to speak and acquire simple skills, although developmental milestones are significantly delayed. The corneal opacities may diminish during the first 6 months of life, but they never clear enough to permit normal vision. Severe disruption of the anterior chamber can lead to cataracts and glaucoma at birth, but these complications usually present later. Corneal transplantation for severe bilateral corneal opacification prior to age 3 to 6 months to prevent amblyopia is performed in severe cases. Simple separation of corneal adhesions has been successful in mild cases.

ETIOLOGY

This disorder has an autosomal recessive inheritance pattern. Mutations in *B3GALTL*, which encodes the transmembrane protein beta 1,3-galactosyltransferase-like, are responsible for Peters'-plus syndrome which is therefore considered a defect of O-glycosylation. Both loss-of-function mutations and large deletions can occur, leading to an absent or truncated protein with an inactive catalytic domain. Most affected individuals tested to date are homozygous for a hot spot splice site mutation in intron 8 (c.660+1G>A).

COMMENT

Peters anomaly, a defect of the anterior chamber, includes central corneal opacity (leukoma), thinning of the posterior aspect of the cornea, and iridocorneal adhesions attached to the edges of the leukoma. Peters anomaly usually occurs as an isolated defect in an otherwise normal individual. However, it can occur as one feature of a multiple malformation syndrome such as Peters'-plus syndrome.

References

Van Schooneveld MJ, et al: Peters'-plus: A new syndrome, *Ophthal Paediatr Genet* 4:141, 1984.

Saal HM, et al: Autosomal recessive Robinow-like syndrome with anterior chamber cleavage anomalies, *Am J Med Genet* 30:709, 1988.

Hennekam RCM, et al: The Peters'-plus syndrome: Description of 16 patients and review of the literature, *Clin Dysmorphol* 2:283, 1993.

Maillette de Buy Wenniger-Prick LJJM, Hennekam RCM: The Peters' plus syndrome: A review, *Ann Genet* 45:97, 2002.

Lee KW, Lee PD: Growth hormone deficiency (GHD): A new association in Peters' Plus syndrome (PPS), *Am J Med Genet A* 124A:388, 2004.

Saskia AJ, et al: Peters Plus syndrome is caused by mutations in *B3GALTL*, a putative glycosyltransferase, *Am J Hum Genet* 79:562, 2006.

Zaidman GW, Flanagan JK, Furey CC: Long-term visual prognosis in children after corneal transplant surgery for Peters anomaly type I, *Am J Ophthalmol* 144:104, 2007.

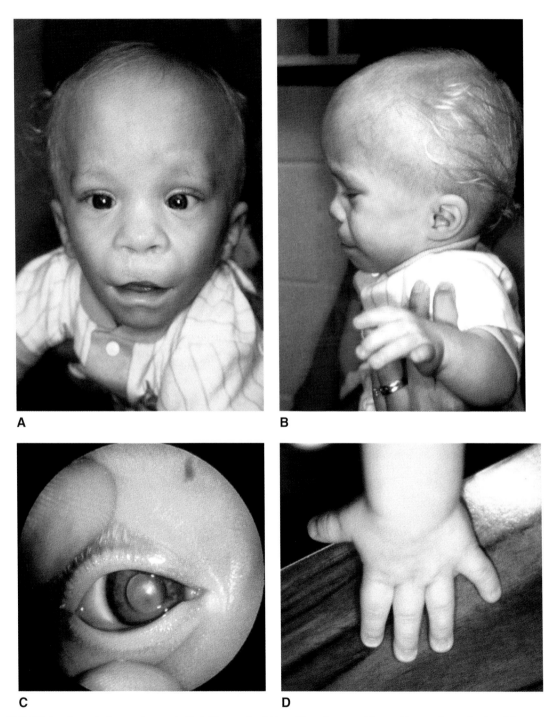

FIGURE 1.   Peters'-plus syndrome. **A–D,** A 15-month-old boy. Note the round face with prominent forehead, long philtrum with cupid-bow shape of upper lip, and thin vermilion border. The corneal opacity noted in the right eye at 4 months **(C)** was markedly decreased by 15 months. (From Hennekam RCM, et al: *Clin Dysmorphol* 2:283, 1993, with permission.)

TORIELLO-CAREY SYNDROME
Agenesis/Hypoplasia of Corpus Callosum, Robin Sequence, Short Palpebral Fissures

Initially described in 1988 by Toriello and Carey, these authors have collected at least 45 cases, 27 males and 17 females and 1 of unknown sex, aged 1 to 14 years. They have provided an excellent review of the associated features in 2003.

ABNORMALITIES

Growth. Prenatal growth deficiency (15%), postnatal growth deficiency in most cases.

Performance. Hypotonia, moderate intellectual disability (IQ 43–60).

Craniofacial. Microcephaly, occasionally present prenatally but most frequently of postnatal onset; large fontanels with delayed closure; telecanthus (lateral displacement of medial canthi) and/or hypertelorism; short palpebral fissures; sparse eyebrows, especially the medial half; sparse eyelashes; short/small nose, anteverted nares, and depressed nasal bridge; thin lips, downturned corners of mouth, cleft hard or soft palate, submucous cleft, high arched palate; micrognathia with or without Robin sequence; full cheeks; malformed ears (cupped, simple, thick helix, posteriorly rotated, low-set); short neck; excess nuchal skin.

Central Nervous System. Complete or partial agenesis/hypoplasia of corpus callosum (82%), cerebellar hypoplasia, Dandy-Walker malformation, cerebral atrophy, dilated ventricles.

Cardiovascular. Defects in approximately 80%, including atrial septal defect, ventricular septal defect, patent ductus arteriosus, pulmonary valve stenosis, tetralogy of Fallot, hypoplastic left heart, atretic mitral valve, double-outlet right heart with type B interrupted aortic arch, coarctation of the aorta, cardiomyopathy, endocardial fibroelastosis.

Other. Laryngeal/hypopharyngeal hypoplasia with stridor and laryngomalacia, abnormal rib number, brachydactyly, clinodactyly of fifth fingers, proximally placed/adducted thumb, camptodactyly, joint hypermobility, cryptorchidism, hypospadias, genital hypoplasia.

OCCASIONAL ABNORMALITIES

Dolichocephaly, brachycephaly, trigonocephaly, craniosynostosis, hydrocephalus, colpocephaly, electroencephalograph abnormalities, speech delay, conductive and/or sensorineural hearing loss, anotia, hypoplasia of optic disc, sparse, thin hair, hyperkeratosis on dorsum of hands, downslanting palpebral fissures, ptosis, Duane anomaly, vertebral defects, clavicular defects, narrow chest, pectus deformities, hypoplastic/dysplastic nails, pes varus, calcaneovalgus, metatarsus adductus, hypermobile joints, increased gap between first and second toes, ureteropelvic junction obstruction, kidney hypoplasia, pelvic kidney, omphalocele, diaphragmatic hernia/eventration, pyloric stenosis, intestinal malrotation, Hirschsprung disease, micropenis, anteriorly placed anus, inguinal and/or umbilical hernias, hypopituitarism, hypothyroidism, eczema.

NATURAL HISTORY

Respiratory distress and obstructive apnea associated with the Robin sequence as well as the laryngeal/hypopharyngeal anomalies lead frequently to serious airway compromise. Early death, mostly within the first months, has occurred in 35%. The survivors, who range from 1 year to 14 years, are all developmentally delayed.

ETIOLOGY

An autosomal recessive inheritance pattern is most likely. The causal gene remains unknown.

References

Toriello HV, Carey JC: Corpus callosum agenesis, facial anomalies, Robin sequence, and other anomalies: A new autosomal recessive syndrome, *Am J Med Genet* 31:17, 1988.

Czarnecki P, et al: Toriello-Carey syndrome: Evidence for X-linked inheritance, *Am J Med Genet* 65:291, 1996.

Chinen Y, et al: Two sisters with Toriello-Carey syndrome, *Am J Med Genet* 87:262, 1999.

Wegner KJ, Hersh JA: Toriello-Carey syndrome: An additional case and summary of previously reported cases, *Clin Dysmorphol* 10:145, 2001.

Toriello HV, et al: Toriello-Carey syndrome: Delineation and review, *Am J Med Genet A* 123A:84, 2003.

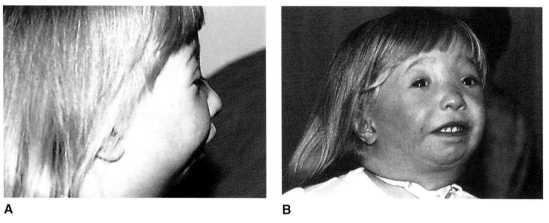

FIGURE 1. Toriello-Carey syndrome. **A** and **B,** A 3-year-old girl. Note the small chin, telecanthus, and thickened helix of the ear. (From Toriello HG, Carey JC: *Am J Med Genet* 31:17, 1988, with permission.)

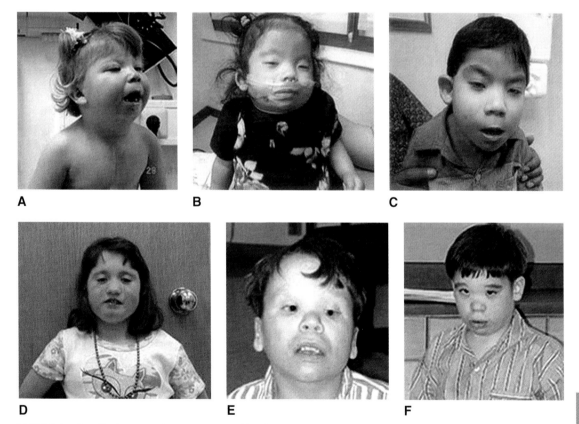

FIGURE 2. Toriello-Carey syndrome. A 3-year-old girl **(A),** an 11-month-old girl **(B),** the 6-year-old brother of the child in **B (C),** a 7-year-old girl **(D),** an 11-year-old boy **(E)** and his 14-year-old brother **(F).** Note the short palpebral fissures, ptosis/blepharophimosis, short small nose, full cheeks, downturned corners of the mouth, and micrognathia. (From Toriello HV, et al: *Am J Med Genet A* 123A:84, 2003, with permission).

T

FINLAY-MARKS SYNDROME (SCALP-EAR-NIPPLE [SEN] SYNDROME)

In 1978, Finlay and Marks reported 10 affected members of a family with defects of the scalp, ears and nipples inherited as an autosomal dominant trait. Since then, more than 30 cases have been reported. Also called scalp-ear-nipple (SEN) syndrome, the abnormally shaped ears and the scalp defect appear to be almost constant features, and the nipple abnormalities are present in more than 50% of cases.

ABNORMALITIES

Craniofacial. Aplasia cutis congenita of scalp; prominent and abnormally shaped ears with hypoplastic tragus, antitragus, and lobule, overfolding of the superior helix, and flattening of the antihelix; telecanthus; broad nasal bridge with excess skin over the glabella; bulbous nasal tip; short columella.

Skin. Rudimentary or absent nipples in both males and females. Mild hypohidrosis with reduced apocrine sweat glands; scanty hair, eyelashes, and eyebrows; reduced pubic and axillary hair.

Nails. Brittle dysplastic nails.

Dentition. Irregular dental eruption and tooth size, widely spaced upper central incisors, irregular alveolar ridges in the newborn.

Extremities. Partial cutaneous syndactyly of third and fourth fingers and second and third toes, camptodactyly of the fifth fingers.

Renal and Urinary Tract. Renal agenesis or hypoplasia, vesicoureteral reflux, pyeloureteral duplication. Secondary renal insufficiency and hypertension.

OCCASIONAL ABNORMALITIES

Rhombencephalosynapsis, coloboma of the lower eyelids and/or iris, congenital cataract, Stahl deformity of the ear, prominent crus of the helix, natal teeth, absence of ear wax, hypospadias, diabetes mellitus, obesity, hair loss, hypertension, loss of libido.

NATURAL HISTORY

The area of aplasia cutis congenita heals over the first year with a lumpy surface consisting of bundles of connective tissue. The scalp hair is sparse in that area. Hypoplastic nipples are common. In some cases, the breasts have not enlarged during pregnancy, nor has lactation occurred. The excess skin in the glabellar region has been excised and seen to be lipomatous. The frequency of urinary defects warrants investigation and follow-up in order to prevent renal failure. Some cases suggest hypertension may also be a primary feature. Diabetes at an early age has been reported in only one family.

ETIOLOGY

Probable autosomal dominant inheritance. Both sporadic and familial cases with vertical transmission have been reported. However, a recent description of siblings born to unaffected parents raises the possibility of germline mosaicism or autosomal recessive inheritance. The defective gene for this syndrome has not been identified.

References

Finlay AY, Marks R: An hereditary syndrome of lumpy scalp, odd ears and rudimentary nipples, *Br J Dermatol* 99:423, 1978.

Plessis G, Le Treust M, Le Merrer M: Scalp defect, absence of nipples, ear anomalies, renal hypoplasia: Another case of Finlay-Marks syndrome, *Clin Genet* 52:231, 1997.

Picard C, et al: Scalp-ear-nipple (Finlay-Marks) syndrome: A familial case with renal involvement, *Clin Genet* 56:170, 1999.

Sobreira NL, et al: Finlay-Marks (SEN) syndrome: A sporadic case and the delineation of the syndrome, *Am J Med Genet A* 140:300, 2006.

Naik P, et al: Finlay-Marks syndrome: Report of two siblings and review of literature, *Am J Med Genet A* 158A:1696, 2012.

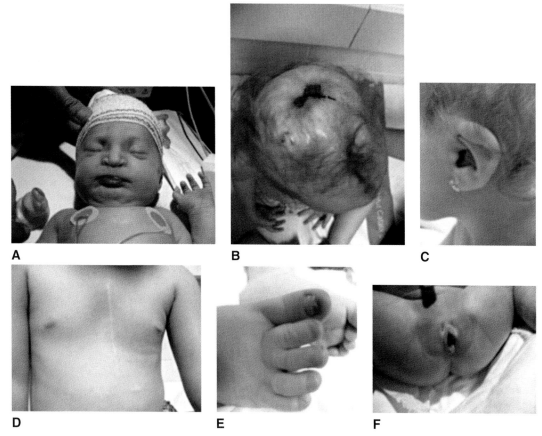

FIGURE 1. Finlay-Marks syndrome. Note the broad nasal bridge with excess skin on the glabella, a bulbous nasal tip, and a short columella **(A)**. Large area of healing aplasia cutis congenita, with a lumpy surface **(B)**. Abnormally shaped ears, hypoplastic tragus, antitragus, and lobule, with overfolding of the superior helix **(C)**. Thorax with areolas present but hypoplastic and a midline thoracic scar from heart surgery **(D)**, partial cutaneous syndactyly of the second and third toes and dysplastic nails **(E)**, and hypoplastic labia majora and clitoris **(F)**.

MOWAT-WILSON SYNDROME
Microcephaly, Distinctive Facies, Hirschsprung Disease

This disorder was initially described in six patients, with a distinctive facies, intellectual disability, and microcephaly, five of whom had Hirschsprung disease. Close to 200 cases have been reported.

ABNORMALITIES

Growth. Postnatal onset of short stature (50%), slender build.

Performance. Moderate-to-severe intellectual disability, early hypotonia, ataxic gait, speech disproportionately delayed relative to comprehension, happy demeanor with frequent smiling, stereotyped behavior, oral behaviors such as chewing or mouthing objects or body parts and grinding teeth, decreased response to pain.

Neurologic. Postnatal onset microcephaly (80%), hypotonia, wide-based gait, elbows held in flexed position with hands up, seizures or abnormal electroencephalograph (73%), total or partial agenesis of corpus callosum (43%), ventriculomegaly.

Facies. High forehead; frontal bossing; square face; sparse hair; large, sparse and medially flared eyebrows; hypertelorism, strabismus, epicanthal folds, deep-set large eyes; broad and low nasal bridge; prominent nasal tip; prominent columella, prominent vertical philtral ridges; full or everted lower lip; upper lip full centrally and thin laterally; posteriorly rotated ears with large, uplifted ear lobes; puffy anterior neck, excess nuchal skin; in late childhood, the face and nose lengthen, the nasal bridge becomes convex and the columella becomes more prominent, the philtrum appears short, and the chin is long and pointed with obvious prognathism.

Cardiac. Defects in 52%, including patent ductus arteriosus, atrial septal defect, ventricular septal defect, tetralogy of Fallot, pulmonary stenosis or atresia, pulmonary artery sling (causing tracheal stenosis), aortic coarctation, bicuspid aortic valve, aortic valve stenosis, and interrupted aortic arch.

Genitourinary. Hypospadias (52%); cryptorchidism (36%); hooding of penis; webbed penis; bifid scrotum; renal anomalies in boys, including vesicoureteral reflux, hydronephrosis, pelvic kidney, duplex kidney.

Other. Hirschsprung disease (46%–57%), constipation, slender tapered fingers, prominent fingertip pads, pes planus, long toes, calcaneovalgus.

OCCASIONAL ABNORMALITIES

Nystagmus, strabismus, ptosis, irregular patches of dark iris pigmentation, microphthalmia, retinal aplasia, iris/retinal/optic disc coloboma, dark pigment clumps in blue irides, iris heterochromia, bifid uvula, submucous cleft palate, cleft lip with or without cleft palate, pyloric stenosis, cerebral atrophy, poor hippocampal formation, pachygyria, cerebellar hypoplasia, prominent interphalangeal joints developing in adolescence, broad hallux, duplicated hallux, deep palmar and plantar creases, supernumerary nipples, skin depigmentation, biliary atresia, vaginal septum.

NATURAL HISTORY

The facial features, particularly the eyebrows and the ear lobes shaped like "orecchiette pasta" are very characteristic and can suggest the diagnosis in a newborn with variable multiple major or minor malformations, with or without Hirschsprung disease. Mean age of walking is 4 years, and those who walk are ataxic. Some remain nonambulatory. Most children develop only limited speech, although some communicate successfully with signing. The age of onset of seizures has varied from several months to over 10 years, and some have been difficult to control.

ETIOLOGY

Most cases have been sporadic, resulting from a de novo deletion (20%) or loss-of-function heterozygous mutation (80%) of the *ZEB2* gene located on chromosome 2q22, which encodes for SIP1 (Smad interacting protein 1). Sibling recurrence is thus likely to be very low but has been reported in at least four pairs of siblings, and both somatic and germline mosaicism in one parent have been proven. From these figures, recurrence risk can be estimated as high as 2.3% (4/175). Patients with large *ZEB2* deletions tend to a more severe phenotype with colon aganglionosis involving longer segments. *ZEB2* appears to be involved in neural crest–derived cells, CNS, heart septation, and midline development.

COMMENT

Because of the wide-based gait, typical stance with arms held flexed at the elbows and hands up, smiling face and lack of speech, this disorder should be considered in patients thought to have Angelman syndrome for whom the diagnosis is not confirmed.

References

Mowat DR, et al: Hirschsprung disease, microcephaly, mental retardation and characteristic facial features: Delineation of a new syndrome and identification of a locus of chromosome 2q22-q23, *J Med Genet* 35:617, 1998.

Wakamatsu N, et al: Mutations in *SIP1,* encoding Smad interacting protein-1, cause a form of Hirschsprung disease, *Nat Genet* 27:369, 2001.

Zweier C, et al: "Mowat-Wilson" syndrome with and without Hirschsprung disease is a distinct, recognizable multiple congenital anomalies-mental retardation syndrome caused by mutations in the zinc finger homeo box 1B gene, *Am J Med Genet* 108:177, 2002.

Mowat DR, et al: Mowat-Wilson syndrome, *J Med Genet* 40:305, 2003.

Wilson MJ, et al: Further delineation of the phenotype associated with heterozygous mutations in *ZFHX1B*, *Am J Med Genet* 119:257, 2003.

Adam MP, et al: Clinical features and management issues in Mowat-Wilson syndrome, *Am J Med Genet A* 140A:2730, 2006.

Garavelli L, Mainardi PC: Mowat-Wilson syndrome, *Orphanet J Rare Dis* 2:42, 2007.

Cecconi M, et al: Recurrence of Mowat-Wilson syndrome in siblings with a novel mutation in the *ZEB2* gene, *Am J Med Genet A* 146A:3095, 2008.

Garavelli L, et al: Mowat-Wilson syndrome: Facial phenotype changing with age: Study of 19 Italian patients and review of the literature, *Am J Med Genet A* 149A:417, 2009.

Ariss M, et al: Ophthalmologic abnormalities in Mowat-Wilson syndrome and a mutation in *ZEB2*, *Ophthalmic Genet* 33:159, 2012.

Evans E, et al: The behavioral phenotype of Mowat-Wilson syndrome, *Am J Med Genet A* 158A:358, 2012.

T

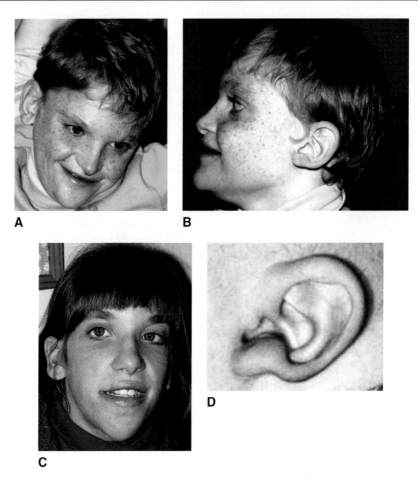

FIGURE 1.   Mowat-Wilson syndrome. **A–D,** Note the prominent nasal tip; upper lip, which is full centrally and thin laterally; posteriorly rotated ears and large uplifted ear lobes; and prognathism, which develops in adolescence. (Courtesy Dr. David Mowat, Sydney Children's Hospital, New South Wales, Australia.)

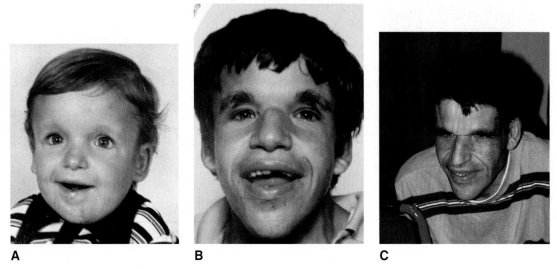

A **B** **C**

FIGURE 2. **A–C,** The same individual at 3 years, 14 years, and 31 years of age, respectively. Note the high forehead, square face, prominent nasal tip, and prognathism. (Courtesy Dr. David Mowat, Sydney Children's Hospital, New South Wales, Australia.)

CEREBRO-COSTO-MANDIBULAR SYNDROME
Rib-Gap Defect with Small Thorax, Severe Micrognathia

This disorder was initially described by Smith and colleagues in 1966. More than 75 cases have been reported.

ABNORMALITIES

Performance. Intellectual disability and speech difficulties are frequent among the survivors.
Growth. Postnatal growth deficiency.
Facies. Severe micrognathia with glossoptosis (the Robin sequence) and short to cleft soft palate.
Thorax. Bell-shaped small thorax with gaps between posterior ossified rib and anterior cartilaginous rib, seen on radiographs, that represent fibrovascular replacement of bone/cartilage, especially fourth to tenth ribs, most frequently at the fifth rib; rudimentary ribs; anomalous rib insertion to vertebrae; missing ribs, most often the twelfth, first, and eleventh; vertebral anomalies.

OCCASIONAL ABNORMALITIES

Microcephaly (25%), short neck, redundant skin including pterygium colli, choanal atresia, dental abnormalities (no tooth buds), indistinct speech, conductive hearing loss, absence of auditory canals, fifth-finger clinodactyly, malformed tracheal cartilages, hypoplastic humerus, elbow hypoplasia, renal cyst or ectopia, clubfoot, scoliosis, congenital hip dislocation, sacral fusion, flask-shaped configuration of pelvis, hypoplastic sternum, clavicles, and pubic rami, epiphyseal stippling of calcaneus, ventricular septal defect, porencephaly, corpus callosal agenesis, dilated lateral ventricles, hydranencephaly, meningomyelocele, omphalocele.

NATURAL HISTORY

Approximately 25% have died in the neonatal period and approximately 56% by 1 year of age, the majority as a result of severe respiratory insufficiency or infection. Of those who survive, feeding and speech difficulties are common, as well as intellectual disability in one third to one half of cases, but no major respiratory difficulties are expected beyond the first year. The rib-gap defects resolve into pseudoarthroses with time. A significantly higher number of rib defects is characteristic of lethal cases.

ETIOLOGY

At least twelve cases of familial inheritance have been reported, five cases involving siblings, four cases involving father and child, and three cases involving mother and child, suggesting both autosomal recessive and autosomal dominant inheritance. The gene is unknown, and mutations in at least four genes (*MYF5, GSC, RUNX2,* and *TCOF1*), causing related craniofacial and thoracic defects, have been ruled out. Clinical manifestations among families suggestive of autosomal recessive and autosomal dominant inheritance are similar.

COMMENT

The clinical manifestations of this disorder in the newborn period are extremely variable and can be limited to the Robin sequence. Thus, cerebro-costo-mandibular syndrome should be considered in newborns with the Robin sequence who show more serious respiratory problems, and the finding of rib gaps and missing ribs will confirm this diagnosis.

References

Smith DW, Theiler K, Schachenmann G: Rib-gap defect with micrognathia, malformed tracheal cartilages, and redundant skin: A new pattern of defective development, *J Pediatr* 69:799, 1966.

Doyle JF: The skeletal defects of the cerebro-costo-mandibular syndrome, *Irish J Med Sci (7th Ser)* 2:595, 1969.

McNicholl B, et al: Cerebro-costo-mandibular syndrome: A new familial developmental disorder, *Arch Dis Child* 45:421, 1970.

Silverman FN, et al: Cerebro-costo-mandibular syndrome, *J Pediatr* 97:406, 1980.

Tachibina K, et al: Cerebro-costo-mandibular syndrome, *Hum Genet* 54:283, 1980.

Leroy JG, et al: Cerebro-costo-mandibular syndrome with autosomal dominant inheritance, *J Pediatr* 99:441, 1981.

Hennekam RCM, et al: The cerebro-costo-mandibular syndrome: Third report of familial occurrence, *Clin Genet* 28:118, 1985.

Burton EM, Oestreich AE: Cerebro-costo-mandibular syndrome with stippled epiphysis and cystic fibrosis, *Pediatr Radiol* 18:365, 1988.

Plötz FB, et al: Cerebro-costo-mandibular syndrome, *Am J Med Genet* 62:286, 1996.

Van den Ende JJ, et al: The cerebro-costo-mandibular syndrome: Seven patients and review of the literature, *Clin Dysmorphol* 7:87, 1998.

Nagasawa H, Yamamoto Y, Kohno Y: Cerebro-costo-mandibular syndrome: Prognosis and proposal for classification, *Congenit Anom (Kyoto)* 50:171, 2010.

Su PH, et al: Exclusion of *MYF5, GSC, RUNX2,* and *TCOF1* mutation in a case of cerebro-costo-mandibular syndrome, *Clin Dysmorphol* 19:51, 2010.

Oestreich AE, Stanek JW: Preautopsy imaging in cerebro-costo-mandibular syndrome, *Pediatr Radiol* 40:S50, 2010.

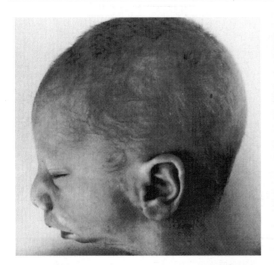

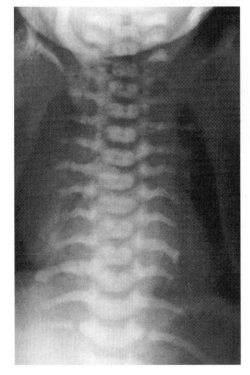

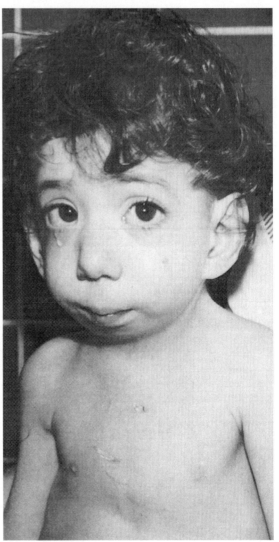

FIGURE 1. Cerebro-costo-mandibular syndrome. *Left*, Newborn showing severe micrognathia and incompletely ossified aberrant ribs. (From Smith DW, et al: *J Pediatr* 69:799, 1966, with permission.) *Right*, A 4-year-old child. (*Right*, From McNicholl B, et al: *Arch Dis Child* 45:421, 1970, with permission.)

T

JARCHO-LEVIN SYNDROME
Spondylothoracic Dysostosis

Jarcho and Levin described this disorder in 1938. Although Jarcho-Levin syndrome has been used as an umbrella term for autosomal recessive dysostosis of the spine and ribs, it should be used specifically for spondylothoracic dysostosis (STD). It occurs most frequently in Puerto Ricans of Spanish descent and is caused by specific recurring mutations in a single gene. The STD phenotype in Puerto Ricans can be more severe, but it is not significantly different from that occurring in other populations, and the causal gene is identical.

ABNORMALITIES

Growth. Short trunk dwarfism of prenatal onset. Average height is 115.7 cm.
Craniofacial. Prominent occiput in infancy that becomes flat with brachycephaly in late childhood; tendency to have broad forehead, wide nasal bridge, anteverted nares, and upslant to palpebral fissures. High palate.
Thorax and Spine. Short thorax with severe shortening of the spine, generalized vertebral segmentation defects (sickle-cell shaped vertebrae), with "crab-like" rib cage, due to ribs that flare in a fan-like pattern with extensive posterior fusion at the vertebrocostal junction, sometimes extending laterally. Anteriorly the ribs appear straight and aligned with no additional points of irregular fusions; irregular and prominent vertebral pedicles, appearing on X-rays like a "tramline," short rigid neck due to cervical vertebral fusions, and low posterior hairline; pectus carinatum; increased anteroposterior chest diameter; lordosis; kyphoscoliosis.
Limbs. Normal with impression of being long.
Other. Protuberant abdomen, inguinal hernia, umbilical hernia.

OCCASIONAL ABNORMALITIES
Cleft soft palate, cryptorchidism, hydronephrosis with ureteral obstruction, double collecting system, bilobed bladder, absent external genitalia, anal and urethral atresia, uterus didelphys, cerebral polygyria, neural tube defects, atrial septal defects, single umbilical artery, talipes equinovarus,

NATURAL HISTORY
Significant thoracic restriction occurs in approximately 60% of newborns, resulting in some type of respiratory distress. Infants with STD have a nearly 44% mortality rate by the end of infancy. For survivors, respiratory infections should be treated vigorously, and orthopedic and surgical management of spine deformities should continue. Scoliosis is not common because of the bilateral symmetric fusion of the ribs at the costovertebral junction, but it can

be severe in some cases. Early motor development can be compromised, but cognition is normal.

ETIOLOGY

This disorder has an autosomal recessive inheritance pattern. Mutations in the mesoderm posterior 2 homologue gene *MESP2* cause spondylothoracic dysostosis. *MESP2* mutations account for approximately 90% of cases in Puerto Rico. All known mutations have occurred in exon 1. Those homozygous for the founder Puerto Rican nonsense mutation, p.Glu103X, seem to have a more severe phenotype than compound heterozygotes (at least one missense mutation) for other common mutations.

COMMENT

Spondylocostal dysostosis is defined by multiple segmentation defects of the vertebrae (at least 10 segments affected) in combination with abnormalities of the ribs, which are malaligned, broadened, bifid, with a variable number of irregular intercostal rib fusions, and sometimes with a reduction in rib number. The condition is less symmetric, the thorax does not display a fan-like configuration, and it is usually less severe in terms of respiratory complications. However, on occasion, it also can be lethal in early life. The inheritance is autosomal recessive, with clinical and genetic heterogeneity. The four genes involved cause somewhat different phenotypes, referred to as SCDO1 through SCDO4. A single family with mutation in *MESP2* (SCDO2), the causal gene for STD, has been reported. *DLL3* (SCDO1), the most frequent causal gene, is associated with abnormal segmentation throughout the entire vertebral column with smooth outlines to the vertebral bodies referred to as the "pebble beach sign" on radiographs seen in late childhood. *LFNG* (SCDO3) causes the most severe shortening of the spine, and *HES7* (SCDO4) causes malsegmentation of the entire spine, with a "tramline sign," leading to a phenotype similar but milder than that seen in STD. These four genes play a significant role in the Notch signaling pathway involved in somitic segmentation.

References

Jarcho S, Levin PM: Hereditary malformations of the vertebral bodies, *Johns Hopkins Med J* 62:216, 1938.

Pérez-Comas A, García-Castro JM: Occipitofacial-cervico-thoracic-abdomino-digital dysplasia: Jarcho-Levin syndrome of vertebral anomalies, *J Pediatr* 85:388, 1974.

Poor MA, et al: Nonskeletal malformations in one of three siblings with Jarcho-Levin syndrome of vertebral anomalies, *J Pediatr* 103:270, 1983.

Karnes PS, et al: Jarcho-Levin syndrome: Four new cases and classification of subtypes, *Am J Med Genet* 40:264, 1991.

Mortier GR, et al: Multiple vertebral segmentation defects: Analysis of 26 new patients and review of the literature, *Am J Med Genet* 61:310, 1996.

Bannykh S, et al: Aberrant Pax1 and Pax9 in Jarcho-Levin syndrome: Report of two Caucasian siblings and literature review, *Am J Med Genet A* 120A:241, 2003.

Turnpenny PD, et al: Novel mutations in *DLL3*, a somitogenesis gene encoding a ligand for the Notch signalling pathway, cause a consistent pattern of abnormal

vertebral segmentation in spondylocostal dysostosis, *J Med Genet* 40:333, 2003.

Cornier AS, et al: Controversies surrounding Jarcho-Levin syndrome, *Curr Opin Pediatr* 15:614, 2003.

Cornier AS, et al: Phenotype characterization and natural history of spondylothoracic dysplasia syndrome: A series of 27 new cases, *Am J Med Genet A* 128A:120, 2004.

Turnpenny PD, et al: Abnormal vertebral segmentation and the notch signaling pathway in man, *Dev Dyn* 236:1456, 2007.

Cornier AS, et al: Mutations in the *MESP2* gene cause spondylothoracic dysostosis/Jarcho-Levin syndrome, *Am J Hum Genet* 82:1334, 2008.

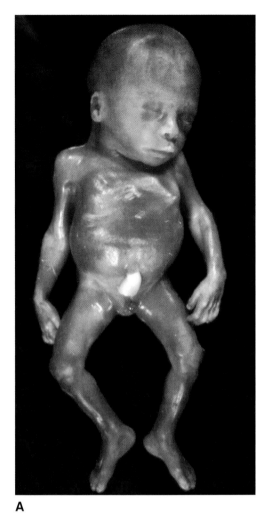

A

B

FIGURE 1.   Jarcho-Levin syndrome. **A** and **B,** Affected neonate with radiograph. (**A,** From Bannykh SI, et al: *Am J Med Genet* 120:241, 2003, with permission; **B,** from Pérez-Comas A, García-Castro JM: *J Pediatr* 85:388, 1974.)

MANDIBULOACRAL DYSPLASIA
Short Stature, Mandibular Hypoplasia, Acro-Osteolysis

Described initially by Cavallazzi and colleagues as an atypical form of cleido-cranial dysostosis, this disorder has now been reported in more than 100 patients. Onset of phenotype commonly occurs between 3 and 14 years and is slowly progressive, but it can occur earlier and evolve faster depending on the causal gene involved.

ABNORMALITIES

Growth. Postnatal onset of growth deficiency.

Craniofacial. Prominent scalp veins, thin beak-like nose with alar hypoplasia, hypoplastic facial bones with prominent eyes, mandibular hypoplasia, difficulty opening mouth.

Limbs. Short, contracted fingers with short bulbous distal phalanges of fingers and toes, with acro-osteolysis, and broad interphalangeal joints; dystrophic nails; generalized joint limitations.

Skin, Hair, Teeth. Thin, mottled, hyperpigmented skin mostly in groin and axillae; progressive thinning and atrophy of skin; prominently visible superficial vasculature; premature loss of teeth; dental crowding and malocclusion; sparse, thin hair.

Imaging. Wormian bones, widened cranial sutures, clavicular hypoplasia, acro-osteolysis, hypoplastic distal phalanges, bell-shaped chest.

Adipose tissue. Type A pattern lipodystrophy with marked loss of subcutaneous fat from the extremities and milder in the face, with normal or slight excess in the neck and truncal regions. Type B pattern generalized lipodystrophy involves the face more severely, as well as the trunk and extremities.

Other. Metabolic syndrome, insulin resistance, glucose intolerance, diabetes mellitus, hypertriglyceridemia, acanthosis nigricans.

OCCASIONAL ABNORMALITIES

Neonatal tooth eruption, amorphous calcific deposits, submetaphyseal erosions, vertebral beaking, cortical osteoporosis, scoliosis, and delayed healing of fracture. Cataracts, hypospadias, delayed puberty, hypogonadism, hepatomegaly, renal failure secondary to focal mesangial scleroses, congenital myopathy.

NATURAL HISTORY

Affected children are normal at birth. Characteristic features of ocular proptosis, micrognathia, loss of facial fat, and short bulbous distal phalanges usually develop between 3 and 14 years and can lead to early suspicion of the disorder. Later, growth deficiency and progressive skeletal changes, involving primarily the clavicles, and digits with acro-osteolysis of the medial end of the clavicles and the distal phalanges (occurring earliest in the second digit). Loss of subcutaneous fat leading to a prematurely aging appearance occurs. Most health complications arise from insulin resistance and diabetes mellitus, as well as glomerulopathy.

ETIOLOGY

Mandibuloacral dysplasia (MAD) has an autosomal recessive inheritance pattern. A mutation in the lamin A/C gene (*LMNA*), which maps to chromosome 1q21, was initially identified in all individuals affected with this disorder. The most common defect is a homozygous missense mutation (p.R527H) in the C-terminal domain of lamin A/C, but different homozygous or compound heterozygous patients have been reported. The *LMNA* gene is responsible for MAD in those families with partial lipodystrophy (type A), but a second gene, *ZMPSTE24*, is responsible for cases of MAD with earlier onset (before 1 year of age). Those children have a more rapidly progressive course, with a generalized pattern of lipodystrophy (type B), severe glomerulopathy, more extensive skeletal changes, and subcutaneous calcifications. *ZMPSTE24* encodes a zinc metalloproteinase involved in post-translational proteolytic cleavage of carboxy terminal residues of farnesylated prelamin A to form mature lamin A. Retention of unprocessed farnesylated prelamin A in the nucleus is toxic to cells.

COMMENT

A broad range of disorders are caused by mutations in the *LMNA* or the *ZMPSTE24* gene, including Hutchinson-Gilford syndrome (progeria), which is caused by *LMNA* mutations and restrictive dermopathy. The latter is lethal early in life and occurs with null mutations in *ZMPSTE24*, leading to absent residual function of the enzyme. At least some residual enzyme activity is usually present in mandibuloacral dysplasia, which explains the milder phenotype.

References

Cavallazzi C, et al: Si du caso di disostosi cleido-cranica, *Rev Clin Pediatr* 65:313, 1960.

Teuconi R, et al: Another Italian family with mandibuloacral dysplasia: Why does it seem more frequent in Italy? *Am J Med Genet* 24:357, 1986.

Toriello HV: Mandibulo-acral dysplasia: Heterogeneity versus variability, *Clin Dysmorphol* 4:12, 1995.

Novelli G: Mandibuloacral dysplasia is caused by a mutation in *LMNA*-encoding lamin A/C, *Am J Hum Genet* 71:426, 2002.

Agarwal AK, et al: Zinc metalloproteinase, *ZMPSTE24,* is mutated in mandibuloacral dysplasia, *Hum Mol Genet* 12:1995, 2003.

Simha V, et al: Genetic and phenotypic heterogeneity in patients with mandibuloacral dysplasia-associated lipodystrophy, *J Clin Endocrinol Metab* 88:2821, 2003.

Garavelli L, et al: Mandibuloacral dysplasia type A in childhood, *Am J Med Genet A* 149A:2258, 2009.

Cunningham VJ, et al: Skeletal phenotype of mandibuloacral dysplasia associated with mutations in *ZMPSTE24,* *Bone* 47:591, 2010.

Ahmad Z, et al: Early onset mandibuloacral dysplasia due to compound heterozygous mutations in *ZMPSTE24,* *Am J Med Genet A* 152A:2703, 2010.

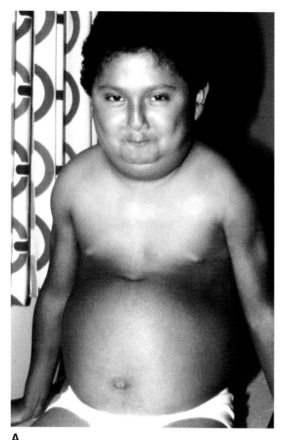

A

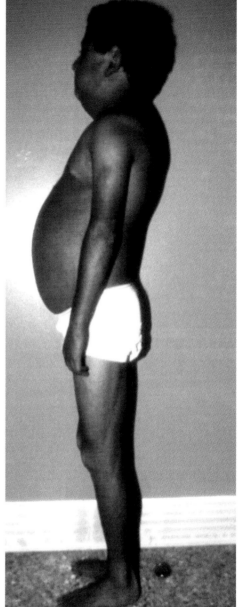

B

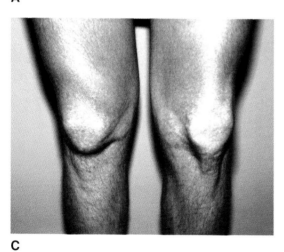

C

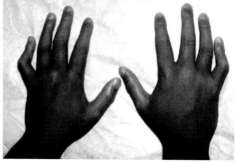

D

FIGURE 1.   Mandibuloacral dysplasia. **A–D,** A 10-year-old boy with a thin, beaked nose with alar hypoplasia; hyperpigmented skin; loss of subcutaneous fat in the extremities; fat accumulation in the trunk, face, and submental region; bell-shaped chest; and camptodactyly. (Figures **1B, 1C, 1E,** and **1F** in Ahmad Z et al, *Am J Med Genet A* 152A:2703, 2010.)

BERARDINELLI-SEIP CONGENITAL LIPODYSTROPHY SYNDROME
(CONGENITAL GENERALIZED LIPODYSTROPHY)
Lipoatrophy, Phallic Hypertrophy, Hepatomegaly, Hyperlipemia

Berardinelli reported this unusual lipodystrophic syndrome in 1954.

ABNORMALITIES

Performance. Mild-to-moderate intellectual disability is a variable feature, dependent on the specific genetic etiology.

Growth. Accelerated growth and maturation during early childhood, final height is normal or slightly above normal, slight enlargement of hands and feet, phallic enlargement, muscle hyperplasia, lack of metabolically active adipose tissue from early life with relative sparing of mechanical adipose tissue (i.e., in orbits, palms and soles, crista galli, buccal region, tongue, scalp, breasts, perineum, periarticular regions, and epidural areas).

Craniofacial. Prominent supraorbital ridges, prognathism, macroglossia. Progressive facial lipoatrophy with prominent bony cheeks, thin nose.

Skin. Coarse with hyperpigmentation, especially in axillae; variable acanthosis nigricans.

Hair. Hirsutism with curly scalp hair, low frontal and posterior scalp hairlines, not following a secondary sexual pattern.

Heart. Hypertrophic cardiomyopathy.

Vascular. Large superficial veins mostly seen in the limbs.

Liver. Hepatomegaly with excess neutral fat and glycogen and eventual cirrhosis.

Plasma. Hyperlipidemia, hypertriglyceridemia, insulin-resistant diabetes mellitus.

Other. Umbilical hernia.

OCCASIONAL ABNORMALITIES

Corneal opacities, hyperproteinemia, hyperinsulinemia, epiphyseal and metaphyseal bone cysts, percussion myxedema, hyperhidrosis, clitoromegaly, amenorrhea, polycystic ovaries, precocious puberty in females.

NATURAL HISTORY

Severe forms of this disorder may have prenatal onset growth retardation. However, in most cases, prenatal growth is normal, and accelerated growth, voracious appetite, and increased metabolic rate occur in early childhood. Muscle hypertrophy and lipoatrophy cause an athletic appearance, even in young children. Hyperinsulinemia and elevated serum triglycerides occur even in infancy, resulting in chylomicronemia, eruptive xanthomas, and acute pancreatitis. Low levels of high-density lipoprotein cholesterol occur. Abnormal glucose tolerance and diabetes appear during puberty. In the absence of functional adipocytes, lipid is stored in other tissues, including muscle and liver. Fatty infiltration of the liver may lead to cirrhosis, and esophageal varices may become a fatal complication. Early onset of diabetes mellitus and dyslipidemia may result in atherosclerosis. Diabetic nephropathy and retinopathy occur. Hypertrophic cardiomyopathy occurs in 25% of cases and is a significant cause of early mortality. Restriction of total fat intake maintains normal triglyceride serum concentration. Treatment with leptin is effective for the control of hypertriglyceridemia and diabetes.

ETIOLOGY

Berardinelli-Seip Congenital Lipodystrophy (BSCL) has an autosomal recessive inheritance pattern. Mutations in the AGPAT2 gene encoding 1-acylglycerol-3-phosphate O-acyltransferase 2, located at 9q34, and BSCL2 encoding protein seipin, which is of unknown function, are responsible for 95% of cases. AGPAT2 is responsible for BSCL type 1 and BSCL2 for BSCL type 2. Individuals with BSCL type 2 have lower serum leptin levels, a much higher prevalence of intellectual disability, more frequent cardiomyopathy, and an earlier onset of diabetes than those with BSCL type 1.

COMMENT

Congenital generalized lipodystrophy types 3 and 4, caused by mutation in two additional genes (*CAV1* and *PTRF*, respectively), can be distinguished due to the presence of myopathy with elevation of serum creatine kinase.

References

Berardinelli W: An undiagnosed endocrinometabolic syndrome: Report of two cases, *J Clin Endocrinol Metab* 14:193, 1954.

Seip M, Trygstad O: Generalized lipodystrophy, *Arch Dis Child* 38:447, 1963.

Senior B, Gellis SS: The syndromes of total lipodystrophy and of partial lipodystrophy, *Pediatrics* 33:593, 1964.

Oserd S, et al: Decreased binding of insulin to its receptor in patients with congenital generalized lipodystrophy, *N Engl J Med* 296:245, 1977.

Garg A, et al: Peculiar distribution of adipose tissue in patients with congenital generalized lipodystrophy, *J Clin Endocrinol Metab* 75:358, 1991.

Klein S, et al: Generalized lipodystrophy: In vivo evidence of hypermetabolism and insulin-resistant lipid, glucose and amino acid kinetic, *Metabolism* 41:893, 1992.

Garg A, et al: Lipodystrophies, *Am J Med* 108:143, 2000.

Agarwal AA, et al: Phenotypic and genetic heterogeneity in congenital generalized lipodystrophy, *J Clin Endocrinol Metab* 88:4840, 2003.

Boutet E, et al: Seipin deficiency alters fatty acid delta9 desaturation and lipid droplet formation in Berardinelli-Seip congenital lipodystrophy, *Biochimie* 91:796, 2009.

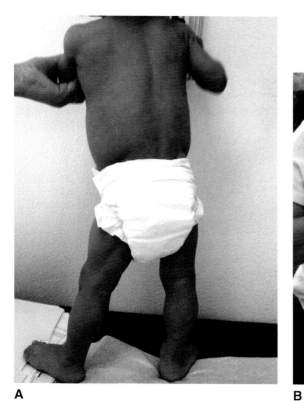

A

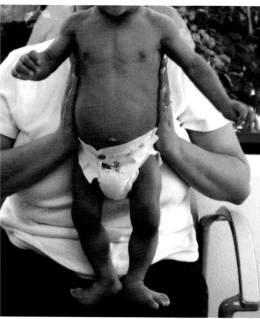

B

FIGURE 1. Berardinelli-Seip Lipodystrophy syndrome. **A** and **B,** A 2-year-old boy showing hypertrophied muscle and relative lack of subcutaneous fat. (Courtesy Dr. Lynne M. Bird, Children's Hospital, San Diego.)

DISTICHIASIS-LYMPHEDEMA SYNDROME
Double Row of Eyelashes, Lymphedema

ABNORMALITIES

Eyes. Distichiasis, an extra row of eyelashes (complete or partial), arising from meibomian glands (95%).

Limbs. Lymphedema, predominantly from knee downward (80% by age 30), often asymmetric, can be unilateral; varicose veins (50%); yellowish, discolored nails.

Other. Vertebral anomalies, epidural cysts, cardiac defects, ptosis.

OCCASIONAL ABNORMALITIES

Short stature, microphthalmia, strabismus, partial ectropion of lower lid, epicanthal folds, pterygium colli, chylothorax, cleft palate (4%), bifid uvula, micrognathia, Robin sequence, scoliosis/kyphosis, cryptorchidism, double uterus, renal anomalies, cardiac arrhythmia.

NATURAL HISTORY

The extra eyelashes may cause irritative ocular problems, photophobia, and recurrent conjunctivitis. The lymphedema usually becomes evident between the ages of 5 and 20 years, especially at the time of adolescence and sometimes for the first time during pregnancy. Only in rare cases is it present in newborns. Males develop lymphedema earlier and are more prone to cellulitis. Varicosities are prominent in half of the patients and require surgery. Some degree of venous valve incompetence appears to be present in all patients. The possibility of epidural cysts with secondary neurologic or other complications must always be considered in this disorder. Eyelash removal or surgery for the lymphedema is difficult to accomplish with good results; hence, treatment is generally symptomatic and withheld unless grossly indicated. Lubrication, cryotherapy, and other methods can improve ocular symptoms. Stockings or bandages for the lymphedema may improve discomfort. Antibiotics should be used promptly when injuries occur to prevent cellulitis.

ETIOLOGY

This disorder has an autosomal dominant inheritance pattern with marked variability of expression and occasional non-penetrance for lymphedema or distichiasis. Mutations in the forkhead family gene *FOXC2* located on chromosome 16q23 are responsible for at least 95% of families studied, but genetic heterogeneity may be present, since no mutation or linkage to the region has been found in a few familial cases. Diagnosis in sporadic cases is often difficult, because affected individuals might have only one of the characteristic features.

COMMENT

Unlike other lymphedema syndromes that are characterized by a failure in development of lymphatic structures, patients with distichiasis-lymphedema syndrome have an increased number of lymphatic vessels and inguinal lymph nodes, which do not appear to function normally.

References

Falls HF, Kertesz ED: A new syndrome combining pterygium colli with developmental anomalies of the eyelids and lymphatics of the lower extremities, *Trans Am Ophthalmol Soc* 62:248, 1964.

Robinow M, Johnson GF, Verhagen AD: Distichiasis-lymphedema: A hereditary syndrome of multiple congenital defects, *Am J Dis Child* 119:343, 1970.

Hoover RE, Kelley JS: Distichiasis and lymphedema: A hereditary syndrome with possible multiple defects—a report of a family, *Trans Ophthalmol Soc* 69:293, 1971.

Holmes LB, Fields JP, Zabriskie JB: Hereditary late-onset lymphedema, *Pediatrics* 61:575, 1978.

Schwartz JF, O'Brien MS, Hoffman JC: Hereditary spinal arachnoid cysts, distichiasis, and lymphedema, *Ann Neurol* 7:340, 1980.

Temple IK, Collin JRO: Distichiasis-lymphoedema syndrome: A family report, *Clin Dysmorphol* 3:139, 1994.

Fang J, et al: Mutations in *FOXC2* (MFH-1), a forkhead family transcription factor, are responsible for the hereditary lymphedema-distichiasis syndrome, *Am J Hum Genet* 67:1382, 2000.

Finegold DN, et al: Truncating mutations in *FOXC2* cause multiple lymphedema syndromes, *Hum Mol Genet* 10:1185, 2001.

Brice G, et al: Analysis of the phenotypic abnormalities in lymphoedema-distichiasis syndrome in 74 patients with *FOXC2* mutations or linkage to 16q24, *J Med Genet* 39:478, 2002.

Mellor RH, et al: Mutations in *FOXC2* are strongly associated with primary valve failure in veins of the lower limb, *Circulation* 115:1912, 2007.

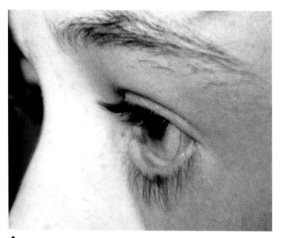

A

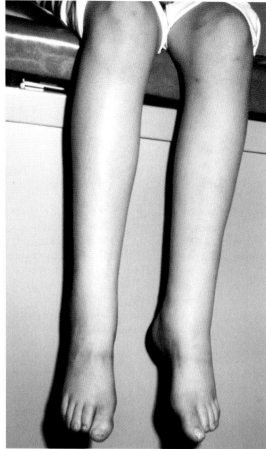

B

FIGURE 1.   Distichiasis-lymphedema syndrome. Distichiasis in the eye of this teenage girl (A) and lymphedema in her leg (B).

T

VICI SYNDROME
Agenesis of the Corpus Callosum, Hypopigmentation, Immunodeficiency

Initially described in 1988 by Vici et al, del Campo et al reported four additional patients in 1999, among them affected male and female siblings, suggesting autosomal recessive inheritance. Twelve patients have been reported to date, with a consistently severe phenotype.

ABNORMALITIES

Growth. Postnatal onset growth retardation, often with severe failure to thrive.

Performance. Profound developmental delay; poor interaction with the environment; often unable to acquire social smile or head control; hypotonia; seizures, with irregular spikes and wave complexes in temporal, parietal, and occipital areas, as well as hypsarrhythmia, on EEG. Profound cervicoaxial hypotonia with hyperextended neck posture, flexed lower limbs, and clenched fists.

Brain. Agenesis of the corpus callosum and septum pellucidum, cerebral atrophy with enlarged ventricles, hypoplasia of the cerebellar vermis and pons, gyral anomalies such as heterotopias or other forms of non-lissencephalic cortical dysplasia, schizencephaly, delayed myelination, opercular hypoplasia, hypoplasia of optic nerves and chiasma.

Craniofacial. Postnatal onset microcephaly, ptosis, depressed nasal bridge, high palate, tented upper lip, mild micrognathia. Mild coarsening of facial features over time.

Ocular. Congenital or acquired cataracts, hypopigmented retina and iris, hypoplasia of macula and optic disk, horizontal nystagmus, marked visual disturbance, lack of light reflex, inconsistent visual fixation and tracking, slow or absent visual evoked potentials, photophobia.

Hearing. Sensorineural hearing loss. Startle responses to noise are usually present.

Skin and Hair. Hypopigmentation of the skin, ranging from lighter complexion to complete albinism. Fair, fine hair, sometimes silvery, which tends to stand on end.

Renal. Renal tubular acidosis.

Cardiac. Cardiomegaly or dilated cardiomyopathy. Elevation of serum cardiac enzymes.

Immune System. Broad spectrum of defects ranging from a combined immunodeficiency to a nearly normal immunity. Lymphopenia associated with different combinations of specific T-cell subset defects; unprotective antibody responses to vaccination; neutropenia; hypogammaglobulinemia; lack of skin responses to several recall antigens.

Muscle. Myopathic changes, including fiber type disproportion, type 1 fiber atrophy, and prominent central nuclei in atrophic fibers noted on muscle biopsy. Increase in glycogen content. On electron microscopy, redundancy of basal lamina with material between layers suggesting exocytosis of debris, vacuole-like areas and dense bodies possibly of lysosomal origin. Myofibrils lacking in many fibers. Mitochondria of variable size, distribution, and morphology.

OCCASIONAL ABNORMALITIES

Cleft lip and palate, hypospadias, hypotelorism, hypertelorism, ostium secundum atrial septal defect, lung hypoplasia.

NATURAL HISTORY

Survival beyond the first 4 years of life is unusual. Sucking and swallowing difficulties with frequent regurgitation lead to failure to thrive. Disturbance of sleep-wakefulness circadian rhythms and impairments in phasic REM sleep parameters occur frequently. Multiple infections, including those of the respiratory, urinary, and gastrointestinal tracts, as well as conjunctivitis and skin and perineal abscesses occur. Infections with *Candida* and *Pseudomonas*, as well as progressive cardiomyopathy, are the main causes of early death. Seizures can be resistant to anticonvulsant therapy. No patient has been able to walk or acquire expressive language other than babbling. Early treatment with beta-blockers may slow the progression of cardiac deterioration. Intellectual disability has been consistently severe, with little progression.

ETIOLOGY

A mutation in *KIAA1632*, on chromosome 18q12.3-q21.1, is responsible. *KIAA1632* is the human homologue of the metazoan-specific autophagy gene epg-5, encoding a key autophagy regulator implicated in the formation of autolysosomes. Autophagy is an evolutionary highly conserved lysosomal degradation pathway. Analysis of 15 families showed mutations in 13. The cases without mutations appeared to have longer survival and no cardiomyopathic manifestations. Vici syndrome is the first example of a human multisystem disorder associated with defective autophagy.

References

Vici CD, et al: Agenesis of the corpus callosum, combined immunodeficiency, bilateral cataract, and hypopigmentation in two brothers, *Am J Med Genet* 29:1, 1988.

del Campo M, et al: Albinism and agenesis of the corpus callosum with profound developmental delay: Vici syndrome, evidence for autosomal recessive inheritance, *Am J Med Genet* 85:479, 1999.

Miyata R, et al: Sibling cases of Vici syndrome: Sleep abnormalities and complications of renal tubular acidosis, *Am J Med Genet A* 143:189, 2007.

McClelland V, et al: Vici syndrome associated with sensorineural hearing loss and evidence of neuromuscular involvement on muscle biopsy, *Am J Med Genet A* 152A:741, 2007.

Finocchi A, et al: Immunodeficiency in Vici syndrome: A heterogeneous phenotype, *Am J Med Genet A* 158A:434, 2012.

Said E, et al: Vici syndrome—A rapidly progressive neurodegenerative disorder with hypopigmentation, immunodeficiency and myopathic changes on muscle biopsy, *Am J Med Genet A* 158A:440, 2012.

Cullup T, et al: Recessive mutations in *KIAA1632* cause Vici syndrome, a multisystem disorder with defective autophagy, *Nat Genet* 45:83, 2013.

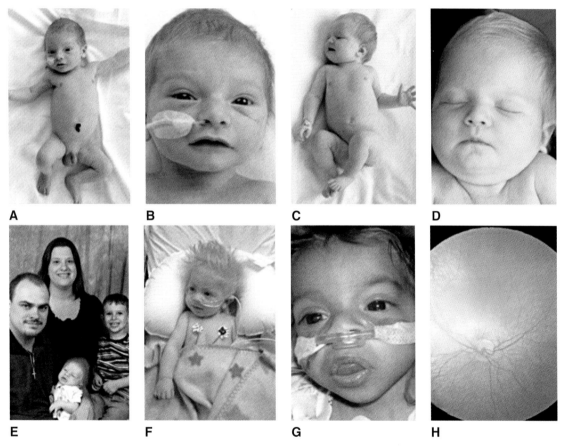

FIGURE 1.   Vici syndrome. **A–G,** Clinical photographs from affected patients. There is marked generalized hypopigmentation relative to the ethnic background **(E, F).** Coarsening of facial features with full lips and macroglossia is noted in some older children **(G).** There is marked retinal hypopigmentation on fundoscopy **(H).** (Reprinted from Cullup T, et al: *Nat Genet* 45:83, 2013.)

LATERALITY SEQUENCES

In addition to reversal of the sides, with partial to complete situs inversus, there can be bilateral left- or right-sidedness. The primary defect in both is a failure of normal asymmetry in morphogenesis. The basic problem would presumably be present before 30 days of development. Figure 1 sets forth the differences as well as the similarities between the patterns predominantly caused by left-sided bilaterality and by right-sided bilaterality. Among other differences, the spleen dramatically reflects the variant laterality in the two. With left-sided bilaterality, there is polysplenia (usually bilateral spleens plus rudimentary extra splenic tissue), and with right-sided bilaterality there is asplenia or a hypoplastic spleen.

Left-right axis malformations are usually isolated but can occur as one feature of a multiple malformation syndrome, the most common of which is immotile cilia syndrome. As a result of defective cilia and flagella, chronic respiratory tract infections occur commonly, and infertility in males, chronic ear infections, and decreased or absent smell occur variably. The cilia are functionally abnormal and, on electron microscopy, have absent or abnormal dynein arms connecting the nine pairs of microtubules. A subgroup of the immotile cilia syndrome is Kartagener syndrome, an autosomal recessive disorder associated with partial to complete situs inversus with gross defects in cardiac septation (50%) in addition to the other features of immotile cilia syndrome.

BILATERAL LEFT-SIDEDNESS SEQUENCE
Bilateral left-sidedness sequence is also known as polysplenia syndrome. The gender incidence is about equal. The cardiac anomalies are usually not as severe as those with bilateral right-sidedness.

BILATERAL RIGHT-SIDEDNESS SEQUENCE
Bilateral right-sidedness sequence is also known as asplenia syndrome, Ivemark syndrome, triad of spleen agenesis, defects of heart and vessels, and situs inversus. The sequence is two to three times more common in males than in females. The complex cardiac anomalies, usually giving rise to cyanosis and early cardiac failure, are the major cause of early death. The possibility of gastrointestinal problems must also be considered, especially as related to the aberrant mesenteric attachments. Renal anomalies are also more frequent (25%). Survivors have had an increased frequency of cutaneous, respiratory, and other infections, possibly

related to the asplenia. Tests to detect asplenia include evaluation of red blood cells for Howell-Jolly bodies and Heinz bodies.

OCCASIONAL ABNORMALITIES

Intestinal malrotation, biliary atresia, anomalous portal and hepatic vessels, intestinal obstruction, anal atresia/stenosis, urinary tract defects including renal agenesis/hypoplasia and ureteral malformations, meningomyelocele, cerebellar hypoplasia, arrhinencephaly.

ETIOLOGY

The defect in lateralization leading to the failure of normal asymmetry in morphogenesis is most likely etiologically heterogeneous. As such, although usually sporadic, autosomal dominant, autosomal recessive, and X-linked recessive inheritance have all been documented. At present, only 10% of cases are caused by mutations of known genes, although additional candidate genes have emerged from studies of left-right axis development in vertebrates. Mutations in *ZIC3*, an X-linked zinc-finger transcription factor located at Xq26.2, which are frequently associated with hindgut anomalies in addition to the failure in normal symmetry, are responsible for a small number of cases. Mutations in *NODAL*, which are associated with a higher frequency of pulmonary valve atresia, and *ACVR2B* account for the majority of known genetic cases. In addition, mutations of *LEFTY A*, on chromosome 1q42, *CFC1, CCDC11, GDF1,* and *NKX2-5* have been responsible for rare cases.

COMMENT

Both bilateral left-sidedness (polysplenia) and bilateral right-sidedness (asplenia) have been documented in different persons in the same family, indicating that the two conditions represent different manifestations of a primary defect in lateralization leading to failure of normal body asymmetry.

The molecular determinants of normal body asymmetry are beginning to emerge. In the mouse, motile embryonic cilia generate directional flow of extraembryonic fluid surrounding the node located at the tip of the embryo in the midline. This flow concentrates left-right determinants to one side of the node activating asymmetric gene expression at the node and beyond. In the chick, *activin* on the right side of the primitive streak represses expression of the gene sonic hedgehog (*Shh*). The remaining expression of *Shh* on the left induces *nodal* on the left, leading to the normal looping of the heart tube to the right.

References

Freedom RM: The asplenia syndrome, *J Pediatr* 81:1130, 1972.

Van Mierop LHS, et al: Asplenia and polysplenia syndromes, *Birth Defects* 8:74, 1972.

Afzelius AB: Kartagener's syndrome and abnormal cilia, *N Engl J Med* 297:1011, 1977.

U

Mathias RS, et al: X-linked laterality sequence: Situs inversus, complex cardiac defects, splenic defects, *Am J Med Genet* 28:111, 1987.

Mikkila SP, et al: X-linked laterality sequence in a family with carrier manifestations, *Am J Med Genet* 49:435, 1994.

Levin M, et al: A molecular pathway determining left-right asymmetry in chick embryogenesis, *Cell* 82:803, 1995.

Casey B: Two rights make a wrong: Human left-right malformations, *Hum Mol Genet* 7:1565, 1998.

McGrath J, Brueckner M: Cilia are at the heart of vertebrate left-right asymmetry, *Curr Opinion Genet Devel* 13:385, 2003.

Mohapatra B, et al: Identification and functional characterization of *NODAL* rare variants in heterotaxy and isolated cardiovascular malformations, *Hum Mol Genet* 18:861, 2009.

Ma L, et al: Mutations in *ZIC3* and *ACVR2B* are a common cause of heterotaxy and associated cardiovascular anomalies, *Cardiol Young* 22:194, 2012.

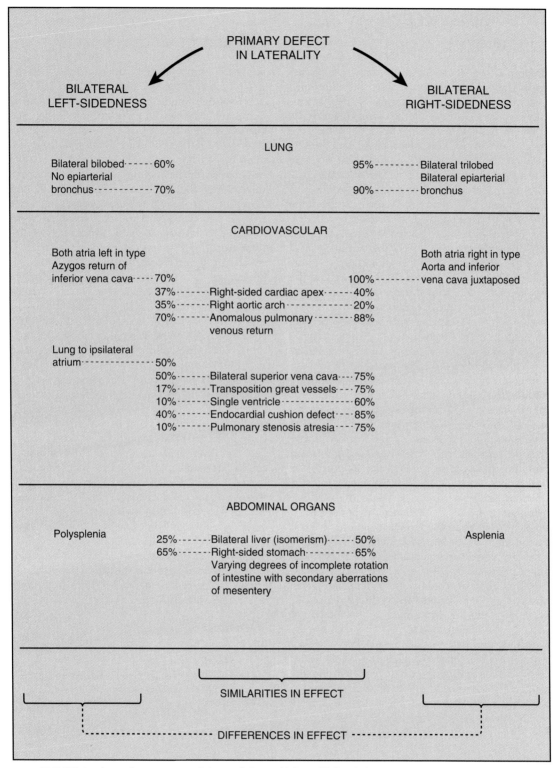

FIGURE 1.   Laterality sequences. Primary defects of bilateral left-sidedness and bilateral right-sidedness.

HOLOPROSENCEPHALY SEQUENCE
Arrhinencephaly-Cebocephaly-Cyclopia: Primary Defect in Prechordal Mesoderm

Holoprosencephaly results from incomplete cleavage of the prosencephalon between the eighteenth and twenty-eighth day of gestation. Neuroanatomically it is divided—based on the extent to which the forebrain has failed to separate—into alobar (the most severe type), semilobar, lobar, and middle interhemispheric type (the mildest type). In the alobar type, the prosencephalon fails to cleave sagittally into cerebral hemispheres, transversely into telencephalon and diencephalon, and horizontally into olfactory tracts and bulbs. As a consequence of, and associated with, these severe defects in brain development, varying degrees of midline facial development occur. Cyclopia represents a severe deficit in early midline facial development, and the eyes become fused, the olfactory placodes consolidate into a single tube-like proboscis above the eye, and the ethmoid and other midline bony structures are missing. Less severe deficits result in hypotelorism and varying degrees of inadequate midfacial and incomplete forebrain development that are more common than cyclopia and frequently include midline cleft lip and palate. The important clinical point is that incomplete midline facial development—such as hypotelorism, absence of the philtrum or nasal septum, a single central incisor, congenital nasal pyriform aperture stenosis, and/or a missing frenulum of the upper lip—suggests the possibility of a serious anomaly in brain development and function. Endocrine disorders, including diabetes insipidus, adrenal hypoplasia, hypogonadism, thyroid hypoplasia, and growth hormone defects, are common. In addition, seizures and autonomic instability affecting temperature control, heart rate, and respiration have been reported. Finally ptosis, coloboma, choanal atresia, cleft lip and palate, genitourinary and renal anomalies, including micropenis, cryptorchidism, and ambiguous genitalia, as well as cardiac defects occur.

Although the defect is isolated in the vast majority of cases, holoprosencephaly is etiologically heterogeneous with both genetic and environmental causes identified. Aneuploidy syndromes—including trisomies 13 and 18, as well as several structural chromosome aberrations, including del2p21, dup3pter, del7q36, del13q, del18p, and del21q22.3—should be considered. Autosomal dominant mutations in a number of genes have been identified in "nonsyndromic" holoprosencephaly. Mutations in four genes that have been identified in both sporadic and familial cases are responsible for the majority of these nonsyndromic cases. These four genes are *SHH, ZIC2, SIX3,* and *TGIF.* Sonic hedgehog (*SHH*), responsible for 12% of cases, is associated with wide variability of expression and is located at 7q36. Mutations in *ZIC2,* located at 13q32, occur in 9% of cases and are associated with a specific facial phenotype, including bitemporal narrowness, upslanting palpebral fissures, a flat nasal bridge, a short nose with anteverted nares, a broad and deep philtrum, and large ears. Mutations in *SIX3,* located at 2p21 and associated with an increase in renal anomalies, occur in up to 5% of cases, and mutations in *TGIF,* located at 18p11.3, occur in 1% to 2% of cases. Mutations in a number of genes involved in signaling pathways important for brain development, including *PATCHED1* and *GLI2,* as well as *TDGF1* and *FAST1,* which are involved in the Nodal/transforming growth factor β (TGF-β) pathway, occur far less frequently. Parents of an affected child should be checked for mild manifestations such as a single central incisor, a missing upper lip frenulum, and absence of the nasal cartilage. Finally, holoprosencephaly has been seen as one feature of multiple malformation syndromes such as Meckel-Gruber syndrome and Smith-Lemli-Opitz syndrome, in the offspring of diabetic women, and as an occasional feature in fetal alcohol spectrum disorder. The prognosis for central nervous system function in individuals with this type of defect is very poor.

References

Adelmann HB: The problem of cyclopia. Part II, *Q Rev Biol* 11:284, 1936.

DeMeyer W, et al: The face predicts the brain: Diagnostic significance of median facial anomalies for holoprosencephaly (arrhinencephaly), *Pediatrics* 34:256, 1964.

Cohen MM: An update on the holoprosencephalic disorders, *J Pediatr* 101:865, 1982.

Siebert JR, et al: *Holoprosencephaly: An Overview and Atlas of Cases*, New York, 1990, Wiley-Liss.

Gurrieri F, et al: Physical mapping of the holoprosencephaly critical region on chromosome 7q36, *Nat Genet* 3:247, 1993.

Muenke M, et al: Linkage of a human brain malformation, familial holoprosencephaly, to chromosome 7 and evidence for genetic heterogeneity, *Proc Natl Acad Sci U S A* 91:8102, 1994.

Ming JE, Muenke M: Multiple hits during early embryonic development: Digenic diseases and holoprosencephaly, *Am J Hum Genet* 71:1017, 2002.

Cohen MM: Holoprosencephaly: Clinical, anatomic, and molecular dimensions, *Birth Defects Res A Clin Mol Teratol* 76:658, 2006.

Dubourg C, et al: Holoprosencephaly, *Orphanet J Rare Dis* 2:8, 2007.

Solomon BD, et al: Analysis of genotype-phenotype correlations in human holoprosencephaly, *Am J Med Genet C Semin Med Genet* 154C:133, 2010.

Solomon BD, et al: Genotype and phenotype analysis of 396 individuals with mutation in sonic hedgehog, *J Med Genet* 49:473, 2012.

U

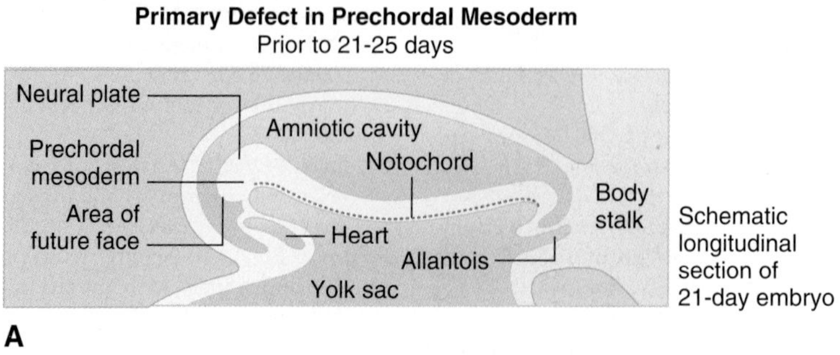

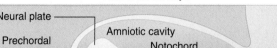

Primary Defect in Prechordal Mesoderm
Prior to 21-25 days

FIGURE 1.   Holoprosencephaly sequence. **A,** Schematic longitudinal section of 21-day embryo.

Continued

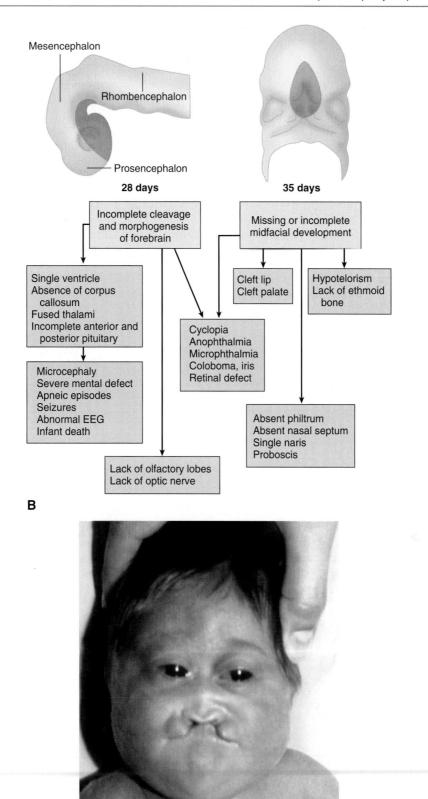

Mesencephalon

Rhombencephalon

Prosencephalon

28 days

35 days

Incomplete cleavage
and morphogenesis
of forebrain

Missing or incomplete
midfacial development

Single ventricle
Absence of corpus
  callosum
Fused thalami
Incomplete anterior and
  posterior pituitary

Cleft lip
Cleft palate

Hypotelorism
Lack of ethmoid
  bone

Microcephaly
Severe mental defect
Apneic episodes
Seizures
Abnormal EEG
Infant death

Cyclopia
Anophthalmia
Microphthalmia
Coloboma, iris
Retinal defect

Absent philtrum
Absent nasal septum
Single naris
Proboscis

Lack of olfactory lobes
Lack of optic nerve

B

C

FIGURE 1, cont'd.   B, Developmental pathogenesis of the sequence. **C,** Affected individual.

U

MENINGOMYELOCELE, ANENCEPHALY, INIENCEPHALY SEQUENCES
Primary Defect in Neural Tube Closure

The initiating malformation appears to be a defect in closure of the neural groove to form an intact neural tube, which is normally completely fused by 28 days. Anencephaly represents a defect in closure at the anterior portion of the neural groove. The secondary consequences are these: (1) The unfused forebrain develops partially and then tends to degenerate; (2) the calvarium is incompletely developed; and (3) the facial features and auricular development are secondarily altered to a variable degree, including cleft palate and frequent abnormality of the cervical vertebrae.

Defects of closure at the mid or caudal neural groove can give rise to meningomyelocele and other secondary defects, as depicted. Of greatest concern relative to outcome for independence and survival is the hydrocephalus and other manifestations of the Chiari II malformation, which is present if virtually all cases.

Defects of closure in the cervical and upper thoracic region can culminate in the iniencephaly sequence, in which secondary features may include retroflexion of the upper spine with short neck and trunk, cervical and upper thoracic vertebral anomalies, defects of thoracic cage, anterior spina bifida, diaphragmatic defects with or without hernia, and hypoplasia of lung and/or heart. Evidence suggesting that there may be four sites of anterior neural tube closure explains the variations observed in their location, recurrence risk, and etiology. Most commonly, no specific etiology is appreciated and the recurrence risk is 1.9% for parents who have had one affected child. Measurement of alpha fetoprotein (AFP) in maternal serum in conjunction with detailed ultrasonography allows prenatal diagnosis in the vast majority of cases.

The U.S. Public Health Service has recommended that women of childbearing age should consume 0.4 mg of folic acid daily to reduce their risk of conceiving a child with a neural tube defect. For women who previously have had an affected infant, it has been recommended that 4.0 mg daily of folic acid should be consumed from 1 month before conception through 3 months of pregnancy.

References

Giroud A: Causes and morphogenesis of anencephaly. Ciba Foundation Symposium on Congenital Malformations, 1960, pp 199–218.

Lemire RJ, et al: Caudal myeloschisis (lumbo-sacral spina bifida cystica) in a five millimeter (horizon XIV) human embryo, *Anat Rec* 152:9, 1965.

Lemire RJ, Beckwith JB, Shepard TH: Iniencephaly and anencephaly with spinal retroflexion, *Teratology* 6:27, 1972.

Centers for Disease Control and Prevention: Recommendations for use of folic acid to reduce number of spina bifida cases and other neural tube defects, *JAMA* 269:1233, 1993.

Van Allen MI, et al: Evidence for multi-site closure of the neural tube in humans, *Am J Med Genet* 47:723, 1993.

Golden JA, Chernoff GF: Multiple sites of anterior neural tube closure in humans: Evidence from anterior neural tube defects (anencephaly), *Pediatrics* 95:506, 1995.

McLone DG, Dias MS: The Chiari II malformation: Cause and impact, *Childs Nerv Syst* 19:540, 2003.

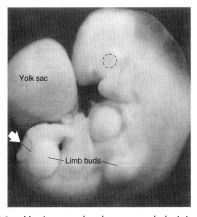
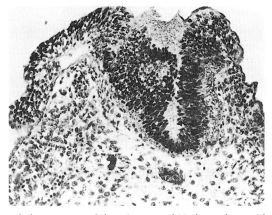

FIGURE 1.   Meningomyelocele, anencephaly, iniencephaly sequences. Otherwise normal 28-day embryo with incomplete closure of the posterior neural groove (*arrow*), which shows aberrant growth of cells to the side in a transverse section (*right*). Had this embryo survived, it would presumably have developed a meningomyelocele. (From Lemire R: *Anat Rec* 152:9, 1965. Copyright © 1965. Reprinted with permission of Wiley-Liss, Inc., a subsidiary of John Wiley & Sons, Inc.)

DEFECTS IN CLOSURE OF NEURAL TUBE

Dorsal View of Normal Embryo of 23 Days

Cephalad neural groove

Caudad neural groove

Somite

Neural tube
(normally completely
closed by 28 days)

DEFECT IN CLOSURE OF
ANTERIOR NEURAL TUBE

DEFECT IN CLOSURE

Neural tube

Somite

1. Incomplete development of
   brain, with degeneration
2. Incomplete development of
   calvaria
3. Alteration in facies
   +/– auricle

Neural deficit
caudal to lesion

Meningomyelocele

Defect in
spinous process

+/– Clubfoot

+/– Hydrocephalus

Spina bifida

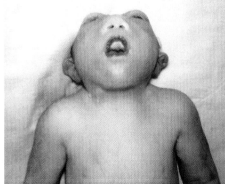

Anencephaly

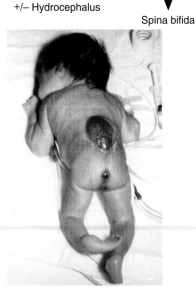

Meningomyelocele with partially
epithelialized sac

FIGURE 2. Developmental pathogenesis of anencephaly and meningomyelocele.

OCCULT SPINAL DYSRAPHISM SEQUENCE
(TETHERED CORD MALFORMATION SEQUENCE)

Following closure of the neural groove at approximately 28 days, the cell mass caudal to the posterior neuropore tunnels downward and forms a canal in a process that gives rise to the most distal portions of the spinal cord—the filum terminale and conus medullaris. Failure of normal morphogenesis in this region leads to a spectrum of structural defects that cause orthopedic or urologic symptoms through tethering or compression of the sacral nerve roots, with restriction of the normal cephalic migration of the conus medullaris. Defects involve structures derived from both mesodermal and ectodermal tissue and include mesodermal hamartomas, sacral vertebral anomalies, hyperplasia of the filum terminale, and structural alterations of the distal cord itself. In most situations, there is a cutaneous marker at the presumed junction between the caudal cell mass and the posterior neuropore in the region of L2-L3. Markers consist of tufts of hair, skin tags, dimples, lipomata, and aplasia cutis congenita. Cutaneous markers such as a pit at the tip of the coccyx are extremely common and are not usually associated with a tethered cord.

The recognition of the surface manifestations of such a malformation sequence at birth should ideally lead to further evaluation and management. Roentgenograms of the spine may or may not show any abnormality. Ultrasound to document normal movement of the spinal cord with respiration, followed by magnetic resonance imaging in questionable cases, is usually sufficient to document the defect. Early management will prevent neuromuscular lower limb or urologic problems such as retention, incontinence, or infection secondary to continued tractional tethering of the cord and nerve roots. If the physician waits for signs of such serious complications, the neurologic damage may not be reversible. A 4% incidence of open neural tube defects has been documented in first-degree relatives of probands.

References

Anderson FM: Occult spinal dysraphism: Diagnosis and management, *J Pediatr* 73:163, 1968.

Carter CO, et al: Spinal dysraphism: Genetic relation to neural tube malformations, *J Med Genet* 13:343, 1976.

Tavafoghi V, et al: Cutaneous signs of spinal dysraphism, *Arch Dermatol* 114:573, 1978.

Higginbottom MC, et al: Aplasia cutis congenita: Cutaneous marker of occult spinal dysraphism, *J Pediatr* 96:687, 1980.

Soonawala N, et al: Early clinical signs and symptoms in occult spinal dysraphism: A retrospective case study of 47 patients, *Clin Neuro Neurosurg* 101:11, 1999.

Hughes JA, et al: Evaluation of spinal ultrasound in spinal dysraphism, *Clin Radiol* 58:227, 2003.

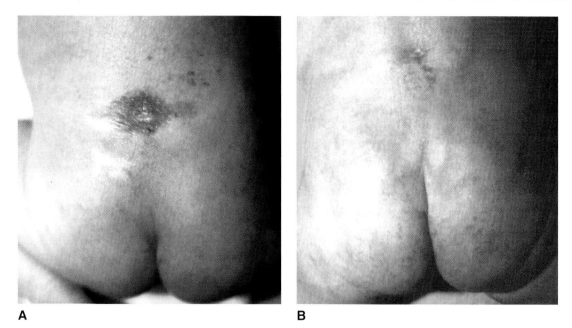

A   **B**

FIGURE 1.   Occult spinal dysraphism sequence. Note the location of these lesions, which were the clues that resulted in surgical correction of tethered cord in early infancy. In addition to the flat hemangioma **(A),** the mound of connective tissue **(B),** and the localized absence of skin (**A** and **B**), surface anomalies may consist of lipomas, deep dimples, hair tufts, and skin tags. (From Higginbottom MC, et al: *J Pediatr* 96:687, 1980, with permission.)

U

SEPTO-OPTIC DYSPLASIA SEQUENCE

De Morsier recognized the association between the absence of the septum pellucidum and hypoplasia of the optic nerves and called it septo-optic dysplasia. The clinical spectrum of altered development and function arising from this defect has been reported by Hoyt and others to include hypopituitary dwarfism. The presumed developmental pathogenesis is depicted to the right.

ABNORMALITIES

Eyes. Hypoplastic optic nerves, chiasm, and infundibulum with pendular nystagmus and visual impairment, occasionally including field defects.

Endocrine. Low levels of growth hormone, thyroid-stimulating hormone, luteinizing hormone, follicle-stimulating hormone, and antidiuretic hormone; hypoglycemia.

Other. Agenesis of septum pellucidum in approximately 50% of cases, agenesis of corpus callosum, microcephaly, schizencephaly.

OCCASIONAL ABNORMALITIES

Cleft lip and/or palate; trophic hormone hypersecretion, including growth hormone, corticotropin, and prolactin; sexual precocity; strabismus; hemiplegia; spasticity; athetosis; epilepsy; autism; cranial nerve palsy; intellectual disability; learning defects; attention deficit disorders; neonatal intrahepatic cholestasis; micropenis; cryptorchidism.

NATURAL HISTORY

Visual impairment, including partial to complete amblyopia, is frequent, and funduscopic evaluation discloses hypoplastic optic disks. Hypopituitarism of hypothalamic origin is a frequent feature and merits hormone replacement therapy. Affected newborns can develop hypoglycemia, jaundice, apnea, hypotonia, or seizures. In an affected child with absence of the septum pellucidum and hypoplasia of the optic nerves who has no other associated defects of central nervous system development, prognosis relative to intellectual performance is good. However, intellectual disability does occur, particularly when associated central nervous system defects are present. Onset of puberty is variable.

Features of the septo-optic dysplasia sequence may occur as a part of a broader pattern of early brain defect, such as the holoprosencephaly type of defect, in which case the prognosis for brain function and survival is poor.

ETIOLOGY

This disorder is etiologically heterogeneous. Most cases are sporadic, with several etiologies suggested. These include teratogens, including intrauterine viral infection, valproic acid (Depakote), and prenatal alcohol exposure, as well as vascular disruption and both homozygous (autosomal recessive) and heterozygous (autosomal dominant) mutations of four genes. These four genes are *HESX1,* located at chromosome 3p21.1-21.2, mutations of which are responsible for some sporadic as well as familial cases (1% of cases), as well as *SOX2, SOX3,* located at Xq27, and *OTX2.* All four of these genes are transcription factors that are essential for forebrain and pituitary development.

References

de Morsier G: Études sur les dysraphies crânio-encéphaliques. III. Agénésie du septum lucidum avec malformation du tractus optique: La dysplasie septo-optique, *Schweiz Arch Neurol Neurochir Psychiatry* 77:267, 1956.

Hoyt WF, et al: Septo-optic dysplasia and pituitary dwarfism, *Lancet* 1:893, 1970.

Brook CGD, et al: Septo-optic dysplasia, *BMJ* 3:811, 1972.

Haseman CA, et al: Sexual precocity in association with septo-optic dysplasia and hypothalamic hypopituitarism, *J Pediatr* 92:748, 1978.

Blethen SL, Weldon VV: Hypopituitarism and septo-optic "dysplasia" in first cousins, *Am J Med Genet* 21:123, 1985.

Margalith D, et al: Congenital optic nerve hypoplasia with hypothalamic-pituitary dysplasia, *Am J Dis Child* 139:361, 1985.

Morgan SA, et al: Absence of the septum pellucidum: Overlapping clinical syndromes, *Arch Neurol* 42:769, 1985.

Hanna CE, et al: Puberty in the syndrome of septo-optic dysplasia, *Am J Dis Child* 143:186, 1989.

Dattani MT, et al: Mutations in the homeobox gene *HESX1/Hesx1* associated with septo-optic dysplasia in human and mouse, *Nat Genet* 19:125, 1998.

Dattani MT, Robinson IC: *HESX1* and septo-optic dysplasia, *Rev Endocr Metab Disord* 3:289, 2002.

Webb EA, Dattani MT: Septo-optic dysplasia, *Eur J Hum Genet* 18:393, 2010.

McCabe MJ, et al: Septo-optic dysplasia and other midline defects: The role of transcription factors: HESX1 and beyond, *Best Pract Res Clin Endocrinol Metab* 25:115, 2011.

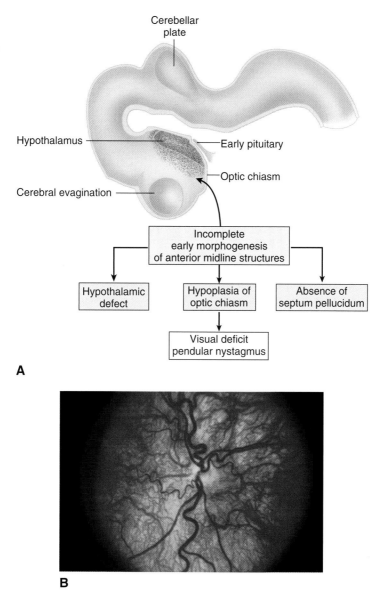

Cerebellar
plate

Hypothalamus ——————   ———— Early pituitary

                                   ——— Optic chiasm

Cerebral evagination ———————

```
            Incomplete
       early morphogenesis
    of anterior midline structures
```

| Hypothalamic defect | Hypoplasia of optic chiasm | Absence of septum pellucidum |

Visual deficit
pendular nystagmus

A

B

FIGURE 1. Septo-optic dysplasia sequence. **A,** Presumed localization of early single defect (stippled area) as shown in sagittal view of 38-day brain. **B,** Photo of retina of 4-year-old patient with the septo-optic dysplasia sequence who had reduced vision, pendular nystagmus, and growth deficiency secondary to pituitary growth hormone deficiency. Note the hypoplastic optic nerve heads and aberrant vascular arrangement.

U

KLIPPEL-FEIL SEQUENCE
Short Neck with Low Hairline and Limited Movement of Head: Primary Defect—Early Development of Cervical Vertebrae

In this malformation sequence, originally described by Klippel and Feil in 1912, the cervical vertebrae are usually fused, although hemivertebrae and other defects may also be found. There may also be secondary webbed neck, torticollis, and/or facial asymmetry. The frequency is approximately 1 in 42,000 births, and 65% of patients are female. The sequence may be a part of a serious problem in early neural tube development, as is found in iniencephaly, cervical meningomyelocele, syringomyelia, or syringobulbia. Primary or secondary neurologic deficits may occur, such as paraplegia, hemiplegia, cranial or cervical nerve palsies, and synkinesia (mirror movements). A strong association exists between mirror movements and cervicomedullary neuroschisis. Three types of Klippel-Feil sequence (KFS) have been described.

Type 1: Cervical spine fusion in which elements of many vertebrae are incorporated into a single block

Type 2: Cervical fusion in which complete segmentation fails at only one or two cervical levels and may include occipitoatlantal fusion

Type 3: Type 1 or type 2 fusion with coexisting segmentation errors in the lower dorsal or lumbar spine

The following defects have occurred in a nonrandom association in patients with KFS: deafness, either conductive or sensorineural, noted in as many as 30% of cases; ear anomalies; congenital heart defects, the most common being a ventricular septal defect; supra-aortic arch anomalies; intellectual disabilities; cleft palate; vocal impairment, rib defects; Sprengel anomaly; posterior fossa dermoid cysts; scoliosis; carpal and tarsal fusion renal abnormalities.

Lateral flexion-extension radiographs of the cervical spine should be performed on all patients to determine the motion of each open interspace. Clinically, flexion-extension is often maintained if a single functioning open interspace is maintained. Those with hypermobility of the upper cervical segment are at risk of developing neurologic impairment. They should be evaluated at least annually and should avoid violent activities. Affected individuals with hypermobility of the lower cervical segment are at increased risk for degenerative disk disease and should be treated symptomatically. Approximately one third of cases have cervical spine–related symptoms. The majority have axial symptoms and they are primarily associated with type 1 patients, whereas predominant radicular and myelopathic symptoms occur in type 2 and type 3 patients.

ETIOLOGY
Usually a sporadic occurrence of unknown etiology, this sequence has rarely been found in siblings. A close evaluation of the immediate family is indicated, because autosomal dominant inheritance with variable expression in affected individuals has been noted, although this is presumably rare. Initially identified in a large autosomal dominant family, mutations in *GDF6*, located at 8q, have been identified in both familial and sporadic KFS patients in which carpal and tarsal fusion has been an associated feature

References

Klippel M, Feil A: Un cas d'absence des vertèbres cervicales, avec cage thoracique remontant jusqu'à la base du crâne (cage thoracique cervicale), *Mouv Inconogr Salpêt* 25:223, 1912.

Morrison SG, Perry LW, Scott LP III: Congenital brevicollis (Klippel-Feil syndrome) and cardiovascular anomalies, *Am J Dis Child* 115:614, 1968.

Palant DJ, Carter BL: Klippel-Feil syndrome and deafness, *Am J Dis Child* 123:218, 1972.

Hensinger RW, et al: Klippel-Feil syndrome; a constellation of associated anomalies, *J Bone Joint Surg Am* 56:1246, 1974.

Dickey W, et al: Posterior fossa dermoid cysts and the Klippel-Feil syndrome, *J Neurol Neurosurg Psychiatry* 54:1016, 1991.

Pizzutillo PD, et al: Risk factors in Klippel-Feil syndrome, *Spine* 19:2110, 1994.

Royal SA, et al: Investigations into the association between cervicomedullary neuroschisis and mirror movements in patients with Klippel-Feil syndrome, *AJNR Am J Neuroradiol* 23:724, 2002.

Samartzis D, et al: Classification of congenitally fused cervical patterns in Klippel-Feil patients, *Spine* 31:E798, 2006.

Sudhakar A, et al: Klippel-Feil syndrome and supra-aortic arch anomaly: A case report, *Int J Angiol* 17:109, 2008.

Tassabehji M, et al: Mutations in *GDF6* are associated with vertebral segmentation defects in Klippel-Feil syndrome, *Hum Mutat* 29:1017, 2008.

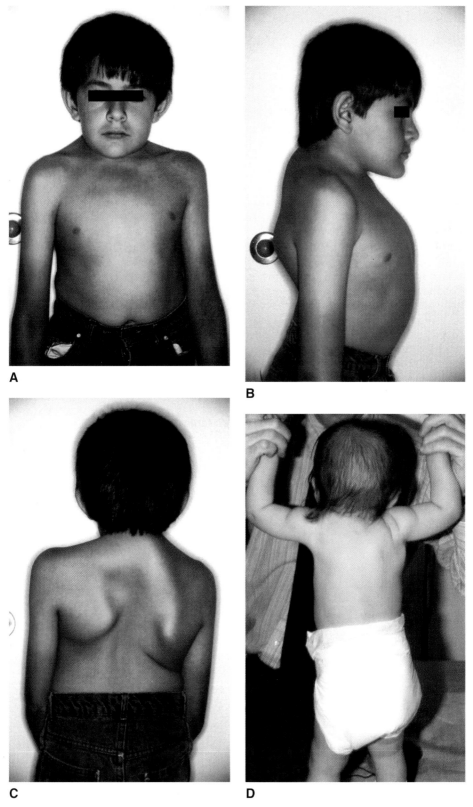

FIGURE 1.   **A–D,** Two children with the Klippel-Feil sequence. Note the Sprengel anomaly in **D.**

U

EARLY URETHRAL OBSTRUCTION SEQUENCE
(PRUNE BELLY SYNDROME)

Early urethral obstruction is most commonly the consequence of urethral valve formation during the development of the prostatic urethra. Less commonly, it is due to urethral atresia, bladder neck obstruction, or distal urethral obstruction. With urine formation occurring, by 7 to 8 weeks of fetal life, there is a progressive back-up of urine flow, leading to the consequences shown in the flow diagram. The male-to-female ratio of 20:1 in this disorder is a result of the predominant malformations being in the development of the prostatic urethra. Cryptorchidism occurs secondary to the bulk of the distended bladder, preventing full descent of the testes. The back-pressure usually limits full renal morphogenesis and may result in dilatation of the renal tubules, which in all cases shows mixed cystic and dysplastic changes. Hypoplasia of the prostate is an essential feature of the disorder and is most likely a primary event in the pathogenesis of the urethral obstruction. The compressive mass of the bladder may limit full rotation of the colon and may even compress the iliac vessels to the point of causing partial defects or vascular disruption of the lower limb(s). The oligohydramnios will give rise to all the secondary phenomena of the oligohydramnios deformation sequence.

Severe early urethral obstruction is often lethal by mid to late fetal life unless the bladder ruptures and is thereby decompressed. The bladder rupture may occur through a patent urachus, an obstructing urethral "valve," or the wall of the bladder or ureter. Following decompression, the fetus will be left with a "prune belly."

Unfortunately, most of those who survive to term have incurred severe renal damage and are unable to live long after birth. Those who do survive may be assisted by urologic procedures to aid urinary drainage and control urinary tract infection. Respiration and bowel movements may be eased by wrapping the abdomen with a "belly binder." With advancing age, the hypoplastic abdominal musculature will usually improve in volume and strength to the point of being no serious problem.

The recurrence risk for the disorder is dependent on the mechanism responsible for the distended bladder. For those cases in which it is due to urethral obstruction, recurrence risk is usually negligible and the defect most commonly occurs in an otherwise normal individual. Although more than one affected child has been reported in some families, it appears that bladder distention in those cases is not the result of mechanical obstruction. A genetic etiology has been identified for some of these conditions. For example, *ACTA2* mutations have resulted in megacystis as one feature in individuals with global smooth muscle dysfunction. A frameshift mutation in muscarine acetylcholine receptor M3 (*CHRM3*) in a familial bladder malformation associated with a prune belly–like syndrome has been reported. Finally, mutations of *HPSE2* have been described in Ochoa (urofacial) syndrome, which is associated with a poorly emptying bladder leading to a prune belly–like syndrome.

In some cases, the early urethral obstruction sequence may be the result of an intrauterine vascular accident. Support for this is based on its occurrence in one member of a monozygotic twin pair as well as its association with single umbilical artery, prenatal exposure to cocaine, and younger maternal age.

Early fetal diagnosis is possible, because sonography will show the distended bladder by 10 weeks post-conception.

References

Stumme EG: Über die symmetrischen kongenitalen Bauchmuskel defeckte und über die Kombination dersel- ben mit anderen Bildunganomalien des Rumfes, *Mitt Grenzigebeite Med Chir* 6:548, 1903.

Silverman FN, Huang N: Congenital absence of the abdominal muscles, *Am J Dis Child* 80:91, 1950.

Lattimer JK: Congenital deficiency of abdominal musculature and associated genitourinary anomalies, *J Urol* 79:343, 1958.

Pagon RA, et al: Urethral obstruction malformation complex: A cause of abdominal muscle deficiency and the "prune belly," *J Pediatr* 94:900, 1979.

Popek EJ, et al: Prostate development in prune belly syndrome (PBS) and posterior urethral valves (PUV): Etiology of PBS lower urinary tract obstruction or primary mesenchymal defect? *Pediatr Pathol* 11:1, 1991.

Jones KL, et al: Vascular steal associated with single umbilical artery: A mechanism responsible for the urethral obstruction malformation sequence, *Proc Greenwood Genet Clinic* 19:85, 2000.

Weber AS, et al: Muscarine acetylcholine receptor m3 mutation causes urinary bladder disease and a prune-belly-like syndrome, *Am J Hum Genet* 89:668, 2011.

Richer J, et al: r179h mutation in *ACTA2*: Expanding the phenotype to include prune belly sequence and skin manifestations, *Am J Med Genet* 158:664, 2012.

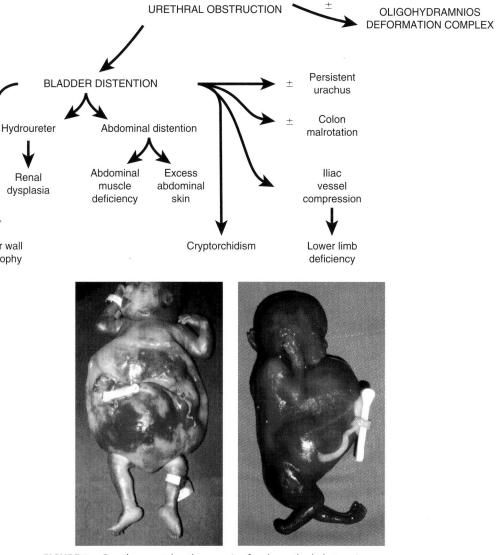

FIGURE 1.   Developmental pathogenesis of early urethral obstruction sequence.

U

EXSTROPHY OF BLADDER SEQUENCE
Primary Defect in Infraumbilical Mesoderm

Normally the bladder portion of the cloaca and the overlying ectoderm are in direct contact (the cloacal membrane) until the infraumbilical mesenchyme migrates into the area at approximately the sixth to seventh week of fetal development, giving rise to the lower abdominal wall, genital tubercles, and pubic rami. A failure of the infraumbilical mesenchyme to invade the area allows for a breakdown in the cloacal membrane, in similar fashion to that which normally occurs at the oral, anal, and urogenital areas, where mesoderm does not intercede between ectoderm and endoderm. Thus, the posterior bladder wall is exposed, in conjunction with defects in structures derived from the infraumbilical mesenchyme.

This malformation sequence, estimated to occur in approximately 1 in 30,000 births, is more likely to occur in males and to the offspring of older mothers. Most cases (71%) have no additional malformations. However, when they occur, associated malformations include renal (26%) and genital anomalies, omphalocele (34%), anal defects (21%), neural tube closure defects (18%), and cardiac defects (15%). This sequence occurs as one feature in some multiple malformation syndromes including 18 trisomy syndrome, XXY syndrome, CHARGE syndrome, and pentalogy of Cantrell.

In most cases, the defect can be closed within the first few days of life. In one study, continence was achieved in 77% of adults, 65% of adolescents, and 12% of children. Adult quality of life (QOL) was globally lower than that of the general population. Children's QOL was also globally lower than that of the general population except for relations with family and school work. In another study of 13 affected individuals older than 17 years of age, 12 reported sexual experiences, 6 were married, 13 attended college, and 7 were employed. All were considered well adjusted. However, for both the parents and affected child, intervention from a multidisciplinary team during different stages of childhood is advised. With respect to fertility, 66% of affected women who had tried to conceive were successful.

The recurrence risk for unaffected parents who have had a child with bladder exstrophy or epispadias is less than 1% (1 in 275). For the offspring of a parent with bladder exstrophy or epispadias, recurrence risk is approximately 1 in 70 live births.

References

Wyburn GM: The development of the infraumbilical portion of the abdominal wall, with remarks on the aetiology of ectopia vesicae, *J Anat* 71:201, 1937.

Muecke EC: The role of the cloacal membrane in exstrophy: The first successful experimental study, *J Urol* 92:659, 1964.

Shapiro E, et al: The inheritance of the exstrophy-epispadias complex, *J Urol* 132:308, 1984.

Jeffs RD: Exstrophy, epispadias, and cloacal and urogenital sinus abnormalities, *Pediatr Clin North Am* 34:1233, 1987.

Stjernqvist K, Kockum CC: Bladder exstrophy: Psychological impact during childhood, *J Urol* 162:2125, 1999.

Reutter H, et al: Seven new cases of familial isolated bladder exstrophy and epispadias complex (BEEC) and review of the literature, *Am J Med Genet A* 120A:215, 2003.

Jochault-Ritz S, et al: Short and long-term quality of life after reconstruction of bladder exstrophy in infancy: Preliminary results of the QUALEX (QUAlity of Life bladder EXstrophy) study, *J Pediatr Surg* 45:1693, 2010.

Siffel C, et al: Bladder exstrophy: An epidemiologic study from the International Clearinghouse for Birth Defects Surveillance and Research and an overview of the literature, *Am J Med Genet C Semin Med Genet* 157:321, 2011.

Deans R, et al: Reproductive outcomes in women with classic bladder exstrophy: An observational cross-sectional study, *Am J Obstet and Gynecol* 206:496e1, 2012.

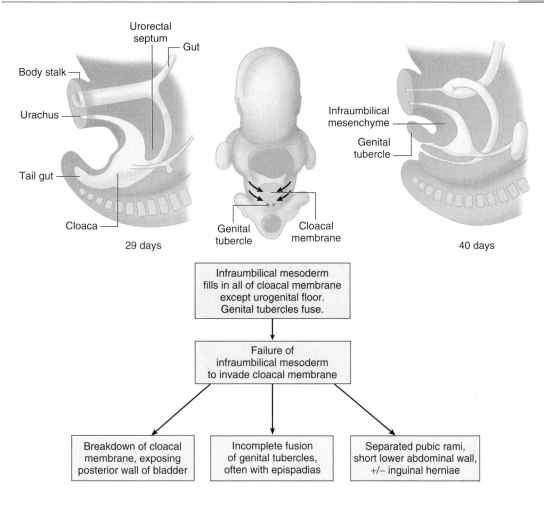

Infraumbilical mesoderm fills in all of cloacal membrane except urogenital floor. Genital tubercles fuse.

Failure of infraumbilical mesoderm to invade cloacal membrane

| Breakdown of cloacal membrane, exposing posterior wall of bladder | Incomplete fusion of genital tubercles, often with epispadias | Separated pubic rami, short lower abdominal wall, +/– inguinal herniae |

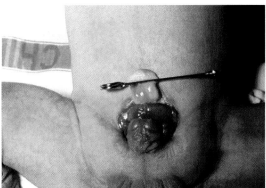

FIGURE 1.   Developmental pathogenesis of exstrophy of bladder sequence.

EXSTROPHY OF CLOACA SEQUENCE (OEIS COMPLEX)

Primary Defect—Early Mesoderm That Will Contribute to Infraumbilical Mesenchyme, Cloacal Septum, and Lumbosacral Vertebrae

Occurring in approximately 1 in 400,000 births, the remarkable similarity among otherwise normal individuals with this bizarre type of defect suggests a similar mode of developmental pathology having its inception as a single localized defect, theoretically in the early development of the mesoderm, which will later contribute to the infraumbilical mesenchyme, cloacal septum, and caudal vertebrae. The consequences are (1) failure of cloacal septation, with the persistence of a common cloaca into which the ureters, ileum, and a rudimentary hindgut open; (2) complete breakdown of the cloacal membrane with exstrophy of the cloaca, failure of fusion of the genital tubercles and pubic rami, and often omphalocele; and (3) incomplete development of the lumbosacral vertebrae with herniation of a grossly dilated central canal of the spinal cord (hydromyelia), yielding a soft, cystic, skin-covered mass over the sacral area, sometimes asymmetric in its positioning. Tethering of the cord is frequently recognized, and scoliosis is common. Bladder function, bladder neck continence, lower extremity function, and erectile capacity all relate, at least partially, to neurologic function. The rudimentary hindgut may contain two appendices, and there is no anal opening. The small intestine may be relatively short. Cryptorchidism is a usual finding in the male. Urinary tract anomalies, including pelvic kidney, renal agenesis, multicystic kidney, and ureteral duplication, occur commonly. Affected females have unfused müllerian elements with completely bifid uterine horns and short, duplicated, or atretic vaginas. Most patients have a single umbilical artery, and anomalies of the lower limbs occasionally occur and include congenital hip dislocation, talipes equinovarus, and agenesis of a limb. The term *OEIS complex* (*o*mphalocele, cloacal *e*xstrophy, *i*mperforate anus, and *s*pinal defects) is an acronym to indicate the common defects associated with cloacal exstrophy.

Additional malformations not felt to be related to the primary defect include rib anomalies, diaphragmatic hernia, abnormal ears, hydrocephaly, microcephaly, encephalocele, anencephaly, cardiac defects (ventricular and atrial septal defects, pulmonary stenosis), ectrodactyly, arthrogryposis, esophageal atresia, and tracheoesophageal fistula.

Long term survival following surgical repair is now the rule. Although the "short bowel syndrome" is a significant problem in early years, the bowel usually adapts and nutritional status stabilizes. Continence of urine, mainly by catheterization, and of stool, mainly by enema washouts, is achievable in most patients. Gender assignment and psychological aspects relating to gender have become a major issue. Previously, many affected children with a 46XY karyotype have undergone gender reassignment. Recent evidence indicates that this may not necessarily be the correct approach. Although quality of life is described as similar among those who have been raised female whether they have an XY or XX karyotype, those with XY chromosomes who have been raised female consistently scored lower on measurements of social adjustment and relationships with family and peers as well as on overall body appearance.

Although the vast majority of cases are sporadic, rare recurrence has been documented in families. In addition, cloacal exstrophy has been reported in 18 trisomy syndrome, del 9q34.1-qter, del(3)(q2.2-q13.2), del 1p36, and a mitochondrial 125rRNA mutation.

References

Spencer R: Exstrophia splanchnica (exstrophy of the cloaca), *Surgery* 57:751, 1965.

Beckwith JB: The congenitally malformed. VII. Exstrophy of the bladder and cloacal exstrophy, *Northwest Med* 65:407, 1966.

Hurwitz RS, et al: Cloacal exstrophy: A report of 34 cases, *J Urol* 138:1060, 1987.

Jeffs RD: Exstrophy, epispadias, and cloacal and urogenital sinus abnormalities, *Pediatr Clin North Am* 34:1233, 1987.

Lund DP, et al: Cloacal exstrophy: A 25-year experience with 50 cases, *J Pediatr* 36:68, 2001.

Schober JM, et al: The ultimate challenge of cloacal exstrophy, *J Urol* 167:300, 2002.

Feldkamp ML, et al: Cloacal exstrophy: An epidemiologic study from the International Clearinghouse for Birth Defects Surveillance and Research, *Am J Med Genet C Semin Med Genet* 157:333, 2011.

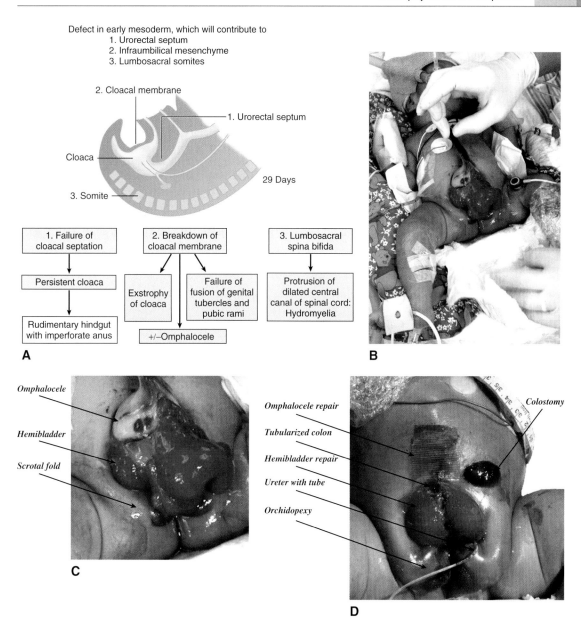

FIGURE 1. **A,** Developmental pathogenesis of exstrophy of cloaca sequence. **B** and **C,** Before surgery. **D,** Following first stage of surgical repair. (**B–D,** Courtesy Dr. Kurt Benirschke, University of California, San Diego.)

U

URORECTAL SEPTUM MALFORMATION SEQUENCE

In 1987, Escobar and colleagues reported six patients with this disorder and reviewed a number of previously reported cases, many of whom had been diagnosed as female pseudohermaphrodites. The principal features include the following: striking ambiguity of the external genitalia with a short phallus-like structure that lacks corpora cavernosa and absent urethra and vaginal openings; imperforate anus; bladder, vaginal, and rectal fistulas; and müllerian duct defects. Other common associated findings include cystic dysplasia/agenesis of kidneys, vertebral anomalies, cardiac defects, tracheoesophageal fistula, talipes equinovarus, and single umbilical artery.

It has been suggested that this pattern of malformation is due to two related events in the development of the urorectal septum. Normally, by the sixth week of development, the urorectal septum divides the cloacal cavity into a urogenital sinus anteriorly and a rectum posteriorly and fuses with the cloacal membrane. At the same time that the urorectal septum fuses with the cloacal membrane, the membrane breaks down, leaving an open urogenital sinus and rectum. Failure of the urorectal septum to divide the cloaca or fuse with the cloacal membrane leads in a cascading fashion to the urorectal septum malformation sequence. Because the cloacal membrane has failed to break down, the median raphe, which represents fusion of the labioscrotal folds in an XY fetus, is not present.

Long-term survival of affected individuals is extremely rare. Virtually all patients are stillborn or die in the neonatal period secondary to respiratory complications of oligohydramnios or renal failure.

Recurrence risk for isolated cases of the urorectal septum malformation sequence is negligible. However, when it occurs as one feature in a multiple malformation syndrome, recurrence risk is for that disorder.

References

Escobar LF, et al: Urorectal septum malformation sequence: Report of six cases and embryological analysis, *Am J Dis Child* 141:1021, 1987.

Wheeler PG, et al: Urorectal septum malformation sequence: Report of thirteen additional cases and review of the literature, *Am J Med Genet* 73:456, 1997.

Qi BQ, et al: Clarification of the process of separation of the cloaca into rectum and urogenital sinus in the rat embryo, *J Pediatr Surg* 35:1810, 2000.

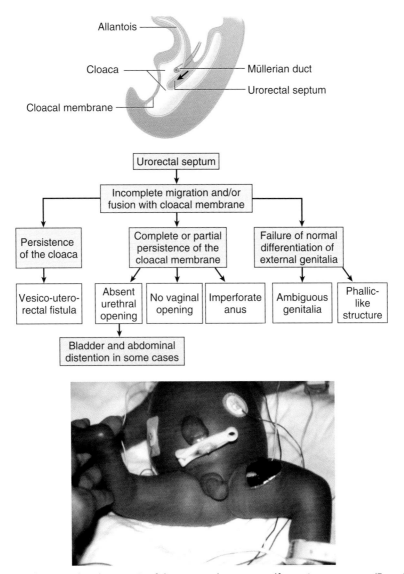

FIGURE 1.   *Top,* Developmental pathogenesis of the urorectal septum malformation sequence. (From Escobar LF, et al: *Am J Dis Child* 141:1021, 1987, with permission. Copyright 1987, American Medical Association.) *Bottom,* 46XX individual with urorectal septum malformation sequence. Note the phallus-like structure, absent urethral and vaginal opening, and imperforate anus.

U

OLIGOHYDRAMNIOS SEQUENCE (POTTER SYNDROME)
Primary Defect—Development of Oligohydramnios

Renal agenesis, which must occur before 31 days of fetal development, will secondarily limit the amount of amniotic fluid and thereby result in further anomalies during prenatal life. The renal agenesis may be the only primary defect, or it may be one feature of a more extensive caudal axis anomaly. Other types of urinary tract defects, such as polycystic kidneys or obstruction, may also be responsible for oligohydramnios and its consequences. Another cause is chronic leakage of amniotic fluid from the time of midgestation. Regardless of the cause, the secondary effects of oligohydramnios are the same and would appear to be the result of compression of the fetus, as depicted subsequently. The cause of death is respiratory insufficiency, with a lack of the late development of alveolar sacs. A similar lag in late development of the lung is observed in association with diaphragmatic hernia and asphyxiating thoracic dystrophy. In each of those situations, there is external compression of the developing lung leading to pulmonary hypoplasia. In addition to the features set forth in the figure, compression also results in large ears (>97%), which are flattened against the head, and loose skin.

When the oligohydramnios is secondary to agenesis or dysgenesis of both kidneys or agenesis of one kidney and dysgenesis of the other, renal ultrasonographic evaluation of both parents and siblings of affected infants should be performed, because 9% of first-degree relatives had asymptomatic renal malformations in a study by Roodhooft and colleagues.

References

Potter EL: Bilateral renal agenesis, *J Pediatr* 29:68, 1946.

Bain AD, Scott JS: Renal agenesis and severe urinary tract dysplasia: A review of 50 cases with particular reference to the associated anomalies, *BMJ* 1:841, 1960.

Thomas IT, Smith DW: Oligohydramnios, cause of the nonrenal features of Potter's syndrome, including pulmonary hypoplasia, *J Pediatr* 84:811, 1974.

Roodhooft AM, et al: Familial nature of congenital absence and severe dysgenesis of both kidneys, *N Engl J Med* 310:1341, 1984.

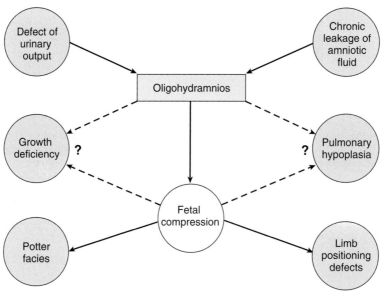

FIGURE 1.   Depiction of the origin and effects of oligohydramnios. The oligohydramnios sequence is implied to be secondary to fetal compression.

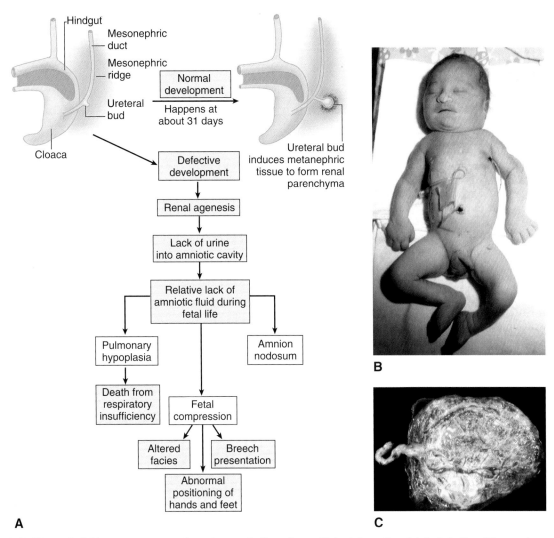

A

B

C

FIGURE 2. **A–C,** The consequences of renal agenesis. Note the multiple deformational defects in **B** and the amnion nodosum (brown-yellow granules from vernix that have been rubbed into defects of the amnionic surface) in **C.**

U

SIRENOMELIA SEQUENCE

This defect was previously thought to be the consequence of a wedge-shaped early deficit of the posterior axis caudal blastema, allowing for fusion of the early limb buds at their fibular margins with absence or incomplete development of the intervening caudal structures. However, Stevenson and colleagues showed that sirenomelia and its commonly associated defects are produced by an alteration in early vascular development. Rather than blood returning to the placenta through the usual paired umbilical arteries arising from the iliac arteries, blood returns to the placenta through a single large vessel, a derivative of the vitelline artery complex, which arises from the aorta just below the diaphragm. The abdominal aorta distal to the origin of this major vessel is always subordinate and usually gives off no tributaries, especially renal or inferior mesenteric arteries, before it bifurcates into iliac arteries. This vascular alteration leads to a "vitelline artery steal" in which blood flow and thus nutrients are diverted from the caudal structures of the embryo to the placenta. Resultant defects include a single lower extremity with posterior alignment of knees and feet, arising from failure of the lower limb bud field to be cleaved into two lateral masses by an intervening allantois; absence of sacrum and other defects of vertebrae; imperforate anus and absence of rectum; absence of external and internal genitalia; renal agenesis; and absence of the bladder. Based on the variable alterations that could exist in blood flow, a variable spectrum of abnormalities occurs in structures dependent on the distal aorta for nutrients. Thus, as with other disruptive vascular defects, no two cases of sirenomelia are ever the same.

References

Wolff E: Les bases de la tératogénèse expérimentale des vertèbres amniotes, d'après les résultats de méthodes directes, *Arch Anat Histol Embryol (Strasb)* 22:1, 1936.

Stevenson RE, et al: Vascular steal: The pathogenic mechanism producing sirenomelia and associated defects of the viscera and soft tissues, *Pediatrics* 78:451, 1986.

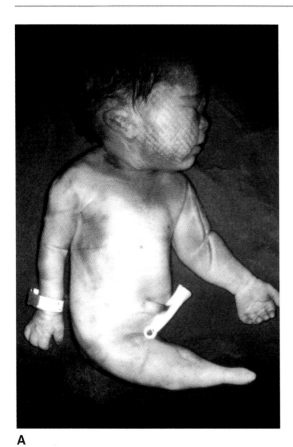

A

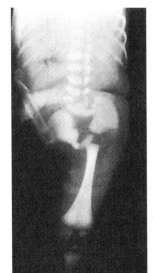

B

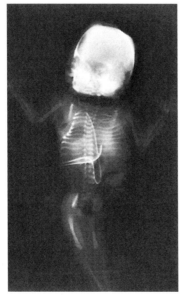

C

FIGURE 1.   A, Stillborn infant with sirenomelia. **B** and **C,** The bones in the single leg vary from completely separate to a single broad femur with two distal ossification centers and a broad tibia with two ossification centers.

CAUDAL DYSPLASIA SEQUENCE (CAUDAL REGRESSION SYNDROME)

This disorder was previously grouped with sireno-melia, which was thought to represent its most severe form. Recent evidence suggests that the two are pathogenetically unrelated. Whereas sirenome-lia and its associated defects are produced by an early vascular alteration leading to a "vitelline artery steal," the caudal dysplasia sequence is most likely heterogenous with respect to its etiology and devel-opmental pathogenesis.

Structural defects of the caudal region observed in this pattern of malformation include the follow-ing (to variable degrees): incomplete development of the sacrum and, to a lesser extent, the lumbar vertebrae; absence of the body of the sacrum, leading to flattening of the buttocks, shortening of the intergluteal cleft and dimpling of the buttocks; dis-ruption of the distal spinal cord, leading second-arily to neurologic impairment, varying from incontinence of urine and feces to complete neuro-logic loss; and extreme lack of growth in the caudal region resulting from decreased movement of the legs secondary to neurologic impairment. A high incidence of unilateral renal agenesis in combina-tion with vesico-ureteric reflux may well contribute to a high risk for impaired renal function. The most severely affected infants have flexion and abduction at the hips and popliteal webs secondary to lack of movement. Talipes equinovarus and calcaneovalgus deformities are common.

Occasional abnormalities include imperforate anus, cleft lip, cleft palate, microcephaly, and meningomyelocele.

NATURAL HISTORY
In the most severely affected individuals, prognosis is poor. Urologic and orthopedic management is required in the vast majority of those who survive.

ETIOLOGY
The cause of this disorder is unknown. Sixteen percent have occurred in offspring of diabetic mothers. Although usually sporadic, a few instances of affected siblings born to unaffected parents have been described.

COMMENT
A pattern of malformation with similar features, the Currarino syndrome—consisting of partial sacral agenesis, a presacral mass (teratoma, anterior meningocele, rectal duplication, or a combination thereof), and anorectal malformations, usually anal stenosis—is due to mutations of the motor neuron and pancreas homeobox 1 (*MNH1,* formerly *HLXB9*) gene located at 7q36 or to microdeletions of 7q36. No pathologic mutations of *HLXB9* have been iden-tified in 48 cases of caudal dysplasia sequence

References

Rusnak SL, Driscoll SG: Congenital spinal anomalies in infants of diabetic mothers, *Pediatrics* 35:989, 1965.

Passarge E, Lenz W: Syndrome of caudal regression in infants of diabetic mothers: Observations of further cases, *Pediatrics* 37:672, 1966.

Gellis SS, Feingold M: Picture of the month: Caudal dys-plasia syndrome, *Am J Dis Child* 116:407, 1968.

Price DL, et al: Caudal dysplasia (caudal regression syn-drome), *Arch Neurol* 23:212, 1970.

Finer NN, et al: Caudal regression anomalad (sacral agen-esis in siblings), *Clin Genet* 13:353, 1978.

Stewart JM, Stoll S: Familial caudal regression anomalad and maternal diabetes, *J Med Genet* 16:17, 1979.

Ross AJ, et al: A homeobox gene, *HLXB9,* is the major locus for dominantly inherited sacral agenesis, *Nat Genet* 20:358, 1998.

Merello E, et al: *HLXB9* homeobox gene and caudal regres-sion syndrome, *Birth Defects Res A Clin Mol Teratol* 76:205, 2006.

Torre M, et al: Long-term urologic outcome in patients with caudal regression syndrome, compared with meningomyelocele and spinal cord lipoma, *J Pediatr Surg* 43:530, 2008.

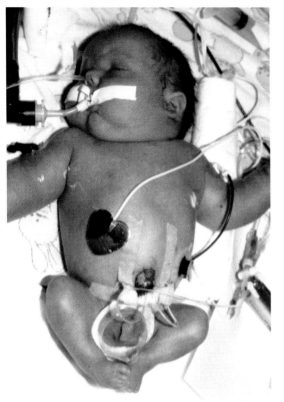

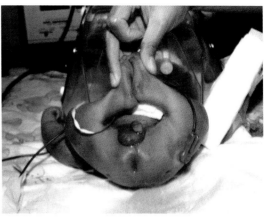

FIGURE 1. Caudal dysplasia sequence. **A,** Newborn male infant with a normal upper body and a short lower segment. **B,** Note the pterygia in the popliteal region, which are secondary to neurologically related flexion contractures at the knees.

A

U

AMNION RUPTURE SEQUENCE

Although the structural defects consequent to amnion rupture were reported by Portal in 1685, it was not until 1965 that the full spectrum of defects that can occur was delineated by Torpin as well as by others. Secondary to amnion rupture, small strands of amnion can encircle developing structures (usually the limbs), leading to annular constrictions, pseudosyndactyly, intrauterine amputations, and umbilical cord constriction. In addition to these disruptive defects, deformational defects can occur secondary to decreased fetal movement, the result of tethering of a limb by an amniotic band; or constraint, the result of decreased amniotic fluid. The decreased fetal activity may result in scoliosis or foot deformities. It may also cause edema, hemorrhage, and resorptive necrosis. Defects of internal organs almost never occur. As is the case with all disruptive defects, no two affected fetuses will have exactly the same features, and there is no single feature that consistently occurs. Examination of the placenta and membranes is diagnostic. Aberrant bands or strands of amnion are noted, or there may be the rolled-up remnants of the amnion at the placental base of the umbilical cord.

Incorrectly, throaco- and/or abdominoschisis, exencephaly and/or encephalocele, usually associated with amnion adhesions and sometimes complicated by rupture of the amnion with amputation defects, have been considered part of the amnion rupture sequence. This pattern of defects, now referred to as the limb–body wall complex, is due to a different pathogenetic mechanism.

NATURAL HISTORY AND MANAGEMENT

The natural history varies with the severity of the problem. Amnion constrictive bands or amputations of the limb in an otherwise normal child occur most commonly. Occasionally, plastic surgery may be indicated, especially for the partially constrictive, deep residual groove that encircles a limb and is associated with partial limitation of vascular or lymphatic return from the distal limb. In such instances, a Z-plasty of the skin may be done to relieve the partial constriction. If there has been chronic amnion leakage, the neonate may show features of the oligohydramnios deformation sequence, including incomplete development of the lung, with respiratory insufficiency. Every attempt should be made to oxygenate and support such an infant, since, with continued lung morphogenesis, the prognosis can be excellent. Because the result of amnion rupture is external compression or disruption, internal anomalies do not occur. Hence, the features evident by surface examination are usually the only abnormalities.

ETIOLOGY

The etiology of this disorder has been, with rare exceptions, idiopathic. Those rare exceptions are known or presumed to be caused by trauma and include two examples of attempted early termination of pregnancy by using a coat hanger and one incident of a woman falling from a horse while pregnant. It has generally been a sporadic event in an otherwise normal family, and hence the recurrence risk is usually stated as being negligible. Although the disruptive defect resulting from amniotic bands may occur at any time during gestation, amnion rupture most likely occurs before 12 weeks' gestation. Before that time, the amnion and chorion are completely separate membranes and, as such, it has been suggested that the amnion is vulnerable to rupture.

References

Portal P: *La Pratique des Accouchements*. Paris, 1685.

Torpin R: Amniochorionic mesoblastic fibrous strings and amniotic bands: Associated constricting fetal malformations of fetal death, *Am J Obstet Gynecol* 91:65, 1965.

Torpin R: *Fetal Malformations Caused by Amnion Rupture during Gestation*, Springfield, Ill, 1968, Charles C Thomas.

Kalousek DK, Bamforth S: Amnion rupture sequence in previable fetuses, *Am J Med Genet* 31:63, 1988.

Moerman P, et al: Constrictive amniotic bands, amniotic adhesions, and limb-body wall complex: Discrete disruption sequences with pathogenetic overlap, *Am J Med Genet* 42:470, 1992.

Martínez-Frías ML, et al: Epidemiological characteristics of amniotic band sequence (ABS) and body wall complex (BWC): Are they different entities? *Am J Med Genet* 73:176, 1997.

Werler MM, et al: Epidemiologic analysis of maternal factors and amniotic band defects, *Birth Defects Res A Clin Mol Teratol* 67:68, 2003.

Jamsheer A, et al: Comparative study of clinical characteristics of amniotic rupture sequence with and without body wall defect: Further evidence for separation, *Birth Defects Res A Clin Mol Teratol* 85:211, 2009.

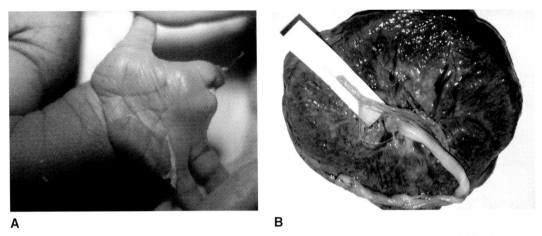

A   **B**

FIGURE 1.   Amnion rupture sequence. **A,** Amputation of the fingers by strands of amnion. **B,** The child's placenta. Note the amnion that has stripped off the left side of the fetal surface of the placenta and is rolled up at the base of the umbilical cord.

U

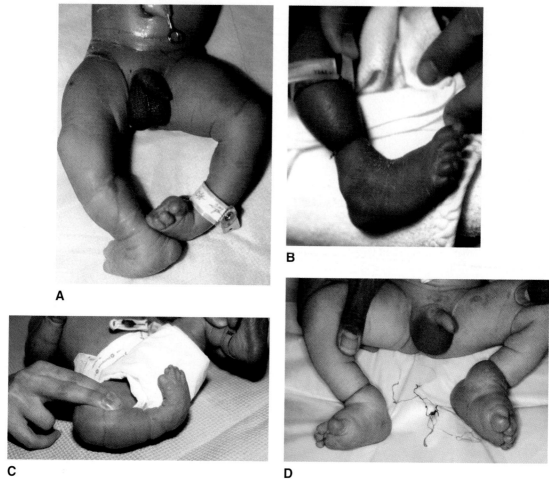

FIGURE 2. Variable limb anomalies secondary to aberrant bands. **A–D,** Bands constricting the ankle, leading to deformational defects and amputation. (**A–F,** From Jones KL, et al: *J Pediatr* 84:90, 1974, with permission.)

Continued

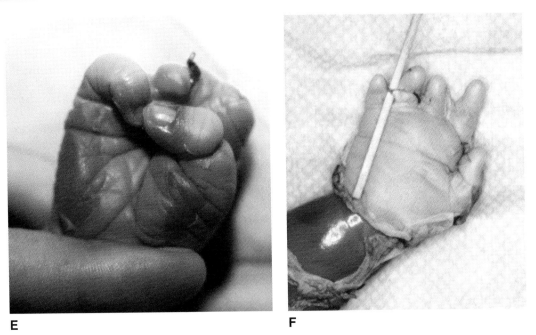

E

F

FIGURE 2, cont'd. E and F, Pseudosyndactyly, amputation, and disruption of finger morphogenesis.

LIMB–BODY WALL COMPLEX

The limb–body wall complex consists of thoraco- or abdominoschisis and limb defects frequently associated with exencephaly/encephalocele and facial clefts. The vast majority of cases are spontaneously aborted; the remainder are stillborn.

Thoraco-abdominoschisis involves an anterolateral body wall defect with evisceration of thoracic or abdominal organs into a persistent extraembryonic coelom. The extraembryonic coelom, the space between the amnion and chorion, is obliterated normally by 60 days' gestation. Failure of the ventral body wall to fuse because of damage to part of the body wall or failure of normal ventral folding of the embryo leads to a persistence of the extraembryonic coelom. The amnion is continuous with the skin at the edge of the defect and the umbilical cord is short and partially devoid of its normal amniotic membrane covering. Limb defects similar to those seen in the amnion rupture sequence, such as amputations secondary to ring constrictions and pseudosyndactyly, occur occasionally. However, other limb defects, such as single forearm or lower leg bones, ectrodactyly, radioulnar synostosis, and polydactyly (defects that cannot be explained on the basis of constriction or tethering by amniotic bands), occur more frequently. The encephaloceles are usually anterior, often multiple, and occasionally attached to the amnion. The facial clefts do not conform to the usual lines of closure of the facial processes and are frequently associated with disruption of the frontonasal processes.

In addition, there is a high incidence of associated anomalies of the internal organs, including the heart, lungs (lobation defects), diaphragm (absent), intestine (nonrotation, atresia, shortened), gallbladder, kidney (absent, hydronephrotic, dysplastic), and genitourinary tract (abnormal external genitalia or uterus, absent gonad, streak ovaries, bladder exstrophy).

The developmental pathogenesis, as well as the etiology of limb–body wall complex, is controversial. Incorrectly it has been included in the past as part of the spectrum of the amnion rupture sequence, a concept that is clearly untenable based on the observation that the amniotic membrane is intact in some cases.

Van Allen and colleagues suggested that an early systemic alteration of embryonic blood supply between 4 and 6 weeks' gestation leads to disruptive vascular defects to the developing embryo, including facial clefts, damage to the calvaria or brain resulting in neural tube–like defects, many of the limb reduction defects, and the internal visceral anomalies. Adhesion of the amnion to these necrotic areas could lead secondarily to amniotic adhesive bands. Failure of the ventral body wall to close because of vascular compromise could lead to persistence of the extraembryonic coelom. Features typical of the amnion band rupture sequence such as constriction bands are secondary to rupture of the amnion that is not adequately supported because the extraembryonic coelom has not been obliterated.

Streeter suggested that this complex was due to very early defects of the embryonic disc, and Hartwig et al later modified Streeter's ideas suggesting that limb–body wall complex is due to defects in the ectodermal placodes, which, it was thought, led to a deficiency of mesoderm.

In 2011, Hunter et al concluded that this complex originates at the embryonic disc stage. They suggested that a defect or deficiency of the ectoderm of the embryonic disc was responsible for most of the malformations seen in this complex.

References

Graham JM, et al: Limb reduction anomalies and early in-utero limb compression, *J Pediatr* 96:1052, 1980.

Miller ME, et al: Compression-related defects from early amnion rupture: Evidence for mechanical teratogenesis, *J Pediatr* 98:292, 1981.

Van Allen ME, et al: Limb-body wall complex: I. Pathogenesis, *Am J Med Genet* 28:529, 1987.

Van Allen ME, et al: Limb-body wall complex II. Limb and spine defects, *Am J Med Genet* 28:549, 1987.

Luebke HJ, et al: Fetal disruptions: Assessment of frequency, heterogeneity, and embryologic mechanisms in a population referred to a community-based stillbirth assessment program, *Am J Med Genet* 36:56, 1990.

Moerman P, et al: Constrictive amniotic bands, amniotic adhesions, and limb-body wall complex: Discrete disruption sequences with pathogenetic overlap, *Am J Med Genet* 42:470, 1992.

Russo R, et al: Limb body wall complex: A critical review and a nosological proposal, *Am J Med Genet* 47:893, 1993.

Martínez-Frías ML: Clinical and epidemiological characteristics of infants with body wall complex with and without limb deficiency, *Am J Med Genet* 73:170, 1997.

Hunter AGW, et al: Limb-body wall defect. Is there a defensible hypothesis and can it explain all the associated anomalies? *Am J Med Genet* 155:2045, 2011.

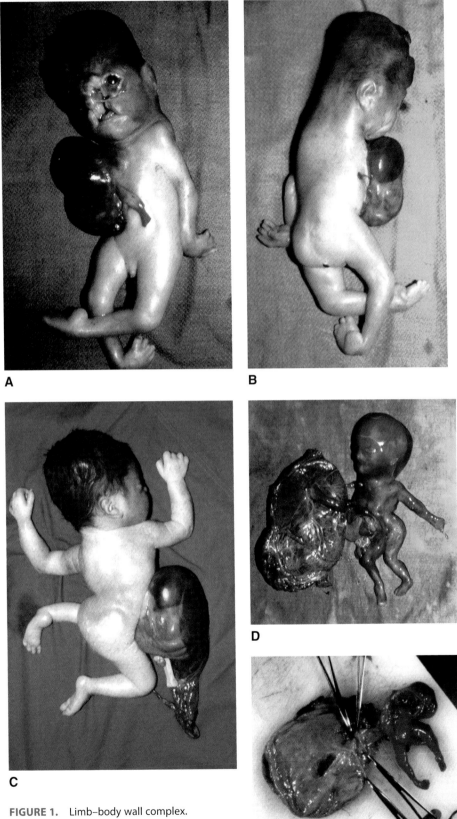

FIGURE 1. Limb–body wall complex.
A–E, Affected fetuses with multiple involvement of limbs, body wall, and craniofacial area.

U

OCULO-AURICULO-VERTEBRAL SPECTRUM
(FIRST AND SECOND BRANCHIAL ARCH SYNDROME, FACIO-AURICULO-VERTEBRAL SPECTRUM, HEMIFACIAL MICROSOMIA, GOLDENHAR SYNDROME)

The predominant defects in this spectrum represent problems in morphogenesis of the first and second branchial arches, sometimes accompanied by vertebral anomalies, renal defects, or ocular anomalies. The occurrence of epibulbar dermoid with this pattern of anomaly, especially when accompanied by vertebral anomalies, was designated as the Goldenhar syndrome, and the predominantly unilateral occurrence was designated as hemifacial microsomia. However, the occurrence of various combinations and gradations of this pattern of anomalies, both unilateral and bilateral, with or without epibulbar dermoid, and with or without vertebral anomalies, has suggested that hemifacial microsomia and the Goldenhar syndrome may simply represent variable manifestations of a similar error in morphogenesis. The frequency of occurrence is estimated to be 1 in 3000 to 1 in 5000, and there is a slight (3:2) male predominance.

ABNORMALITIES

Variable combinations of the following, tending to be asymmetric and 70% unilateral.

Face. Hypoplasia of malar, maxillary, or mandibular region, especially ramus and condyle of mandible and temporomandibular joint; lateral cleft-like extension of the corner of the mouth (macrostomia); hypoplasia of facial musculature; hypoplasia of depressor anguli oris.

Ear. Microtia, accessory preauricular tags or pits, most commonly in a line from the tragus to the corner of the mouth; middle ear anomaly with variable deafness.

Oral. Diminished to absent parotid secretion, anomalies in function or structure of tongue, malfunction of soft palate.

Vertebral. Hemivertebrae or hypoplasia of vertebrae, most commonly cervical but may also be thoracic or lumbar.

Central Nervous System. Hydrocephalus, Arnold-Chiari malformation, occipital encephalocele, agenesis of corpus callosum, calcification of falx cerebri, hypoplasia of septum pellucidum, enlarged ventricles, intracranial dermoid cyst, lipoma in corpus callosum, polymicrogyria.

OCCASIONAL ABNORMALITIES

Eye. Epibulbar dermoid, lipodermoid, notch in upper lid, strabismus, microphthalmia.

Ear. Inner ear defect.

Oral. Cleft lip, cleft palate.

Cardiac. Ventricular and atrial septal defects, patent ductus arteriosus, tetralogy of Fallot, conotruncal defects, and coarctation of aorta, in decreasing order of frequency.

Genitourinary. Ectopic or fused kidneys, renal agenesis, vesicoureteral reflux, ureteropelvic junction obstruction, ureteral duplication, and multicystic dysplastic kidney.

Other. Intellectual disability (IQ below 85 in 13%), speech delay, autism, abnormal caruncles, branchial cleft remnants in anterior-lateral neck, laryngeal anomaly, hypoplasia to aplasia of lung, esophageal atresia, tracheomalacia caused by extrinsic vascular compression, radial and/or rib anomalies, prenatal growth deficiency, low scalp hairline.

NATURAL HISTORY

Reconstructive surgery is strongly indicated. Most of these patients are of normal intelligence. Intellectual disability is more common in association with microphthalmia. Deafness should be tested for at an early age.

ETIOLOGY

The cause of this disorder is unknown; cases are usually sporadic. Estimated recurrence in first-degree relatives is approximately 2%, although minor features of this disorder may be more commonly noted in relatives. When unilateral, it tends to be right-sided. Maternal diabetes has been associated in some cases. Del 22q11.2 has been reported in three cases. Based on studies utilizing an animal model, Poswillo concluded that this disorder was due to interference with vascular supply and focal hemorrhage in the developing first and second branchial arch.

COMMENT

This spectrum occurs more frequently in one member of a monozygotic twin pair and has been seen in increased frequency following assisted reproductive techniques.

References

Goldenhar M: Associations malformatives de l'oeil et de l'oreille, *J Genet Hum* 1:243, 1952.

Summitt RL: Familial Goldenhar syndrome, *Birth Defects* 5:106, 1969.

Pashayan H, et al: Hemifacial microsomia-oculo-auriculo-vertebral dysplasia: A patient with overlapping features, *J Med Genet* 7:185, 1970.

Baum JL, Feingold M: Ocular aspects of Goldenhar's syndrome, *Am J Ophthalmol* 75:250, 1973.

Poswillo D: The pathogenesis of the first and second branchial arch syndrome, *Oral Surg* 35:302, 1973.

Rollnick BR, et al: Oculoauriculovertebral dysplasia and variants: Phenotypic characteristics of 294 patients, *Am J Med Genet* 26:631, 1987.

Cohen MM Jr, et al: Oculoauriculovertebral spectrum: An updated critique, *Cleft Palate J* 26:276, 1989.

Ritchey ML, et al: Urologic manifestations of Goldenhar syndrome, *Urology* 43:88, 1994.

Nijhawan N, et al: Caruncle abnormalities in the oculo-auriculo-vertebral spectrum, *Am J Med Genet* 113:320, 2002.

Wang R, et al: Infants of diabetic mothers are at increased risk for the oculo-auriculo-vertebral sequence: A case-based and case-control approach, *J Pediatr* 141:611, 2002.

Strömland K, et al: Oculo-auriculo-vertebral spectrum: Associated anomalies, functional deficits and possible developmental risk factors, *Am J Med Genet* 143:1317, 2007.

Wieczorek D, et al: Reproduction abnormalities and twin pregnancies in parents of sporadic patients with oculo-auriculo-vertebral spectrum/Goldenhar syndrome, *Hum Genet* 121:369, 2007.

Digilio MC, et al: Congenital heart defects in patients with oculo-auriculo-vertebral spectrum (Goldenhar syndrome), *Am J Med Genet* 146:1815, 2008.

Digilio MC, et al: Three patients with oculo-auriculo-vertebral spectrum and microdeletion 22q11.2, *Am J Med Genet A* 149A:2860, 2009.

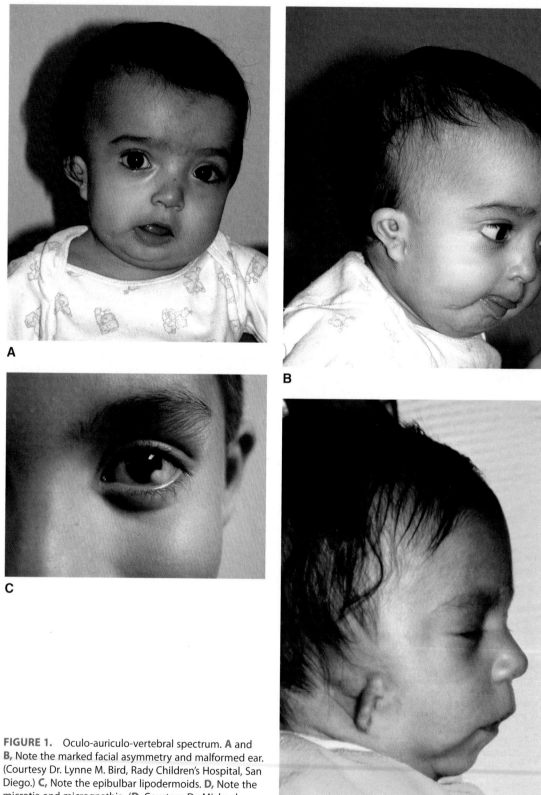

FIGURE 1.   Oculo-auriculo-vertebral spectrum. **A** and
B, Note the marked facial asymmetry and malformed ear.
(Courtesy Dr. Lynne M. Bird, Rady Children's Hospital, San
Diego.) **C,** Note the epibulbar lipodermoids. **D,** Note the
microtia and micrognathia. (**D,** Courtesy Dr. Michael
Cohen, Dalhousie University, Halifax, Nova Scotia.)

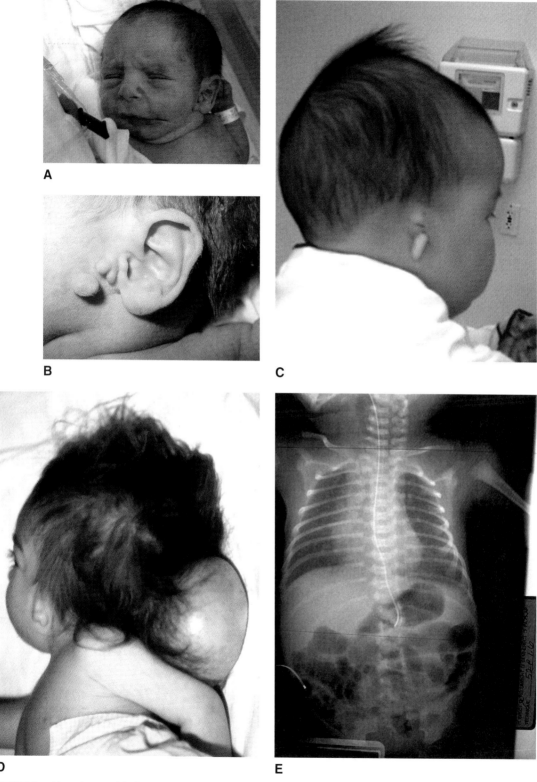

FIGURE 2. Note the variable features including the lateral cleft-like extension of the mouth (**A**), preauricular tags (**B**), and microtia (**C**). (Courtesy Dr. Lynne Bird, Rady Children's Hospital, San Diego.) **D,** Encephalocele. (Courtesy Dr. Michael Cohen, Dalhousie University, Halifax, Nova Scotia.) **E,** Vertebral anomalies.

OROMANDIBULAR-LIMB HYPOGENESIS SPECTRUM
(HYPOGLOSSIA-HYPODACTYLY SYNDROME, AGLOSSIA-ADACTYLY SYNDROME,
GLOSSOPALATINE ANKYLOSIS SYNDROME, FACIAL-LIMB DISRUPTIVE SPECTRUM)
Limb Deficiency, Hypoglossia, Micrognathia

In 1932, Rosenthal described aglossia and associated malformations. Kaplan and colleagues emphasized a "community" or spectrum of disorders and suggested common elements in modes of developmental pathogenesis.

ABNORMALITIES

Various combinations from among the following features:

Craniofacial. Small mouth, micrognathia, hypoglossia, variable clefting or aberrant attachments of tongue; mandibular hypodontia; complete bony fusion of the maxilla and mandible, choanal atresia, cleft palate; cranial nerve palsies, including Moebius sequence; broad nose; telecanthus; lower eyelid defect; facial asymmetry.

Limbs. Hypoplasia of varying degrees, to point of adactyly; syndactyly, angel-shaped phalanx.

Other. Brain defects, especially of cranial nerve nuclei, causing Moebius sequence; splenogonadal fusion, hypoplasia of atlas with craniocervical junction malformation, gastroschisis.

NATURAL HISTORY

Early feeding and speech difficulties may occur. Orthopedic and/or plastic surgery may be indicated for the limb problems. Intelligence and stature are generally normal. Serious problems with hyperthermia can occur in children with four-limb amputation.

ETIOLOGY

The cause of this disorder is unknown; cases are usually sporadic. The hypothesis that the abnormalities are the disruptive consequence of hemorrhagic lesions has experimental backing from the studies of Poswillo. The presumed vascular problem is more likely to occur in distal regions, such as the distal limbs, tongue, and occasionally parts of the brain. Chorionic villus sampling, particularly when performed between 56 and 66 days of gestation, has been associated with this disorder, as has the use of misoprostol as an abortifacient, giving further credence to a disruptive vascular pathogenesis.

References

Rosenthal R: Aglossia congenita: A report of the condition combined with other congenital malformations, *Am J Dis Child* 44:383, 1932.

Poswillo D: The pathogenesis of the first and second branchial arch syndrome, *Oral Surg* 35:302, 1973.

Kaplan P, et al: A "community" of face-limb malformation syndromes, *J Pediatr* 89:241, 1976.

Pauli RM, Greenlaw A: Limb deficiency and splenogonadal fusion, *Am J Med Genet* 13:81, 1982.

Lipson AH, Webster WS: Transverse limb deficiency, oromandibular limb hypogenesis sequences, and chorionic villus biopsy: Human and animal experimental evidence for a uterine vascular pathogenesis, *Am J Med Genet* 47:1141, 1993.

Knoll B, et al: Complete congenital bony syngnathia in a case of oromandibular limb hypogenesis, *J Craniofac Surg* 11:398, 2000.

Kiliç N, et al: Oromandibular limb hypogenesis and gastroschisis, *J Pediatr Surg* 36:E15, 2001.

Camera G, et al: "Angel-shaped phalanx" in a boy with oromandibular-limb hypogenesis, *Am J Med Genet* 119:87, 2003.

Al Kaissi AA, et al: Cervicocervical junction malformation in a child with oromandibular-limb hypogenesis-Möbius syndrome, *Orphanet J Rare Dis* 2:2, 2007.

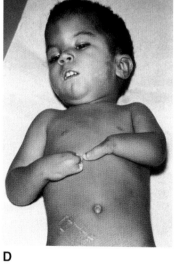

A

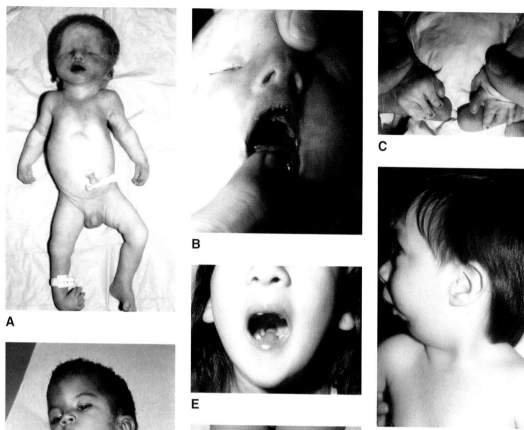

B

C

E

F

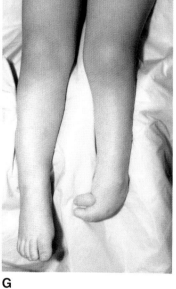

D

G

FIGURE 1. Oromandibular-limb hypogenesis spectrum. No one instance is the same as the next. There are varying degrees of limb deficiency, hypoglossia, or micrognathia. **A–C,** Necropsy photograph of a newborn. **D,** Note that the child has Moebius sequence as an associated feature. **E–G,** This child has splenogonadal fusion as an associated feature.

V

CONGENITAL MICROGASTRIA–LIMB REDUCTION COMPLEX
(MICROGASTRIA, LIMB DEFECTS, SPLENIC ABNORMALITIES)

Robert described the first patient with this disorder in 1842. Subsequently, 16 additional cases have been described.

ABNORMALITIES

Gastrointestinal.   Microgastria,   intestinal malrotation.

Limb. Varying degrees of radial and ulnar hypoplasia, bilateral in 40% of cases; isolated absence of thumbs (20%); terminal transverse defects of humerus (10%); phocomelia (10%); oligodactyly.

Spleen. Abnormalities in 70%, including asplenia, hyposplenia, or splenogonadal fusion.

Other. Renal anomalies in 50%, including pelvic kidney in two cases and unilateral renal agenesis and bilateral cystic dysplasia in one patient each; defects in laterality; cardiac defects in 20% (secundum atrial septal defect and type I truncus arteriosus); central nervous system defects in 20% (arrhinencephaly, fused thalami, polymicrogyria, agenesis of corpus callosum, and hydrocephalus).

OCCASIONAL ABNORMALITIES

Congenital megacolon, esophageal atresia, anal atresia, abnormal lung lobation, anophthalmia and porencephalic cyst, amelia, cryptorchidism, bicornuate uterus, horseshoe kidney, and absent gallbladder.

NATURAL HISTORY

Microgastria usually presents with gastroesophageal reflux and failure to thrive. Death before 6 months of age has occurred in almost 50% of cases. Surgical intervention to create a gastric reservoir improves the ability of patients to tolerate normal feeding volumes.

ETIOLOGY

The cause of this disorder is unknown. All cases have represented sporadic events in otherwise normal families. The occurrence of three cases in which discordance for this disorder has occurred in twins is noteworthy.

References

Robert HLF: Hummungsbildung des Magens, Mangel der Milz und des Netzes, *Arch Anat Physiol Wissenschaftliche Med* 57, 1842.

Lueder GT, et al: Congenital microgastria and hypoplastic upper limb anomalies, *Am J Med Genet* 32:368, 1989.

Meinecke P, et al: Microgastria–hypoplastic upper limb association: A severe expression including microphthalmia, single nostril and arrhinencephaly, *Clin Dysmorphol* 1:43, 1992.

Cunniff C, et al: Congenital microgastria and limb reduction defects, *Pediatrics* 91:1192, 1993.

Lurie IW, et al: Microgastria–limb reduction complex with congenital heart disease and twinning, *Clin Dysmorphol* 4:150, 1995.

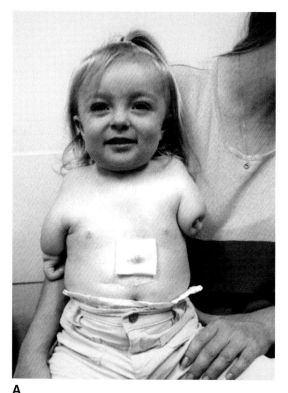

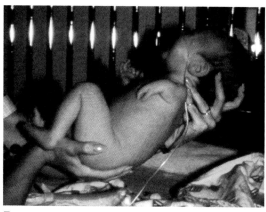

B

A

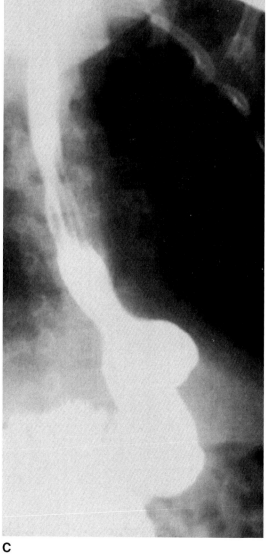

FIGURE 1.   Congenital microgastria–limb reduction complex. **A–C,** Note the limb reduction anomalies and, on the barium-contrast roentgenogram, microgastria and intestinal malrotation.

C

STERNAL MALFORMATION–VASCULAR DYSPLASIA SPECTRUM

In 1985, Hersh and colleagues described two patients with this disorder and summarized the findings in 13 previously reported cases. The principal features include cleft of the sternum that is covered with atrophic skin; a median abdominal raphe extending from the sternal defect to the umbilicus; and cutaneous craniofacial hemangiomata.

In 13 of the cases, the hemangiomata were localized to cutaneous structures, while in one the upper respiratory tract was involved and in another there were multiple hemangiomata in the mucosa of the small bowel, mesentery, and pancreas. The sternal defect varies from a complete cleft to a partial cleft involving the upper one third of the sternum.

Occasional abnormalities have included absent pericardium anteriorly, unilateral cleft lip, micrognathia, glossoptosis and areas of linear hypopigmentation.

A significant morbidity is related to respiratory compromise, gastrointestinal bleeding, and infection, as rapid expansion of the vascular lesion leads to tissue hypoxia and necrosis.

All reported cases of this disorder have been sporadic events in otherwise normal families with the exception of a male with asternia and a facial hemangioma who had a sister with isolated asternia. The etiology of this condition is unknown.

An overlap exists between this disorder and the PHACE syndrome, a term applied to the association of *p*osterior fossa brain abnormalities, *h*emangiomas, *a*rterial anomalies in the cranial vasculature, *c*oarctation of the aorta/cardiac defects, and *e*ye abnormalities. Sternal clefting and supraumbilical raphe can also be present. Thus, all children with the sternal malformation–vascular dysplasia spectrum should undergo a complete neurologic examination, four limb blood pressures, echocardiography, magnetic resonance imaging of the brain, and ophthalmologic evaluation.

References

Hersh JH, et al: Sternal malformation/vascular dysplasia association, *Am J Med Genet* 21:177, 1985.

James PA, McGaughran J: Complete overlap of PHACE syndrome and sternal malformation–vascular dysplasia association, *Am J Med Genet* 110:78, 2002.

Mazereeuw-Hautier J, et al: Sternal malformation/vascular dysplasia syndrome with linear hypopigmentation, *Br J Dermatol* 155:192, 2006.

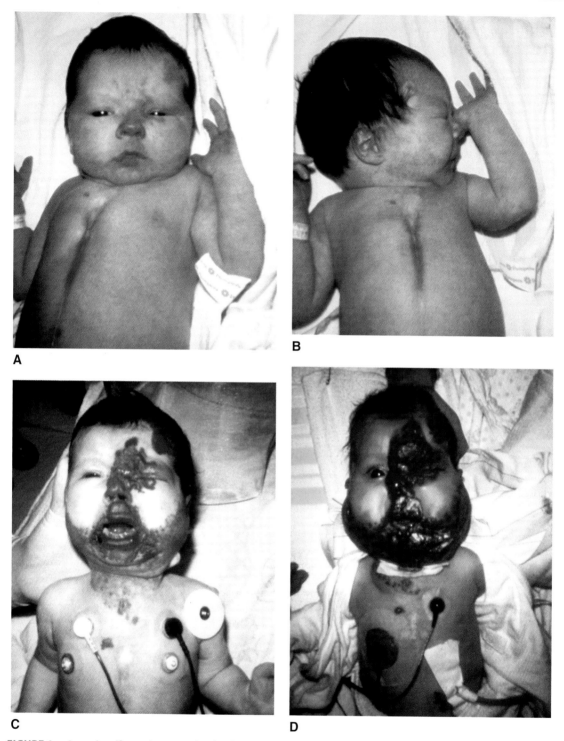

FIGURE 1.   Sternal malformation–vascular dysplasia spectrum. **A** and **B,** Affected child in newborn period. **C,** At 6 weeks. **D,** At 4 months. Note the capillary hemangiomata over the face and the cleft of the upper one third of the sternum, which is covered with atrophic skin. (From Hersh JH: *Am J Med Genet* 21:177, 1985, with permission from Wiley-Liss, a division of John Wiley & Sons.)

V

MONOZYGOTIC TWINNING AND STRUCTURAL DEFECTS—GENERAL

Monozygotic (MZ) twinning occurs in approximately 1 in 200 births and, as such, represents the most common aberration of morphogenesis noted in humans. The frequency of MZ twin conceptuses is probably appreciably higher than 1 in 200. Livingston and Poland found a threefold excess of MZ twins among spontaneous abortuses versus liveborn twins, with the ratio of MZ to dizygotic (DZ) being 17:1 in the abortuses versus 0.8:1 in the liveborn twins. Most of these MZ aborted twins had structural defects and may represent the early lethal effect of the types of structural defects that have been noted to occur with excess frequency in MZ twins.

Structural defects occur two to three times more commonly in liveborn MZ twins than in DZ twins or singletons. The origin and nature of these defects are summarized in Table 1-1, and the first three categories are individually set forth in the following subsections. The fourth category of deformation, caused by in utero crowding, which is not increased in MZ versus DZ twins, is set forth in *Smith's Recognizable Patterns of Human Deformation* by John M. Graham, Jr. (3rd ed, Philadelphia, 2007, Saunders) and will not be detailed here.

MZ twinning may occur soon after conception, and this type may even have separate placentas with dichorionic-diamnionic membranes. The development of two embryonic centers in the blastocyst by 4 to 5 days of gestation yields twins with monochorionic-diamnionic membranes, the most common type of MZ twinning. The final potential timing for the induction of MZ twinning is by 15 to 16 days of development, with the formation of more than one Hensen node and primitive streak in the embryonic plate. This will result in monochorionic-monoamnionic twins, who account for approximately 4% of MZ twins.

In addition to the problems that were alluded to concerning MZ twins, there appears to be an increased likelihood of fetal death in one or more of MZ twins who develop in a monoamnionic sac, at least partially because of cord entanglements leading to vascular problems. There is also an overall excess of perinatal mortality in MZ twins. The primary cause is prematurity, but the excess of structural defects also contributes to this high mortality.

The value and importance of examining the placenta for the condition of the membranes, vascular interconnections between the twins, and evidence of a deceased twin should be obvious.

The etiologies for MZ twinning are largely unknown. A single-gene, dominant type of inheritance has been implicated in an occasional family. Experimental studies have implied environmental factors, such as late fertilization of the ovum in the rabbit and vincristine administration in the rat.

MONOZYGOTIC TWINS AND EARLY MALFORMATIONS

The excess of early types of malformation among MZ twins may be the consequence of the same etiology that gave rise to the MZ twinning aberration of morphogenesis. For example, Stockard was able to produce both MZ twinning and early malformation such as cyclopia by early environmental insults (alterations of oxygen level and temperature) to the developing Atlantic minnow (*Fundulus*). The findings of Schinzel and colleagues confirm this hypothesis. They found that the malformations in MZ twins were predominantly early defects, presumably engendered at the same time as the MZ twinning. The incidence of associated early malformations was greatest in the monochorionic-monoamnionic cases, which would usually have been induced at the

Table 1-1 ORIGIN AND TYPES OF STRUCTURAL DEFECTS IN MONOZYGOTIC TWINS	
Origin	**Types of Defects**
A. The same causative factor that gave rise to MZ twinning	Early malformations or malformation sequences
B. Incomplete twinning	Conjoined twins

C. Consequence of vascular placental shunts
  1. Artery-artery
  2. Artery-vein
  3. Death of one twin leading to decreased blood flow and hypoxia
	Disruptions, including acardiac and amorphous twins
	Twin-twin transfusion, causing unequal size, unequal hematocrit, or other problems

D. Constraint in fetal life	Deformations caused by uterine constraint

time of embryonic plate development and hence would theoretically be more likely to have associated early malformations. The early types of defects that have been considered to be of excess frequency in MZ twins are the following:

1. Sacrococcygeal teratoma
2. Sirenomelia sequence (see Subchapter 1U)
3. The VACTERL association (see Subchapter 1W)
4. Exstrophy of the cloaca sequence (see Subchapter 1U)
5. Holoprosencephaly sequence (see Subchapter 1U)
6. Anencephaly (see Subchapter 1U)

Approximately 5% to 20% of such cases are concordant; thus, the majority of cases are discordant. When one twin has the more severe degree of a malformation sequence, the other twin may show lesser degrees of the same type of initiating defect.

These early defects are presented individually in this text. Most are early lethals and cause spontaneous abortion. This is probably a partial explanation of the excess of MZ twins among spontaneous abortuses.

Recurrence risk counseling should involve the total problem, namely, the MZ twinning plus the associated malformation sequence. To our knowledge, this risk is of low to negligible magnitude, although the specific etiologies for this type of problem are unknown.

CONJOINED TWINS

Conjoined twins may be viewed as examples of incomplete twinning and occur in approximately 1% of MZ twins. Although it is feasible that two closely placed embryonic centers in the 4- to 5-day-old blastocyst could result in conjoined twins, it seems more likely that they originate at the primitive streak stage of the embryonic plate (15 to 17 days). Current experimental techniques in animals have not been successful in producing conjoined twins.

The most common type of conjoined twins is termed *thoracopagus*, in which the twins are joined at the thorax. Juncture at the head, buttocks, and, less commonly, other anatomic sites also occurs. Partial to complete duplication of only the upper or lower body parts may also take place.

As with MZ twins in general, there is a higher incidence of early malformations in conjoined twins. Disregarding the incidence of anomalies related to the sites of juncture, there is a 10% to 20% occurrence of major early defects. As with separate MZ twins, the malformations in conjoined twins are often not concordant. The high frequency of associated malformations in conjoined twins may relate to the timing of the defect, which is presumed to be at the embryonic plate-primitive streak stage of development.

The likelihood of particular types of early malformation occurring in certain kinds of conjoined twins is increased nonrandomly. For example, the dicephalic-conjoined twin frequently has anencephaly, most commonly affecting only one of the heads. Whether this relates to differences in early blood flow to the respective heads remains to be determined. Furthermore, the right-sided twin of a dicephalic conjoined twin pair virtually always has situs inversus. The recurrence risk for conjoined twins appears to be negligible.

PLACENTAL VASCULAR SHUNTS IN MONOZYGOTIC TWINS—GENERAL

Benirschke has indicated that the great majority of monochorionic (single placenta) twins have a conjoined placenta with vascular interconnections. These develop on a chance basis and are usually evident on the fetal surface of the placenta where the major vessels course between the fetuses and the major cotyledons. The magnitude of intertwin vascular shunts may be judged by the caliber of the connecting vessels, which relates to the amount of flow they have carried. Much of the early in utero mortality and excess of structural defects in MZ twins may well relate to the secondary consequences of these vascular connections between the twins. Some of the types of shunts and their adverse effects on one or both of the MZ twins are set forth subsequently.

Artery-Artery Twin Disruption Sequence

Benirschke emphasized the dire consequences that could result from a sizable artery-artery placental shunt, usually accompanied by a vein-vein shunt. The tendency will be for the arterial pressure of one twin to overpower that of the other, usually early in morphogenesis. The "defeated" recipient then has reverse flow from the co-twin. This sends "used" arterial blood from the donor into the iliac vessels of the recipient, perfusing the lower part of the body more than the upper part. The results are a host of disruptions, with deterioration of previously existing tissues as well as incomplete morphogenesis (malformation) of tissues that are in the process of formation. The variably missing tissues include the head, heart, upper limbs, lungs, pancreas, and upper intestine. Rudiments of early disrupted tissues may be found in the residuum. The extent of disruption may be even broader, leaving as the residuum an "amorphous" twin. There is every gradation, from amorphia to acardia to less severe degrees of disruption, with no one case being identical to another. Examples of some of the gradations of severity are shown in Figure 3.

The donor twin may have an excessive cardiac load resulting in cardiomegaly and even cardiac decompensation, with secondary liver dysfunction, hypoalbuminemia, and edema. Sometimes this may progress to the level of hydrops.

Artery-Vein Twin Transfusion Sequence

Artery-vein transfusion may result in problems such as those summarized in Table 1-2. The excessive volume in the recipient twin not only tends to lead to increased growth and an enlarged heart but also causes increased kidney size and excess urine output, with resultant polyhydramnios. The high hematocrit may constitute a serious risk of vascular problems and merits early postnatal management. The donor twin, being hypovolemic, tends to have diminished renal blood flow, smaller kidneys, and oligohydramnios (when the twins are diamnionic). There may even be evidence of transient renal insufficiency in the smaller twin during the first days after birth, as the kidneys have been hypofunctional since before birth.

Tan and colleagues have found that 18% of MZ twins are discrepant in size and hematocrit at birth; hence, this is not a rare occurrence. Treatment may be warranted soon after birth to provide each affected twin with a more normal hematocrit.

Complications in a Monozygotic Twin from the in utero Death of the Co-twin

Benirschke first implicated death of an MZ co-twin (stillborn or fetus papyraceus) as a potential cause for problems in the surviving twin. Decreased blood flow caused by hemodynamic changes with consequent hypoxia is the most likely mechanism. The resultant areas of ischemia and disruption, with subsequent loss of tissue, lead to disruptive vascular defects in the co-twin of the deceased MZ twin, some of which are the following:

1. Disseminated intravascular coagulation
2. Aplasia cutis
3. Porencephalic cyst to hydranencephaly
4. Limb amputation
5. Intestinal atresia
6. Gastroschisis

Melnick has concluded, from the Collaborative Perinatal Project (50,000 deliveries), that approximately 3% of near-term MZ twins have a deceased co-twin, and about one third of the survivors, or 1% of MZ twin births, have severe brain defects as a consequence of the foregoing mechanisms. The surviving infants with porencephalic cysts or hydranencephaly are usually severely mentally deficient with microcephaly, spastic diplegia, and seizures.

Table 1-2 **PROBLEMS SECONDARY TO ARTERIOVENOUS TWIN-TWIN TRANSFUSION**		
Feature	**Donor Twin**	**Recipient Twin**
Growth	Smaller size	Larger size
Hematocrit	Low	High
Blood volume	Hypovolemia	Hypervolemia
Renal blood flow and renal size	Diminished	Increased
Amnionic fluid	Oligohydramnios	Polyhydramnios
Heart size	Diminished	Increased

References

General

Stockard CR: Developmental rate and structural expression: An experimental study of twins, "double monsters," and single deformities and the interaction among embryonic organs during their origin and development, *Am J Anat* 28:115, 1921.

Benirschke K: Twin placenta in perinatal mortality, *NY State J Med* 61:1499, 1961.

Benirschke K, Driscoll SG: The placenta in multiple pregnancy, *Handbuch Pathol Histol* 7:187, 1967.

Bomsel-Helmreich O: Delayed ovulation and monozygotic twinning in the rabbit, *Acta Genet Med Gemellol* 23:19, 1974.

Myrianthopoulos NC: Congenital malformations in twins, *Acta Genet Med Gemellol* 24:331, 1976.

Harvey MAS, Huntley RM, Smith DW: Familial monozygotic twinning, *J Pediatr* 90:246, 1977.

Kaufman MH, O'Shea KS: Induction of monozygotic twinning in the mouse, *Nature* 276:707, 1978.

Schinzel AAGL, et al: Monozygotic twinning and structural defects, *J Pediatr* 95:921, 1979.

Livingston JE, Poland BJ: A study of spontaneously aborted twins, *Teratology* 21:139, 1980.

Early Malformations in Monozygotic Twins

Stockard CR: Developmental rate and structural expression: An experimental study of twins, "double monsters," and single deformities and the interaction among embryonic organs during their origin and development, *Am J Anat* 28:115, 1921.

Gross RE, et al: Sacrococcygeal teratomas in infants and children, *Surg Gynecol Obstet* 92:341, 1951.

Mohr HP: Missbilundugen bei Zwillingen, *Ergeb Inn Med Kinderheilkd* 33:1, 1972.

Davies J, Chazen E, Nance WE: Symmelia in one of monozygotic twins, *Teratology* 4:367, 1976.

Smith DW, et al: Monozygotic twinning and the Duhamel anomalad (imperforate anus to sirenomelia): A nonrandom association between two aberrations in morphogenesis, *Birth Defects* 12:53, 1976.

Schinzel AAGL, et al: Monozygotic twinning and structural defects, *J Pediatr* 95:921, 1979.

Livingston JE, Poland BJ: A study of spontaneously aborted twins, *Teratology* 21:139, 1980.

Conjoined Twins

Riccardi VM, Bergmann CA: Anencephaly with incomplete twinning (diprosopus), *Teratology* 16:137, 1977.

Schinzel AAGL, et al: Monozygotic twinning and structural defects, *J Pediatr* 95:921, 1979.

Vascular Shunts between Monozygotic Twins

Confalonieri C: Gravidanza gemellare monocoriale biamniotica con feto papiraceo ed atresia intestinale congenita nell'altro feto, *Riv Ost Ginec Prat* 33:199, 1951.

Naeye RL: Human intrauterine parabiotic syndrome and its complications, *N Engl J Med* 268:804, 1963.

Hague IU, Glassauer FE: Hydranencephaly in twins, *NY State J Med* 69:1210, 1969.

Moore CM, et al: Intrauterine disseminated intravascular coagulation: A syndrome of multiple pregnancy with a dead twin fetus, *J Pediatr* 74:523, 1969.

Saier F, et al: Fetus papyraceus: An unusual case with congenital anomaly of the surviving fetus, *Obstet Gynecol* 45:271, 1975.

Balvour RP: Fetus papyraceus, *Obstet Gynecol* 47:507, 1976.

Weiss DB, et al: Gastroschisis and fetus papyraceus in double ovum twins, *Harefuah* 91:392, 1976.

Benirschke K, Harper V: The acardiac anomaly, *Teratology* 15:311, 1977.

Mannino FL, et al: Congenital skin defects and fetus papyraceus, *J Pediatr* 91:599, 1977.

Melnick M: Brain damage in survivor after death of monozygotic co-twin, *Lancet* 2:1287, 1977.

Schinzel AAGL, et al: Monozygotic twinning and structural defects, *J Pediatr* 95:921, 1979.

Tan KL, et al: The twin transfusion syndrome, *Clin Pediatr* 18:111, 1979.

Jones KL, Benirschke K: The developmental pathogenesis of structural defects: The contribution of monozygotic twins, *Semin Perinatol* 7:239, 1983.

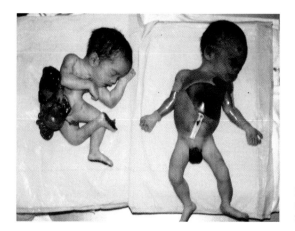

FIGURE 1.   MZ twins discordant for limb–body wall complex. (Courtesy Dr. Kurt Benirschke, University of California, San Diego.)

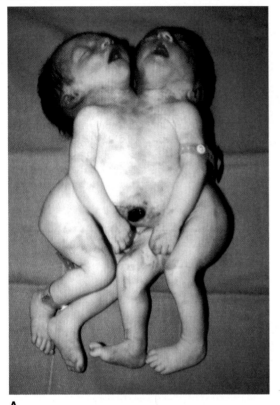

A

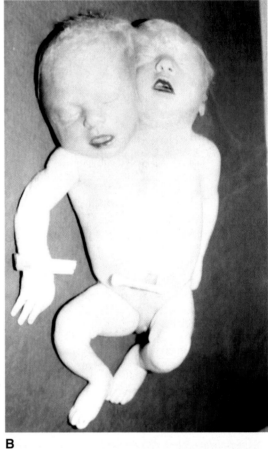

B

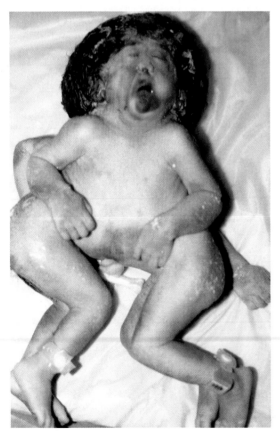

C

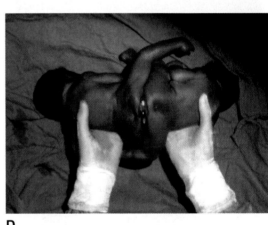

D

FIGURE 2. Varying degrees of conjoined twins.
A, Attached at the chest (thoracopagus), which is the
most common type. **B,** Dicephalus (two heads).
C, Cephalothoracopagus. **D,** Joined at the buttocks.
(Courtesy Dr. Kurt Benirschke, University of California,
San Diego.)

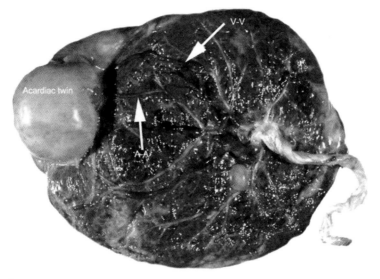

A

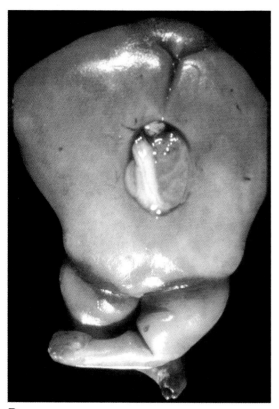

B

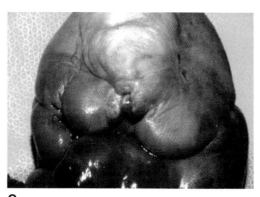

C

FIGURE 3. Artery-artery twin disruption sequence. **A,** Amorphous acardiac twin partially embedded in the placenta. Note the artery-artery vascular anastomosis (*left arrow*) and the vein-vein vascular anastomosis (*right arrow*), which have led to the reversal of blood flow. **B** and **C,** Acardiac twin with upper limb deficiency, marked disruption of the craniofacial area and upper body, and relative sparing of the lower body caused by artery-artery shunt and reverse circulation from co-twin. (Courtesy Dr. Kurt Benirschke, University of California, San Diego.)

V

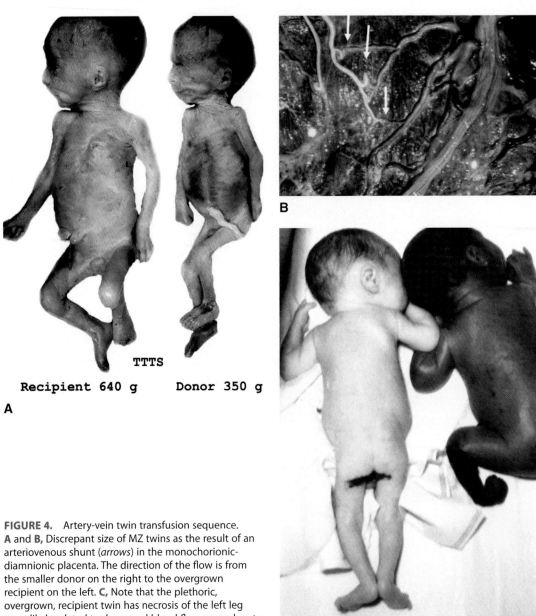

FIGURE 4. Artery-vein twin transfusion sequence.
A and **B,** Discrepant size of MZ twins as the result of an arteriovenous shunt (*arrows*) in the monochorionic-diamnionic placenta. The direction of the flow is from the smaller donor on the right to the overgrown recipient on the left. **C,** Note that the plethoric, overgrown, recipient twin has necrosis of the left leg most likely related to decreased blood flow secondary to polycythemia. (Courtesy Dr. Kurt Benirschke, University of California, San Diego.)

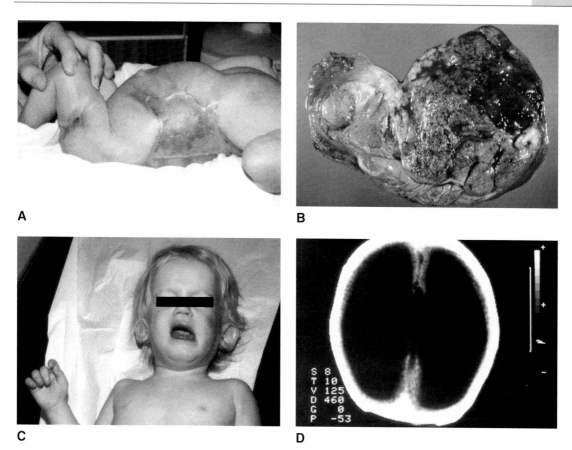

FIGURE 5.   Impact of death of MZ twin on surviving co-twin. **A** and **B,** A newborn infant with aplasia cutis congenita related to the in utero death of his MZ co-twin, who can be seen embedded in the left of the placental membranes. **C** and **D,** Child with hypertonic diplegia, seizures, and developmental deficiency, who had hydranencephaly. At birth, there was a macerated 30-cm co-twin of the same sex.

VACTERL ASSOCIATION

An association is a term used to designate the non-random tendency of some malformations to occur together more commonly than would be expected by chance, without being components of a syndrome. VACTERL is an acronym that stands for *v*ertebral, *a*nal, *c*ardiac, *t*racheal, *e*sophageal, *r*enal, and *l*imb. VACTERL association defects include vertebral defects, anal atresia, cardiac defects, tracheoesophageal fistula with esophageal atresia, renal dysplasia, and limb/radial defects. Prenatal growth deficiency and single umbilical artery are also nonrandom features of this pattern of anomalies. The general spectrum of the pattern in 34 cases is presented subsequently, as summarized by Temtamy and Miller. Initially described as VATER association, another "R" was added when renal anomalies were included, followed by a "C" for cardiac "L" for limb eventually replaced the "R" for radial anomaly.

ABNORMALITIES

Vertebral anomalies	70%
Cardiac defects	53%
Anal atresia with or without fistula	80%
Tracheoesophageal fistula with esophageal atresia	70%
Renal anomaly	53%
Radial dysplasia, including thumb or radial hypoplasia, preaxial polydactyly, syndactyly	65%
Single umbilical artery	35%

OTHER LESS FREQUENT DEFECTS
Prenatal growth deficiency, postnatal growth deficiency, laryngeal stenosis, bronchial anomalies, ear anomaly, large fontanels, defect of lower limb (23%), rib anomaly, defects of external genitalia, occult spinal dysraphia with tethered cord.

NATURAL HISTORY
Although many of these patients may fail to thrive and have slow developmental progress in early infancy related to their defects, the majority of them have normal brain function. Adults with VACTERL association have a number of difficulties often related to the primary malformations. Those with vertebral defects often experience significant back, shoulder, and/or neck pain. Sequelae of anal anomalies include constipation and obstruction as well as functional stooling problems. Following surgical repair of tracheoesophageal fistula, dysphagia, choking, and reflux, as well as reactive airway disease and tracheomalacia, can occur. Nephrolithiasis and urinary tract infections are common sequelae of renal defects.

ETIOLOGY
This pattern of malformation has generally been a sporadic occurrence in an otherwise normal family. The etiology is unknown. It has more frequently appeared in the offspring of diabetic mothers. In addition, it occurs more frequently in individuals who have Fanconi anemia, particularly in association with complementation groups D1, E, and F. Because Fanconi anemia has an autosomal recessive mode of inheritance, with a 25% recurrence risk, it is critical to be aware of that possibility. Chromosomal breakage studies to rule out Fanconi anemia should be seriously considered in all cases of VACTERL association, particularly those cases in which additional features, including skin pigmentation abnormalities, growth retardation, and microcephaly, are present. Features of this association may occur in an otherwise normal child or as a part of a broader pattern, such as the trisomy 18 or del(13q) syndromes, in which case the prognosis is not favorable. It is also important to recognize that VACTERL association is not in and of itself a diagnosis, but rather a nonrandom association of defects. As such, when one of the associated features is identified, careful evaluation for other VACTERL association defects should be undertaken. In cases in which a malformation not usually encountered with VACTERL association defects is identified, further investigation is warranted.

COMMENT
A distinct, genetically determined disorder referred to as VACTERL with hydrocephalus (VACTERL-H) has been reported. Both autosomal and X-linked recessive inheritance have been documented for that disorder. No clinical distinction is possible to differentiate between autosomal and X-linked recessive families. Although a poor prognosis is the rule, survival with a relatively good outcome has been noted in some cases. An association with Fanconi anemia is stronger than is seen in VACTERL association without hydrocephalus. Mutations or deletions of the *FANCB* gene, which is responsible for Fanconi anemia complementation group B, are common in X-linked recessive VACTERL-H. Similarly, a

diagnosis of Fanconi anemia and autosomal recessive VACTERL-H has been documented.

References

Say B, Gerald PS: A new polydactyly, imperforate anus, vertebral anomalies syndrome, *Lancet* 2:688, 1968.

Say D, et al: A new syndrome of dysmorphogenesis–imperforate anus associated with polyoligodactyly and skeletal (mainly vertebral) anomalies, *Acta Paediatr Scand* 60:197, 1971.

Quan L, Smith DW: The VATER association. Vertebral defects, Anal atresia, T-E fistula with esophageal atresia, Radial and Renal dysplasia: A spectrum of associated defects, *J Pediatr* 82:104, 1973.

Temtamy SA, Miller JD: Extending the scope of the VATER association: Definition of a VATER syndrome, *J Pediatr* 85:345, 1974.

Evans JA, et al: VACTERL with hydrocephalus: Further delineation of the syndrome(s), *Am J Med Genet* 34:177, 1989.

James HE, et al: Distal spinal cord pathology in the VATER association, *J Pediatr Surg* 29:1501, 1994.

Botto L, et al: The spectrum of congenital anomalies of the VATER association: An international study, *Am J Med Genet* 71:8, 1997.

Källén K, et al: VATER non-random association of congenital malformations: Study based on data from four malformation registers, *Am J Med Genet* 101:26, 2001.

Faivre L, et al: Should chromosomal breakage studies be performed in patients with VACTERL association? *Am J Med Genet* 137:55, 2005.

Kanu A, et al: Bronchial anomalies in VACTERL association, *Pediatr Pulmonol* 43:930, 2008.

Solomon BD, et al: Evidence for inheritance in patients with VACTERL association, *Hum Genet* 127:731, 2010.

McCauley J, et al: X-linked VACTERL with hydrocephalus syndrome: Further delineation of the phenotype caused by *FANCB* mutations, *Am J Med Genet* 155:2370, 2011.

Raam MS, et al: Long-term outcomes of adults with features of VACTERL association, *Eur J Med Genet* 54:34, 2011.

W

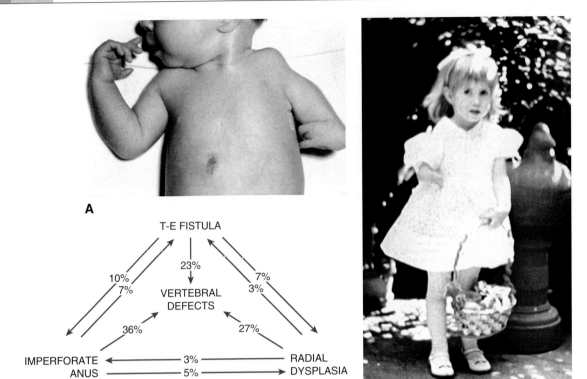

A

T-E FISTULA

10%
7%

23%

7%
3%

VERTEBRAL
DEFECTS

36%

27%

IMPERFORATE
ANUS

3%
5%

RADIAL
DYSPLASIA

C

B

FIGURE 1. VATERR association as initially set forth. **A,** Young infant with vertebral anomalies, anal atresia, esophageal atresia with tracheoesophageal fistula, radial aplasia on the left, and thumb hypoplasia on the right. **B,** Same patient at 2 years of age, with normal intelligence. **C,** Relative frequencies of some of the other VATER association defects when the patient is ascertained by virtue of having one of the defects. (From Quan L, Smith DW: *J Pediatr* 82:104, 1973, with permission.)

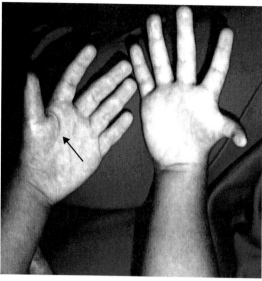

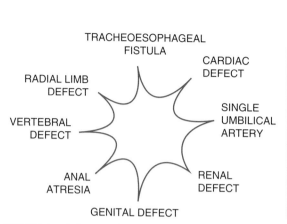

TRACHEOESOPHAGEAL
FISTULA

CARDIAC
DEFECT

RADIAL LIMB
DEFECT

SINGLE
UMBILICAL
ARTERY

VERTEBRAL
DEFECT

ANAL
ATRESIA

RENAL
DEFECT

GENITAL DEFECT

FIGURE 2.   *Left,* Expanded VACTERL association of defects. *Right,* Note the relatively severe thumb (radial) defect of the right hand and the much more subtle "radial" defect of the left hand (*arrow*). The *arrow* depicts a hypoplastic thenar eminence and crease.

W

MURCS ASSOCIATION
Müllerian Duct, Renal and Cervical Vertebral Defects

The MURCS association, as described in 30 patients by Duncan and colleagues in 1979, consists of a nonrandom association of müllerian duct aplasia, renal aplasia, and cervicothoracic somite dysplasia.

ABNORMALITIES

Growth. Small stature.

Skeletal. Cervicothoracic vertebral defects, especially from C5–T1 (80%), sometimes to the extent of comprising the Klippel-Feil malformation sequence.

Genitourinary. Absence of proximal two thirds of vagina and absence to hypoplasia of uterus (96%, but there is an ascertainment bias for this defect; sometimes referred to as the Rokitansky malformation sequence); renal agenesis or ectopy (88%).

OCCASIONAL ABNORMALITIES

Moderate frequency of rib anomalies, occipitoatlantoaxial junction malformation, early-onset senile ankylosing vertebral hyperostosis, upper limb anomalies (primarily reduction defects although duplicated thumb has occurred), and Sprengel scapular anomaly. Infrequent features include deafness, cerebellar cyst, external ear defects, facial asymmetry, cleft lip and palate, micrognathia, gastrointestinal defects, anorectal malformations, defects of laterality, abnormal lung lobation, and occipital encephalocele.

NATURAL HISTORY

Most patients are ascertained because of primary amenorrhea or infertility associated with normal secondary sexual characteristics. Rarely, the MURCS association may be diagnosed in the course of an investigation for a renal malformation or because of multiple malformations. Small stature is frequent, with adult stature usually being less than 152 cm.

ETIOLOGY

The etiology of this disorder is unknown; it is usually a sporadic disorder in an otherwise normal family.

COMMENT

The Mayer-Rokitansky-Küster-Hauser anomaly, one of the defects that comprise the MURCS association, is characterized by an incomplete to atretic vagina and a rudimentary to bicornuate uterus. The fallopian tubes and ovaries are usually nearly normal with normal secondary sexual characteristics, except for a lack of menstruation. The lower vagina, which is derived from an outpouching from the urogenital sinus, is usually present as a blindly ending pouch. The cause is unknown. Although most cases are sporadic, approximately 4% of cases have been familial, with affected female siblings.

References

Rokitansky K: Über sog. Verdoppelung des Uterus, *Med Jahrb des Osterreich Staates* 26:39, 1838.

Byran AL, et al: One hundred cases of congenital absence of the vagina, *Surg Gynecol Obstet* 88:79, 1949.

Duncan PA: Embryologic pathogenesis of renal agenesis associated with cervical vertebral anomalies (Klippel-Feil phenotype), *Birth Defects* 13(3D):91, 1977.

Duncan PA, et al: The MURCS association: Müllerian duct aplasia, renal aplasia, and cervicothoracic somite dysplasia, *J Pediatr* 95:399, 1979.

Greene RA, et al: MURCS association with additional congenital anomalies, *Hum Pathol* 17:88, 1986.

Mahajan P, et al: MURCS association—a review of 7 cases, *J Postgrad Med* 38:109, 1992.

Suri M, et al: MURCS association with encephalocele: Report of a second case, *Clin Dysmorph* 9:31, 2000.

Lopez AG, et al: MURCS association with duplicated thumb, *Clin Genet* 61:308, 2002.

Gunsar C, et al: MURCS association and rectovestibular fistula: Case report of a patient treated with one-stage posterior sagittal anorectoplasty and sigmoid loop vaginoplasty, *J Pediatr Surg* 38:262, 2003.

Kaissi AA, et al: Occipitoatlantoaxial junction malformation and early onset senile ankylosing vertebral hyperostosis in a girl with MURCS association, *Am J Med Genet* 149:470, 2009.

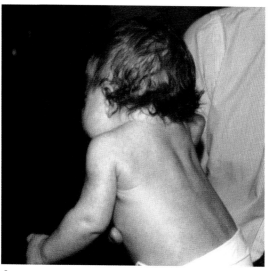

A

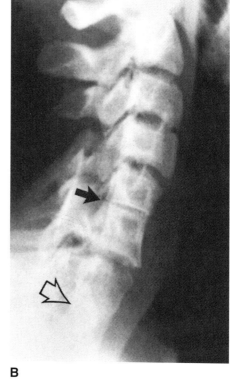

B

FIGURE 1. MURCS association. **A,** Child with short neck secondary to cervical vertebral defects. **B,** An example is depicted in the radiograph. Note the partial to complete cervical vertebral fusion (*arrows*).

W

CHAPTER 2

Morphogenesis and Dysmorphogenesis

Knowledge of normal morphogenesis may assist in the interpretation of structural defects, and the study of structural defects may assist in the understanding of normal morphogenesis. Each anomaly must have a logical mode of development and cause. When interpreting a structural defect, the clinician is looking back to an early stage in development with which he or she has often had little acquaintance. This chapter sets forth some of the phenomena of morphogenesis and the normal stages in early human development, followed by the types of abnormal morphogenesis and the relative timing of particular malformations.

NORMAL MORPHOGENESIS

Phenomena of Morphogenesis

The genetic information that guides the morphogenesis and function of an individual is all contained within the zygote. After the first few cell divisions, differentiation begins to take place, presumably through activation or inactivation of particular genes, allowing cells to assume diverse roles. The entire process is programmed in a timely and sequential order with little allowance for error, especially in early morphogenesis.

Although little is known about the fundamental processes that control morphogenesis, it is worthwhile to mention some of the normal phenomena that occur and to give examples of each.

Cell Migration

The proper migration of cells to a predestined location is critical in the development of many structures. For example, the germ cells move from the yolk sac endoderm to the urogenital ridge, where they interact with other cells to form the gonad.

Control over Mitotic Rate

The size of particular structures, as well as their form, is largely the consequence of control over the rates of cell division.

Interaction between Adjacent Tissues

The optic cup induces the morphogenesis of the lens from the overlying ectoderm, the ureteric bud gives rise to the development of the kidney from the adjacent metanephric tissue, the notochord is essential for normal development of the overlying neural tissue, and the prechordal mesoderm is important for the normal morphogenesis of the overlying forebrain. These are but a few examples of the many interactions that are essential features in morphogenesis.

Adhesive Association of Like Cells

In the development of a structure such as long bone, the early cells tend to aggregate closely in condensations, a membrane comes to surround them, and only later do they resemble cartilage cells. The association of like cells is dramatically demonstrated by admixing trypsinized liver and kidney cells in vitro and observing them reaggregate with their own kind.

Controlled Cell Death

Controlled cell death plays a role in normal morphogenesis. Examples include death of tissue between the digits resulting in separation of the fingers and recanalization of the duodenum. The dead cellular debris is engulfed by large macrophages, leaving no trace of the tissue.

Hormonal Influence over Morphogenesis

Androgen effect is one example of a hormonal influence over morphogenesis—in this case, that of the external genitalia. Normally, the individual with a Y chromosome has testosterone from the fetal testicle that induces enlargement of the phallus, closure of the labia minora folds to form a penile urethra, and fusion of the labioscrotal folds to form a scrotum. Before 8 weeks' gestation, the genitalia appear female in type and will remain so unless androgenic hormone is present.

857

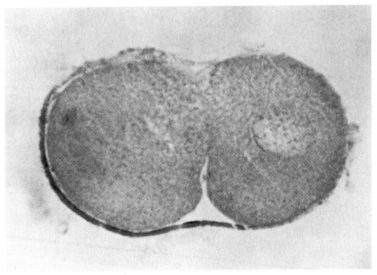

FIGURE 2-1.   Two-cell specimen, within zona pellucida. (From the Department of Embryology, Carnegie Institution of Washington, DC, Baltimore.)

Mechanical Forces

Mechanical forces play a major role in morphogenesis. The size, growth, and form of the brain and its early derivatives, for example, have a major function in the formation of the calvarium and upper face. The alignment of collagen fibrils and bone trabeculae relates directly to the direction of forces exerted on these tissues. The role of mechanical factors in development is covered in the text *Smith's Recognizable Patterns of Human Deformation.*

Normal Stages in Morphogenesis

The general steps in normal morphogenesis as set forth here are illustrated in Figures 2-1 to 2-16. The first week is a period of cell division without much enlargement, the conceptus being dependent on the cytoplasm of the ova for most of its metabolic needs. By 7 to 8 days, the zona pellucida is gone, and the outlying trophoblast cells invade the endometrium and form the early placenta that must function both to nourish the parasitic embryo and to maintain the pregnancy via its endocrine function. During this time, a relatively small inner cell mass has become a bilaminar disk of ectoderm and endoderm, each with its own fluid-filled cavity, the amniotic sac and yolk sac, respectively. By the end of the second week, a small mound, a primitive node, has developed in the ectoderm, and behind it a primitive streak forms. The embryo now has an axis to which further morphogenesis will relate. Cells migrate forward from the node between the ectoderm and endoderm to form an elastic cord, the notochord, which temporarily provides axial support for the embryo as well as influencing the

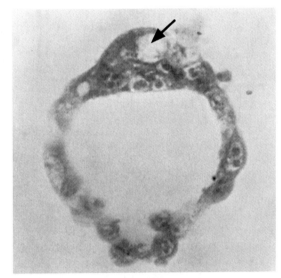

FIGURE 2-2.   A 4- to 5-day-old blastocyst. The embryonic cell mass *(arrow)*. (From the Department of Embryology, Carnegie Institution of Washington, DC, Baltimore.)

adjacent morphogenesis. Ectodermal cells migrate through the node and the primitive streak to specific areas between the ectoderm and endoderm, becoming the mesoderm. One of the early mesodermal derivatives is a circulatory system: During the third week, the heart begins to develop, vascular channels form in situ, and blood cells are produced in the yolk sac. By the end of the third week, the heart is pumping, a neural groove has formed anterior to the node, the para-axial mesoderm has begun to be segmented into somites, the anterior and

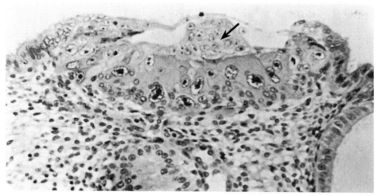

FIGURE 2-3.   Seven days. The major part of the conceptus, the cytotrophoblast, has invaded the endometrium, and the embryo *(arrow)* is differentiating into two diverse cell layers, the ectoderm and endoderm. The amniotic cavity is beginning to form. (From the Department of Embryology, Carnegie Institution of Washington, DC, Baltimore.)

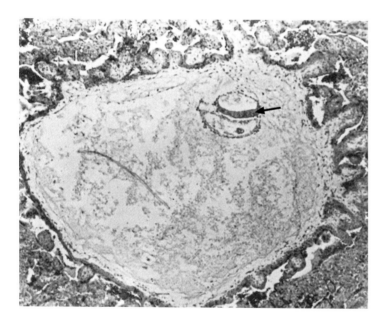

FIGURE 2-4.   Fourteen to sixteen days. The thicker ectoderm *(arrow)* has its continuous amniotic sac, whereas the underlying endoderm has its yolk sac. Major changes will now begin to take place.

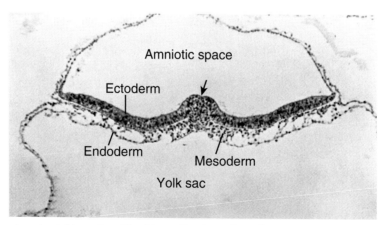

FIGURE 2-5.   Seventeen to eighteen days. Mesoblast cells migrate from the ectoderm through the node (the hillock marked by the *arrow*) and the primitive streak to specific locations between the ectoderm and endoderm, constituting the highly versatile mesoderm. Anterior to the node the notochordal process develops, providing axial support and influencing subsequent development such as that of the overlying neural plate.

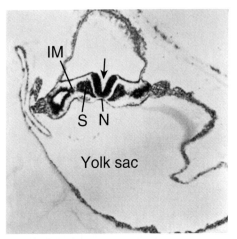

FIGURE 2-6.   Twenty-one to twenty-three days. The midaxial ectoderm has thickened and formed the neural groove *(arrow)*, partially influenced by the underlying notochordal plate *(N)*. Lateral to it, the mesoblast has now segmented into somites *(S)*, intermediate mesoderm *(IM)*, and somatopleure and splanchnopleure as intervening steps toward further differentiation. Vascular channels are developing in situ from mesoderm, blood cells are being produced in the yolk sac wall, and the early heart is beating. Henceforth, development is extremely rapid, with major changes each day.

posterior regions of the embryo have begun to curl under, and the foregut and hindgut pouches become distinct. The stage is now set for the period of major organogenesis, which is best considered in relation to individual structures.

Early morphogenesis is set forth in the accompanying figures. As noted in the illustrations found on the inside front cover and inside back cover of this book, each stage of development represents a synchronous syndrome of characteristics.

ABNORMAL MORPHOGENESIS

As mentioned in the introduction, there are four general types of developmental pathology leading to structural defects. The first type is malformation, which is poor formation of the tissue. The second is deformation, caused by altered mechanical forces on a normal tissue. Deformation may be secondary to extrinsic forces, such as uterine constraint on a normal fetus, or to intrinsic forces related to a more primary malformation. The third type of pathology is disruption, which is a result of the breakdown of previously normal tissue. An example of this is

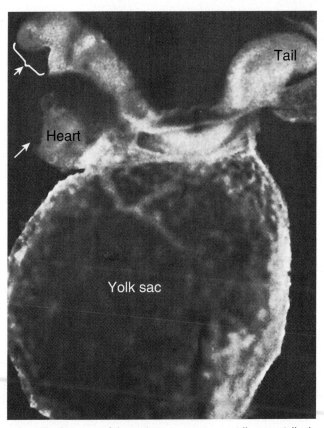

FIGURE 2-7.   Twenty-four days. The fore part of the embryo is growing rapidly, especially the anterior neural plate. The cardiac tube *(long arrow)*, under the developing face *(short arrow)*, is functional. (From the Department of Embryology, Carnegie Institution of Washington, DC, Baltimore.)

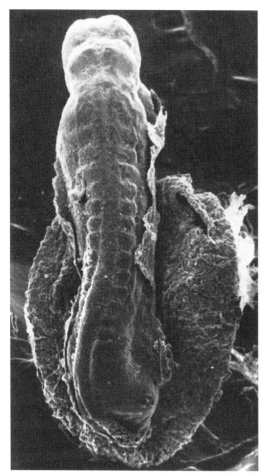

FIGURE 2-8. Scanning electron microscope photograph of human embryo of about 23 to 25 days' gestation, with the amnion largely stripped away. This dorsal view beautifully shows the developing brain (anterior) and spinal cord just after neural tube formation and the orderly bilateral segmentation of the somites. (Courtesy Dr. Jan E. Jirásek, Prague, Czech Republic.)

porencephalic cyst of vascular causation. The fourth mechanism of abnormal morphogenesis is dysplasia, in which there is a lack of normal organization of cells into tissue. Hamartomas are examples of this mechanism. These anomalies represent an organizational defect leading to an abnormal admixture of tissues, often with a tumor-like excess of one or more tissues. Some have malignant potential. Examples of hamartomas are hemangiomas, melanomas, fibromas, lipomas, adenomas, and some strange admixtures that defy traditional classification.

Extrinsic deformation is set forth in a separate text, *Smith's Recognizable Patterns of Human Deformation*. A few disruption patterns of anomaly are considered in this book, as well as some dysplasias, with the major emphasis being on patterns of malformation, including malformation sequences. However,

it is very important for the reader to appreciate that many of the anomalies in a given malformation sequence or syndrome are actually deformations that are engendered by the altered mechanical forces resulting from the more primary malformation. For example, most minor anomalies represent deformations, often secondary to a malformation.

Malformations may be broken down into a number of subcategories in terms of the nature of the poor formation.

Types of Malformation

Incomplete Morphogenesis

These are anomalies that represent incomplete stages in the development of a structure; they include the following subcategories, with one example listed for each.

Lack of development: renal agenesis secondary to failure of ureter formation
Hypoplasia: micrognathia
Incomplete separation: syndactyly (cutaneous)
Incomplete closure: cleft palate
Incomplete septation: ventricular septal defect
Incomplete migration of mesoderm: exstrophy of bladder
Incomplete rotation: malrotation of the gut
Incomplete resolution of early form: Meckel diverticulum
Persistence of earlier location: cryptorchidism

Aberrant Form

An occasional anomaly may be interpreted as an aberrant form that never exists in any stage of normal morphogenesis. An example is the pelvic spur in the nail-patella syndrome. Such an anomaly may be more specific for a particular clinical syndrome entity than anomalies of incomplete morphogenesis.

Accessory Tissue

Accessory tissue such as polydactyly, preauricular skin tags, and accessory spleens may be presumed to have been initiated at approximately the same time as the normal tissue, developing into finger rays, auricular hillocks of His, and spleen, respectively.

Functional Defects

Function is a necessary feature in joint development; hence, joint contractures, such as clubfoot, may be caused by a functional deficit in the use of the lower limb resulting from a more primary malformation.

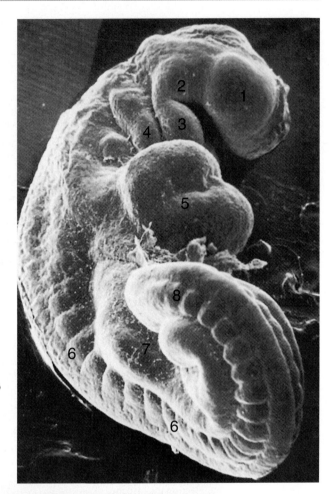

FIGURE 2-9. Scanning electron microscope photograph of a 28- to 30-day-old human embryo with the amnion removed, showing the following features: *1,* early optic vesicle outpouching; *2,* maxillary swelling; *3,* mandibular swelling; *4,* hyoid swelling; *5,* heart; *6,* somites, with adjacent spinal cord; *7,* early rudiments of upper limb bud; and *8,* tail. (Courtesy Dr. Jan E. Jirásek, Prague, Czech Republic.)

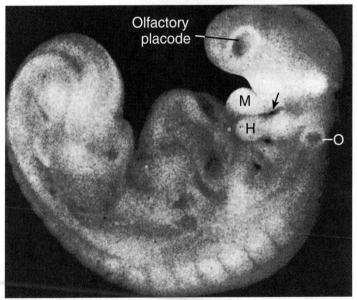

FIGURE 2-10. Twenty-eight to thirty days. The optic cup has begun to invaginate. Between it and the mandibular process is the area of the future mouth, where the buccopharyngeal membrane, with no intervening mesoderm, has broken down. Within the recess of the mandibular *(M)* and hyoid *(H)* processes, the future external auditory meatus will develop *(arrow),* and dorsal to it the otic vesicle *(O)* forms the inner ear. The relatively huge heart must pump blood in the yolk sac and developing placenta as well as to the embryo proper. Foregut outpouchings and evaginations will now begin to form various glands and the lung and liver primordia. Foregut and hindgut are now clearly delineated from the yolk sac. The somites, which will differentiate into myotomes (musculature), dermatomes (subcutaneous tissue), and sclerotomes (vertebrae), are evident on into the tail bud.

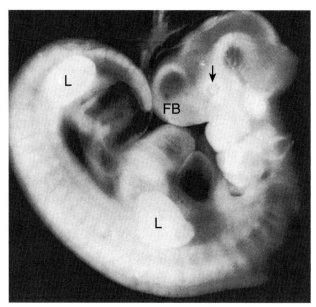

FIGURE 2-11. Approximately 30 to 31 days. The brain is rapidly growing, and its early cleavage into bilateral future cerebral hemispheres is evident in the telencephalic outpouching of the forebrain *(FB)*. To the right of this is the developing eye with the optic cup *(arrow)* and the early invagination of the future lens from surface ectoderm. The limb swellings *(L)* have developed from the somatopleura. The loose mesenchyme of the limb bud, interacting with the thickened ectodermal cells at its tip, carries all the potential for the full development of the limb. The liver is now functional and will be a source of blood cells. The mesonephric ducts, formed in the mesonephric ridges, communicate to the cloaca, which is beginning to become septated, and the yolk sac is regressing.

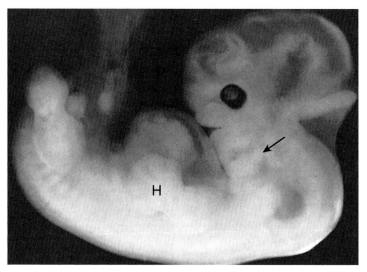

FIGURE 2-12. Thirty-six days. The retina is now pigmented, still incompletely closed at its inferomedial margin. Closure of the retinal fissure is nearly complete. The auricular hillocks are forming the early auricle *(arrow)* from the adjacent borders of the mandibular and hyoid swellings. The hand plate *(H)* has formed with condensation of mesenchyme into the five finger rays. The lower limb lags behind the upper limb in its development. The ventricular septum is partitioning the heart. The ureteral bud from the mesonephric duct has induced a kidney from the mesonephric ridge, which is also forming gonads and adrenal glands. Cloacal septation is nearly complete; the infraumbilical mesenchyme has filled in all the cloacal membrane except the urogenital area; and the genital tubercles are fused, whereas the labioscrotal swellings are unfused. The gut is elongating, and a loop of it may be seen projecting out into the body stalk.

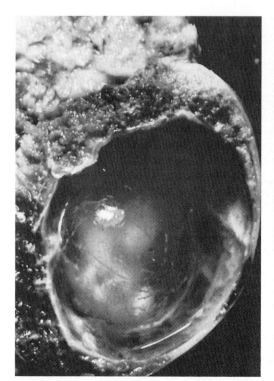
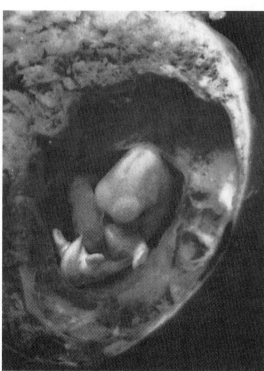

FIGURE 2-13. Forty-two days. In situ embryo *(left)* with the amnion removed *(right)* to show the phenomenal extent of early brain development with formation of the cerebral hemispheres, large heart, still "paddle-like" limbs, and the regressing tail. (Courtesy Dr. Jan E. Jirásek, Prague, Czech Republic.)

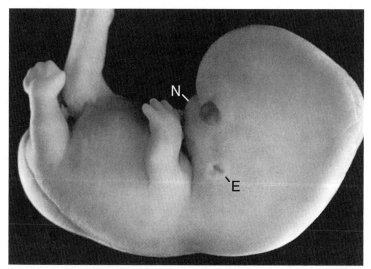

FIGURE 2-14. Forty-five days. The nose *(N)* is relatively flat, and the external ear *(E)* is gradually shifting in relative position as it continues to grow and develop. A neck area is now evident, the anterior body wall has formed, and the thorax and abdomen are separated by the septum transversum (diaphragm). The fingers are now partially separated, and the elbow is evident. The major period of cardiac morphogenesis and septation is complete. The urogenital membrane has now broken down, yielding a urethral opening. The phallus and lateral labioscrotal folds are the same for both sexes at this age.

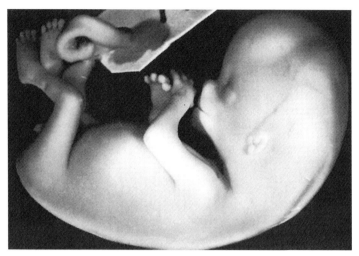

FIGURE 2-15.   A 10-week-old boy. The eyelids have developed and fused, not to reopen until 4 to 5 months. Muscles are developed and functional, normal morphogenesis of joints is dependent on movement, and primary ossification is occurring in the centers of developing bones. In the male, the testicle has produced androgen and masculinized the external genitalia, with enlargement of the genital tubercle, fusion of the labioscrotal folds into a scrotum, and closure of the labia minora folds to form a penile urethra, these structures being unchanged in the female. The testicle does not descend into the scrotum until 8 or 9 months.

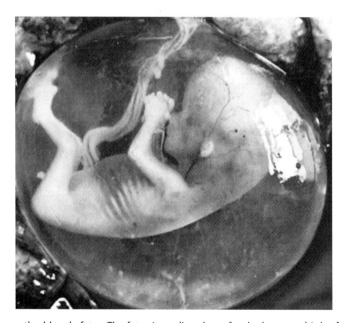

FIGURE 2-16.   A 3½-month-old male fetus. The fetus is settling down for the last two thirds of prenatal life. The morphogenesis of the lung, largely solid at this point in development, will not have progressed to the capacity for aerobic exchange for another 3 to 4 months. The skin is increasing in thickness, and its accessory structures are differentiating. The form of the palmar surface of the hand and foot, especially the character of the prominent apical and other pads, will influence the patterning of parallel dermal ridges that form transversely to the relative lines of growth stress on the palms and soles between 16 and 19 weeks. Subcutaneous tissue is thin, and adipose tissue does not develop until 7 to 8 months.

RELATIVE TIMING OF MALFORMATIONS

Malformations resulting from incomplete morphogenesis usually have their origin before the time when normal development would have proceeded beyond the form represented by the malformation. This type of developmental timing should not be construed as indicating that something happened at a particular time; all one can say is that a problem existed before a particular time. Serious errors in early morphogenesis seldom allow for survival; hence, only a few malformation problems are seen that can be said to have occurred before 23 days. The cyclopia-cebocephaly type of defect appears to be the consequence of a defect in the prechordal

mesoderm, and presumably developed before 23 days. Aside from this example, the vast majority of serious malformations represent errors that occur after 3 weeks of development.

Table 2-1 sets forth the relative timing as well as the presumed developmental error for some of the

Table 2-1   RELATIVE TIMING AND DEVELOPMENTAL PATHOLOGY OF CERTAIN MALFORMATIONS

Tissues	Malformation	Defect in	Causes Prior to	Comment
Central nervous system	Anencephaly	Closure of anterior neural tube	26 days	Subsequent degeneration of forebrain
	Meningomyelocele	Closure in a portion of the posterior neural tube	28 days	80% lumbosacral
Face	Cleft lip	Closure of lip	36 days	42% associated with cleft palate
	Cleft maxillary palate	Fusion of maxillary palatal shelves	10 weeks	
	Branchial sinus or cyst	Resolution of branchial cleft	8 weeks	Preauricular and along the line anterior to sternocleidomastoid
Gut	Esophageal atresia plus tracheoesophageal fistula	Lateral septation of foregut into trachea and foregut	30 days	
	Rectal atresia with fistula	Lateral septation of cloaca into rectum and urogenital sinus	6 weeks	
	Duodenal atresia	Recanalization of duodenum	7–8 weeks	Associated incomplete or aberrant mesenteric attachments
	Malrotation of gut	Rotation of intestinal loop so that cecum lies to the right	10 weeks	
	Omphalocele	Return of midgut from yolk sac to abdomen	10 weeks	
	Meckel diverticulum	Obliteration of vitelline duct	10 weeks	May contain gastric or pancreatic tissue
	Diaphragmatic hernia	Closure of pleuroperitoneal canal	6 weeks	
Genitourinary system	Exstrophy of bladder	Migration of infraumbilical mesenchyme	30 days	Associated müllerian and wolffian duct defects
	Bicornuate uterus	Fusion of lower portion of müllerian ducts	10 weeks	
	Hypospadias	Fusion of urethral folds (labia minora)	12 weeks	
	Cryptorchidism	Descent of testicle into scrotum	7–9 months	
Heart	Transposition of great vessels	Directional development of bulbus cordis septum	34 days	
	Ventricular septal defect	Closure of ventricular septum	6 weeks	
	Patent ductus arteriosus	Closure of ductus arteriosus	9–10 months	
Limb	Aplasia of radius	Genesis of radial bone	38 days	Often accompanied by other defects of radial side of distal limb
	Syndactyly, severe	Separation of digital rays	6 weeks	
Complex	Cyclopia, holoprosencephaly	Prechordal mesoderm development	23 days	Secondary defects of midface and forebrain

malformations that appear to represent incomplete stages in morphogenesis.

References

Ebert JD, Sussex I: Interacting Systems in Development, New York, 1970, Holt, Rinehart & Winston.

Gilbert SF: Developmental Biology, ed 7, Sunderland, Mass, 2003, Sinauer Associates.

Graham JM: Smith's Recognizable Patterns of Human Deformation, ed 2, Philadelphia, 1988, WB Saunders.

Hamilton WJ, Boyd JD, Mossman HW: Human Embryology, Baltimore, 1962, Williams & Wilkins.

Millen JW: Timing of human congenital malformations, Dev Med Child Neurol 5:343, 1963.

Moore KL, Persaud TVN: The Developing Human: Clinically Oriented Embryology, ed 7, Philadelphia, 2004, WB Saunders.

Moore KL, Persaud TVN, Shiota K: Color Atlas of Human Embryology, Philadelphia, 1994, WB Saunders.

Nilsson L, Ingelman-Sundberg A, Wirsen C: A Child Is Born, New York, 1986, Dell Books.

O'Rahilly R, Muller F: Human Embryology and Teratology, New York, 1992, Wiley-Liss.

Sadler TW: Langman's Medical Embryology, ed 11, Baltimore, 2010, Lippincott Williams & Wilkins.

Streeter GL: Developmental Horizons in Human Embryo: Age Groups XI to XXIII, Washington, DC, 1951, Carnegie Institute of Washington.

Willis RA: The Borderland of Embryology and Pathology, Washington, DC, 1962, Butterworth.

CHAPTER 3

Genetics, Genetic Counseling, and Prevention

The basic process of morphogenesis is genetically controlled. However, the ability of an individual to reach his or her genetic potential with respect to structure, growth, or cognitive development is affected by environmental factors in both prenatal and postnatal life. Review of the etiologies of those structural abnormalities and syndromes for which an etiology is known indicates that the majority of malformations and syndromes appear to be genetically determined. The purpose of this chapter is to outline the most prevalent mechanisms through which genetic abnormalities impact morphogenesis, to discuss the techniques that are currently available for genetic testing, to suggest genetic counseling for each of these abnormalities, and to discuss approaches to prevention.

The haploid human genome contains just over 20,000 protein-coding genes, which are far fewer than had been expected before sequencing. Only about 1.5% of the genome codes for proteins. The rest consists of noncoding RNA genes, regulatory sequences, introns, and noncoding DNA.

Genes come in pairs. The great majority of these genes are distributed in the 46 chromosomes that are found in the nucleus of the cell. A few genes reside in the cytoplasm inside the mitochondria, the energy-producing apparatus of the cell. Genetic abnormalities may be grossly divided into those that affect gene dosage (chromosomal and genomic abnormalities), those that involve changes (mutations) in the actual genes themselves (single-gene disorders), and those that create a susceptibility to developmental errors that is then modified by other genes and factors in the environment (polygenic and multifactorial inheritance). The frequency with which each of these genetic mechanisms contributes to malformation and disease depends on the time in development at which inquiry is made. For example, roughly half of all first-trimester miscarriages are a consequence of chromosomal abnormalities, whereas only 6 of 1000 live-born infants are similarly affected. Figure 3-1 provides a perspective as to the frequency with which each mechanism

contributes to birth defects or human disease over the lifetime of a population. Each of these problems is considered separately as it relates to malformation, especially multiple defect syndromes. Recommended genetic counseling is presented at the end of each section.

GENETIC IMBALANCE CAUSED BY GROSS CHROMOSOMAL ABNORMALITIES AND SUBMICROSCOPIC GENOMIC IMBALANCE

The 46 normal chromosomes consist of 22 homologous pairs of autosomes plus an XX pair of sex chromosomes in the female or an XY pair in the male. Normal development is dependent not only on the gene content of these chromosomes but on the gene balance as well. An altered number of chromosomes most commonly arises because of fault in chromosome distribution at cell division. During the gametic meiotic reduction division (Fig. 3-2), one of each pair of autosomes and one of the sex chromosomes are distributed randomly to each daughter cell, whereas during mitosis (Fig. 3-3), each replicated chromosome is separated longitudinally at the centromere so that each daughter cell receives an identical complement of genetic material. Abnormal segregation in meiosis or mitosis will lead to an incorrect number of chromosomes (aneuploidy) in daughter cells. In addition, a piece of a chromosome can be deleted, duplicated, inverted, or exchanged between two chromosomes.

Identifying Visible Chromosome Abnormalities: The Karyotype

Figure 3-4 shows the natural appearance of the stained chromosomes at early, middle, and later stages of mitosis. It would obviously be difficult to count these chromosomes or to distinguish their individual structure from such preparations. To

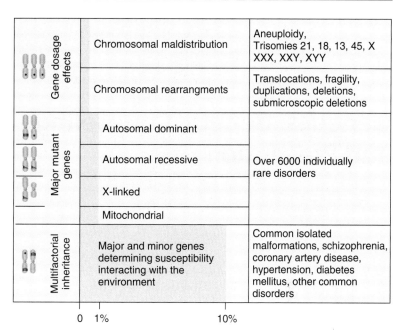

FIGURE 3-1. The scale at the base represents the percentage of individuals born who have, or will have, a problem in life secondary to a genetic difference. The three categories of genetic aberration are depicted to the left. The *dots* within the chromosomes represent "normal" genes, the *bar* represents a dominant mutant gene, the *hash-bar* represents a recessive mutant gene, and the *triangles* denote major and minor genes that confer susceptibility to a given process.

Gene dosage effects	Chromosomal maldistribution	Aneuploidy, Trisomies 21, 18, 13, 45, X XXX, XXY, XYY	
	Chromosomal rearrangments	Translocations, fragility, duplications, deletions, submicroscopic deletions	
Major mutant genes	Autosomal dominant	Over 6000 individually rare disorders	
	Autosomal recessive		
	X-linked		
	Mitochondrial		
Multifactorial inheritance	Major and minor genes determining susceptibility interacting with the environment	Common isolated malformations, schizophrenia, coronary artery disease, hypertension, diabetes mellitus, other common disorders	

0 1%   10%

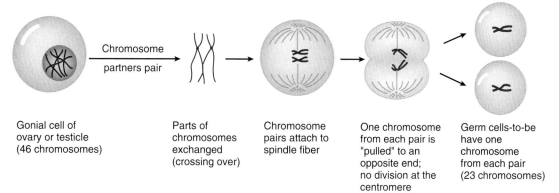

Chromosome partners pair

| Gonial cell of ovary or testicle (46 chromosomes) | Parts of chromosomes exchanged (crossing over) | Chromosome pairs attach to spindle fiber | One chromosome from each pair is "pulled" to an opposite end; no division at the centromere | Germ cells-to-be have one chromosome from each pair (23 chromosomes) |

FIGURE 3-2. Meiotic reduction division in development of gametes (sex cells). One pair of chromosomes is followed through the cycle.

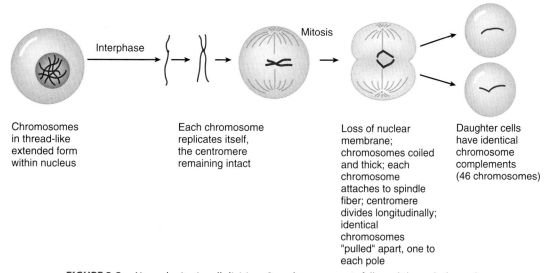

Interphase   Mitosis

| Chromosomes in thread-like extended form within nucleus | Each chromosome replicates itself, the centromere remaining intact | Loss of nuclear membrane; chromosomes coiled and thick; each chromosome attaches to spindle fiber; centromere divides longitudinally; identical chromosomes "pulled" apart, one to each pole | Daughter cells have identical chromosome complements (46 chromosomes) |

FIGURE 3-3. Normal mitotic cell division. One chromosome is followed through the cycle.

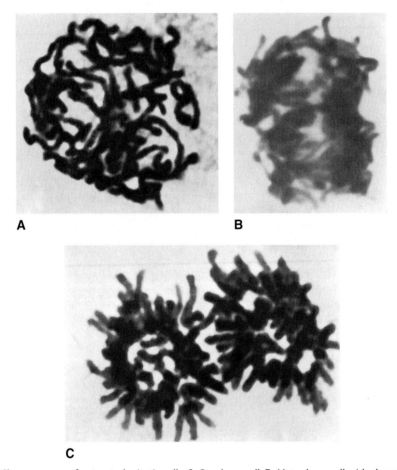

FIGURE 3-4. Chromosomes of untreated mitotic cells. **A,** Prophase cell. **B,** Metaphase cell with chromosomes attached to the spindle fibers and beginning to separate. **C,** Anaphase cell with identical chromosomal complements having been "pulled apart" toward the development of two daughter cells.

obtain adequate preparations for the study of chromosome number and morphology, the cultured cells are treated with an agent that blocks the spindle formation and thus leads to the accumulation of cells at the metaphase of mitosis. These cells are then exposed to a hypotonic solution that spreads the unattached chromosomes, allowing for preparations such as those shown in Figure 3-5. Various techniques, such as trypsin treatment and Giemsa staining, can be used to allow for the identification of individual chromosomes. The development of synchronized culture techniques that allow evaluation of chromosomes in prophase and prometaphase have greatly enhanced the ability to detect subtle abnormalities and have expanded our understanding of the impact of chromosomal rearrangement on morphogenesis. A chromosome analysis using this technique is a high-resolution analysis (Fig. 3-6). Banding techniques applied on metaphase or prometaphase preparations allow the recognition of each of the individual chromosomes, aneuploidies, and loss or gain of chromosome

fragments larger than 5 Mb in standard resolution and 3 Mb in high-resolution karyotypes. All chromosome studies require cell culture in advance.

Identifying Smaller Genomic Imbalance: FISH, CGH, Arrays, and MLPA

Two technologies that allow detection of more subtle changes in copy number in the genome are fluorescence in situ hybridization (FISH) and comparative genomic hybridization (CGH). In FISH, fluorescent-labeled probes of known DNA sequence are hybridized to chromosomes that are fixed on a slide and denatured in place (in situ), allowing the probe to attach to its complementary sequence. When viewed with a wavelength of light that excites the fluorescent dye, a colored signal is generated, allowing localization of the probe. FISH probes may consist of contiguous genomic sequences, parts of chromosomes, or whole chromosomes. Depending on the probe and the clinical question, FISH may be performed on interphase instead of metaphase cells;

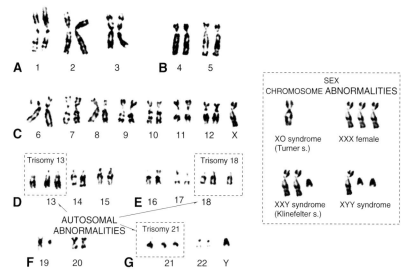

FIGURE 3-5. Giemsa-stained chromosomes arranged into a karyotype by letter grouping and number designation on the basis of length of the chromosome, position of the centromere, and banding patterns. The most common types of aneuploidy are shown within the boxes.

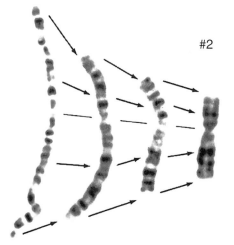

#2

FIGURE 3-6. Giemsa-stained chromosome number 2 harvested at different points in the cell cycle. The prometaphase appearance is on the *left,* while the metaphase is on the *right.* Note the dramatic increase in detail visible in the prometaphase chromosome. (Courtesy Dr. James T. Mascarello, Children's Hospital, San Diego.)

this would offer advantages in some clinical situations such as prenatal diagnosis. Interphase FISH obviates the need for cell culture and may be performed rapidly; however, it will not locate a targeted DNA sequence in a specific chromosomal region. CGH is based on FISH technology. DNA from one sample is labeled with a red fluorescent dye while DNA from another is labeled with green. The two are mixed in equal amounts and "painted" on normal human chromosome preparations. The ratio of red-to-green fluorescence along each chromosome is measured. Deviations from the expected 1:1 ratio of red to green will be detected as a change in the color signal in that region documenting gain or loss of copy number. Chromosomal CGH has been used to identify the chromosomal origin of small chromosome fragments of unknown origin (markers). It has also been used to identify visible extra bands in a karyotype that cannot be identified based on the banding pattern itself. Even greater resolution can be achieved using known DNA sequences instead of whole chromosomes as hybridization targets. DNA sequences can be printed on a chip such that small fragments of DNA may be interrogated. If the printed sequences overlap, in a so-called tiling-path array, coverage of the entire genome may be achieved. A variety of different probes are in clinical usage, including large ones derived from bacterial artificial chromosomes (BAC array), small ones consisting of oligonucleotide sequences (oligo-array), and very small single nucleotide polymorphisms (SNPs) containing sequences (SNP array). Array technology does not require cell culture. Small amounts of DNA can suffice, as DNA can undergo preamplification (Fig. 3-7).

Multiple ligation probe amplification (MLPA), a variation of the multiplex polymerase chain reaction (PCR), permits up to 40 targets to be amplified with only a single primer pair. MLPA is often used to interrogate dosage of multiple fragments in a specific genomic region known to have variable size deletions, or in all the subtelomeres in one reaction. Because it costs much less than chromosomal

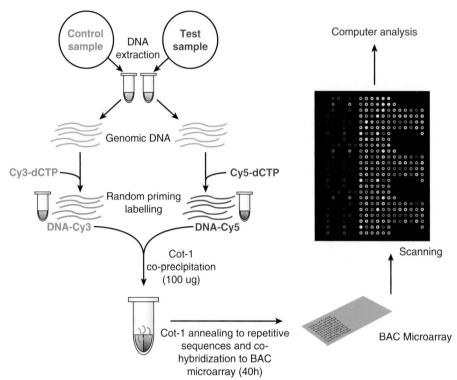

FIGURE 3-7. Array CGH implies labeling of control and test samples with distinct fluorescence, and hybridization to a BAC microarray where genomic fragments derived from BAC clones have been previously printed. The analysis of fluorescence will establish the differential dose of each point, which, after computer analysis, will be able to identify deletions and duplications in the test sample. (Courtesy Prof. Pérez Jurado, Universitat Pompeu Fabra, Barcelona.)

microarrays, MPLA is used to confirm array results and to verify the presence or absence of an abnormality in a parent.

The Impact of Chromosomal and Genomic Imbalance during Development

Figure 3-8 illustrates some of the mechanisms that can lead to genetic imbalance (too many or too few copies of normal genes) as a consequence of chromosomal rearrangement and maldistribution. Such cytogenetically visible abnormalities occur in at least 4% of recognized pregnancies. Most of these imbalances have such an adverse effect on morphogenesis that the conceptus does not survive. Smaller imbalances more likely result in surviving individuals with variable dysmorphology and developmental disability. Figure 3-9 summarizes the frequency and types of visible chromosomal abnormalities found in newborns and spontaneous abortuses. Approximately 50% of these have a chromosome abnormality compared to 0.5% of live-born babies. The nature of the abnormalities detected in live-born infants differs from those seen in abortuses, with sex chromosomal aneuploidy and trisomy 21 (Down syndrome) accounting for most of the anomalies observed in live-born infants because

these are least likely to have an early lethal effect. It has been estimated that only approximately 1 in 500 45,X conceptuses survives to term compared to 4% of trisomies 18 and 13, and 20% of trisomy 21 conceptuses. There are some data to suggest that survival is impacted by the presence of a normal, as well as an aneuploid, cell line (mosaicism). The Human Genome Project has identified that the genome is in clumps with some chromosomes (such as 19 with 1621 known genes) being gene-rich and others (such as the Y with 251 genes) gene-poor. Autosomes 21, 18, and 13 are relatively gene-poor, perhaps contributing to their in utero survival. In general, smaller genomic imbalances will more often be viable, presenting with major and/or minor malformations, intellectual disability, and/or abnormal behavior. Microdeletions and microduplications as a group are found more often than aneuploidy in children presenting postnatally with delayed psychomotor development.

Abnormal Number of Chromosomes (Aneuploidy)

Although much is being learned about the etiology of faulty chromosomal distribution, one clear recognized factor is older maternal age. This applies

Chromosomal Maldistribution

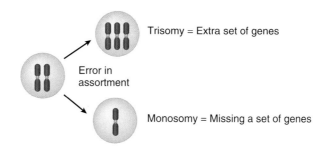

Trisomy = Extra set of genes

Error in assortment

Monosomy = Missing a set of genes

Chromosomal Breakage

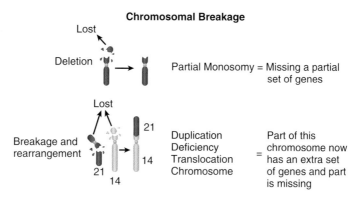

Lost

Deletion → Partial Monosomy = Missing a partial set of genes

Lost

Breakage and rearrangement

Duplication
Deficiency
Translocation
Chromosome

= Part of this chromosome now has an extra set of genes and part is missing

Maldivision at Centromere

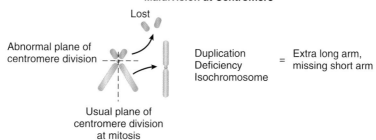

Lost

Abnormal plane of centromere division

Duplication
Deficiency
Isochromosome

= Extra long arm, missing short arm

Usual plane of centromere division at mitosis

FIGURE 3-8. Types of chromosomal abnormalities leading to genetic imbalance.

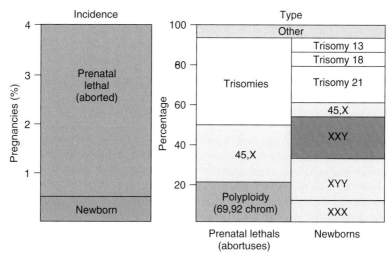

FIGURE 3-9. Incidence and types of chromosomal abnormalities.

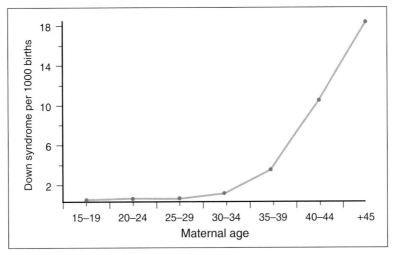

FIGURE 3-10.   Increasing incidence of the Down syndrome during the later portion of a woman's reproductive period. (From Smith DW: *Am J Obstet Gynecol* 90:1055, 1964, with permission.)

especially to the autosomal trisomy syndromes and to the sex chromosome aneuploidy, XXX and XXY. Figure 3-10 shows the progressive increase in the frequency of live-born infants with Down syndrome during the later period of a woman's reproductive life. The frequency of aneuploidy detected by amniocentesis at 14 to 16 weeks' gestation is appreciably higher because some of the aneuploid conceptuses detected at this early stage in gestation would normally abort spontaneously or die in utero later in pregnancy.

The timing of the error in chromosome distribution can seldom be stated with assurance from a routine karyotype, although molecular techniques, as is discussed subsequently, have permitted detailed investigation of this issue in certain aneuploidy states. Numerical errors may result from altered chromosomal segregation in the cells that will give rise to the germ cells (gonadal mosaicism), or in either the first or second division of meiosis leading to an abnormal chromosome number in the egg or sperm (nondisjunction), or during the first divisions of the newly formed zygote. Errors in the assortment of chromosomes may also occur later in embryogenesis, giving rise to somatic mosaic individuals who have two populations of cells from the standpoint of chromosome number. Mosaicism also develops when a trisomic conceptus "self-corrects" and loses one copy of the trisomic chromosome in early cell division, thus establishing a normal cell line along with the aneuploid cell line. This process has been termed "trisomic rescue." Individuals who are mosaic for a condition show every gradation of the phenotype associated with that chromosomal abnormality, from a pattern indistinguishable from complete aneuploidy to

near-normal appearance and function. In general, the degree of mosaicism present in the peripheral blood is not, in and of itself, that helpful in predicting prognosis. Detection of mosaicism may require the sampling of more than one tissue. Identification of the parent of origin of individual chromosomes has shed some light on the source of the extra or deleted chromosome and the stage of cell division during which accidents leading to aneuploidy occur. In conceptuses and live-born individuals with 45,X, the chromosome that is deleted is usually paternal in origin. This is consistent with the observation that maternal age is not related to a 45,X karyotype in the fetus. By contrast, the extra chromosome in trisomy 21 is of maternal origin in 95% of cases. Most of the maternal errors involve nondisjunction in meiosis I. Of the paternally derived chromosomes, most represent errors in meiosis II. Similarly, the extra X chromosome in 47,XXX females is usually maternally derived. In 47,XXY the source of the extra chromosome appears to be equally divided. In those cases of 47,XXY and 47,XXX with a maternally derived extra chromosome, increasing maternal age correlates with errors in the first meiotic cell division but not with errors in meiosis II or in postzygotic events. The precise etiology of nondisjunction is unknown; however, evidence is accumulating that mammalian trisomies may be a consequence of abnormal levels or positioning of meiotic crossovers (recombination events). Between 1% and 5% of sperm from chromosomally normal men are aneuploid. Indirect estimates from spontaneous abortions and studies of embryos from in vitro fertilization clinics have suggested an aneuploidy rate of nearly 25% in oocytes.

Structural Chromosomal and Genomic Rearrangements

In addition to resulting from errors in chromosome number, genetic imbalance can result from chromosomal rearrangement (see Fig. 3-8). A break in one chromosome may result in loss or gain of information (deletion or duplication). If more than one chromosome breaks, rearrangement of the resulting pieces may take place, creating a translocation. Reciprocal translocations always involve two chromosomal fragments, including two different telomeres, and can be recognized with techniques that will identify the unique subtelomeric sequences of each chromosome, such as subtelomeric FISH or MLPA. Robertsonian translocations occur among acrocentric chromosomes, in which the small arms that contain redundant genetic sequences are lost in the rearrangement, leading to a derivative chromosome containing the long arms of two different chromosomes in a karyotype with 45 chromosomes. The genome is still functionally balanced. An individual can have a translocation between chromosomes with no evident problem as long as he or she has a balanced set of genes. Only in cases in which the breakpoints cause a cryptic deletion or involve an important exonic or regulatory sequence will the "balanced" rearrangement be associated with an altered phenotype. However, as illustrated in Figure 3-11, a balanced carrier of

a translocation has a significant risk of producing unbalanced germ cells during the meiotic reduction division, meiosis I. Should a germ cell receive the translocation chromosome as well as the normal 21 chromosome from the same parent, the resulting zygote would be trisomic for most of chromosome 21. Such individuals generally have Down syndrome. About 4% of patients with Down syndrome have 46 chromosomes, with the extra set being attached to another chromosome. Similarly, a small proportion of patients with the trisomy 18 syndrome or the trisomy 13 syndrome have the extra set of genes attached as part of a translocation chromosome.

Some patterns of malformation result from a deletion (or duplication) of chromosomal material in which the missing (or extra) piece is so small that routine chromosome analysis cannot detect the abnormality. Such conditions are referred to as microdeletion (microduplication) syndromes to denote the fact that the phenotype is a consequence of imbalance in dosage of several genes that lie next to each other along a chromosome. If several genes in the deleted (or duplicated) segment are responsible for the phenotype, the condition may be designated a contiguous gene disorder. However, the phenotypes of some microdeletions (microduplications) are actually the consequence of imbalance in a single gene in the rearranged interval. These deletions/duplications may be considered

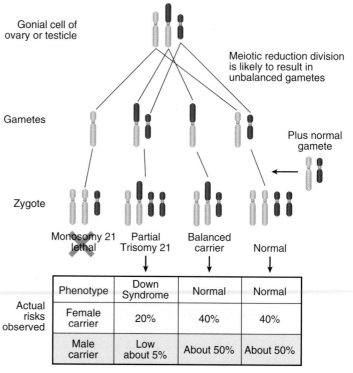

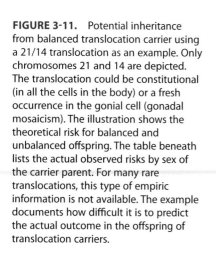

FIGURE 3-11. Potential inheritance from balanced translocation carrier using a 21/14 translocation as an example. Only chromosomes 21 and 14 are depicted. The translocation could be constitutional (in all the cells in the body) or a fresh occurrence in the gonial cell (gonadal mosaicism). The illustration shows the theoretical risk for balanced and unbalanced offspring. The table beneath lists the actual observed risks by sex of the carrier parent. For many rare translocations, this type of empiric information is not available. The example documents how difficult it is to predict the actual outcome in the offspring of translocation carriers.

Gonial cell of ovary or testicle

Meiotic reduction division is likely to result in unbalanced gametes

Gametes

Plus normal gamete

Zygote

Monosomy 21 lethal | Partial Trisomy 21 | Balanced carrier | Normal

Phenotype	Down Syndrome	Normal	Normal
Actual risks observed — Female carrier	20%	40%	40%
Male carrier	Low about 5%	About 50%	About 50%

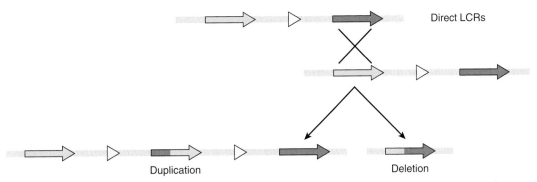

FIGURE 3-12. Malalignment of sequences with high homology called low copy repeats (LCRs) or segmental duplications (*light and darker blue*) can cause nonallelic homologous recombination (NAHR) leading to a duplication or a deletion of the single copy region (*yellow*) of the resulting chromosomes after recombination. (Courtesy Prof. Pérez Jurado, Universitat Pompeu Fabra, Barcelona.)

monogenic disorders. FISH, MLPA, and array technologies are techniques used to identify these submicroscopic rearrangements. Breaks in chromosomes can arise through various mechanisms. However, there are recurrent rearrangements that occur because the regional structure of the genome contains low copy repeats (LCRs), also called segmental duplications, that predispose to nonallelic homologous recombination (NAHR), leading to deletion or duplication of the single copy sequences flanked by these LCRs (Fig. 3-12). NAHR produces some of the most common microdeletion and microduplication syndromes. Many are associated with recognizable patterns not only because they are frequent but also because the deleted (or duplicated) segments are identical.

Another type of chromosomal abnormality that can lead to genetic imbalance is maldivision at the centromere during mitosis, leading to the formation of an isochromosome (see Fig. 3-8). The cell receiving the isochromosome has an extra dose of either the long or short arm of the parent chromosome and is missing the set of genes on the opposite arm. Isochromosome Xq accounts for roughly 10% of the cases of Turner syndrome in live-born female infants.

Incidence of Chromosomal Abnormalities and Genomic Rearrangements in Patients with Intellectual Disability

Surveys of the incidence of visible chromosomal abnormalities in newborns have documented that roughly 1 in 520 normal individuals has a balanced structural chromosomal rearrangement, whereas 1 in 1700 newborns has an unbalanced rearrangement. The incidence of microdeletions/duplications in the general population is unknown. Systematic surveys of undiagnosed children with intellectual disability and multiple structural defects have

documented an 8% incidence of visible chromosome abnormalities. High-resolution chromosome analysis identifies an additional 1.1% of patients evaluated for similar indications. A 7.4% detection rate for submicroscopic chromosome rearrangements among individuals with moderate to severe intellectual disability of unknown etiology and a 0.5% rate for mild intellectual disability have been documented based on the use of FISH or MLPA probes, which recognize the unique subtelomeric sequences of each chromosome. More recently array technologies have increased the detection rate of pathogenic genomic rearrangements to 14% to 20%, depending on whether these numbers are assessed in patients with previous genetic testing or no previous genetic testing.

Interpretation of the Causality of Genomic Imbalance

Whereas the loss or gain of visible chromosome fragments containing hundreds of genes is almost always the cause of an abnormal phenotype, smaller imbalances are most often part of human normal variation. The frequency of copy number variants (CNVs) in the genome is very high and, in most cases, reflects normal dosage variation not associated with phenotype. Knowledge of the consequences of dosage imbalance throughout the genome is currently incomplete. This often makes the interpretation of array findings very difficult. In addition to the medical literature, web-based tools such as DECIPHER may be of assistance in determining if CNV is benign or pathologic.

Indications and Sequence of Chromosomal and Genomic Studies

The utility of array technology as a "first round" test has been firmly established, with recognition of a

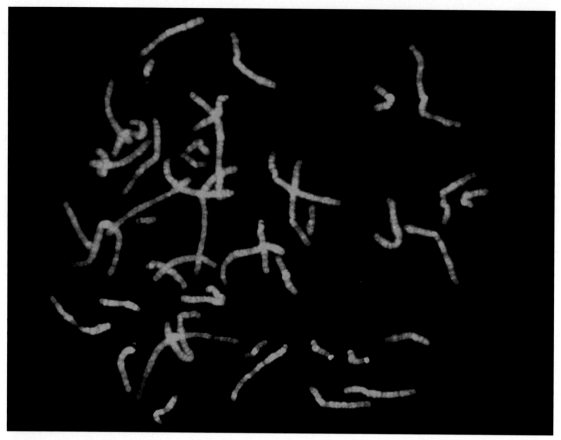

FIGURE 3-13. FISH analysis for the DiGeorge critical region in a patient with deletion 22q11.2 syndrome. Two fluorescent probes are used. One hybridizes with the telomere of chromosome 22, allowing ready identification of both chromosomes. The second probe identifies the DiGeorge critical region. In this patient, only one signal is visible, consistent with a submicroscopic deletion in the other chromosome. (Courtesy Dr. James T. Mascarello.)

much higher detection rate of pathogenic genomic imbalance than that revealed by even high-resolution chromosome analysis. Because of its lower cost, standard karyotype remains the preferred test in specific situations such as clinical suspicion of specific aneuploidies or syndromes associated with large genomic rearrangements. In addition, a karyotype is needed for the identification of balanced rearrangements (translocations and inversions), which are not detected by any technology addressing dosage. FISH with unique sequence probes is still the least costly way to confirm the diagnosis in well-known phenotypes such as Williams syndrome (del 7q11.2) shown in Figure 3-13 or the velocardiofacial syndrome (del 22q11.2). Multitelomere FISH remains the optimal way to diagnose small reciprocal translocations. With respect to mosaicism, arrays are not able to detect levels below roughly 20%. Karyotyping or FISH may be required, including examining several different tissues and scoring large numbers of cells.

GENETIC COUNSELING FOR CHROMOSOMAL AND GENOMIC ABNORMALITIES

Autosomal Trisomy Syndromes

Chromosomal studies are warranted on all individuals suspected of having an autosomal trisomy syndrome to determine whether full trisomy (47 chromosomes) or an unbalanced robertsonian translocation is involved. If a full trisomy is identified, the risk for recurrence is roughly 1%. For women 35 years of age and older, the risk is based on the maternal age at delivery in the subsequent pregnancy. For trisomy 21, parental karyotypes are suggested only if a second child in the same sibship has an identical trisomy. In this rare circumstance, mosaicism in one of the parents may be detected in as much as 38% of families if a diligent search is made. The presence of a second- or third-degree relative with a similar trisomy can be accounted for by chance alone and does not appear to increase the risk for recurrence.

Should an unbalanced robertsonian translocation be identified, both parents must be evaluated to determine if either one is a balanced translocation carrier, a finding in approximately one third of cases. The recurrence risk for parents with normal chromosomes is very small (probably less than 1%) and reflects the unlikely possibility of gonadal mosaicism that cannot be identified by peripheral blood karyotype. The recurrence risk for a carrier parent is obviously increased, but it is often different, depending on the gender of the carrier parent, and less of a risk than the theoretical possibilities might indicate because of the frequent prenatal lethality of autosomal trisomies (see Fig. 3-11).

Other Chromosomal Disorders

45,X Syndrome

Chromosome analysis is still the optimal way to diagnose Turner syndrome. Although a wide variety of chromosomal rearrangements are known to produce the phenotype (including X/XX and X/XY mosaicism, X, iso X, or X, deleted X), the recurrence risk for these arrangements is low to negligible. The finding of a Y-bearing cell line suggests an increased risk for malignant tumor in the dysgenetic gonad, which should be removed.

Any Case with a Visible Deletion, Duplication, or Unbalanced Translocation

In this situation, chromosome studies should be done on both parents to rule out a rearrangement such as a pericentric inversion, a balanced translocation, or, in rare cases, an insertion, that could predispose to recurrence of the abnormality. If parental karyotypes are normal, as is the case in the majority of families, the recurrence risk is low. If a parental rearrangement is identified, the theoretical risk for recurrence is increased. Other family members may be at risk. For some of the more common rearrangements, empiric risk figures are available in the literature. The actual risks often do not coincide with the theoretical risk as has been previously reviewed (see Fig. 3-11). In the case of balanced translocation carriers, the previous reproductive experience of the couple must be considered in counseling.

Microdeletion and Microduplication Syndromes

Although microdeletion syndromes are chromosomal abnormalities, because the problem that produces the phenotype is genetic imbalance rather than genetic mutation and because the abnormality is identified using molecular cytogenetic methodology, from a counseling standpoint the conditions behave like dominantly inherited Mendelian disorders. The majority of cases represent de novo events that carry a negligible risk for recurrence for unaffected parents and a 50% risk for the affected individual's offspring. Evaluation of parents using FISH analysis, MLPA, or focused high-resolution cytogenetics is recommended, since vertical transmission of microdeletion syndromes is reported. Many, but not all, parents with microdeletions also express the phenotype to some degree. Recurrence risk for the genomic anomaly in these individuals is 50% for each subsequent pregnancy, but the severity of the phenotype that might ensue is often unpredictable, thus posing a challenge for genetic counseling.

Identification of a new microdeletion or microduplication—neither previously found in the normal population with significant frequency nor previously reported in affected patients with concordant phenotypes—is a challenge for interpretation. In case the CNV contains genes, or has a significant size, parents should be tested. If the CNV is inherited from a normal parent and there are no studies that point to pathogenicity, it is usually considered a benign variant. If de novo, the assumption of causality can only be based on gene content, animal studies, and the concordance of the specific gene loss or duplication with a recognized phenotype. Unfortunately, many microdeletions or microduplications will remain as CNVs of uncertain significance, and future experience will confirm their association with phenotype or their benign nature. The literature and public databases should be searched for previously reported cases before providing the family with significant information on prognosis and natural history.

GENETIC IMBALANCE CAUSED BY SINGLE-GENE DISORDERS

Genes located on the X chromosome are referred to as X-linked genes and those on the autosomes as autosomal genes. A human being is a diploid organism with two sets of chromosomes, one set from each parent. Each pair of chromosomes will have comparable gene determinants located at the same position on each chromosome pair. The pair of genes may be referred to as alleles, or partners, which normally work together. Thus, with the exception of the genes of the X and Y chromosomes in the male and those of the mitochondria, each genetic determinant is present in two doses, one from each parent. Biallelic expression of most genes is the common rule. However, for most genes on the X and for close to a hundred genes on the autosomes, only a single copy of the gene is actively expressed (monoallelic expression). A mutant gene indicates a changed gene. A major mutant gene is herein defined as a genetic determinant that has changed in such a way that it can give rise to an abnormal characteristic. If a mutant gene in a single dose produces an abnormal characteristic despite the presence of a normal allele (partner), it is referred to as "dominant" because it causes abnormality even when counterbalanced by a normal gene partner. A mutant gene that causes an abnormal characteristic when present in double dosage (or single dosage without a normal partner, as for an X-linked mutant gene in the male) is referred to as "recessive." These principles, set forth diagrammatically in Figure 3-14, reflect Mendelian laws of inheritance, which equate the presence of an altered gene or pair of genes with a phenotype or trait. As more is learned about the molecular biology of mutant genes, the distinction between dominant and recessive genes has blurred. Dominant mutations impact

development through a variety of mechanisms. Loss of one copy of the gene (haploinsufficiency) may reduce by half the gene product resulting in functional alteration of development. Mutations may also create proteins with either an increased function (gain of function mutations) or a totally new function (dominant negative mutations) that will interfere with normal development as well. Interestingly, mutations causing haploinsufficiency in the gene may cause one phenotype and those resulting in gain of function, a completely different one. The various forms of osteogenesis imperfecta are good examples of types of dominant mutations. Because collagen is a triple helical molecule, mutations that give rise to one abnormal procollagen molecule will impact the final assembly process and produce a severe skeletal phenotype, whereas mutations that reduce but do not alter the gene product typically result in mild fracturing. Recessive mutations also often serve to reduce the quantity of product made

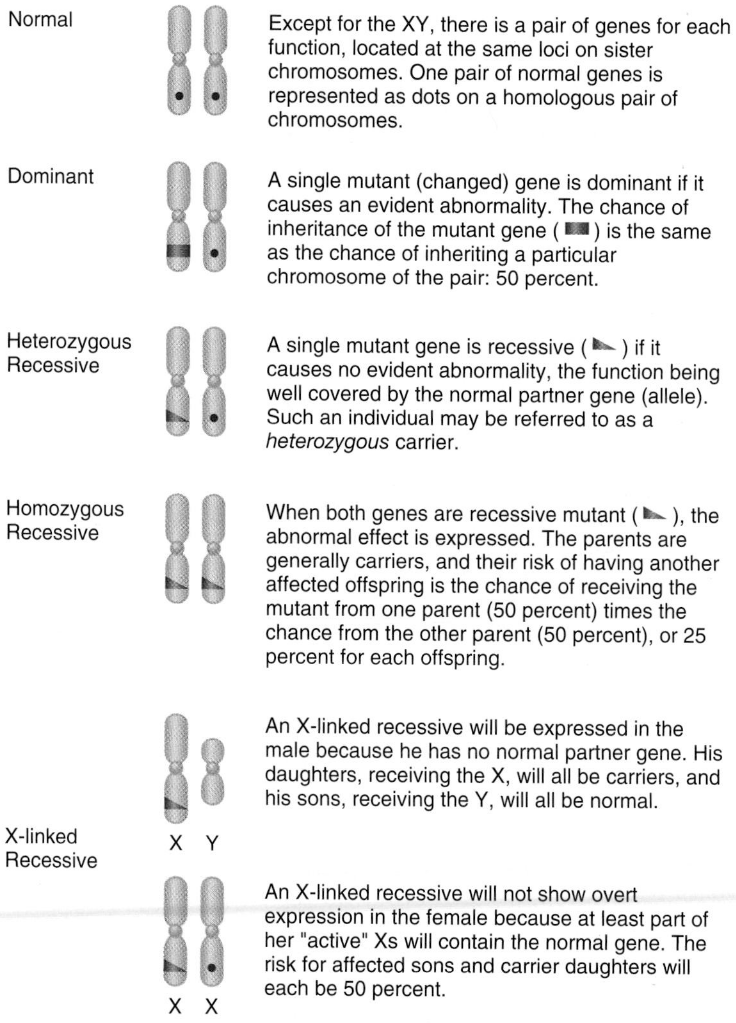

Normal Except for the XY, there is a pair of genes for each function, located at the same loci on sister chromosomes. One pair of normal genes is represented as dots on a homologous pair of chromosomes.

Dominant A single mutant (changed) gene is dominant if it causes an evident abnormality. The chance of inheritance of the mutant gene (▬) is the same as the chance of inheriting a particular chromosome of the pair: 50 percent.

Heterozygous Recessive A single mutant gene is recessive (◣) if it causes no evident abnormality, the function being well covered by the normal partner gene (allele). Such an individual may be referred to as a *heterozygous* carrier.

Homozygous Recessive When both genes are recessive mutant (◣), the abnormal effect is expressed. The parents are generally carriers, and their risk of having another affected offspring is the chance of receiving the mutant from one parent (50 percent) times the chance from the other parent (50 percent), or 25 percent for each offspring.

An X-linked recessive will be expressed in the male because he has no normal partner gene. His daughters, receiving the X, will all be carriers, and his sons, receiving the Y, will all be normal.

X-linked Recessive   X   Y

 An X-linked recessive will not show overt expression in the female because at least part of her "active" Xs will contain the normal gene. The risk for affected sons and carrier daughters will each be 50 percent.

X   X

FIGURE 3-14.   Normal and major mutant gene inheritance (Mendelian inheritance).

by half; however, many biologic systems are forgiving of quantitative decrease in gene function—hence the silence of recessive mutations when present in single copy (heterozygosity). Hurler syndrome is an example. Half of the normal amount of activity of alpha iduronidase has no effect on the individual with the altered gene; however, the enzyme deficiency resulting from a double dose of the altered gene produces a severe phenotype.

"Expression" is a term used to indicate the extent of abnormality that is due to a genetic aberration. The expression may be stated as severe, usual, mild, or no expression, the last being synonymous with lack of penetrance in an individual who has the genetic aberration. Individuals with the same genetic aberration frequently show variance in expression, especially with respect to structural defects.

Traditionally, the mutant gene disorders have been categorized into those caused by genes located on the autosomes (autosomal dominant and autosomal recessive) and those caused by genes on the X chromosome (X-linked dominant and X-linked recessive).

Identifying Sequence Variation: Traditional Sanger Sequencing, Next-Generation Sequencing, Exome Sequencing, Whole Genome Sequencing

DNA sequencing is the process of reading the nucleotide bases in a DNA molecule. It includes any method or technology that is used to determine the order of the four bases, adenine, guanine, cytosine, and thymine, in a strand of DNA. Sanger sequencing has been used clinically for many years to assess sequence of known genes. Although very reliable, the assays are costly and slow. The high demand for low-cost sequencing has driven the development of high-throughput sequencing (next-generation sequencing [NGS]) technologies that parallelize the sequencing process, producing thousands or millions of sequences at once.

The clinical scenario will determine which technique is most appropriate. If a known gene is the only known cause of the condition, direct analysis in search of the mutation through Sanger sequencing will be the approach of choice. Once the mutation is found in the index case, a simple targeted PCR assay will serve to identify other affected or carrier family members. If a condition is genetic heterogeneous (e.g., Noonan syndrome), NGS panels, including all genes known to be causal, would be the optimum strategy. Exome sequencing (including all the protein coding genes) could be considered when the molecular basis of some cases of a certain phenotype is still unknown and in cases of clear unknown etiology. As of this printing, whole

genome sequence remains too costly for routine clinical use. Moreover, knowledge of the impact of variation in nonexonic regions or the exon-intron junctions, is still largely unknown. However, the results of the ENCODE project have established most of our DNA sequence is functional, and this fact speaks for a widespread medical use of whole genome sequencing in the future (Fig. 3-15).

Autosomal Dominant Disorders

Autosomal dominant disorders show a wide variation in expression among affected individuals both between families and among affected family members, presumably because of differences in the normal allele (partner) of the mutant gene as well as other differences in the genetic and environmental background of the affected individual. Figure 3-16 demonstrates the variation in expression for the autosomal dominant disorder ectrodactyly. The risk of the single mutant gene being passed to a given offspring is 50%, yet the risk of a severe defect of hand development is less than 50% because of variation in expression. To use the example of autosomal dominant Waardenburg syndrome type I, the risk of inheritance of the mutant gene, *PAX3*, from an affected individual is 50%, yet only about 20% of affected individuals have deafness. Hence, the risk of deafness in offspring of a parent with Waardenburg syndrome is the risk of receiving the mutant gene (50%) times the likelihood of expression for deafness in the disorder (20%), or 10%.

This dichotomy between the risk of receiving the gene and the risk of a particular expression of the disorder must be utilized in counseling, especially for autosomal dominant conditions. A significant proportion of autosomal dominant patterns of malformation appear to represent fresh gene mutations in the individuals who express the condition. In reproductive counseling for the family, it is important to try to distinguish between (a) lack of expression in the parent caused by variability and (b) fresh gene mutation in the child. Knowledge of both the natural history and the clinical variability of the disorder is extremely helpful in these determinations. Fresh gene mutation is more likely at older paternal age, as has been shown for at least 12 autosomal dominant multiple malformation syndromes. Hence, paternal age should always be noted in the evaluation of disorders that may be the consequence of a single mutant gene.

Autosomal Recessive Disorders

Autosomal recessive disorders generally have less variation in expression among family members than do dominant syndromes. The inheritance is from clinically normal parents who both have the

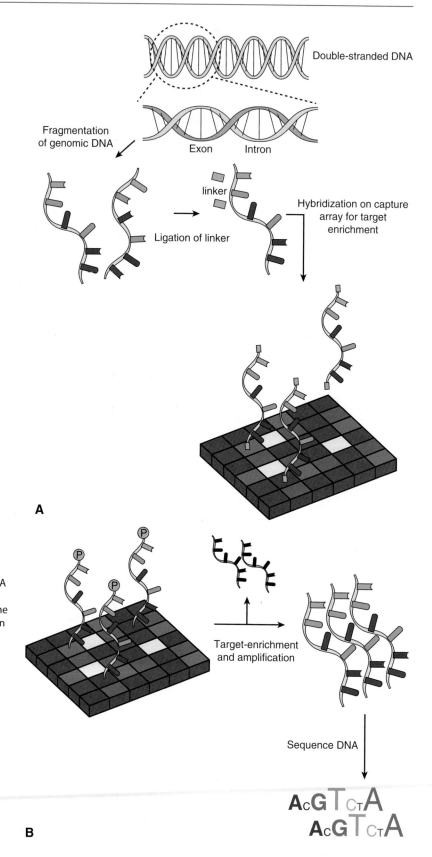

FIGURE 3-15.   A, Exome sequencing workflow: Part 1. Double-stranded genomic DNA is fragmented by sonication. Linkers are then attached to the DNA fragments, which are then hybridized to a capture microarray designed to target only the exons. **B,** Exome sequencing workflow: Part 2. Target exons are enriched, eluted, and then amplified by ligation-mediated PCR. Amplified target DNA is then ready for high-throughput sequencing. (Adapted from http://en.wikipedia.org/wiki/File:Exome_Sequencing_Workflow_1a.png by Sarah Kusala, licensed under the Creative Commons Attribution 3.0 Unported license.)

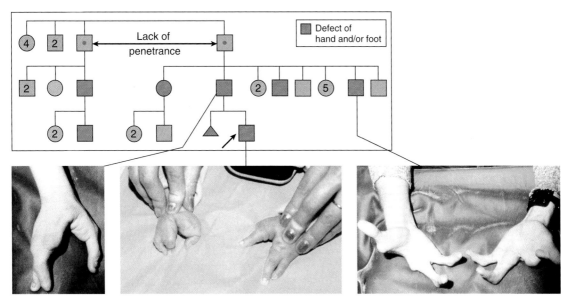

FIGURE 3-16.   Variation in expression for autosomal dominant ectrodactyly among various related individuals. Note also the intraindividual asymmetry of expression in the propositus (*arrow*).

same, or an allelic, recessive mutant gene in single dose. The likelihood of this occurring is enhanced if the parents are related. Hence, the possibility of consanguinity should always be addressed in disorders known to be autosomal recessive as well as when evaluating patterns of malformation of unknown cause.

X-Linked Disorders

Mutations on the X chromosome may be dominant or recessive in nature. Dominant mutations produce obvious clinical effects in XX females and either severe or lethal effects in the XY male who has no normal gene to lessen the impact of the mutation. By contrast, X-linked recessive mutations usually have minimal to no impact on the XX (carrier) female, whereas XY males demonstrate a phenotype. Intermediate situations do occur, in which carrier females are affected to a lesser degree than their male relatives. In X-linked hypohidrotic ectodermal dysplasia, males manifest the full phenotype, while females may have only hypodontia and patchy areas of decreased hair growth. Random X-inactivation in females accounts for this phenomenon. Since half the cells in any tissue will inactivate the normal X and the other half the X with the mutation, a patchy phenotype occurs in females if the disorder has cutaneous manifestation. Severe expression in females can be caused by skewed X-inactivation where the mutated allele lies in the preferentially active X. Severe expression of X-linked recessive disorders may also be seen in females with 45,X syndrome, or Turner syndrome.

Parent-of-Origin Effects

Although it has been assumed that genes inherited from mother and father are equally weighted in terms of expression and effect, observations in a variety of clinical settings have led to the appreciation that this is not invariably the case. Triploid conceptuses, who have an entire extra complement of genes, provide graphic illustration of this point. When triploidy is produced by one maternal and two paternal sets of chromosomes, the pregnancy consists of a large hydatidiform placenta with a small, malformed but proportionate fetus. If two maternal and one paternal set of chromosomes are responsible, the fetus is disproportionately growth-retarded and the placenta is usually extremely small, confirming observations in mouse embryos that paternal genes contribute to placental development, whereas maternal genes tend to define the embryo.

Genomic imprinting is a phenomenon, first described in mice, whereby certain genes are marked differently during male versus female germ cell formation so that apparently identical genes possess dissimilar function depending on whether they are passed from the mother or the father. Imprinting commonly serves to "turn off" a gene or reduce its expression. Less than a hundred genes are known to be imprinted in humans. Imprinting has been shown to play a role in a number of human syndromes, including Prader-Willi syndrome, Angelman syndrome, and Beckwith syndrome. For example, Prader-Willi syndrome occurs if the paternal copies of genes in the q11 region of chromosome 15 are missing through deletion of that region or disomy as discussed subsequently. The inference from this observation is that the maternally inherited genes at this locus are normally imprinted or turned off. Absence for whatever reason of the paternally derived copies produces the phenotype. Current understanding suggests that imprinting involves allele-specific epigenetic modification through a variety of mechanisms, including cytosine methylation and histone acetylation. These modifications are erased in the germ cells and re-established in early embryogenesis. Imprinted genes tend to cluster in the genome and have regional regulation by local imprinting centers, like the X-inactivation center (Xist), which spreads inactivation along one of the X chromosomes.

"Uniparental disomy" is a term that indicates that both members of a chromosome pair or both alleles of a gene pair come from the same parent. This situation usually occurs when an embryo, initially trisomic for a certain chromosome, "self-corrects" by eliminating one of the extra chromosomes. In one third of such cases, the remaining two chromosomes will have the same parent of origin, resulting in uniparental disomy for the genes on that chromosome. The impact of uniparental disomy on morphogenesis is just beginning to be understood. Overgrowth in Beckwith syndrome is caused by a variety of mechanisms that perturb the balance of imprinted growth-promoting and growth-repressing genes in the region 11p15. Paternal disomy is one such mechanism. Moreover, uniparental disomy may account for some of the phenotypic effects occasionally observed in individuals with apparently balanced robertsonian translocations involving chromosome 14 or 15. The implication is that certain chromosomes contain genes that are either paternally or maternally imprinted. Two copies from one parent would disturb the gene balance required for normal development. Uniparental disomy from correction of a trisomic conceptus is one mechanism that is known to produce Prader-Willi syndrome. Unrelated to imprinted genes, uniparental disomy may cause autosomal recessive disorders when only one parent is a carrier if a child inherits both chromosomes from the carrier parent and none from the noncarrier.

Unstable DNA Mutations

Throughout the human genome there are a number of sites in which short triplet repeated sequences of nucleotides normally occur. Although the purpose of these triplet repeats is not always known, the number of repeats at a given site is usually transmitted in a stable fashion from one generation to the next. An unstable DNA mutation occurs when the number of copies of a repeated sequence becomes increased. Expansion in the number of repeats at a locus may produce disease directly, or it may create what has been termed a "premutation." The latter indicates that the expanded sequence has no clinical effects on the individual; however, the sequence is likely to be unstable during meiosis (germ cell formation), resulting in offspring with a full mutation and clinical abnormalities. Although unstable DNA mutations usually expand further during meiosis, contraction of unstable sequences is documented. Unstable DNA mutations account for some observations that seem to defy the laws of single-gene inheritance such as anticipation (a condition getting worse in successive generations) and unaffected transmitting males in X-linked recessive disorders. Parent-of-origin effects are common in unstable mutations, with some expanding only when transmitted through the mother and others showing paternal effects. Several classes of trinucleotide repeat disorders are recognized. Fragile X syndrome is the prototype for conditions caused by expansion of trinucleotide repeats in the noncoding region of the responsible gene. Such expansions typically cause loss of function of the involved gene. Myotonic dystrophy has a similar pathogenesis. A second class of conditions, typically with midlife-onset neurodegeneration, is caused by much smaller expansions of a polyglutamine $(CAG)_n$ track within the exon of a gene. The altered protein resulting from these mutations disrupts protein turnover within the cell, an effect that worsens over time. Strand slippage during DNA replication is thought to be the likely mechanism of formation for these classes of repeats. Expansion within a polyalanine tract has been shown to account for a variety of disorders, including synpolydactyly type II, cleidocranial dysplasia (one family), and holoprosencephaly 5. These expansions typically occur in genes that code for transcription factors. Mutations produce defects by altering the function of downstream target genes.

Mitochondrial Mutations

The DNA of the normal mitochondrion is a circular molecule that contains 37 genes encoding 22 types of transfer RNA, two types of ribosomal RNA, and 13 structural proteins, which are all subunits of the respiratory chain complexes involved in oxidative phosphorylation. Any given cell may contain from a hundred to several thousand mitochondria. Because the mitochondria are the energy-producing apparatus of the cell, many mitochondrial disorders described present postnatally with variable multisystem involvement, including visual loss, progressive myopathy, seizures, encephalopathy, or diabetes, presumably as a consequence of insufficient energy production in a critical tissue. The effects of mitochondrial mutation appear to worsen over time. Mitochondrial mutations commonly affect only a portion of the DNA molecules of each mitochondrion, in variable amounts in different tissues—a phenomenon known as heteroplasmy. Heteroplasmy is responsible for marked variability in expression as a consequence of mitochondrial DNA mutations. It should be noted that the majority of genes involved in mitochondrion energy production are located in the nuclear DNA. Disorders associated with mutations in these genes are usually recessively inherited. Only a minority of mitochondrial disorders are caused by mutations in mitochondrial DNA associated with cytoplasmic, matrilineal inheritance.

GENETIC COUNSELING FOR SINGLE-GENE DISORDERS

For single-gene disorders, it is a good general rule to consult the literature directly before counseling families or affected individuals regarding the availability of testing as it pertains to carrier detection, presymptomatic diagnosis, and prenatal diagnosis, because the nature of the workup that is required to address many of these questions changes dramatically as the level of the understanding of the genetic abnormality becomes more refined. Increasingly, molecular diagnosis is available for single-gene disorders. The U.S. GeneTests website (http://www.genetests.org) and the Orphanet European website (http://www.orpha.net) are excellent sources of information regarding laboratories offering testing on both a clinical and research basis.

Autosomal Dominant Disorders

The parents and siblings of the affected individual should be examined to determine whether any of them show any features of the disorder in question. The nature of the "examination" to exclude clinically the effects of an altered gene varies by disorder from simple assessment of parental stature in achondroplasia to cutaneous examination plus eye evaluation plus cranial and renal imaging in tuberous sclerosis. As genetic tests have become increasingly available and affordable, genetic testing for the mutation in the child and subsequent confirmation in the parents can be a better way to ensure parents do not carry the mutation, especially in conditions with marked variable expression or reduced penetrance. The need for molecular testing will be diagnosis specific. For example, in tuberous sclerosis, a phenotype with great variation in expression, molecular testing can be extremely helpful; however, in achondroplasia, DNA testing is usually not needed since the presence of mutation can be very

easily assessed based on the stature of the individual. More distant relatives do not need to worry about having affected children if the parents are not affected and do not carry the mutation. If neither parent carries the known mutation or shows no features of the condition, it is appropriate to counsel the family that the occurrence in the child likely represents a fresh gene mutation (gene change in one of the germ cells that went to make the baby) for which the risk for recurrence is negligible.

The risk for an affected individual having an affected child is 50% for each offspring. This number represents the risk for vertical transmission of the altered gene; however, it does not predict the severity of the effect in offspring who inherit the mutation. Knowledge of the frequency of various features in affected individuals is helpful in outlining not only the risk for transmission but also the likelihood of particular complications.

In the uncommon circumstance in which a dominant condition is the result of an unstable mutation in DNA, the likelihood of anticipation (increasing severity in subsequent generations) should be addressed if the affected parent is of the gender in which expansion of the unstable sequence is known to occur. For example, congenital myotonic dystrophy occurs only when the altered gene is transmitted through the mother.

Autosomal Recessive Disorders

Inheritance is from clinically normal parents who both have the same, or an allelic, recessive mutant gene in single dose. The risk is obviously enhanced if the parents are related. The possibility of consanguinity should always be addressed in disorders known to be autosomal recessive and when evaluating patterns of malformation of unknown cause. Autosomal recessive disorders generally have less variation in expression among members of the same family than do autosomal dominant conditions.

Recurrence risk from the same parentage is 25% for each subsequent pregnancy. The risk of any relative having an affected child may be calculated by multiplying his or her risk of being a heterozygote (carrier) times the risk of marrying a heterozygote (the general carrier frequency for that gene in the population) times one fourth (the chance of two heterozygotes having an affected offspring).

In counseling parents of individuals with recessive disorders, it is helpful to emphasize that most people are heterozygous for many genes that cause no problem because each is balanced by a normal partner. The normal children of carrier parents have a two out of three chance of being carriers as well. Their risk of randomly marrying another carrier is usually low; thus, their risk for affected offspring is low. However, partners of known carriers should be offered screening in advance of pregnancy if testing is available and affordable. Carrier screening for a number of autosomal recessive disorders is becoming more widely available as NGS allows the development of broad panels for testing. It is likely that ethnic-specific carrier screening panels and whole genome sequencing will change the current paradigm.

X-Linked Recessive Disorders

The X-linked genes in the XY male are present in a single dose with no partner gene. Hence, a single copy of a mutant gene on the X chromosome will express a full recessive disorder. The chance of an XX female having a pair of such X-linked recessive genes and expressing the same disorder as the XY male is very small. The following generalizations apply to this pattern of inheritance: with rare exception, only males are affected; transmission is through unaffected or mildly affected (carrier) females; male-to-male transmission does not occur.

X-linked disorders in the male often represent fresh gene mutation. These disorders present a problem in determining the generation in which the gene mutation arose, for it could be in the patient alone or in the mother or even further back in the family, having been silently passed through carrier females. Although molecular testing is the optimal way to address the question, for some X-linked disorders, such as hypohidrotic ectodermal dysplasia, this dilemma can be resolved clinically by demonstrating the presence or absence of mild (carrier) expression in the females in question. Older paternal age has been noted to be a factor in fresh X-linked mutation; however, the older age effect is seen in the father of the mother (maternal grandfather) of the first affected XY male rather than the boy's father from whom he does not receive his X.

For unstable X-linked mutations, such as those that account for the fragile X syndrome, counseling needs to incorporate knowledge of parent-of-origin effects. Unstable X-linked mutations tend to expand when passed through the mother, accounting for a more severe phenotype in offspring of carrier women who inherit the altered gene.

For X-linked recessive disorders in general, if the mother is not a carrier, the risk for recurrence is low. If the mother is a carrier, she has a 50% risk that any future male will be affected. Normal sons cannot transmit the disorder. All sons of affected males are normal. All daughters of affected males are usually clinically normal carriers.

In general, all daughters of carrier mothers will be clinically normal, although 50% will carry the altered gene and have a risk for vertical transmission. The major exception is the case of unstable DNA mutation in which daughters of carrier mothers who inherit an expanded mutation often show clinical effects.

In cases of intellectual disability or dysmorphic phenotypes of unknown cause in males, there is a chance of an X-linked recessive disorder. The identification of previous affected males related through potential carrier females is a strong argument for X-linked inheritance. X-inactivation studies in the mothers of the affected male may reflect markedly skewed X-inactivation (>95%), which supports this mode of inheritance. NGS panels targeting genes on the X chromosome as well as targeted arrays or MLPA of the X chromosome could be considered if phenotype recognition does not establish a clinical diagnosis.

X-Linked Dominant Inheritance

X-linked dominant disorders show expression in the XX female, usually with more severe, often lethal, effects in the XY male. This type of inheritance is most commonly confused with autosomal dominant inheritance from which it may be discriminated in the following ways: males are more severely affected than females, although affected males are underrepresented in large kindreds, reflecting the male lethality of X-linked dominant conditions; male-to-male transmission is not observed; instead, affected males have normal sons and all of their daughters are affected.

Affected females have a 50% risk for affected daughters. Although the risk that an XY fetus will inherit the gene is also 50%, the probability of a liveborn affected male is usually significantly less because of the selection pressure against affected XY conceptuses. Males born to affected women are usually normal. The affected males represent early miscarriages.

Mothers of daughters with X-linked dominant conditions should be examined closely for evidence of clinical effect. If the mother is normal, fresh gene mutation in the offspring is likely and the risk for recurrence is negligible. Molecular testing is critical if clinical uncertainty exists. If not, counseling is the same as that for affected females mentioned previously.

Mitochondrial Inheritance

Because mitochondria are exclusively maternally inherited, males with disorders caused by mitochondrial mutations have no risk for affected offspring. Females, on the other hand, have a risk that approaches 100%, because the human egg is the source of all of the mitochondria for the offspring. Most affected women have both normal and abnormal mitochondria; thus, any given egg will have both types in different proportions. Random distribution of mitochondria in dividing cells in the early embryo creates different proportions of abnormal to normal mitochondria in different tissues. A clinical phenotype occurs only when a threshold of abnormal to normal mitochondria is exceeded in a critical tissue. Thus, all offspring of affected women may be assumed to have inherited some abnormal mitochondria; however, not all will manifest disease. Clinically unaffected daughters of affected women also have a risk for vertical transmission, because lack of clinical disease does not preclude the possibility that some of the daughter's mitochondria might harbor the mutation.

MULTIFACTORIAL INHERITANCE

In the mid-1960s, a model was advanced to explain the findings emerging from a variety of epidemiologic studies, which suggested that a broad number of common malformations—including cleft lip and palate, isolated cleft palate, neural tube defects, clubfoot, and pyloric stenosis, among others—tended to cluster in families, although the pattern of inheritance did not conform to the laws of gene transmission as set forth by Mendel. The model involved the concept of genetic liability or susceptibility to a given characteristic, governed by many different genes, and a threshold, determined by both genetic and environmental factors. Individuals lying beyond the threshold exhibited the phenotype, whereas those who did not were phenotypically normal. The model converted the normal distribution of a morphogenetic process within a population into an "all-or-none" expression of a structural defect. As initially proposed, the many

genes contributing to susceptibility were given equal weight. The multifactorial/threshold model makes several predictions that in large measure are in accord with the clinical and epidemiologic observations regarding given malformations:

1. Familial clustering is observed. As stated previously, clustering is observed among family groups. In addition, many common malformations have different birth frequencies in different populations. Because numerous subtle genetic differences are presumed to account for some of the normal variation observed among ethnic groups, it is hypothesized that some of these differences may confer susceptibility for certain developmental problems. Thus, the model would predict variation in the prevalence of certain malformations by ethnic groups, a finding that is well documented in population surveys.
2. The risk for first-degree relatives (parents, siblings, and offspring) approximates the square root of the population risk. Table 3-1 lists the frequency of recurrence of the same defect in offspring of normal parents who have had one affected child. For the majority of defects, the risk is 2% to 5%, which is 20 to 40 times the frequency of the problem in the general population. The figures in Table 3-1 are derived from direct observations in clinical populations and correlate well with the numbers predicted by the model.
3. Second-degree relatives (uncles, aunts, half-siblings) have a sharply lower risk than first-degree relatives. This characteristic differentiates multifactorial inheritance from autosomal dominant inheritance in which

Table 3-1 RECURRENCE RISKS FOR SOME DEFECTS			
	RECURRENCE RISK FOR		
Defect	Normal Parents of One Affected Child	Future Males	Future Females
Cleft lip with or without cleft palate	4%–5%*		
Cleft palate alone	2%–6%		
Cardiac defect (common type)	3%–4%		
Pyloric stenosis	3%	4%	2.4%
Hirschsprung anomaly	3%–5%		
Clubfoot	2%–8%		
Dislocation of hip	3%–4%	0.5%	6.3%
Neural tube defects—anencephaly, meningomyelocele	3%–5%		
Scoliosis	10%–15%		

*Range of recurrence risks observed.

the risk drops only by half with each degree of relational distance from the affected individual and from autosomal recessive inheritance in which the major risk is for full siblings.

4. The greater the number is of affected family members, the greater the risk is for recurrence. This pattern of recurrence of multifactorial traits is in contrast to both dominant and recessive inheritance in which the risk for future offspring remains unchanged despite recurrences.

5. Consanguinity increases the risk. This concept relates to the fact that inbreeding increases the number of "susceptibility genes," thus making a developmental problem more likely.

6. The more severe the malformation is, the greater the risk for recurrence. This presumes that the severity of the malformation reflects a greater adverse genetic influence, thereby increasing the risk from the same parentage. Certainly with cleft lip and palate, data support the hypothesis, because the risk for recurrence in subsequent children when an offspring has a severe bilateral cleft lip and palate is 5.7% as contrasted with a 2.5% recurrence risk when the offspring has a less severe degree of defect.

7. The risk for recurrence will be increased for relatives of the least affected gender, if gender differences are noted. The gender difference between the XX and XY genetic background has an appreciable effect on the occurrence of many malformations (Fig. 3-17). Some of the gender differences in malformation occurrence may be explained as the direct effects of structural genital differences, such as hypospadias in the male. Similarly, the marked male predominance of the urethral obstruction sequence may be explained by the fact that the most common site of urethral obstruction is the prostatic urethra. The humoral impact of testosterone, which makes connective tissue tougher in the male, may explain the preponderance of dislocation of the hip, related to connective tissue laxity, in the female. Also, testosterone, which is produced by the male during the first few postnatal months, may enhance the likelihood of muscle hypertrophy and thereby increase the tendency to develop hypertrophic pyloric stenosis. The gender differences related to the incidence of other structural defects would appear to imply that genes on the X or Y chromosome may increase the likelihood of particular anomalies developing during morphogenesis.

One indirect manner in which the genetic background of XX versus XY may influence the frequency of structural defects at birth is simply the growth rate in utero. Thus, with the exception of anomalies related to joint laxity, most late uterine constraint-induced deformations are more common in the male, who is normally growing faster in the last trimester of gestation than the female.

It is hypothesized that if it takes more genetic factors to give rise to an anomaly in the female, then the affected female should pass on more of these genetic factors to her offspring, who would have a higher frequency of the anomaly than would offspring of affected males. Observational studies in pyloric stenosis documenting a 24% risk of transmission from affected mothers compared to 6% from affected fathers bear this out.

8. Concordance in twins. If both twins have a defect, they are concordant for the anomaly. If one twin has the defect and the other does not, they are discordant. The frequency of concordance and discordance in monozygotic and dizygotic twins has been used to argue both for environmental and for single-gene causation of common malformations. For most of these defects, the incidence of concordance in dizygotic twins is similar to that of siblings born of separate pregnancies,

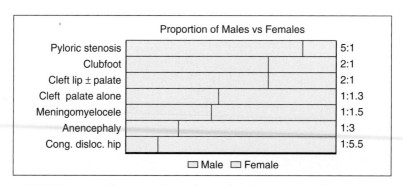

FIGURE 3-17.   Relative gender incidence of single common malformations.

arguing against both a single-gene etiology and a major environmental influence.

Over the past 15 years, numerous investigators have reanalyzed previously published data sets for specific "multifactorial" malformations with respect to a variety of alternative hypotheses. For cleft lip with or without cleft palate, it now seems likely that susceptibility is determined by a small number of genes (two to eight) acting in a multiplicative fashion and interacting with environmental factors. This is likely true with respect to genes that define susceptibility to other common "multifactorial" malformations.

Until recently, SNPs and other sequence variation were recognized as the main source of genetic variation leading to multifactorial diseases or malformations. However, the recent evidence of the great variation in copy number for certain genomic regions has triggered a search for association of CNVs to birth defects and genetic diseases in a multifactorial model. Interestingly, several deletions and their reciprocal duplications (1q21.1, 15q11.2, 15q13.3, 16p11.2, 16p13.3) have been shown to be associated with increased risk of intellectual disability, autism, epilepsy, subtle dysmorphic features, and even specific heart defects such as tetralogy of Fallot. How these CNVs interact with other genetic or environmental factors is still unknown, but they certainly show marked low penetrance in vertical transmission and should be understood in the framework of the multifactorial inheritance model.

Despite the accumulating evidence that suggests that the multifactorial model is probably not strictly biologically true, the empiric data obtained from the observational studies used to construct the model remain the basis for genetic counseling of families. Molecular testing for susceptibility genes will be possible when whole genome sequencing becomes clinically available.

That environmental influences play a role in the determination of common malformations is borne out by many studies such as those of anencephaly and meningomyelocele that document that social class is a variable that impacts birth frequency. Birth-order influences have also been noted, with congenital dislocation of the hip and pyloric stenosis being more likely to occur in firstborn children. One obvious environmental factor is fetal in utero constraint leading to deformation. Such constraint is more common in the firstborn who is the first to distend the uterus and the abdominal wall. Environmental factors such as this probably explain the greater frequency of dislocation of the hip as well as most other deformations in the firstborn.

Studies in experimental animals have dramatically illustrated the profound influence that genetic

background may have on the likelihood of a given environmental teratogen causing malformation. For example, Fraser could regularly produce cleft palate in mouse embryos of the A/Jax strain by giving the mothers a high dose of cortisone during early gestation, whereas the same treatment in a different strain led to only 17% affected offspring. In humans, genetic susceptibility to hydantoin-induced teratogenesis appears to correlate with the genetically determined activity levels of epoxide hydrolase, one of the enzymes necessary for the metabolism of hydantoin. Expression of the phenotype requires both genetic susceptibility and drug exposure.

The search for environmental factors that allow for expression of a single malformation is ongoing. However, just as the genetic differences that contribute to susceptibility are multiple and difficult to characterize, so environmental factors are likely to be multiple and incremental in effect. The total factors combine to approach the threshold for a particular error in morphogenesis, a threshold predominantly set by the genetic makeup of the individual.

GENETIC COUNSELING FOR DEFECTS THAT ARE A RESULT OF MULTIFACTORIAL INHERITANCE

When evaluating a child with a birth defect, a careful physical examination is essential to determine whether that defect is in fact isolated. Only then can multifactorial inheritance be assumed and empiric risk figures used for genetic counseling. For many common single defects, empiric risk figures relative to recurrence of the problem in a subsequent pregnancy are available. The risk is 3% to 5% or less for most of the common single defects, with the exception of scoliosis (see Table 3-1). The risk figures may be slightly increased when the defect in the affected individual is severe in degree, and decreased when the anomaly is mild in degree. If the gender of the child impacts the condition (such as in pyloric stenosis and hip dislocation), gender-specific risks for recurrence may be appropriate. If two offspring are affected, the risk for the next child is two to three times greater, or approximately 10% to 15%. Because recurrence risk figures address the risk for first-degree relatives, the risk that an affected individual will have affected offspring is similar in magnitude to that of the sibling risk (or 3%-5%). As the factors that influence both genetic and environmental susceptibility to multifactorial traits become elucidated, it is expected that more precise counseling will be possible.

The multifactorial model is useful in explaining common malformations to parents, as it dictates that the genetic factors that contribute come from both sides of the family. It is helpful to explain the developmental pathology of the defects so that parents can appreciate that there was only a single localized problem in the early development of their child. A discussion that the localized problem in development must have occurred before a particular time in gestation may be helpful in dispelling any concerns over later gestational events that are likely to have had no impact on the occurrence on the particular malformation. The prognosis of multifactorial traits depends on the amenability of the specific malformation to surgical intervention or, in the case of constraint-related problems, to postural intervention. The prognosis is poor for certain neural tube defects but may be quite good for cardiac malformations and other defects in which advances in therapy have improved both morbidity and mortality.

PRENATAL DIAGNOSIS

Technologic advancement as well as progress in the understanding of the etiology and pathogenesis of many disorders have made the possibility for prenatal diagnosis an increasing reality for many families. For a very few conditions, fetal therapy may be available; however, most prenatal diagnosis is offered to allow parents options for managing their reproductive risk. The subsequent sections present some of the techniques for early fetal evaluation along with indications for their application.

Screening Approaches for the General Pregnant Population

Chromosomal and Genomic Abnormalities

Because the risk for many chromosomal aneuploidy states increases with advancing maternal age, various approaches have been developed to assess fetal karyotypes in older mothers. The most accurate way to address this issue is with direct assessment of the fetal chromosomes, which requires a sample of fetal cells. The traditional method by which this is done is amniocentesis at 15 to 18 weeks of pregnancy. Although highly accurate, the procedure carries a roughly 1 in 400 risk for miscarriage, which is a deterrent to some couples. Chorionic villus sampling (CVS) affords the advantage of earlier diagnosis, as the procedure is done at 11 to 12 weeks of pregnancy. The test carries a slightly increased risk for miscarriage even correcting for the earlier gestational age at which testing is done. In addition, mosaicism in the sampled placental cells is documented in approximately 1% of cases, causing counseling dilemmas. Noninvasive serum

screening during the second trimester using a triple marker screen (maternal age, alpha fetoprotein, human chorionic gonadotropin, and unconjugated estriol) or quad screening (triple markers plus dimeric inhibin A) is a useful way to modify the age-related risk for Down syndrome to determine which women in the general population are at high enough risk that more invasive testing should be offered. Noninvasive first-trimester screening using ultrasound measurement of nuchal translucency with serum marker analysis (pregnancy-associated plasma protein A and human chorionic gonadotropin) has also been used. With combined first- and second-trimester screening results (integrated testing), a 90% Down syndrome detection rate is possible with a less than 1% false-positive rate. The newest noninvasive screening approach for the major autosomal trisomies involves sequencing cell-free fetal DNA in maternal serum. Early reports have documented upward of 95% sensitivity with extremely low false-positive rates. Although not yet validated in low-risk populations, the technique utilized has broad applicability for detection of other copy number abnormalities.

On the other hand, currently available CGH array technology allows for the detection of a wide variety of syndromes caused by genomic imbalance if fetal cells are available for testing. Many microdeletion/microduplication syndromes occur in apparently low-risk pregnancies. Several studies have established the increased detection rate of prenatal arrays in comparison to the standard karyotype, especially in the setting of ultrasound anomalies. In addition, most of these studies also document a significant detection of pathogenic CNVs in low-risk pregnancies. CNVs of uncertain significance pose an even greater counseling challenge in the prenatal context, particularly in the absence of ultrasound findings. However, invasive testing with array CGH may become the approach of choice for couples wishing to avoid the birth of a child with a recognizable pattern of malformation for which testing is possible.

Single-Gene Disorders

Carrier screening has been available only for a number of single-gene disorders that are inherited in an autosomal recessive fashion and that have a high prevalence in certain populations. Examples include Tay-Sachs disease, sickle cell anemia, and cystic fibrosis. However, NGS approaches have allowed the development of fast and affordable testing for large panels of disorder for which an individual may not have an increased risk. The number of conditions for which carrier screening is possible is likely to increase exponentially as the cost of sequencing comes down.

Multifactorial Conditions, Including Apparently Isolated Malformations

The only multifactorial conditions for which population screening is specifically available are the neural tube closure defects. Elevation of alpha fetoprotein, both in the amniotic fluid and in maternal serum, has been associated with the presence of an open defect in the fetus. Serum screening in conjunction with thorough ultrasound evaluation should detect over 90% of affected pregnancies.

Ultrasonography is also an increasingly useful screening tool for a number of other malformations. Even though variations in equipment and operator experience make this an imperfect screening modality as it is currently practiced, the detection rates for many birth defects have increased dramatically in recent years.

Prenatal Diagnostic Approaches for Specific Disorders

Chromosomal and Genomic Abnormalities

Amniocentesis or CVS should be offered in the following situations:

1. Abnormal combined ultrasound and biochemical screening for autosomal trisomies
2. Previous child with trisomy 21 or other trisomy
3. Parental balanced translocation
4. Affected parent with a microdeletion or microduplication syndrome
5. Any de novo abnormality in which the parents, although chromosomally normal, are interested, because this is the only way to exclude recurrence from gonadal mosaicism
6. Isolated or multiple defects or markers identified by ultrasound that require more precise definition of the overall prognosis for the fetus
7. Parental desire to test for as many genomic conditions as possible

Array CGH is likely to replace standard karyotyping in many situations as experience with interpretation of CNVs grows.

Single-Gene Disorders

Prenatal testing for single-gene disorders is more difficult because the approach that is used for any given condition depends on, among other things, the level of understanding of the molecular basis of the disorder in question. Testing can be done at the level of the gene (DNA), the message (RNA), the product (biochemical analysis), or the phenotype produced (gross morphology). Even in situations in which the gene that causes a specific condition is known, direct analysis of the gene is not always the easiest, least costly, and most reliable approach to prenatal testing. The rapidity with which changes occur in this arena dictates that the literature be reviewed at the time prenatal diagnosis is requested. Information available in textbooks will be out of date for some conditions at the time of publication.

1. For conditions in which the specific gene mutation is known, prenatal diagnosis is often possible using amniocentesis or CVS to collect fetal cells for direct mutation analysis. If a common mutation accounts for the majority of the cases (such as achondroplasia) the approach can be relatively straightforward. By contrast, in conditions such as Marfan syndrome, in which multiple different mutations within the same gene produce the same phenotype, prenatal diagnosis using direct DNA analysis is possible only if the family's specific mutation is known.
2. For disorders in which the location of the gene is known, linkage (indirect) analysis may be useful. This technique dictates that DNA samples be obtained on multiple family members and often requires a confirmed diagnosis in more than one family member. Nonpaternity is occasionally discovered in the course of this type of investigation. Recombination leading to misdiagnosis can occur, and the technique should always involve multiple markers in the gene or as close to the gene locus as possible.
3. Biochemical studies may be diagnostic in conditions in which the approach is based on analysis of gene product. Some tests are performed on amniotic fluid directly. Other studies demand cultured fetal cells for enzyme analysis.
4. For X-linked conditions in which neither direct DNA analysis nor linkage is available, prenatal gender determination may be an option. However, 50% of the male offspring of carrier women would be expected to be normal.
5. For conditions in which the diagnosis is made on the clinical phenotype, prenatal diagnosis is dependent on the ability of ultrasound to visualize specific features of the condition such as severe limb shortening in some of the skeletal dysplasias.
6. For conditions with marked variability in expression or incomplete penetrance, identification of a mutation may not be fully predictive of the presence of the phenotype. For

example, in the EEC syndrome caused by mutation in p63, the ultrasound identification of a cleft lip and palate or ectrodactyly may be far more useful than testing for the mutation alone.

7. For abnormalities detected by ultrasound, multiple-gene NGS panels will be developed for groups of birth defects and/or ultrasound markers related to multiple potential genetic causes, for example, a skeletal dysplasia panel or Noonan syndrome panel for large nuchal translucency.

Multifactorial Conditions

For conditions that have neither a chromosomal nor genetic marker, prenatal diagnosis is entirely dependent on the amenability of the specific structural defects to ultrasound imaging. For example, holoprosencephaly is readily visualized with prenatal imaging, whereas isolated cleft palate is not always detected at this time. It is important that clinicians be aware of the limitations of ultrasound. The Eurofetus Study regarding the accuracy of ultrasound detection of fetal malformations in an unselected population documented a roughly 60% overall detection rate, which is also to say that 40% of defects were missed. This is not to downplay the usefulness of ultrasound imaging but rather to foster realistic expectations among families and physicians when this method is used.

Suggested Readings

Antonarakis SE, and the Down Syndrome Collaborative Group: Parental origin of the extra chromosome in trisomy 21 using DNA polymorphism analysis, *N Engl J Med* 324:872, 1991.

Antonarakis SE, et al: The meiotic stage of non-disjunction in trisomy 21: Determination by using DNA polymorphisms, *Am J Hum Genet* 50:544, 1992.

Arenas F, Smith DW: Sex liability to single structural defects, *Am J Dis Child* 132:970, 1978.

Armengol L, et al: Clinical utility of chromosomal microarray analysis in invasive prenatal diagnosis, *Hum Genet* 131:513, 2012.

Ball RH, et al: First- and second-trimester evaluation of risk for Down syndrome, *Obstet Gynecol* 110:10, 2007.

Bianchi DW, et al: Genome-wide fetal aneuploidy detection by maternal plasma DNA sequencing, *Obstet Gynecol* 119:890, 2012.

Breman A, et al: Prenatal chromosomal microarray analysis in a diagnostic laboratory; experience with >1000 cases and review of the literature, *Prenat Diagn* 32:351, 2012.

Brown LY, Brown SA: Alanine tracts: The expanding story of human illness and trinucleotide repeats, *Trends Genet* 20:51, 2004.

Buehler BA, et al: Prenatal prediction of risk of the fetal hydantoin syndrome, *N Engl J Med* 322:1567, 1990.

Caskey CT, et al: Triplet repeat mutations in human disease, *Science* 256:784, 1991.

Church GM: Genomes for all, *Sci Am* 294:46, 2006.

Cooper GM, et al: A copy number variation morbidity map of developmental delay, *Nat Genet* 43:838, 2011.

Cummings CJ, Zoghbi HY: Fourteen and counting: Unraveling trinucleotide repeat diseases, *Hum Mol Genet* 9:909, 2000.

de Vries BB et al: Clinical studies on submicroscopic subtelomeric rearrangements: A checklist, *J Med Genet* 38:145, 2001.

Donnai D: Robertsonian translocations: Clues to imprinting, *Am J Med Genet* 46:681, 1993.

Ewigman BG, et al: Effect of prenatal ultrasound screening on perinatal outcome, *N Engl J Med* 329:821, 1993.

Farrall M, Holder SE: Familial recurrence pattern analysis of cleft lip with or without cleft palate, *Am J Hum Genet* 50:270, 1992.

Feenstra I, et al: European Cytogeneticists Association Register of Unbalanced Chromosome Aberrations (ECARUCA); an online database for rare chromosome abnormalities, *Eur J Med Genet* 49:279, 2006.

Firth HV, et al: DECIPHER: Database of Chromosomal Imbalance and Phenotype in Humans Using Ensembl Resources, *Am J Hum Genet* 84:524, 2009.

Fraser FC: *The use of teratogens in the analysis of abnormal developmental mechanisms. First International Conference on Congenital Malformations*, Philadelphia, 1961, Lippincott.

Golbus MS, et al: Prenatal genetic diagnosis in 3000 amniocenteses, *N Engl J Med* 300:157, 1979.

Graham JM: *Smith's Recognizable Patterns of Human Deformation*, ed 3, Philadelphia, 2007, Elsevier.

Grandjean H, et al: The performance of routine ultrasonographic screening of pregnancies in the Eurofetus Study, *Am J Obstet Gynecol* 181:446, 1999.

Hall N: Advanced sequencing technologies and their wider impact in microbiology, *J Exp Biol* 210:1518, 2007.

Harper P: *Practical Genetic Counseling*, ed 7, London, 2010, Hodder Arnold.

Hassold T, Hunt P: To err (meiotically) is human: The genesis of human aneuploidy, *Nat Rev Genet* 2:280, 2001.

Hassold T, et al: Molecular studies of parental origin and mosaicism in 45,X conceptuses, *Hum Genet* 89:647, 1992.

Hillman SC, et al: Additional information from array comparative genomic hybridization technology over conventional karyotyping in prenatal diagnosis: A systematic review and meta-analysis, *Ultrasound Obstet Gynecol* 37:6, 2011.

Hunt PA, Hassold TJ: Sex matters in meiosis, *Science* 296:2181, 2002.

International Human Genome Sequencing Consortium: Finishing the euchromatic sequence of the human genome, *Nature* 431:931, 2004.

Jones KL, et al: Older paternal age and fresh gene mutation, *J Pediatr* 86:84, 1975.

Jumlongras D, et al: A nonsense mutation in MSX1 causes Witkop syndrome, *Am J Hum Genet* 69:67, 2001.

Kaminsky EB et al. An evidence-based approach to establish the functional and clinical significance of copy number variants in intellectual and developmental disabilities, *Genet Med* 13:777, 2011.

Leung TY, et al: Identification of submicroscopic chromosomal aberrations in fetuses with increased nuchal translucency and apparently normal karyotype, *Ultrasound Obstet Gynecol* 38:314, 2011.

MacDonald M, et al: The origin of 47,XXY and 47,XXX aneuploidy: Heterogeneous mechanisms and role of aberrant recombination, *Hum Mol Genet* 3:1365, 1994.

Malone RD, et al: First-trimester or second-trimester screening, or both, for Down's syndrome, *N Eng J Med* 353:2001, 2005.

Mascarello JT, Hubbard V: Routine use of methods for improved G-band resolution in a population of patients with malformations and developmental delay, *Am J Med Genet* 38:37, 1991.

McFadden DE, Kalousek DK: Two different phenotypes of fetuses with chromosomal triploidy: Correlation with parental origin of the extra haploid set, *Am J Med Genet* 38:535, 1991.

Miller DT, et al: Consensus statement: Chromosomal microarray is a first-tier clinical diagnostic test for individuals with developmental disabilities or congenital anomalies, *Am J Hum Genet* 86:749, 2010.

Mitchell LE, Christensen K: Analysis of the recurrence patterns for nonsyndromic cleft lip with or without cleft palate in the families of 3,073 Danish probands, *Am J Med Genet* 61:371, 1996.

Moore GE, et al: Linkage of an X-chromosome cleft palate gene, *Nature* 326:91, 1987.

Palomaki GE, et al: ENA sequencing of maternal plasma reliably identifies trisomy 18 and 13 as well as Down syndrome: An international collaborative study, *Genet Med* 14:296, 2012.

Pangalos CG, et al: DNA polymorphism analysis in families with recurrence of free trisomy 21, *Am J Hum Genet* 51:1015, 1992.

Pennisi E: ENCODE Project writes eulogy for junk DNA, *Science* 337:1159, 2012.

Phelan MC, et al: Mental retardation in South Carolina. III. Chromosome aberrations, *Proc Greenwood Genet Center* 15:45, 1996.

Sanger F, Coulson AR: A rapid method for determining sequences in DNA by primed synthesis with DNA polymerase, *J Mol Biol* 94:441, 1975.

Sanger F, et al: DNA sequencing with chain-terminating inhibitors, *Proc Natl Acad Sci U S A* 74:5463, 1977.

Schuster SC: Next-generation sequencing transforms today's biology, *Nat Methods* 5:16, 2008.

Shaw CJ, et al: Comparative genomic hybridisation using a proximal 17p BAC/PAC array detects rearrangements responsible for four genomic disorders, *J Med Genet* 4:113, 2004.

Sinden RR, et al: Triplet repeat DNA structures and human genetic disease: Dynamic mutations from dynamic DNA, *J Biosci* 27:53, 2002.

Smith DW, Aase JM: Polygenic inheritance of certain common malformations, *J Pediatr* 76:653, 1970.

Sparks AB, et al: Selective analysis of cell-free DNA in maternal blood for evaluation of fetal trisomy, *Prenat Diag* 32:3, 2012.

Wald NJ, et al: SURUSS in perspective, *Br J Obstet Gynecol* 111:521, 2004.

Wallace DC: Mitochondrial defects in neurodegenerative disease, *Ment Retard Dev Disabil Res Rev* 7:158, 2001.

Walter J, Paulsen M: Imprinting and disease, *Sem Cell Dev Biol* 14:101, 2003.

Yu W, et al: Development of a comparative genomic hybridization microarray and demonstration of its utility with 25 well-characterized 1p36 deletions, *Hum Mol Genet* 12:2145, 2003.

CHAPTER 4

Minor Anomalies: Clues to More Serious Problems and to the Recognition of Malformation Syndromes

Minor anomalies are herein defined as unusual morphologic features that are of no serious medical or cosmetic consequence to the patient. The value of their recognition is that they may serve as indicators of altered morphogenesis in a general sense or may constitute valuable clues in the diagnosis of a specific pattern of malformation. Those who want a more detailed discussion of this subject or those who desire information on a minor malformation not addressed in this chapter are referred to Jon M. Aase's *Diagnostic Dysmorphology*.[2]

Regarding the general occurrence of minor anomalies detectable by surface examination (except for dermatoglyphics), Marden and colleagues[9] found that 14% of newborn babies had a single minor anomaly. This was of little concern because the frequency of major defects in this group was not appreciably increased. However, only 0.8% of the babies had two minor defects, and in this subgroup, the frequency of a major defect was five times that of the general group. Of special importance were the findings in babies with three or more minor anomalies. This was found in only 0.5% of babies,[10] and 90% of them had one or more major defects as well, as depicted in Figure 4-1.

In two additional studies, Mehes and colleagues[10] and Leppig and colleagues[8] demonstrated that 26% and 19.6% of newborn infants with three or more minor anomalies, respectively, had a major malformation, a much lower incidence than that documented in the study by Marden and colleagues and most likely related to differences in study design. Based on these studies, it is concluded that any infant with three or more minor anomalies should be evaluated for a major malformation, many of which are occult.

These minor external anomalies are most common in areas of complex and variable features, such as the face, auricles, hands, and feet. Before ascribing significance to a given minor anomaly in a patient, it is important to note whether it is found in other family members. Almost any minor defect may occasionally be found as a usual feature in a particular family, as noted in Figure 4-2.

Figures 4-3 to 4-8 illustrate certain minor anomalies and allude to their developmental origin and relevance. Many, if not most, minor anomalies represent deformations caused by altered mechanical forces affecting the development of otherwise normal tissue. The reason for the deformation may be purely external uterine constraint. Thus, most minor anomalies of external ear formation at birth are constraint-induced. However, the minor deformational anomaly may be the result of a more primary malformation, and this is the presumed reason for the association between minor anomalies and major malformations.

CALVARIUM

The presence of unusually large fontanels (see standards in Chapter 5) may be a nonspecific indicator of a general lag in osseous maturation.[13] It may, for example, lead to the detection of congenital hypothyroidism in the newborn or young infant, as shown in Figure 4-9.[16] The finding of a large posterior fontanel is especially helpful in this regard, because the posterior fontanel is normally fingertip size or smaller in 97% of full-term neonates. Large fontanels may also be a feature in certain skeletal dysplasias and can, of course, be a sign of increased intracranial pressure.

DERMAL RIDGE PATTERNS (DERMATOGLYPHICS)

The parallel dermal ridges form on the palms and soles of the fetus between weeks 13 and 19. Their patterning appears to be dependent on the surface contours at the time, and the parallel dermal ridges

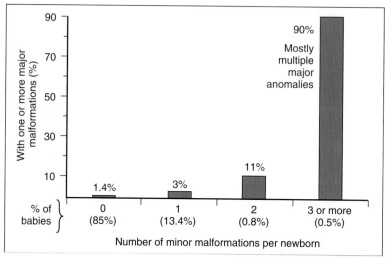

FIGURE 4-1. Frequency of major malformations in relation to the number of minor anomalies detected in a given newborn baby. (From Marden PM, Smith DW, McDonald MJ: *J Pediatr* 64:357, 1964, with permission.)

tend to develop transversely to the planes of growth stress.[11] Curvilinear arrangements occur when there is a surface mound, for example, over the fetal pads that are prominently present during early fetal life on the fingertips, on the palm between each pair of fingers, and occasionally in the hypothenar area. Indirect evidence suggests that a high fetal fingertip pad tends to give rise to a whorl pattern, a low pad yields an arch pattern, and an intermediate pad produces a loop, as illustrated in Figure 4-10*B*. The dermal ridge patterning thereby provides an indelible historical record that indicates the form of the early fetal hand (or foot). Mild to severe alterations in hand morphology occur in a variety of syndromes, and hence it is not surprising that dermatoglyphic alterations have been noted in numerous dysmorphic syndromes. These alterations have seldom been pathognomonic for a particular condition. Rather, they simply provide additional data that, viewed in relation to the total pattern of malformation, may enhance the clinician's capacity to arrive at a specific overall diagnosis. Dermal ridge patterning may be evaluated with a seven-power illuminated magnifying device, such as an otoscope, or a stamp collector's flashlight, which has a wider field of vision. Permanent records may be obtained by a variety of techniques.[3,5,17] There are two general categories of dermatoglyphic alterations: an aberrant pattern and unusual frequency or distribution of a particular pattern on the fingertips.

Aberrant Patterning

Distal Axial Palmar Triradius

Triradii occur at the junction of three sets of converging ridges (Fig. 4-10*A*). There are usually no triradii between the base of the palm and the interdigital areas of the upper palm. However, patterning in the hypothenar area often gives rise to a distal axial triradius located, by definition, greater than 35% of the distance from the wrist crease to the crease at the base of the third finger. This alteration, found in approximately 4% of whites, is a frequent feature in a number of patterns of malformation.

Open Field in Hallucal Area (Arch Tibial)

"Open field" simply means that there is a relative lack of complexity in patterning, and it thereby implies a low surface contour in that area at the time that ridges developed (see Fig. 4-10*A*). The hallucal area of the sole usually has a loop or whorl pattern, and a lack of such a pattern is unusual in the normal individual; however, it is found in approximately 50% of patients with Down syndrome and as an occasional feature in other syndromes.

Lack of Ridges

The failure of development of ridges in an area, most commonly the hypothenar region of the palm, is an occasional but nonspecific feature in de Lange syndrome.

Other Patterns

There are a number of other unusual patterns, especially in the upper palmar, hypothenar, and thenar areas, which may be of clinical significance, but these are so rarely of value in an individual case that they will not be discussed.

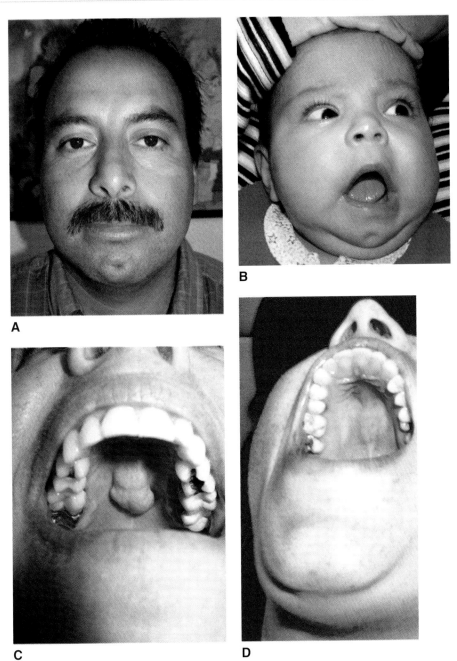

FIGURE 4-2.   An otherwise normal father (A) and daughter (B) with a pit on the chin. An otherwise normal mother (C) and daughter (D) with a torus deformity of the palate. A family history should be obtained before ascribing significance to a given minor anomaly.

Unusual Frequency or Distribution of Patterns on the Fingertips

High Frequency of Low-Arch Configurations

It is unusual to find a normal person with more than six of ten fingertips having a low-arch configuration; however, this is a frequent feature in trisomy 18 syndrome and XXXXY syndrome, presumably reflecting hypoplasia of the fetal fingertip pads in these disorders. High frequency of low arches is nonspecific, being an occasional finding in certain other syndromes and in approximately 0.9% of normal individuals.

High Frequency of Whorl Patterning

It is unusual to find nine or more fingertip whorls in an individual (3% in normal persons). Excessive

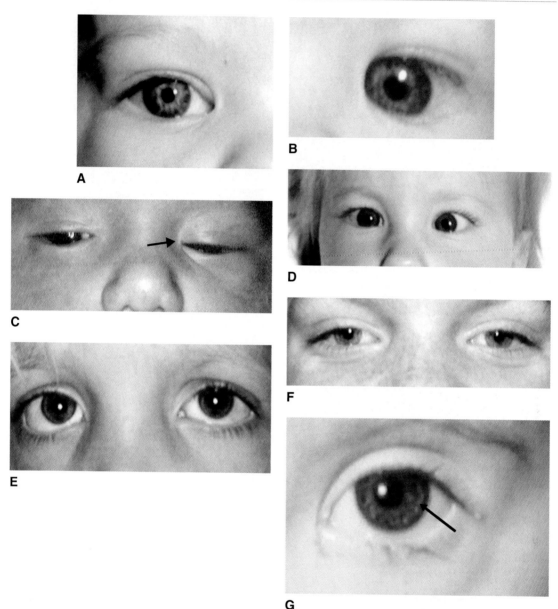

FIGURE 4-3.   Minor anomalies of the ocular region. A and B, Inner epicanthal folds appear to represent redundant folds of skin, secondary to either low nasal bridge (most common) or excess skin, as in cutis laxa. Minor folds are frequent in early infancy, and as the nasal bridge becomes more prominent, they are obliterated. C, A unilateral epicanthal fold (arrow) is indicative of torticollis. (C, From Jones MC: J Pediatr 108:702, 1986, with permission.) Slanting of the palpebral fissures seems to be secondary to the early growth rate of the brain above the eye versus that of the facial area below the eye. For example, the patient with upslanting (D) had mild microcephaly with a narrow frontal area, resulting in the upslant; the patient with downslanting (E) had maxillary hypoplasia, resulting in the downslant. Mild degrees of upslant were noted in 4% of 500 normal children. F, "Ocular hypertelorism" refers to widely spaced eyes. A low nasal bridge will often give rise to a visual impression of ocular hypertelorism. This should always be determined by measurement. Measurement of inner canthal distance, coupled with the visual distinction of whether telecanthus is present, is usually sufficient. G, Brushfield spots are speckled rings about two thirds of the distance to the periphery of the iris. There is relative lack of patterning beyond the ring. These spots are found in 20% of normal newborn babies, but they are found in 80% of babies with Down syndrome.

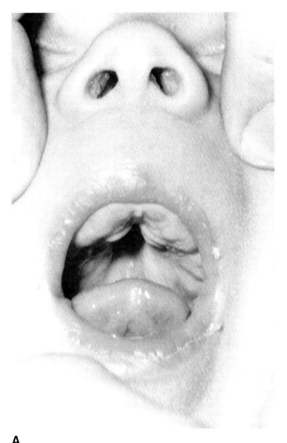

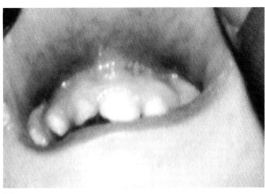

B

FIGURE 4-4.   Minor anomalies of the oral region.
A, Prominent lateral palatal ridges may be secondary to a
deficit of tongue thrust into the hard palate, allowing for
relative overgrowth of the lateral palatal ridges. This ridge
may be a feature in a variety of disorders, especially those
with hypotonia and with serious neurologic deficits
related to sucking. As such, it can be a useful sign of a
long-term deficit in function. B, Lack of lingular frenulum
and single central incisor. Indicative of holoprosencephaly.

A

patterning, presumably reflecting prominent fetal
pads, is more likely to be found in 45X syndrome,
Smith-Lemli-Opitz syndrome, occasionally in other
patterns of malformation, and in some normal
individuals.

Unusual Distribution, Especially of Radial Loop Patterns

Loops opening to the radial side of the hand are
unusual on the fourth and fifth fingers. Radial loop
patterns on these fingers are more common in
people with Down syndrome (12.4%) than in individuals who are normal (1.5%).

HAIR: ORIGIN AND RELEVANCE OF ABERRANT SCALP AND UPPER FACIAL HAIR PATTERNING AND GROWTH

The origin and relevance of hair directional patterning and aberrant hair growth[15] will be considered
individually.

Hair Directional Patterning

Normal Development and Relevance

The origin of the sloping angulation of each hair
follicle, which determines the surface hair directional patterning, is derived from the direction of
stretch on the surface skin during the time the hair
follicle is growing down from it into the loose
underlying mesenchyme, as shown in Figure 4-11.
Over the scalp and upper face, this directional patterning reflects the plane of growth stretch on the
surface skin that was exerted by the growth of
underlying structures during the period of hair follicle downgrowth, which takes place from 10 to 16
weeks of fetal life. Thus the parietal hair whorl, or
crown, is interpreted as representing the focal point
from which the posterior scalp skin was under
growth tension exerted by the dome-like outgrowth
of the early brain during this fetal period (Fig. 4-12).
Its location is normally several centimeters anterior
to the position of the posterior fontanel. Fifty-six
percent of single parietal hair whorls are located to

Text continued on page 904

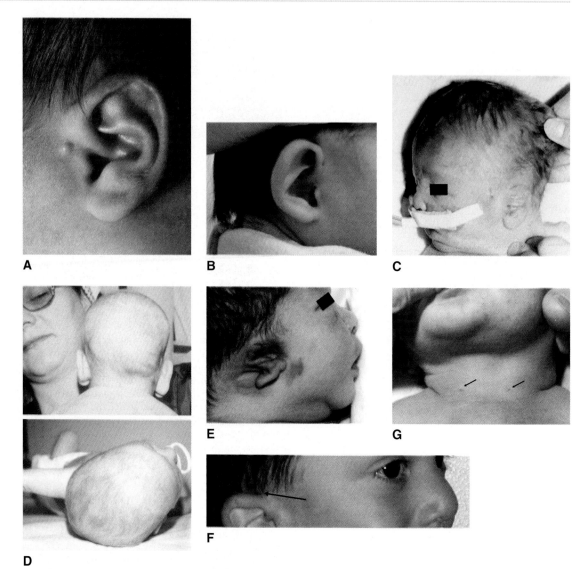

A

B

C

D

E

G

F

FIGURE 4-5. Minor anomalies of the auricular region. A, Preauricular tags, which often contain a core cartilage, appear to represent accessory hillock of His, the hillocks that normally develop in the recess of the mandibular and hyoid arches and coalesce to form the auricle. B, Preauricular pits may be familial, are twice as common in females as in males, and are more common in blacks than in whites. Both pits and tags should initiate evaluation of hearing. C, Large ears are often due to intrauterine constraint, as in this child with oligohydramnios. Asymmetric ear size can be secondary to torticollis as in D. The child's head was positioned constantly on his right side, leading to plagiocephaly and enlargement of the right ear. E, Microtia. This defect should always initiate evaluation for hearing loss. Eighty-five percent of children with unilateral microtia have an ipsilateral hearing loss, and 15% have a contralateral hearing loss as well. F, Low-set ears: This designation is made when the helix meets the cranium at a level below that of a horizontal plane that may be an extension of a line through both inner canthi. This plane may relate to the lateral vertical axis of the head. Ears slanted: This designation is made when the angle of the slope of the auricle exceeds 15 degrees from the perpendicular. Note that the findings of low placement and slanted auricle often go together and usually represent a lag in morphogenesis, since the auricle is normally in that position in early fetal life. It is important to appreciate that deformation of the head secondary to in utero constraint may temporarily distort the usual landmarks.[15] G, Branchial cleft sinuses.

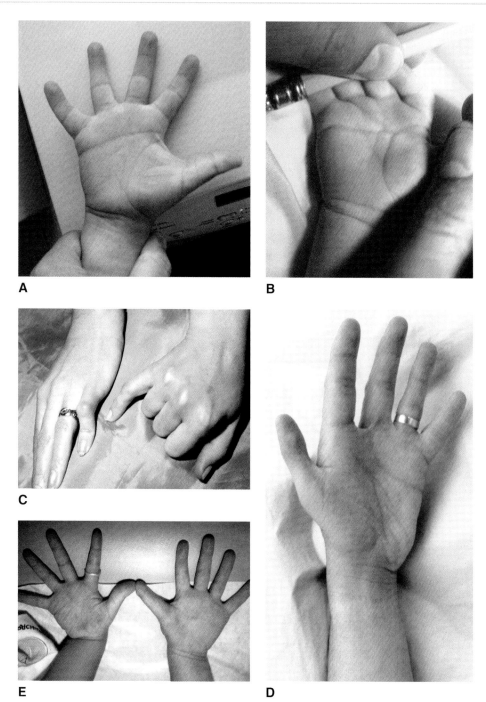

FIGURE 4-6.   Minor anomalies of the hands. A and B, Creases represent the planes of folding (flexion) of the thickened volar skin of the hand. As such, they are simply deep wrinkles. The finger creases relate to flexion at the phalangeal joints, and if there has been no flexion, as in B, there is no crease.[7] Camptodactyly (contracted fingers), depicted in B and C, most commonly affects the fifth, fourth, and third digits in decreasing order of frequency. It is presumably the consequence of relative shortness in the length of the flexor tendons with respect to the growth of the hand. The thenar crease is the consequence of oppositional flexion of the thumb; hence, if there is no oppositional flexion, there will be no crease, as in D and E.

Continued

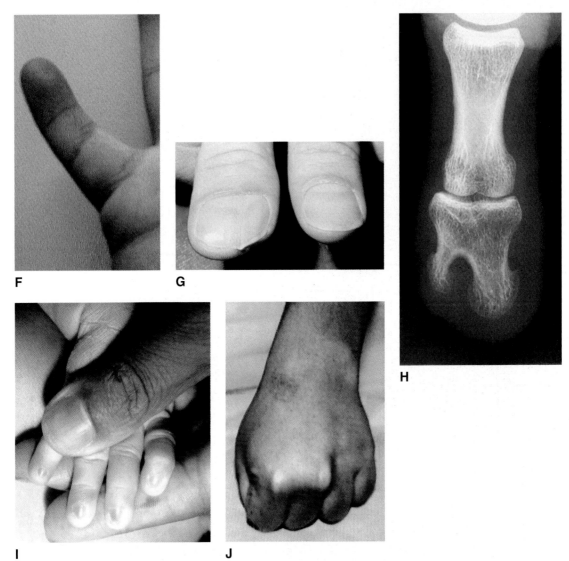

FIGURE 4-6, cont'd.   The slanting upper palmar crease reflects the palmar plane of folding related to the slope of the third, fourth, and fifth metacarpophalangeal joints. The midpalmar crease is the plane of skin folding between the upper palmar crease and the thenar crease. Any alteration in the slope of the third, fourth, and fifth metacarpophalangeal planes of flexion, or relative shortness of the palm, may give rise to but a single midpalmar plane of flexion and thereby the simian crease, as in A. This is found unilaterally in approximately 4% of normal infants and bilaterally in 1%. Davies[6] found the incidence to be 3.7% in newborn babies and noted that the simian crease is twice as common in males as in females. All degrees are found between the normal and the simian crease, including the bridged palmar crease. The creases are evident by 11 to 12 weeks of fetal life; hence, any gross alteration in crease patterning is usually indicative of an abnormality in form or function of the hand prior to 11 fetal weeks.[7] Clinodactyly (curved finger) (F) is most common in the fifth finger and is the consequence of hypoplasia of the middle phalanx, normally the last digital bone to develop. Up to 8 degrees of inturning of the fifth finger is within normal limits. Regardless of which digits are affected (fingers or toes), there is usually incurvature toward the area between the second and third digits. Partial cutaneous syndactyly represents an incomplete separation of the fingers and most commonly occurs between the third and fourth fingers and between the second and third toes. The nails generally reflect the size and shape of the underlying distal phalanx; hence, a bifid nail (G) reflects dimensions of the underlying respective phalanges (H), as does the hypoplastic nail shown in I. Malproportionment or disharmony in the length of particular segments of the hand is not uncommon. The most common is a short middle phalanx of the fifth finger with clinodactyly. F, Another anomaly is relative shortness of the fourth or fifth metacarpal or metatarsal bone. This is best appreciated in the hand by having the patient make a fist and observing the position of the knuckles, as shown in J. The altered alignment of these metacarpophalangeal joints may result in an altered palmar crease, especially the simian crease. It may also yield the impression of partial syndactyly between the third, fourth, and fifth fingers. Such relative shortness of the fourth and fifth metacarpals may develop postnatally by earlier-than-usual fusion of the respective metacarpal epiphyseal plates. When this occurs, it tends to do so in the center of the epiphyseal plate first, yielding the radiographic appearance of a cone-shaped epiphysis. This is a nonspecific anomaly that may occur by itself or as one feature of a number of syndromes.

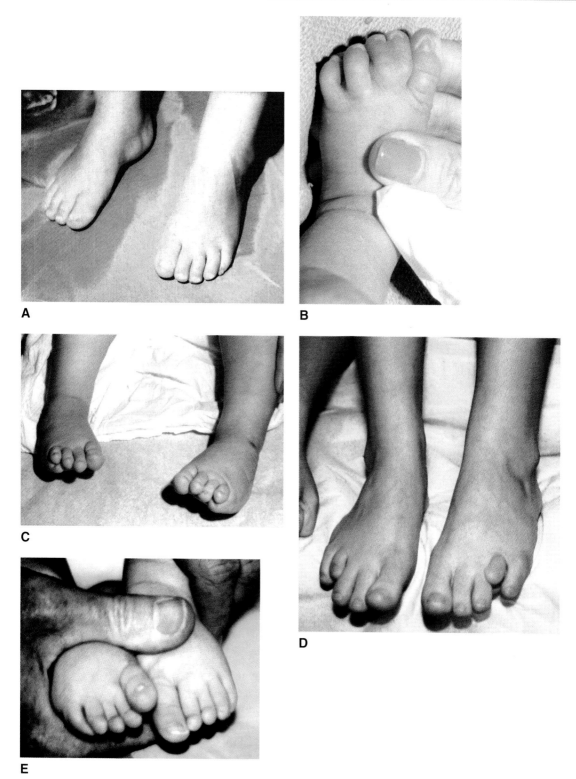

FIGURE 4-7. Minor anomalies of the feet. A and B, Syndactyly (most commonly between digits 2 and 3). If, as in A, its degree is less than one third of the distance from the base of the first phalanx to the distal end of the third, it is considered a variation of normal, whereas in B it is greater than one third of that distance and is thus considered a minor malformation. C, Clinodactyly of the fifth toe with overlapping. D, Short fourth metatarsal making the fourth toe appear short. E, Hypoplasia of nails.

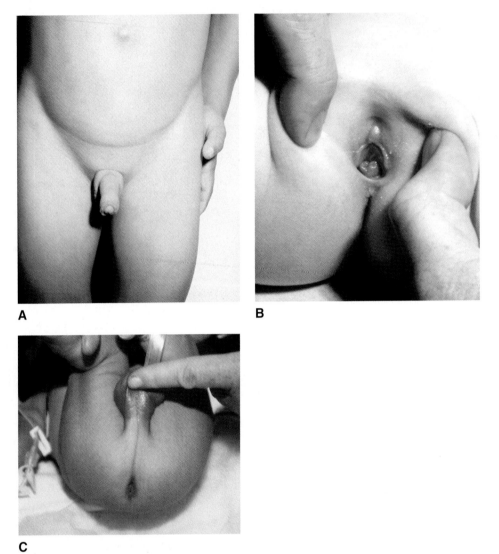

A

B

C

FIGURE 4-8.   Minor anomalies of genitalia. A, Shawl scrotum appears to represent a mild deficit in the full migration of the labial-scrotal folds and, as such, may be accompanied by other signs of incomplete masculinization of the external genitalia. This photo shows a patient with Aarskog syndrome. B, Hypoplasia of the labia, which may in some cases give rise to the false visual impression of a large clitoris. C, Median raphe is due to testosterone-induced fusion of the labioscrotal folds in a normal male. It is never seen in a 46,XX individual unless there has been abnormal secretion of androgen.

the right of the midline; 30% are left-sided, and 14% are midline in location. Five percent of normal individuals have bilateral parietal hair whorls. From the posterior whorl, the parietal hair stream flares out progressively, sweeping anteriorly to the forehead. Over the frontal region, the growth of the forebrain and the upper face results in bilateral frontal hair streams that emanate from the fixed points of the ocular puncta and tend to arc outward in a lateral direction, thereby affecting eyebrow hair directional patterning (Fig. 4-13). The anterior parietal hair stream normally converges with the upsweeping frontal hair stream on the forehead, resulting in a variety of forehead hair patterning, such as converging whorls and quadriradial patterns. If the frontal hair stream meets the parietal hair stream above the forehead, there may be an anterior upsweep of the scalp hair, known as a "cowlick." Mild-to-moderate lateral upsweep or central upsweep of the scalp hair occurs in 5% of normal individuals.

Defects of the calvarium, such as primary craniosynostosis, have not been noted to affect hair patterning, because the calvarium is not yet developed at the time of hair follicle downgrowth.

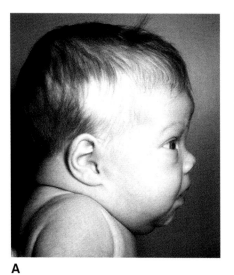
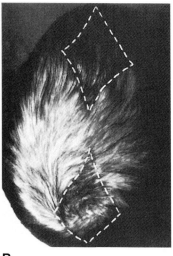

A

B

FIGURE 4-9. A and B, Unusually large fontanels, especially the posterior fontanel, in a 6-week-old baby with athyrotic hypothyroidism. The fetal onset of retarded osseous maturation is also evident in the immature facial bone development. (From Smith DW, Popich G: *J Pediatr* 80:753, 1972, with permission.)

Relevance and Nature of Aberrant Scalp and Upper Facial Hair Directional Patterning

Abnormal size or shape of the brain and upper facial area during the 10- to 16-week fetal period can result in aberrant hair patterning. Severe microcephaly may lead to a lack of a parietal hair whorl (25%) or a frontal upsweep of the scalp hair (70%), as shown in Figure 4-14. This feature appears to relate to the individual who has a narrow and smaller frontal area of the brain.

The parietal whorl is more likely to be midline and posteriorly located in patients with microcephaly, as shown in Figure 4-15. In other gross defects of early brain development, the hair directional patterning may be secondarily altered. In each case, the aberrant scalp hair patterning reflects the altered shape or growth of the early fetal brain. Gross aberrations of hair patterning often imply a serious degree of mental deficiency, because the brain is at such an early stage of development at 10 to 16 weeks (Fig. 4-16). Abnormal eyebrow patterning, such as the unusual outflaring of the medial eyebrows of the patient shown in Figure 4-17, implies that there was abnormal shape or growth in the upper midface before or during the period of hair follicle downgrowth, which occurs from 10 to 16 weeks of fetal development.

Hair Growth Patterns

Normal Development and Relevance

At 18 fetal weeks, when hair first emerges, it grows on the entire face and scalp. Later, the eyebrows and scalp hair predominate, and the growth of hair over the remainder of the face is suppressed. Studies imply that there is a periocular zone of hair growth suppression.

Nature and Relevance of Aberrant Facial Hair Growth Patterns

The V-shaped midline, downward projection of the scalp hair, known as the "widow's peak," is considered to represent an upper forehead intersection of the bilateral fields of periocular hair growth suppression.[14] This may occur because the fields are widely spaced, as in ocular hypertelorism, or because the ocular fields of hair growth suppression are smaller with a low-scalp hairline and low position of intersection, as illustrated in Figure 4-18. In the presence of cryptophthalmos, there may be an abnormal projection of scalp-like hair growth toward the ocular area (Fig. 4-19). The auricle appears to influence hair growth in the region anterior to the ear. With absence of the auricle, there is usually absence of hair growth in the sideburn area (Fig. 4-20) anterior to the ear. When there is a rudimentary ear, such as is often found in Treacher Collins syndrome, there may be an aberrant tongue of hair growth projecting onto the cheek area.

Usually, a short neck or webbed neck may be associated with the secondary feature of a low posterior hairline, especially at the lateral borders, as shown in Figure 4-21.

It is not yet known whether the facial body hirsutism found in patients with de Lange syndrome and in patients with various other failure-to-thrive growth deficiency disorders represents a more

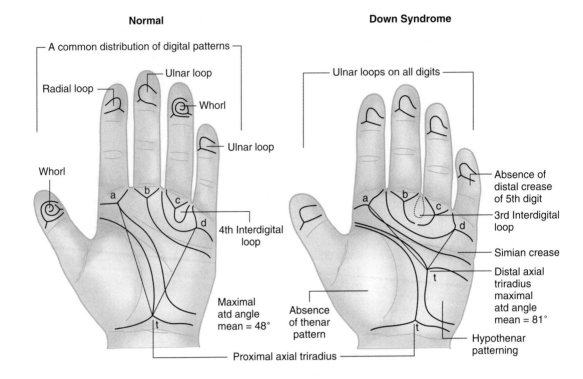

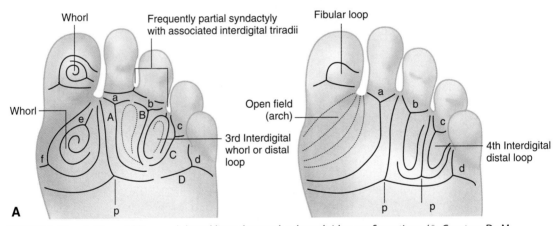

FIGURE 4-10.   A, The solid lines and dotted lines denote the dermal ridge configurations. (**A,** Courtesy Dr. M. Bat-Miriam; prepared by Mr. R. Lee of the Kennedy-Galton Center near St. Albans, England.)

Continued

generalized failure of normal growth suppression in these conditions.

OTHER CUTANEOUS ANOMALIES

Cutaneous features such as unusual dimples and punched-out scalp lesions are shown in Figure 4-22. The skin normally grows in response to the growth of the structure that it invests. Tangential traction on the skin produced by external constraint can lead to redundant skin (Fig. 4-23).[1] Differentiation between talipes equinovarus caused by intrauterine constraint and talipes equinovarus caused by a neurologic problem that limits joint mobility can sometimes be made by observing the skin, which in the latter situation is taut and thin, secondary to early onset of lack of movement in a fetus that has had ample space to move.

Text continued on page 912

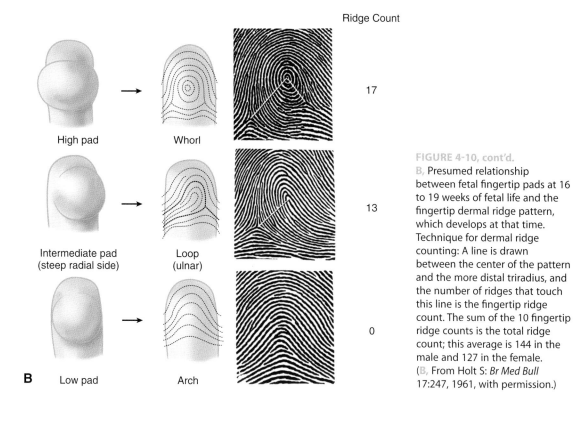

Ridge Count

17

13

0

B

High pad → Whorl

Intermediate pad (steep radial side) → Loop (ulnar)

Low pad → Arch

FIGURE 4-10, cont'd. B, Presumed relationship between fetal fingertip pads at 16 to 19 weeks of fetal life and the fingertip dermal ridge pattern, which develops at that time. Technique for dermal ridge counting: A line is drawn between the center of the pattern and the more distal triradius, and the number of ridges that touch this line is the fingertip ridge count. The sum of the 10 fingertip ridge counts is the total ridge count; this average is 144 in the male and 127 in the female. (B, From Holt S: Br Med Bull 17:247, 1961, with permission.)

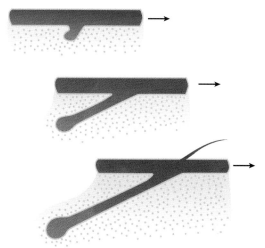

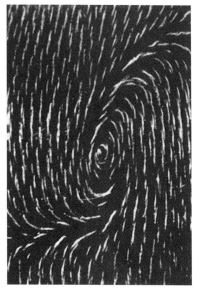

FIGURE 4-11.   Hair follicles over the scalp begin their downgrowth into the loose underlying mesenchyme at 10 fetal weeks. The slope of each hair follicle, and thereby the hair directional patterning, is determined by the direction of growth stretch (arrows) exerted on the surface skin by the development of underlying tissues. For the scalp hair, the patterning relates to the growth in size and form of the underlying brain during the period of 10 to 16 weeks. By 18 weeks, when hairs are extruded onto the surface, their patterning is set. (From Smith DW, Gong BT: Teratology 9:17, 1974. Copyright © 1974. Reprinted with permission of Wiley-Liss, Inc., a subsidiary of John Wiley & Sons, Inc.)

FIGURE 4-12.   Parietal hair whorl at 18 weeks. This appears to be the fixed focal point from which the skin is being stretched by the dome-like outgrowth of the brain between 10 and 16 weeks. (From Smith DW, Gong BT: Teratology 9:17, 1974. Copyright © 1974. Reprinted with permission of Wiley-Liss, Inc., a subsidiary of John Wiley & Sons, Inc.)

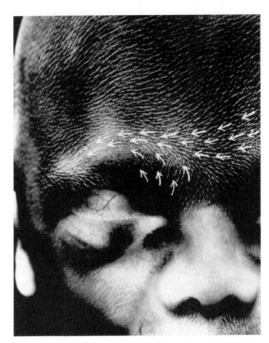

FIGURE 4-13. Frontal hair stream at 18 weeks, arcing laterally from the ocular punctum to meet with the downsweeping parietal hair stream. The frontal hair stream has been influenced by the growth of the underlying upper facial structures and the forebrain. (From Smith DW, Gong BT: *Teratology* 9:17, 1974. Copyright © 1974. Reprinted with permission of Wiley-Liss, Inc., a subsidiary of John Wiley & Sons, Inc.)

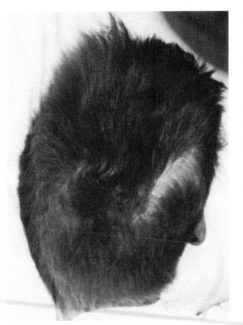 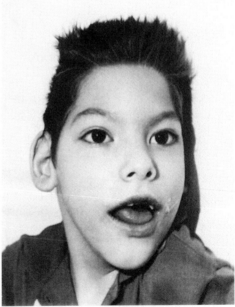

FIGURE 4-14. Hair patterning in a patient with primary microcephaly. The posterior scalp shows a lack of concise whorl, and the anterior scalp shows a marked frontal upsweep. These findings are interpreted as being the consequence of a deficit in growth of the brain before and during the period of hair follicle development and thus imply an early defect in morphogenesis of the brain before 10 to 16 weeks. (From Smith DW, Gong BT: *Teratology* 9:17, 1974. Copyright © 1974. Reprinted with permission of Wiley-Liss, Inc., a subsidiary of John Wiley & Sons, Inc.)

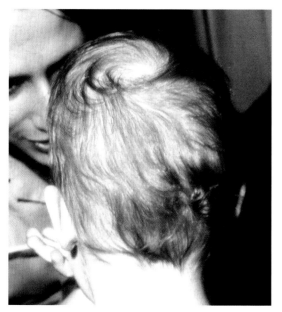

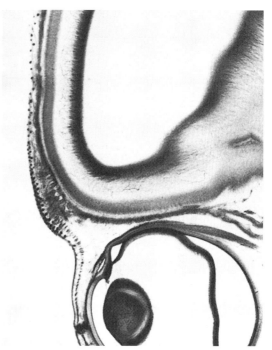

FIGURE 4-15.   Posterior scalp hair of the type more commonly found in mild microcephaly, in this instance, Down syndrome. The parietal whorl tends to be more central and posterior than usual, being over the former position of the posterior fontanel. This is considered secondary to the brain having been smaller and more symmetric than usual at 10 to 16 weeks, the time when the hair follicles develop. (From Smith DW, Gong BT: *Teratology* 9:17, 1974. Copyright © 1974. Reprinted with permission of Wiley-Liss, Inc., a subsidiary of John Wiley & Sons, Inc.)

FIGURE 4-16.   Sagittal section of forebrain area of a 10-week-old fetus, showing the early stage of cerebral cortical development and the lack of any organized calvarium at the time the hair follicles are beginning their downgrowth. (From Smith DW, Gong BT: *Teratology* 9:17, 1974. Copyright © 1974. Reprinted with permission of Wiley-Liss, Inc., a subsidiary of John Wiley & Sons, Inc.)

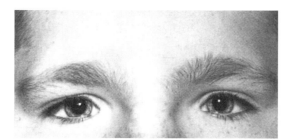

FIGURE 4-17.   Aberrant mid-eyebrow patterning, which implies an aberration in growth or form of underlying facial structures by 10 to 16 fetal weeks. This patient has Waardenburg syndrome, in which aberrant mid-upper facial development is a usual feature.

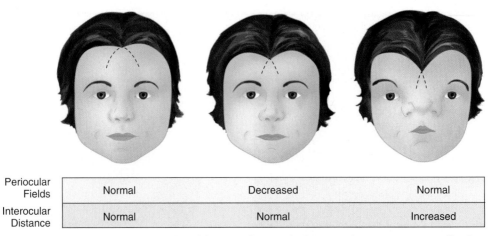

Periocular Fields	Normal	Decreased	Normal
Interocular Distance	Normal	Normal	Increased

FIGURE 4-18.   If the eyes are widely spaced, or if the area of periocular hair growth suppression is smaller than usual, the bilateral zones of periocular hair growth suppression may overlap at a lower point than usual, allowing for the presence of a widow's peak. The drawing on the right is of a patient with the frontonasal dysplasia anomaly. (From Smith DW, Cohen MM Jr: *Lancet* 2:1127, 1973, with permission.)

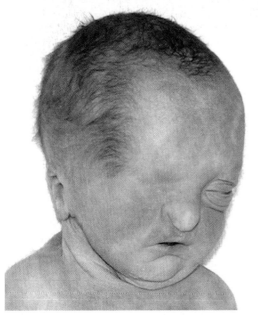

FIGURE 4-19.   Aberrant growth of hair in lateral forehead area, related to the cryptophthalmos anomaly. (From Bergsma D, McKusick VA, editors: National Foundation—Birth Defects, Baltimore, 1973, Williams & Wilkins, p 27, with permission.)

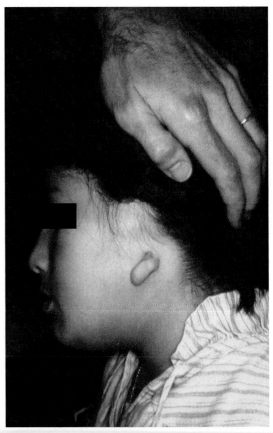

FIGURE 4-20.   Lack of preauricular (sideburn) hair growth in relation to a deficit of auricular development.

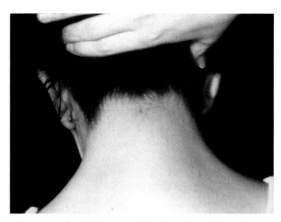

FIGURE 4-21.   Low posterior hairline, usually related to either a short or webbed neck.

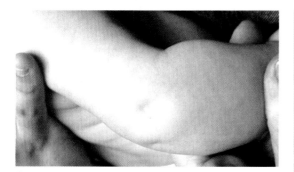

A

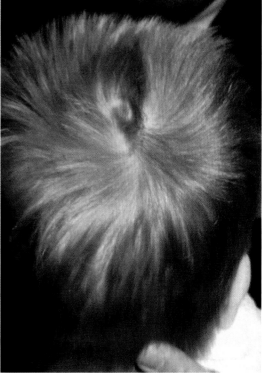

B

FIGURE 4-22.   A, Unusual dimples may occur at a location where there has been a closer than usual proximity between the skin and underlying bony structures during fetal life, resulting in deficient development of subcutaneous tissue at that locus. Such dimples may be secondary either to a deficit in early subcutaneous tissue or to an aberrant bony promontory. They tend to occur at the elbows, at the knees, over the acromion promontories, and over the lower sacrum. B, Punched-out scalp lesions are most commonly found toward the midline in the posterior parietal scalp area. The skin is usually totally lacking, but the crater becomes covered with scar tissue postnatally. The developmental pathology for these lesions is unknown.

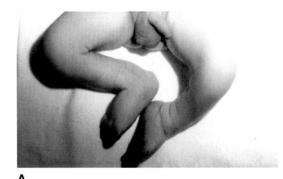

A

FIGURE 4-23. Redundant skin (A) is indicative of tangential traction produced by external constraint. Compare the redundant skin in A to the tight, thin skin over the joints in B, which is indicative of early onset lack of mobility secondary to neurologic impairment.

B

References

1. Aase JM: Structural defects as a consequence of late intrauterine constraint: Craniotabes, loose skin and asymmetric ear size, Semin Perinatol 7:237, 1983.
2. Aase JM: Diagnostic Dysmorphology, New York, 1990, Plenum Medical.
3. Aase JM, Lyons RB: Technique for recording dermatoglyphics, Lancet 1:32, 1971.
4. Davies P: Sex and the single transverse crease in newborn singletons, Dev Med Child Neurol 8:729, 1966.
5. Ford-Walker N: Inkless methods of finger, palm and sole printing, J Pediatr 50:27, 1957.
6. Graham JM: Recognizable Patterns of Human Deformation, ed 2, Philadelphia, 1988, WB Saunders.
7. Jones MC: Unilateral epicanthal folds: Diagnostic significance, J Pediatr 108:702, 1986.
8. Leppig KA, et al: Predictive value of minor anomalies: Association with major malformations, J Pediatr 110:530, 1987.
9. Marden PM, Smith DW, McDonald MJ: Congenital anomalies in the newborn infant, including minor variations, J Pediatr 64:357, 1964.
10. Mehes K, et al: Minor malformation in the neonate, Helv Pediatr Acta 28:477, 1973.
11. Mulvihill J, Smith DW: Genesis of dermal ridge patterning, J Pediatr 75, 1969.
12. Popich GA, Smith DW: The genesis and significance of digital and palmar hand creases: Preliminary report, J Pediatr 77:1917, 1970.
13. Popich GA, Smith DW: Fontanels: Range of normal size, J Pediatr 80:479, 1972.
14. Smith DW, Cohen MM Jr: Widow's peak scalp anomaly, origin and relevance to ocular hypertelorism, Lancet 2:1127, 1973.
15. Smith DW, Gong BT: Scalp hair patterning as a clue to early fetal brain development, J Pediatr 83:374, 1973, and Teratology 9:17, 1974.
16. Smith DW, Popich GA: Large fontanels in congenital hypothyroidism: A potential clue toward earlier recognition, J Pediatr 80:753, 1972.
17. Uchida IA, Soltan HC: Evaluation of dermatoglyphics in medical genetics, Pediatr Clin North Am 10:409, 1963.

CHAPTER 5

Normal Standards

The following compilation of normal measurements is set forth as an aid in determining whether or not a given feature is abnormal. Such data may be especially useful when the visual impression is potentially misleading. For example, when the nasal bridge is low, the visual impression may falsely suggest ocular hypertelorism, and when the patient is obese, the hands may appear to be small. Besides comparing patient measurements with these normal cross-sectional population standards, it may be important to contrast the findings of the patient with those of his parents or siblings in an attempt to determine whether or not a given feature is unusual for that particular family.

These measurements have been obtained predominantly from whites; hence, they may not be accurate for other racial groups. Separate data are presented for males and females, except for features that do not show significant differences between the sexes. For paired structures, the measurements are given for the right side. Many of the charts were kindly supplied by Dr. Murray Feingold from his Boston study of normal measurements. For normal measurements of structures not included in this chapter, the reader is referred to Hall and colleagues' *Handbook of Normal Physical Measurements*.[1]

STANDARDS FOR HEIGHT AND WEIGHT

The growth charts for children (Figs. 5-1 to 5-12) were developed by the National Center for Health Statistics in collaboration with the National Center for Chronic Disease Prevention and Health Promotion.

Notes on Use

1. Weight is preferably taken in the nude; otherwise, the estimated weight of clothing is subtracted before plotting.
2. When a child is born earlier than 37 weeks' gestation, the birth weight is plotted at the appropriate number of weeks on the preterm growth chart. Subsequent weights are plotted in relation to this "conception age"; thus, for a child born at 32 weeks, the 8-weeks-after-birth weight is plotted at B (birth) on the scale, the 12-week weight at 4 weeks after B, and so on. Length is plotted in the same manner.
3. Supine length (up to age 2.0 years) should be taken with the infant lying on a measuring table constructed for this purpose. One person holds the infant's head so that he looks straight upward (the lower borders of the eye sockets and the external auditory meati should be in the same vertical plane) and pulls very gently to bring the top of the head into contact with the fixed measuring board. A second person, the measurer, presses the infant's knees down into contact with the board, and, also pulling gently to stretch the infant out, holds the infant's feet, with the toes pointing directly upward. The measurer brings the movable footboard to rest firmly against the infant's heels and reads the measurement to the last completed 0.1 cm.
4. Standing height should be taken without shoes, the child standing with heels and back in contact with an upright wall or, preferably, a statometer made for this purpose. His head is held so that he looks straight forward, with the lower borders of the eye sockets on the same horizontal plane as the external auditory meati (i.e., head not with nose tipped upward). A right-angled block (preferably counterweighted) is slid down the wall until its bottom surface touches the child's head, and a scale fixed to the wall is read. During this measurement, the child should be told to stretch his neck to be as tall as possible, although care must be taken to prevent his heels from coming off the ground. The measurer should apply gentle but firm upward pressure under the mastoid processes to help the child stretch. In this way, the variation

913

in height from morning to evening is minimized. Standing height should be recorded to the last completed 0.1 cm.

OTHER STANDARDS

The reader will find charts showing normal measurements for head circumference, chest, hand, foot, inner and outer canthal distances, palpebral fissure length, fontanel, ear, penis, and testis (Figs. 5-13 to 5-25) after the growth charts.

Reference

1.   Hall JG, et al: Handbook of Normal Physical Measurements, New York, 1989, Oxford University Press.

CDC Growth Charts: United States

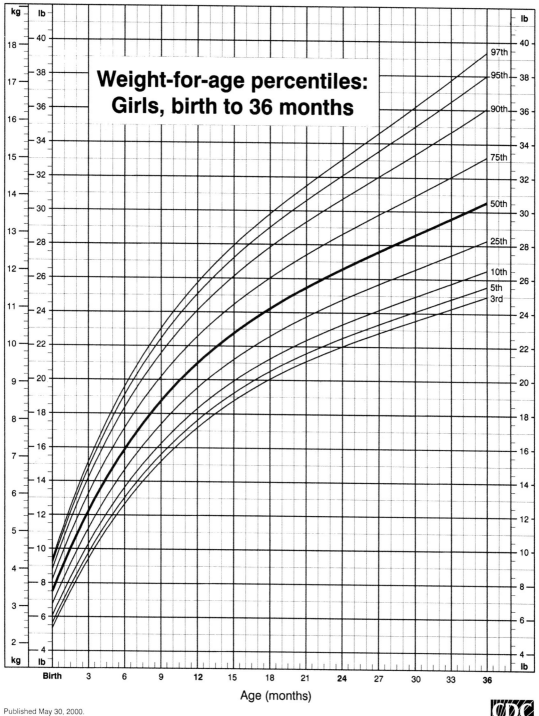

FIGURE 5-1. Weight-for-age percentiles: girls, birth to 36 months. (Developed by the National Center for Health Statistics in collaboration with the National Center for Chronic Disease Prevention and Health Promotion [2000].)

CDC Growth Charts: United States

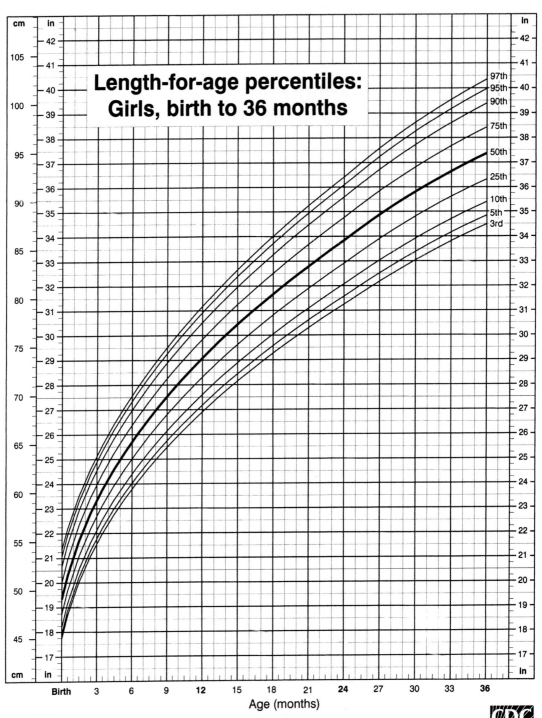

Length-for-age percentiles: Girls, birth to 36 months

Age (months)

Published May 30, 2000.
SOURCE: Developed by the National Center for Health Statistics in collaboration with the National Center for Chronic Disease Prevention and Health Promotion (2000).

SAFER · HEALTHIER · PEOPLE™

FIGURE 5-2. Length-for-age percentiles: girls, birth to 36 months. (Developed by the National Center for Health Statistics in collaboration with the National Center for Chronic Disease Prevention and Health Promotion [2000].)

CDC Growth Charts: United States

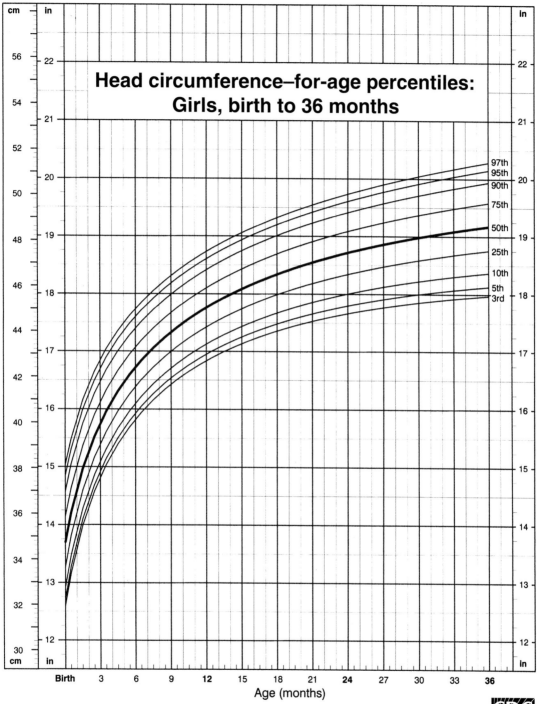

Head circumference–for-age percentiles:
Girls, birth to 36 months

Published May 30, 2000.
SOURCE: Developed by the National Center for Health Statistics in collaboration with
the National Center for Chronic Disease Prevention and Health Promotion (2000).

FIGURE 5-3.   Head circumference–for-age percentiles: girls, birth to 36 months. (Developed by the National Center for Health Statistics in collaboration with the National Center for Chronic Disease Prevention and Health Promotion [2000].)

CDC Growth Charts: United States

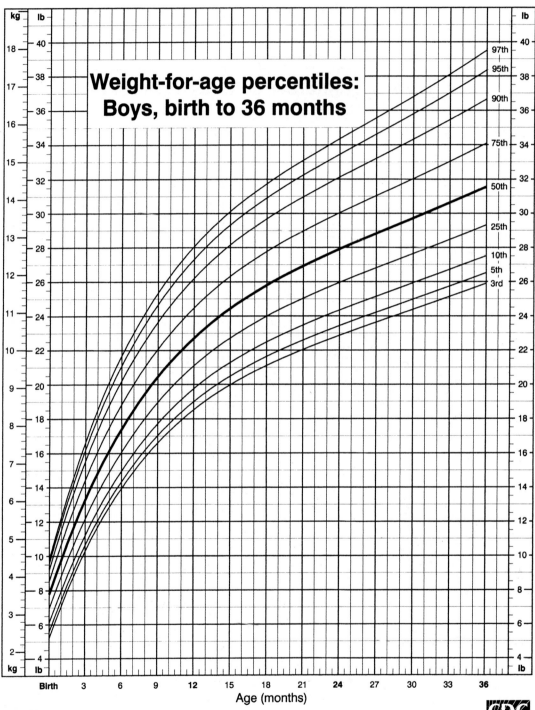

Published May 30, 2000.
SOURCE: Developed by the National Center for Health Statistics in collaboration with
the National Center for Chronic Disease Prevention and Health Promotion (2000).

FIGURE 5-4.   Weight-for-age percentiles: boys, birth to 36 months. (Developed by the National Center for Health Statistics in collaboration with the National Center for Chronic Disease Prevention and Health Promotion [2000].)

CDC Growth Charts: United States

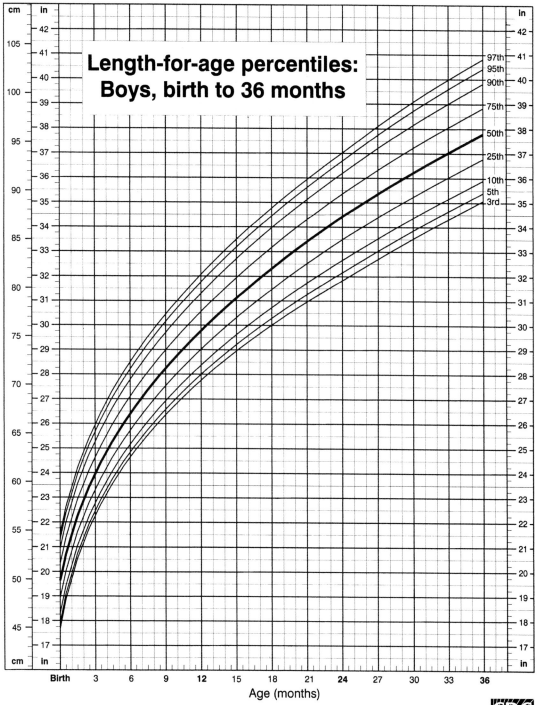

Length-for-age percentiles: Boys, birth to 36 months

Published May 30, 2000.
SOURCE: Developed by the National Center for Health Statistics in collaboration with
the National Center for Chronic Disease Prevention and Health Promotion (2000).

FIGURE 5-5. Length-for-age percentiles: boys, birth to 36 months. (Developed by the National Center for Health Statistics in collaboration with the National Center for Chronic Disease Prevention and Health Promotion [2000].)

CDC Growth Charts: United States

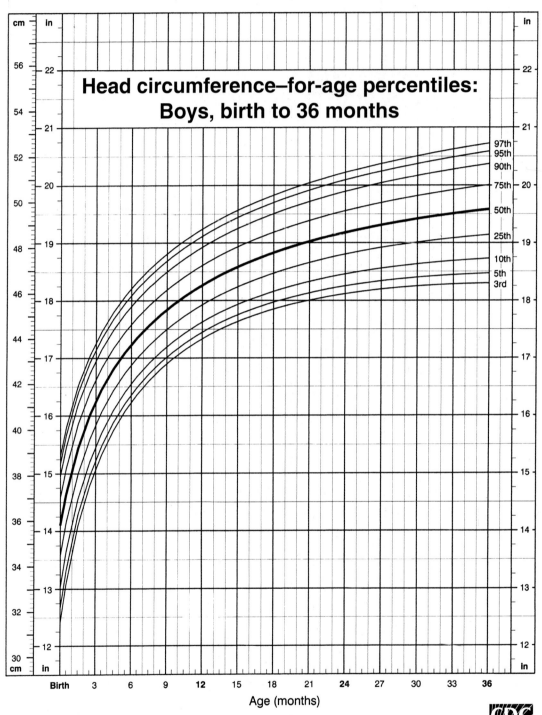

Published May 30, 2000.
SOURCE: Developed by the National Center for Health Statistics in collaboration with
the National Center for Chronic Disease Prevention and Health Promotion (2000).

FIGURE 5-6. Head circumference–for-age percentiles: boys, birth to 36 months. (Developed by the National Center for Health Statistics in collaboration with the National Center for Chronic Disease Prevention and Health Promotion [2000].)

CDC Growth Charts: United States

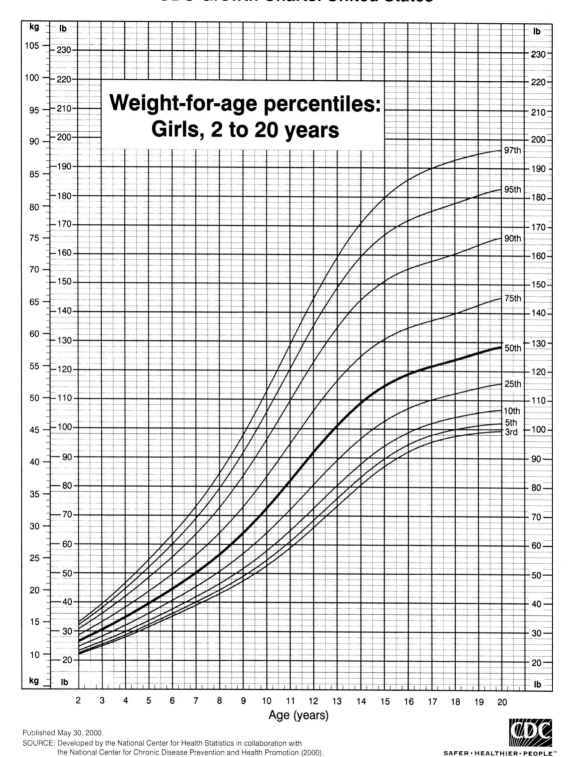

Weight-for-age percentiles: Girls, 2 to 20 years

Published May 30, 2000.
SOURCE: Developed by the National Center for Health Statistics in collaboration with the National Center for Chronic Disease Prevention and Health Promotion (2000).

SAFER·HEALTHIER·PEOPLE™

FIGURE 5-7. Weight-for-age percentiles: girls, 2 to 20 years. (Developed by the National Center for Health Statistics in collaboration with the National Center for Chronic Disease Prevention and Health Promotion [2000].)

CDC Growth Charts: United States

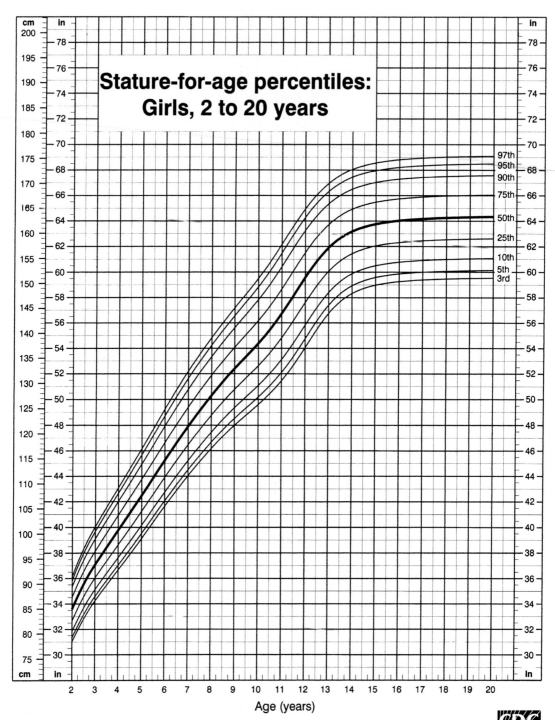

Stature-for-age percentiles:
Girls, 2 to 20 years

Published May 30, 2000.
SOURCE: Developed by the National Center for Health Statistics in collaboration with
the National Center for Chronic Disease Prevention and Health Promotion (2000).

SAFER · HEALTHIER · PEOPLE™

FIGURE 5-8. Stature-for-age percentiles: girls, 2 to 20 years. (Developed by the National Center for Health Statistics in collaboration with the National Center for Chronic Disease Prevention and Health Promotion [2000].)

CDC Growth Charts: United States

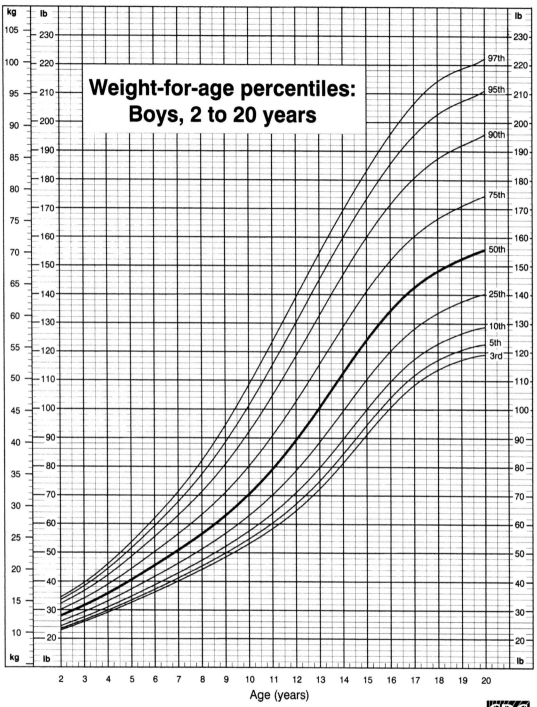

Weight-for-age percentiles: Boys, 2 to 20 years

Age (years)

Published May 30, 2000.
SOURCE: Developed by the National Center for Health Statistics in collaboration with the National Center for Chronic Disease Prevention and Health Promotion (2000).

SAFER·HEALTHIER·PEOPLE™

FIGURE 5-9. Weight-for-age percentiles: boys, 2 to 20 years. (Developed by the National Center for Health Statistics in collaboration with the National Center for Chronic Disease Prevention and Health Promotion [2000].)

CDC Growth Charts: United States

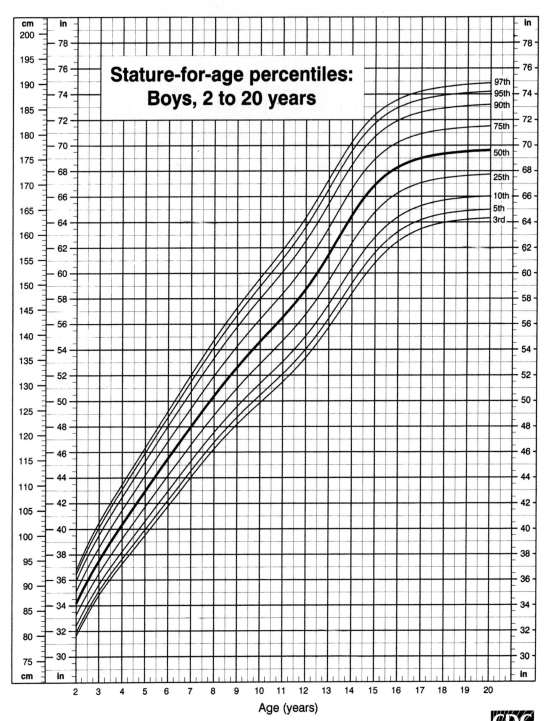

Stature-for-age percentiles: Boys, 2 to 20 years

Published May 30, 2000.
SOURCE: Developed by the National Center for Health Statistics in collaboration with
the National Center for Chronic Disease Prevention and Health Promotion (2000).

SAFER · HEALTHIER · PEOPLE™

FIGURE 5-10. Stature-for-age percentiles: boys, 2 to 20 years. (Developed by the National Center for Health Statistics in collaboration with the National Center for Chronic Disease Prevention and Health Promotion [2000].)

CDC Growth Charts: United States

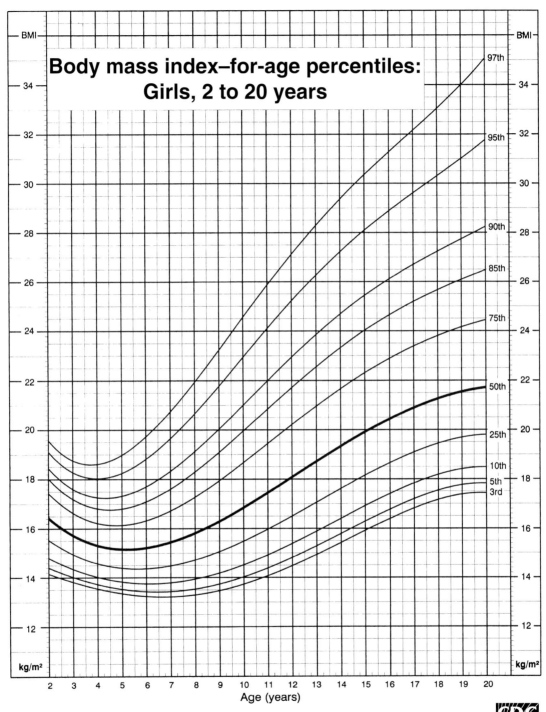

FIGURE 5-11.   Body mass index–for-age percentiles: girls, 2 to 20 years. (Developed by the National Center for Health Statistics in collaboration with the National Center for Chronic Disease Prevention and Health Promotion [2000].)

CDC Growth Charts: United States

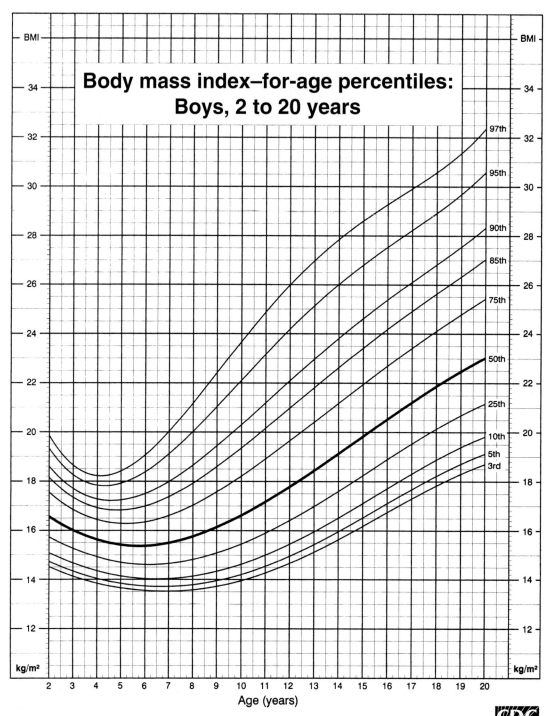

Body mass index–for-age percentiles: Boys, 2 to 20 years

Published May 30, 2000.
SOURCE: Developed by the National Center for Health Statistics in collaboration with the National Center for Chronic Disease Prevention and Health Promotion (2000).

SAFER·HEALTHIER·PEOPLE™

FIGURE 5-12. Body mass index–for-age percentiles: boys, 2 to 20 years. (Developed by the National Center for Health Statistics in collaboration with the National Center for Chronic Disease Prevention and Health Promotion [2000].)

HEAD CIRCUMFERENCES

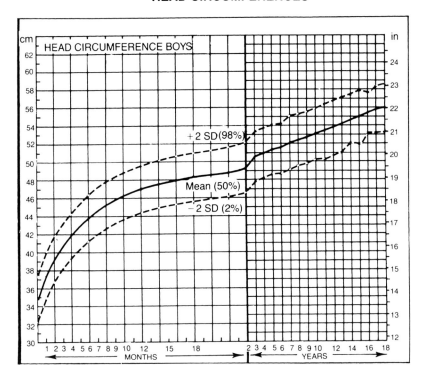

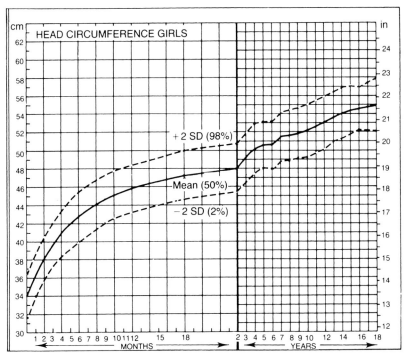

FIGURE 5-13.   Head circumferences. (From Nellhaus G: *Pediatrics* 41:106, 1968. University of Colorado Medical Center Printing Services.)

CHEST MEASUREMENTS

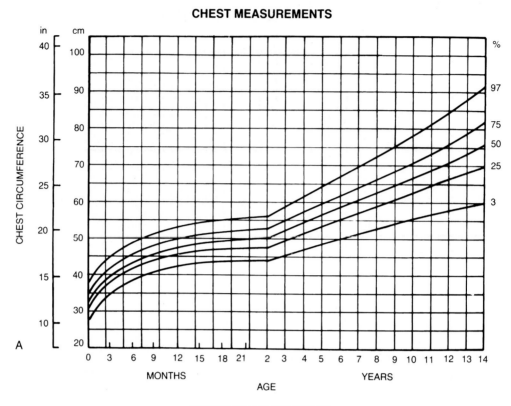

A

CHEST MEASUREMENTS

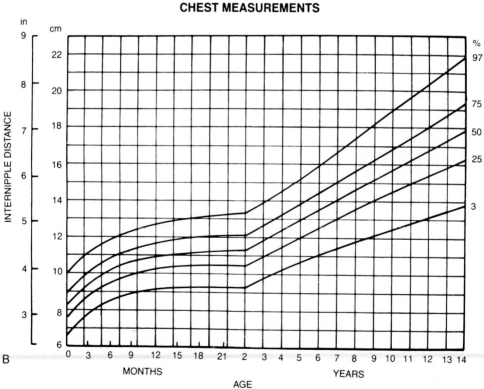

B

FIGURE 5-14.   Chest circumference (A) and internipple distance (B). (From Feingold M, Bossert WH: *Birth Defects* 10[Suppl 13], 1974. With permission of the copyright holder, March of Dimes Birth Defects Foundation.)

HAND MEASUREMENTS

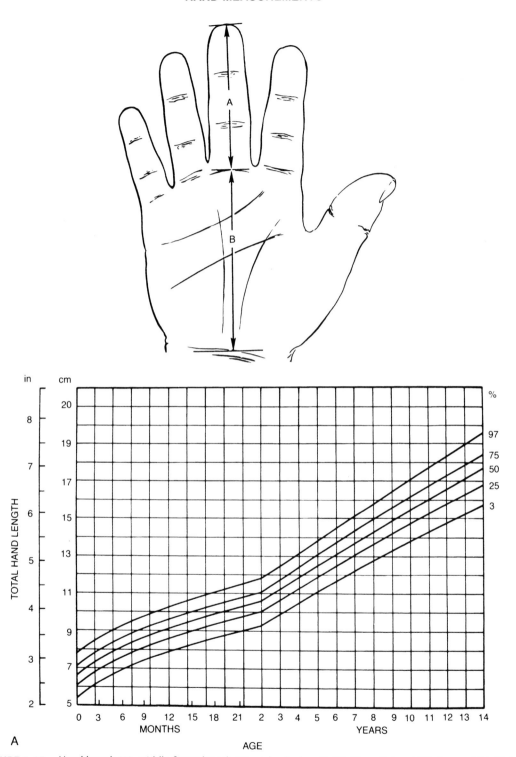

FIGURE 5-15.   Hand length (A), middle finger length (B), and palm length (C). (From Feingold M, Bossert WH: *Birth Defects* 10[Suppl 13], 1974. With permission of the copyright holder, March of Dimes Birth Defects Foundation.)

Continued

HAND MEASUREMENTS

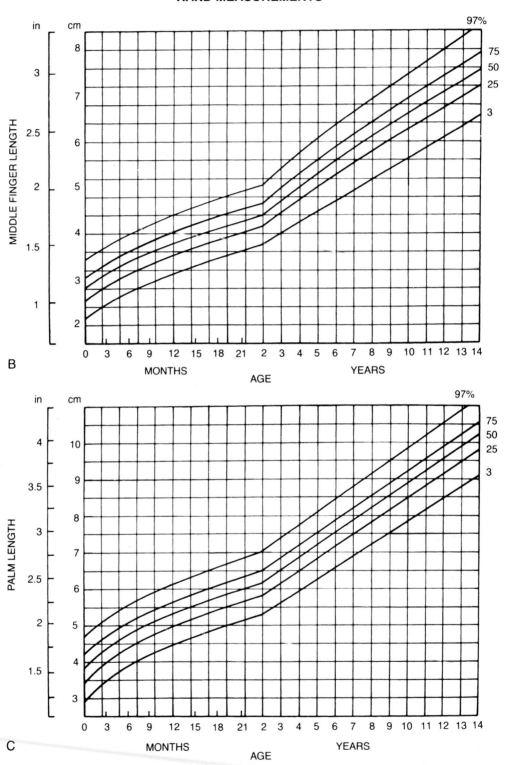

FIGURE 5-15, cont'd

HAND MEASUREMENTS

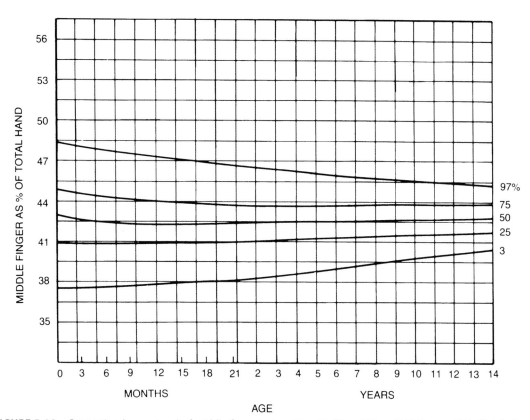

FIGURE 5-16.   Proportion (percentage) of middle finger to hand length. (From Feingold M, Bossert WH: *Birth Defects* 10[Suppl 13], 1974. With permission of the copyright holder, March of Dimes Birth Defects Foundation.)

FOOT LENGTH

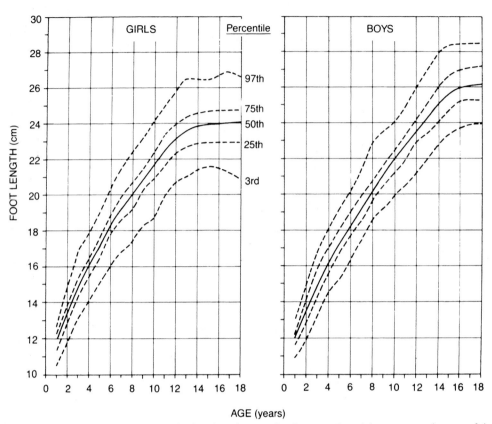

AGE (years)

FIGURE 5-17. Mean and percentile values for foot length. Note that because the adolescent growth spurt of the foot usually begins prior to the general linear growth spurt and ends before final height attainment, the foot growth spurt is a good early indicator of adolescence. (Adapted from Blais MM, Green WT, Anderson M: *J Bone Joint Surg Am* 38-A:998, 1956, with permission.)

FACIAL MEASUREMENTS

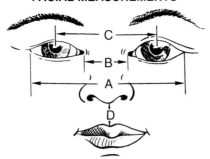

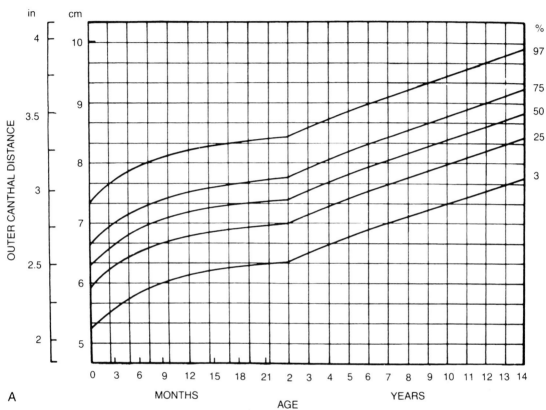

A

Continued

FACIAL MEASUREMENTS

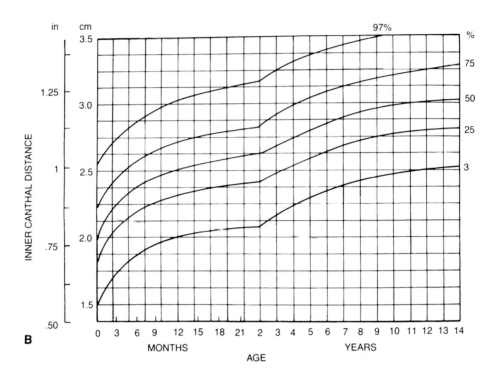

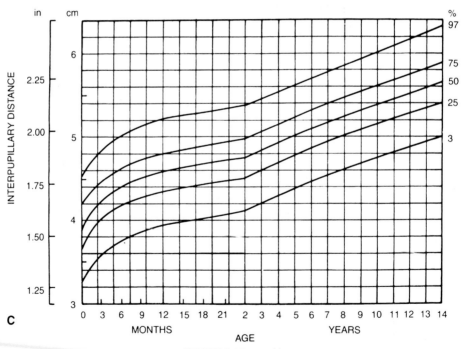

FIGURE 5-18, cont'd

EYE MEASUREMENTS

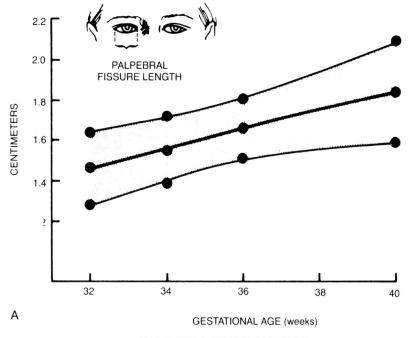

A

GESTATIONAL AGE (weeks)

PALPEBRAL FISSURE LENGTH

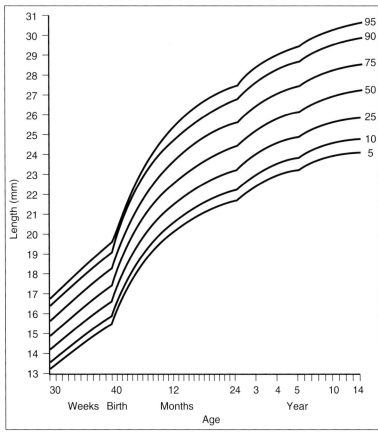

FIGURE 5-19.   A, Palpebral fissure length, 32 to 40 weeks. (From Jones KL et al: *J Pediatric* 92:787, 1978, with permission.) B, Relationship of palpebral fissure length to age in white American children. (From Thomas IT, Gaitantzis YA, Frias JL: *J Pediatr* 111:267–268, 1987, with permission.)

B

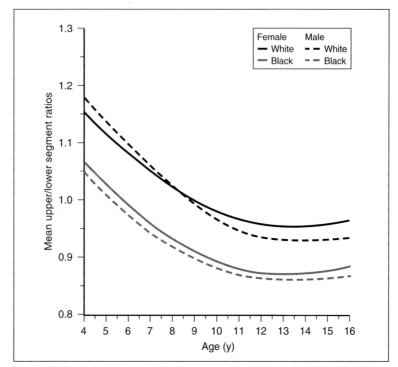

FIGURE 5-20.   Ethnic differences in mean upper-to-lower segment ratios. (Data from McKusick VA: *Heritable Disorders of Connective Tissue*, ed 4, St. Louis, 1971, Mosby.)

EAR LENGTH

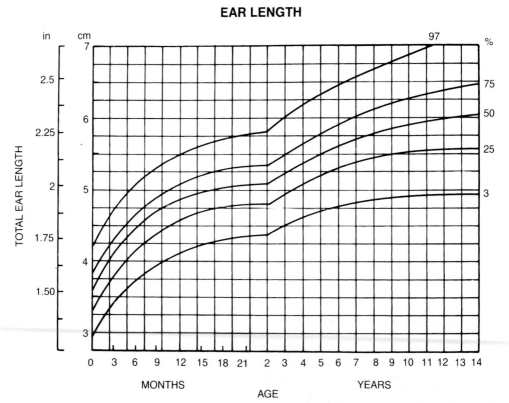

FIGURE 5-21.   Maximum ear length. (From Feingold M, Bossert WH: *Birth Defects* 10[Suppl 13], 1974. With permission of the copyright holder, March of Dimes Birth Defects Foundation.)

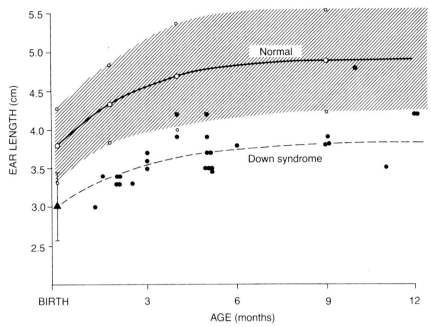

FIGURE 5-22. Ear length in normal babies during the first year, showing mean and 2 standard deviations in the hatched area, as contrasted with ear length in Down syndrome, showing mean and 2 standard deviations for 26 affected newborns and individual values (*black dots*) during the first year. (From Aase JM et al: *J Pediatr* 82:845, 1973, with permission.)

PENILE LENGTH

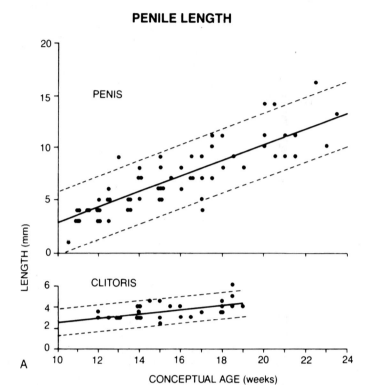

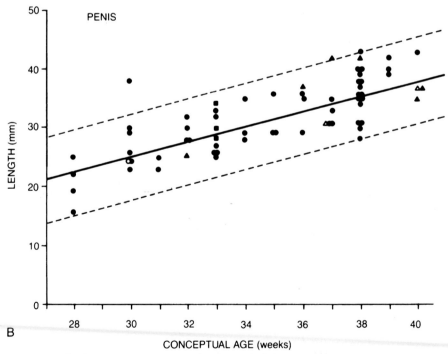

FIGURE 5-23.   **A,** Growth of the penis contrasted with growth of the clitoris from formalin-fixed fetuses. **B,** Penile stretched length (from pubic bone to tip of glans) in the newborn. The mean full-term length is 3.5 cm with a 2 standard deviation range, from 2.8 to 4.2 cm. The *solid line* approximates the mean values, and the *broken lines* the 2 standard deviation values. (From Feldman KW, Smith DW: *J Pediatr* 86:395, 1975, with permission.)

PENILE AND TESTICULAR GROWTH

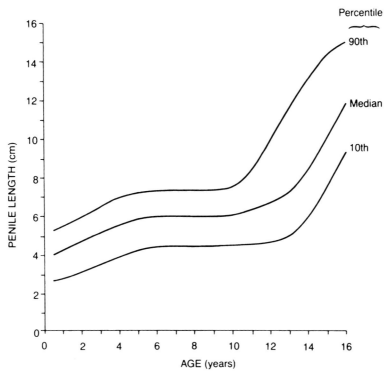

FIGURE 5-24. Penile growth in stretched length (from the pubic ramus to the tip of the glans) from infancy into adolescence. (From Schonfeld WA: *Am J Dis Child* 65:535, 1943, with permission.)

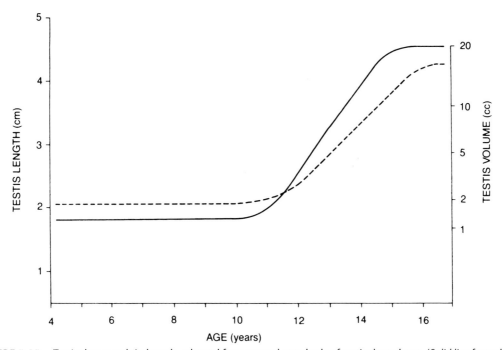

FIGURE 5-25. Testicular growth in length, adapted from normal standards of testicular volume. (*Solid line* from data of A. Prader, Zurich; broken line from data of Laron A, Zilka E: *J Clin Endocrinol Metab* 29:1409, 1969.)

Pattern of Malformation Differential Diagnosis by Anomalies

The following lists were developed from the syndromes delineated in Chapter 1. Listed for each anomaly are the syndromes in which this defect is a frequent feature, as well as those syndromes in which it is an occasional feature. Characteristics such as mental or growth deficiency are not considered because they are frequent features in a large number of disorders.

The anomalies are set forth under the following headings:

1. Central Nervous System Dysfunction Other Than Mental Deficiency
2. Deafness
3. Brain: Major Anomalies
4. Cranium
5. Scalp and Facial Hair Patterning
6. Facies
7. Ocular Region
8. Eye
9. Nose
10. Maxilla and Mandible
11. Oral Region and Mouth
12. Teeth
13. External Ears
14. Neck, Thorax, and Vertebrae
15. Limbs
16. Limbs: Nails, Creases, Dermatoglyphics
17. Limbs: Joints
18. Skin and Hair
19. Cardiac
20. Abdominal
21. Renal
22. Genital
23. Endocrine and Metabolism
24. Immune Deficiency
25. Hematology-Oncology
26. Unusual Growth Patterns

1. Central Nervous System Dysfunction Other Than Mental Deficiency

Hypotonicity

Frequent in

Achondroplasia	454
Acrocallosal S.	304
Angelman S.	270
Axenfeld-Rieger S.	768
Bannayan-Riley-Ruvalcaba S.	686
Blepharophimosis-Ptosis-Epicanthus Inversus S. (variable)	312
Börjeson-Forssman-Lehmann S.	756
Cardio-Facio-Cutaneous S.	172
Cerebro-Oculo-Facio-Skeletal (COFS) S.	234
Coffin-Lowry S.	372
Coffin-Siris S.	752
Cohen S.	280
Curry-Jones S.	544
Deletion 3p S.	34
Deletion 4p S.	38
Deletion 4q S.	40
Deletion 9p S.	46
Deletion 11q S.	56
Deletion 18p S.	62
Deletion 18q S.	64
Deletion 22q13 S.	112
Down S.	7
Ehlers-Danlos S.	624
FG S.	376
Gómez–López-Hernández S. (central)	246
Hypophosphatasia	506
Johanson-Blizzard S.	144
Kabuki S.	156
Killian/Teschler-Nicola S. (infancy)	282
Langer-Giedion S.	384
Lenz Microphthalmia S.	366
Macrocephaly-Capillary Malformation S.	674
Marden-Walker S.	300
Marfan S.	612
Marshall-Smith S.	216
Matthew-Wood S.	288
Microdeletion 1Q41Q42 S.	88
Microdeletion 1Q43Q44 S.	90
Microdeletion 15q24 S.	106
Microdeletion 16p11.2p12.2 S.	108
Microdeletion 17q21 S.	110
Microdeletion 22q11.2 S.	358
Miller-Dieker S.	254
Mowat-Wilson S.	776
Mulibrey Nanism S.	136
9q34.3 Subtelomeric Deletion S.	102
1p36 Deletion S.	84
Opitz G/BBB S.	182
Osteogenesis Imperfecta S., Type II	638
Pitt-Hopkins S.	268
Prader-Willi S. (infancy)	274
Shprintzen-Goldberg S.	620
Simpson-Golabi-Behmel S.	222
Sotos S.	206
Spondyloepiphyseal Dysplasia Congenita	472
Stickler S.	378
Thanatophoric Dysplasia	448
3C S.	306
Toriello-Carey S.	772
Vici S.	794
X-Linked α-Thalassemia/Mental Retardation S. (infancy)	374
Xq Distal Duplication or Disomy	114

3. Brain: Major Anomalies

Anencephaly/ Meningomyelocele

Encephalocele

Holoprosencephaly

Frontal Bossing or Prominent Central Forehead

Frequent in
Achondroplasia 454
Acrocallosal S. 304
Acromesomelic Dysplasia 468
Antley-Bixler S. 554
Apert S. 536
Boomerang Dysplasia 442
Cardio-Facio-Cutaneous S. 172
Cleidocranial Dysostosis 526
Cranioectodermal Dysplasia 714
Craniofrontonasal Dysplasia 546
Crouzon S. 540
Deletion 2q37 S. 96
Deletion 22q13 S. 114
Fetal Valproate S. 736
FG S. 376
Freeman-Sheldon S. 294
GAPO S. 718
Gómez–López–Hernández S. 246
Gorlin S. 692
Greig Cephalopolysyndactyly S. 552
Hallermann-Streiff S. 150
Hypohidrotic Ectodermal Dysplasia 704
Jarcho-Levin S. 782
Killian/Teschler-Nicola S. 282
Larsen S. 564
Lenz-Majewski Hyperostosis S. 522
Leroy I-Cell S. 594
Macrocephaly-Capillary Malformation S. 674
Marshall-Smith S. 216
Melnick-Needles S. 762
Microdeletion 1q41Q42 S. 88
Microdeletion 1Q43Q44 S. 90
Microdeletion 17q21 S. 110
Mowat-Wilson S. 776
Mucopolysaccharidosis I H, I H/S, I S 596
Mulibrey Nanism S. 136
1p36 Deletion S. 84
Opitz G/BBB S. 182
Osteopetrosis: Autosomal Recessive—Lethal 518
Oto-Palato-Digital S., Type I 368
Oto-Palato-Digital S., Type II 370
Peters'-Plus S. 770
Pfeiffer S. 534
Pyknodysostosis 524
Rapp-Hodgkin Ectodermal Dysplasia 708
Robinow S. 178
Rubinstein-Taybi S. 124
Russell-Silver S. 128
Schinzel-Giedion S. 302
Shprintzen-Goldberg S. 620
Smith-Magenis S. 262
3C S. 306
3-M S. 134

Tricho-Dento-Osseous S. 710
Trisomy 8 S. 24
Wiedemann-Rautenstrauch S. 192

Occasional in
Beals S. 618
Hypochondroplasia 462
Laurin-Sandrow S. 348
Oral-Facial-Digital S. 352
Rothmund-Thomson S. 198
Sotos S. 206

5. Scalp and Facial Hair Patterning

Anterior Upsweep, Scalp

Frequent in
Fetal Aminopterin/ Methotrexate S. 740
FG S. 376
Johanson-Blizzard S. 144
Rubinstein-Taybi S. 124
Trisomy 13 S. 20

Occasional in
Campomelic Dysplasia 452
Prader-Willi S. 274

Posterior Midline Scalp Defects

Frequent in
Adams-Oliver S. 416
Curry-Jones S. 544
Deletion 4p S. 38
Finlay-Marks S. 774
Johanson-Blizzard S. 144
Trisomy 13 S. 20

6. Facies

"Flat" Facies

Frequent in
Achondroplasia 454
Alagille S. 758
Apert S. 536
Autosomal Recessive Chondrodysplasia Punctata 504
Campomelic Dysplasia 452
Carpenter S. 550
Chondrodysplasia Punctata, X-Linked Dominant Type 500
Desbuquois Dysplasia 592
Down S. 7
Duplication 10q S. 52
Escobar S. 406
Kniest Dysplasia 476
Larsen S. 564
Lethal Multiple Pterygium S. 236
Marshall S. 338
Microdeletion 16p11.2p12.2 S. 108
Schwartz-Jampel S. 298
Smith-Magenis S. 262

Spondyloepiphyseal Dysplasia Congenita 472
Stickler S. 378
XXXXX S. 76
XXXY and XXXXY S. 72
Zellweger S. 290

Occasional in
Cleidocranial Dysostosis 526
Crouzon S. 540
Deletion 4p S. 38
Freeman-Sheldon S. 294
Gorlin S. 692
Leroy I-Cell S. 594
Marshall-Smith S. 216
Trisomy 13 S. 20
Waardenburg S. 332

"Round" Facies

Frequent in
Aarskog S. 176
Albright Hereditary Osteodystrophy 588
Amyoplasia Congenita Disruptive Sequence 224
Deletion 2q37 S. 96
Deletion 5p S. 42
Deletion 18p S. 62
Desbuquois Dysplasia 592
Geleophysic Dysplasia 486
Microdeletion 1Q43Q44 S. 90
Peters'-Plus S. 770
Prader-Willi S. 274

Occasional in
Bardet-Biedl S. 764
Cleidocranial Dysostosis 526
Down S. 7
Spondylocarpotarsal Synostosis S. 562
XXXXX S. 76
XXXY and XXXXY S. 72
Zellweger S. 290

"Broad" Facies

Frequent in
Apert S. 536
Carpenter S. 550
Crouzon S. 540
Gorlin S. 692
Mowat-Wilson S. 776

Occasional in
Bardet-Biedl S. 764
Cleidocranial Dysostosis 526
Prader-Willi S. 274
Sotos S. 206
Spondylocarpotarsal Synostosis S. 562
XXXY and XXXXY S. 72

"Triangular" Facies

Frequent in
Distal Arthrogryposis S., Type 2B 228

8. Eye

Myopia

Blue Sclerae

Microphthalmos

Colobomata of Iris

Oral Frenula (Webs)

Cleft or Irregular Tongue

Macroglossia

Microglossia

13. External Ears

Low-Set Ears

Malformed Auricles

Sternal Malformation–Vascular
Dysplasia Spectrum 840
Sturge-Weber Sequence 646
Tuberous Sclerosis S. 660
Xeroderma Pigmentosa S. 722

Occasional in
Antley-Bixler S. 554
Baller-Gerold S. (facial
hemangioma) 558
Bannayan-Riley-Ruvalcaba S. 686
Cardio-Facio-Cutaneous S. 172
Coffin-Siris S. 752
Diastrophic Dysplasia
(midface) 490
Fetal Alcohol S.
(hemangiomata) 728
45X S. 78
Leroy I-Cell S.
(hemangiomata) 594
Microdeletion 17q21 S.
(eczema) 110
Radial Aplasia–
Thrombocytopenia S.
(glabellar hemangioma) 428
Rubinstein-Taybi S. 124
Schinzel-Giedion S. (facial
hemangioma) 302
Simpson-Golabi-Behmel S.
(hemangiomatosis) 222
Trisomy 13 S. (hemangiomata) 20
Trisomy 18 S. 14

Photosensitive Dermatitis

Frequent in
Bloom S. 140
Cockayne S. 194
Rothmund-Thomson S. 198
Xeroderma Pigmentosa S. 722

Occasional in
Prader-Willi S. 274

**Deep Sacral Dimple,
Pilonidal Cyst**

Frequent in
Bloom S. 140
Carpenter S. 550
Chondrodysplasia Punctata,
X-Linked Dominant Type 500
Deletion 4p S. 38
Fetal Hydantoin S. 734
FG S. 376
Robinow S. 178
Smith-Lemli-Opitz S. 152

Occasional in
Deletion 22q13 S. 112
Dubowitz S. 138
Microdeletion 16p11.2p12.2
S. 108
Miller-Dieker S. 254
Okihiro S. 424
Zellweger S. 290

Other Dimples

Frequent in
Amyoplasia Congenita
Disruptive Sequence 224
Campomelic Dysplasia 452
Caudal Dysplasia Sequence
(buttock) 824
Deletion 18q S. 64
Distal Arthrogryposis S.,
Type 1 228
Duplication 9p S. 48
Freeman-Sheldon S. (chin) 294
Hypophosphatasia 506
Pena-Shokeir Phenotype 232

Unusual Acne

Frequent in
Apert S. 536
XYY S. 68

Occasional in
Gorlin S. (milia) 692
Oral-Facial-Digital S. (milia) 352

Hirsutism

Frequent in
Berardinelli-Seip Congenital
Lipodystrophy S. 790
Brachmann–de Lange S. 118
Cantú S. 578
Cerebro-Oculo-Facio-Skeletal
(COFS) S. 234
Coffin-Siris S. 752
Duplication 3q S. 36
Fetal Hydantoin S. 734
Frontometaphyseal Dysplasia 514
Hajdu-Cheney S. 508
Hunter S. 600
Marshall-Smith S. 216
Mucopolysaccharidosis I H,
I H/S, I S 596
Schinzel-Giedion S. 302
Trisomy 18 S. 14

Occasional in
Bardet-Biedl S. 764
Bloom S. 140
Costello S. 168
Deletion 2q37 S. 96
Fetal Alcohol S. 728
Floating-Harbor S. 186
45X S. 78
Greig Cephalopolysyndactyly
S. 552
Hypomelanosis of Ito 658
Microdeletion 1Q43Q44 S. 90
Microdeletion 2q31.1 S. 92
Rubinstein-Taybi S. 124

**Alopecia (Sparse to
Absent Hair)**

Frequent in
CHILD S. 408
Clouston S. 712

Cockayne S. 194
Coffin-Siris S. (sparse scalp
hair) 752
Costello S. 168
Cranioectodermal Dysplasia 714
Deletion 2q37 S. (hair and
eyebrows) 96
Dubowitz S. 138
Encephalocraniocutaneous
Lipomatosis (focal) 680
Finlay-Marks S. 774
GAPO S. 718
Gómez–López-Hernández S.
(parietal-occipital) 246
Hallermann-Streiff S. 150
Hay-Wells S. of Ectodermal
Dysplasia 394
Hypohidrotic Ectodermal
Dysplasia 704
Incontinentia Pigmenti S. 654
Johanson-Blizzard S. 144
Killian/Teschler-Nicola S. 282
Langer-Giedion S. 384
Lenz-Majewski Hyperostosis
S. (infancy) 522
Linear Sebaceous Nevus
Sequence (spotty alopecia) 650
Menkes S. 266
Metaphyseal Dysplasia,
McKusick Type 498
Mowat-Wilson S. 776
Nablus Mask-Like Facial S. 258
Oculodentodigital S. 362
Progeria S. 188
Rapp-Hodgkin Ectodermal
Dysplasia 708
Tricho-Rhino-Phalangeal S.,
Type I 388
Vici S. (fair and fine) 794
Wiedemann-Rautenstrauch S. 192
Yunis-Varón S. 590

Occasional in
Cardio-Facio-Cutaneous S. 172
Chondrodysplasia Punctata,
X-Linked Dominant Type 500
Chondroectodermal Dysplasia 488
Deletion 2q37 S. 96
Deletion 18p S. 62
Down S. 7
FG S. 376
Goltz S. 698
Hypomelanosis of Ito 658
Linear Sebaceous Nevus
Sequence 650
Microcephalic Primordial
Dwarfing S. 146
Neu-Laxova S. 238
Oral-Facial-Digital S. 352
Pachyonychia Congenita S. 720
Popliteal Pterygium S. 404
Rapp-Hodgkin Ectodermal
Dysplasia 708
Roberts S. 396

Hepatomegaly

Frequent in

Achondrogenesis, Types IA and IB	432
Berardinelli-Seip Congenital Lipodystrophy S.	790
Cantú S.	578
Geleophysic Dysplasia	486
Hunter S.	600
Leroy I-Cell S.	594
Morquio S.	606
Mucopolysaccharidosis I H, I H/S, I S	596
Mucopolysaccharidosis VII	610
Mulibrey Nanism S.	136
Osteopetrosis: Autosomal Recessive—Lethal	518
Sanfilippo S.	604
Zellweger S.	290

Occasional in

Aase S.	430
Beckwith-Wiedemann S.	218
Cardio-Facio-Cutaneous S.	172
Cockayne S.	194
GAPO S.	718
Klippel-Trenaunay S.	672
Mandibuloacral Dysplasia	786
Mucopolysaccharidosis I H, I H/S, I S	596
Noonan S.	164
Simpson-Golabi-Behmel S.	222

Pyloric Stenosis

Frequent in

Apert S.	536
Brachmann–de Lange S.	118
Deletion 11q S.	56
Down S.	7
Fetal Hydantoin S.	734
FG S.	376
Marden-Walker S.	300
Menkes S.	266
Miller S.	342
Pitt-Hopkins S.	268
Simpson-Golabi-Behmel S.	222
Smith-Lemli-Opitz S.	152
Trisomy 18 S.	14
Ulnar-Mammary S.	402
Zellweger S.	290

Incomplete Rotation of Colon (Malrotation)

Frequent in

Congenital Microgastria–Limb Reduction Complex	838
Curry-Jones S.	544
Deletion 2q37 S.	96
Early Urethral Obstruction Sequence	812
Fryns S.	286
Limb–Body Wall Complex	830

Occasional in

Aarskog S.	176
Brachmann–de Lange S.	118
Cardio-Facio-Cutaneous S.	172
Cat-Eye S.	66
Coffin-Siris S.	752
Down S.	7
Duplication 10q S.	52
Fanconi Pancytopenia S.	426
FG S.	376
Fraser S.	322
Goltz S.	698
Hajdu-Cheney S.	508
Kabuki S.	156
Killian/Teschler-Nicola S.	282
Laterality Sequences	796
Lethal Multiple Pterygium S.	236
Marfan S.	612
Matthew-Wood S.	288
Meckel-Gruber S.	242
Miller S.	342
Simpson-Golabi-Behmel S.	222
Smith-Lemli-Opitz S.	152
3C S.	306
Triploidy S. and Diploid/Triploid Mixoploidy S.	30
Trisomy 13 S.	20
Trisomy 18 S.	14
Zellweger S.	290

Duodenal Atresia

Occasional in

Deletion 2q37 S.	96
Down S.	7
Fanconi Pancytopenia S.	426
Fetal Hydantoin S.	734
Fryns S.	286
Matthew-Wood S.	288
Opitz G/BBB S. (stricture)	182
Townes-Brocks S.	346

Hirschsprung Aganglionosis

Frequent in

Down S.	7
Mowat-Wilson S.	776
Smith-Lemli-Opitz S.	152
Waardenburg S.	332

Occasional in

Aarskog S.	176
Cat-Eye S.	66
Deletion 13q S.	58
Fryns S.	286
Jeune Thoracic Dystrophy	450
Metaphyseal Dysplasia, McKusick Type	498
Nager S.	344
Okihiro S.	424
Pitt-Hopkins S.	268
Rubinstein-Taybi S.	124
Senter-KID S.	724
Toriello-Carey S.	772

Tracheoesophageal-Fistula/Esophageal Atresia

Frequent in

Methimazole/Carimazole Embryopathy	744
VACTERL Association	850

Occasional in

Apert S.	536
CHARGE S.	330
Congenital Microgastria–Limb Reduction Complex	838
Down S.	7
Fanconi Pancytopenia S.	426
Metaphyseal Dysplasia, McKusick Type	498
Microdeletion 22q11.2 S.	358
Monozygotic Twinning and Structural Defects—General	842
Mycophenolate Mofetil Embryopathy	746
Opitz G/BBB S.	182
Pfeiffer S.	534
Trisomy 18 S.	14
Waardenburg S.	332

Diaphragmatic Hernia

Frequent in

Donnai-Barrow S.	328
Fryns S.	286
Matthew-Wood S.	288
Microdeletion 1Q41Q42 S.	88

Occasional in

Apert S.	536
Autosomal Recessive Chondrodysplasia Punctata	504
Beckwith-Wiedemann S. (eventration)	218
Brachmann–de Lange S.	118
Coffin-Siris S.	752
Craniofrontonasal Dysplasia	546
Deletion 2q37 S.	96
Deletion 9p S.	46
Ehlers-Danlos S.	624
Escobar S.	406
Hydrolethalus S.	250
Kabuki S. (eventration)	156
Killian/Teschler-Nicola S.	282
Lethal Multiple Pterygium S.	236
Levy-Hollister S.	422
Marfan S.	612
Matthew-Wood S.	288
Meningomyelocele, Anencephaly, Iniencephaly Sequences	804
Microdeletion 15q24 S.	106
Microdeletion 22q11.2 S.	358
Microphthalmia–Linear Skin Defects S.	702
Miller S.	342
Mycophenolate Mofetil Embryopathy	746

Other Bleeding Tendency

Occasional in

Ehlers-Danlos S.	624
Hereditary Hemorrhagic Telangiectasia	688
Noonan S.	164

Leukocytosis

Occasional in

Down S.	7
Radial Aplasia– Thrombocytopenia S.	428

Lymphoreticular Malignancy

Occasional in

Bloom S.	140
Down S.	7
Dubowitz S.	138
Fanconi Pancytopenia S.	426
Noonan S.	164

Other Malignancies

Frequent in

Aniridia–Wilms Tumor Association (Wilms tumor, gonadoblastoma)	54
Beckwith-Wiedemann S.	218
Bloom S.	140
Deletion 4p S. (myelodysplastic syndrome)	38
Gorlin S.	692
Hay-Wells S. of Ectodermal Dysplasia	394
Multiple Endocrine Neoplasia, Type 2B (medullary thyroid carcinoma)	690
Neurocutaneous Melanosis Sequence (melanoma)	648
Pallister-Hall S. (hypothalamic hamartoblastoma)	244
Peutz-Jeghers S. (colon carcinoma)	684
Xeroderma Pigmentosa S.	722

Occasional in

Alagille S. (hepatocellular)	758
Blepharophimosis-Ptosis-Epicanthus Inversus S.	312
Cockayne S. (basal cell tumors)	194
Costello S.	168
Deletion 13q S. (retinoblastoma)	58
Dubowitz S.	138
Incontinentia Pigmenti S. (subungual keratotic tumors)	654
Linear Sebaceous Nevus Sequence (nephroblastoma, basal cell epithelioma)	650
Macrocephaly-Capillary Malformation S.	674
Maffucci S.	682

Metaphyseal Dysplasia, McKusick Type	498
Microcephalic Primordial Dwarfing S. (osteosarcoma)	146
Monozygotic Twinning and Structural Defects—General (sacrococcygeal teratoma)	842
Mulibrey Nanism S. (Wilms tumor, ovarian tumor)	136
Multiple Exostoses S. (bone sarcoma)	568
Neurocutaneous Melanosis Sequence	648
Neurofibromatosis S.	664
Proteus S.	678
Rothmund-Thomson S.	198
Russell-Silver S.	128
Schinzel-Giedion S. (embryonal tumors)	302
Senter-KID S. (squamous carcinoma)	724
Simpson-Golabi-Behmel S. (embryonal tumors)	222
Sotos S.	206
Trisomy 8 S.	24
Trisomy 18 S. (Wilms tumor)	14
Tuberous Sclerosis S.	660
Weaver S. (neuroblastoma, ovarian tumor, sacrococcygeal teratoma)	212
XXY S., Klinefelter S. (germ cell tumors, breast cancer, lung cancer)	70

26. Unusual Growth Patterns

Obesity

Frequent in

Albright Hereditary Osteodystrophy	588
Bardet-Biedl S.	764
Börjeson-Forssman-Lehmann S.	756
Carpenter S.	550
Cohen S.	280
Deletion 2q37 S.	96
45X S.	78
Killian/Teschler-Nicola S.	282
9q34.3 Subtelomeric Deletion S.	102
1p36 Deletion S.	84
Prader-Willi S.	274

Occasional in

Carpenter S.	550
Down S.	7
Finlay-Marks S.	774
Kabuki S.	156
Metaphyseal Dysplasia, McKusick Type	498
Microdeletion 15q24 S.	106
9q34.3 Subtelomeric Deletion S.	102

Ulnar-Mammary S.	402
Williams S.	160
XXXY and XXXXY S.	72
XXY S., Klinefelter S.	70

Hydrops Fetalis

Frequent in

Achondrogenesis, Types IA and IB	432
Fibrochondrogenesis	436
45X S.	78
Monozygotic Twinning and Structural Defects— General	842
Osteogenesis Imperfecta S., Type II	638

Occasional in

Chondrodysplasia Punctata, X-Linked Dominant Type	500
Down S.	7
Lethal Multiple Pterygium S.	236
Morquio S.	606
Mucopolysaccharidosis VII	610
Noonan S.	164
Short Rib–Polydactyly S., Type II (Majewski Type)	444
Type II Achondrogenesis-Hypochondrogenesis	434

Early Macrosomia, Overgrowth

Frequent in

Beckwith-Wiedemann S.	218
Berardinelli-Seip Congenital Lipodystrophy S.	790
Cantú S.	578
Macrocephaly-Capillary Malformation S.	674
Marshall-Smith S.	216
Simpson-Golabi-Behmel S.	222
Sotos S.	206
Weaver S.	212

Occasional in

Acrocallosal S.	304
Bannayan-Riley-Ruvalcaba S.	686
Fragile X S.	202
Fryns S.	286
Killian/Teschler-Nicola S.	282
Proteus S.	678

Asymmetry

Frequent in

Cervico-Oculo-Acoustic S. (facial)	340
CHILD S. (limbs)	408
Chondrodysplasia Punctata, X-Linked Dominant Type (limbs)	500
Craniofrontonasal Dysplasia (craniofacial)	546

Index

Note: Page numbers followed by f indicate figures; those followed by t indicate tables.

FETAL DEVELOPMENT

AGE weeks	LENGTH cm — C–R	LENGTH cm — Tot.	WT gm	GROSS APPEARANCE	CNS	EYE, EAR	FACE, MOUTH	CARDIO-VASCULAR	LUNG
7½	2.8				Cerebral hemisphere; Infundibulum, Rathke's	Lens nearing final shape	Palatal swellings; Dental lamina, Epithel	Pulmonary vein into left atrium	
8	3.7				Primitive cereb. cortex; Olfactory lobes; Dura and pia mater	Eyelid; Ear canals	Nares plugged; Rathke's pouch detach.; Sublingual gland	A–V bundle; Sinus venosus absorbed into right auricle	Pleuroperitoneal canals close; Bronchioles
10	6.0				Spinal cord histology; Cerebellum	Iris; Ciliary body; Eyelids fuse; Lacrimal glands; Spiral gland different	Lips, Nasal cartilage; Palate		Laryngeal cavity reopened
12	8.8				Cord—cervical & lumbar enlarged, Cauda equina	Retina layered; Eye axis forward; Scala tympani	Tonsillar crypts; Cheeks; Dental papilla	Accessory coats, blood vessels	Elastic fibers
16	14				Corpora quadrigemina; Cerebellum prominent; Myelination begins	Scala vestibuli; Cochlear duct	Palate complete; Enamel and dentine	Cardiac muscle condensed	Segmentation of bronchi complete
20						Inner ear ossified	Ossification of nose		Decrease in mesenchyme; Capillaries penetrate linings of tubules
24		32	800		Typical layers in cerebral cortex; Cauda equina at first sacral level		Nares reopen; Calcification of tooth primordia		Change from cuboidal to flattened epithelium; Alveoli
28		38.5	1100		Cerebral fissures and convolutions	Eyelids reopen; Retinal layers complete; Perceive light			Vascular components adequate for respiration
32		43.5	1600	Accumulation of fat		Auricular cartilage	Taste sense		Number of alveoli still incomplete
36		47.5	2600						
38		50	3200		Cauda equina, at L–3; Myelination within brain	Lacrimal duct canalized	Rudimentary frontal maxillary sinuses	Closure of foramen ovale, ductus arteriosus, umbilical vessels, ductus venosus	
First postnatal year +					Continuing organization of axonal networks; Cerebrocortical function, motor coordination; Myelination continues until 2–3 years	Iris pigmented, 5 months; Mastoid air cells; Coordinate vision, 3–5 months; Maximal vision by 5 years	Salivary gland ducts become canalized; Teeth begin to erupt 5–7 months; Relatively rapid growth of mandible and nose	Relative hypertrophy left ventricle	Continue adding new alveoli